# LGBTQ-Parent Families

Abbie E. Goldberg • Katherine R. Allen
Editors

# LGBTQ-Parent Families

Innovations in Research
and Implications for Practice

Second Edition

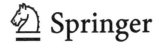

*Editors*
Abbie E. Goldberg
Department of Psychology
Clark University
Worcester, MA, USA

Katherine R. Allen
Department of Human Development
and Family Science
Virginia Tech
Blacksburg, VA, USA

ISBN 978-3-030-35609-5          ISBN 978-3-030-35610-1    (eBook)
https://doi.org/10.1007/978-3-030-35610-1

This Springer imprint is published by the registered company Springer Nature Switzerland AG
The registered company address is: Gewerbestrasse 11, 6330 Cham, Switzerland

*Dedication*
*To the pioneers of LGBTQ-parent family scholarship, the*
*emerging generation of new scholars, and our students*

# Preface

Since the first edition of this book was published in 2013, there has been a significant expansion in the range and depth of research on LGBTQ-parent families. Many of the topics covered in the first edition—for example, gay fathers and surrogacy, bisexual parents, transgender parents, race and ethnicity for sexual minority parents and their children, and research methods with LGBTQ populations—have been the subject of increased scholarly attention, warranting updated and expanded coverage. Furthermore, various topics that were not covered in the first edition have emerged as important research areas—for example, poverty in LGBTQ-parent families, LGBTQ-parent families and health, LGBTQ foster parents, religion and LGBTQ-parent families, and siblings and family of origin relationships—demanding inclusion in this edition. Indeed, of the 30 chapters in this book, 12 are devoted to topics that were not included in the first edition. The remaining 18 chapters have been substantially revised and updated to reflect growth in the field.

As in the first edition, all of the chapters in this second edition aim to address intersectionality and context. What this means, in action, is that the chapter authors aim to highlight research that explores sexual orientation in concert with other key social locations and identities, including gender, race, class, and nationality. In addition, the authors have sought to explicitly acknowledge and ideally explore the range of sexual identities and genders within and beyond "LGBTQ." In some cases, as in the chapters on asexuality and immigration, the research is very much in its infancy—and, in turn, the authors must present the general research on asexuality and immigration, respectively, propose its relevance for LGBTQ-parent families, and also highlight and make predictions about relevant directions for further research. Another new feature of this second edition is that all authors explicitly aimed to expand their coverage of international research, thus capturing the field of LGBTQ-parent families across diverse nations and cultures. Finally, all of the chapters in the second edition attend to the theoretical frameworks evident in the body of work associated with their topics.

The book begins with overview chapters that cover topics that have received the most scholarly attention. These chapters address the research on LGBTQ parenting in the context of family building route (parenting post-heterosexual divorce and separation, donor insemination, adoption), as well as how LGBTQ parenting intersects with specific identities and social locations (bisexuality, race/ethnicity) and how LGBTQ parents and their families fare in certain broad domains (economic well-being, health). The latter two chapters are new chapters entirely and represent areas of key policy relevance and great public interest.

The book then moves to chapters on relatively understudied topics—namely, important emerging research areas that have thus far received more limited attention. These chapters cover LGBTQ-parent families in the context of their route to parenthood (surrogacy, foster parenting) and their relational, sexual, and gender identities (polyamory, asexuality, trans parents). Some chapters address key social locations that intersect with LGBTQ parenting (religion, immigration), as well as important intergenerational relationships in the lives of LGBTQ parents and their families (LGBTQ parents and LGBTQ children, sibling relationships). Some chapters focus explicitly on contextual factors in LGBTQ-parent families (workplace, schools, community context, non-Western geographic regions). Finally, two new chapters focus on difficult and even painful transitions in the lives of LGBTQ-parent families (separation and divorce, loss and death of a child). The inclusion of these last two chapters is an important marker of the field's growth. That is, individual scholars and the field of LGBTQ parenting as a whole are now willing to engage with truly difficult and once invisible topics that may occur within LGBTQ-parent families, without fear that acknowledging and addressing such challenging issues will only further stigmatize the LGBTQ community.

The book also addresses applied topics to aid scholars and practitioners in focusing on legal, clinical, and educational concerns relevant to LGBTQ-parent families. Namely, we include a set of chapters that address LGBTQ-parent families and the law, clinical work with LGBTQ parents and prospective parents, clinical work with children of LGBTQ parents, and pedagogy and LGBTQ-parent families. A final set of chapters focuses on the growing sophistication of research methodology in the study of LGBTQ-parent families. Specifically, these chapters address multilevel modeling approaches to quantitative dyadic data analysis, the use of multiple qualitative approaches in studying the complexity of LGBTQ-parent families, the expansion of representative datasets relevant to the study of LGBTQ-parent families, and methods, recruitment, and sampling issues, particularly with the novel options increasingly available through social media in LGBTQ-parent family research.

Much has happened since 2013—or, really, 2012—when the first edition went to press. In 2012, marriage equality was not yet a federal reality across the United States. No US states or territories banned conversion therapy. The World Health Organization (WHO) regarded being transgender as a mental illness. As of this writing, marriage equality is a reality across the United States, 20 US states and territories have banned conversion therapy, and the WHO has stopped classifying trans people as mentally ill. Yet these favorable changes have been accompanied by changes that are widely regarded by LGBTQ community members, activists, and researchers as quite negative. For example, the current US president's administration has proposed many pieces of legislation that severely curtail the rights and freedom of LGBTQ people in areas as diverse as the military to public accommodations to adoption. The United States has also seen escalating violence against trans people—especially trans women of color. And beyond the United States, same-sex relations are often criminalized: indeed, 69 countries currently criminalize gay sex (Greenhalgh, 2019).

These changes, positive and negative, inevitably shape the daily lives and experiences of LGBTQ people and their families and differentially affect LGBTQ-parent families based on where they live and their access to resources and privilege, given their particular configuration of intersecting identities (e.g., racial, gender, nationality). Research must account for the social and political context in which LGBTQ-parent families are living their lives and carefully consider the personal and contextual resources that enable families to survive and thrive or that undermine their functioning and resilience. All of the chapters in this book attend to context, examining the broader systemic forces (e.g., national immigration policies, lack of employment discrimination protections) that marginalize, erase, or explicitly stigmatize sexual and gender minorities and their families. Yet the chapters—and, more specifically, their authors and the families about whom they write—also acknowledge the agency, resourcefulness, and resilience of LGBTQ-parent family members amidst broader injustices and stigma. These chapters set the stage for further research that meaningfully describes the experiences of LGBTQ-parent families *in context* (historical, geographic, social, political, and familial) and, in turn, pushes for changes that will improve these families' lives. Indeed, if LGBTQ people and their families suffer—if they experience depression or abuse substances, engage in turbulent relationships, or have difficulty maintaining employment—we must critically examine the structural forces of racism, sexism, heterosexism, and the like, which contribute to social inequities and disproportionately create or exacerbate the personal challenges that individuals experience within the context of family life. The tools of scholarship—research, theory, and application—can facilitate this type of critical examination and thus provide a powerful vehicle for understanding, advocacy, and social change.

Worcester, MA, USA                                              Abbie E. Goldberg
Blacksburg, VA, USA                                             Katherine R. Allen

## Reference

Greenhalgh, H. (2019, June 28). *Stonewall 50. Where next for LGBT+lives?* Retrieved from https://www.weforum.org/agenda/2019/06/stonewall-50-where-next-for-lgbt-lives-by-thomson-reuters-foundation/

# Contents

# About the Editors

**Abbie E. Goldberg** is a Professor in the Department of Psychology at Clark University in Worcester, Massachusetts, USA. She received her BA in Psychology from Wesleyan University and her MA in Psychology and PhD in Clinical Psychology from the University of Massachusetts Amherst. Her research examines diverse families, including lesbian- and gay-parent families and adoptive parent families. A central theme of her research is the decentering of any "normal" or "typical" family, sexuality, or gender to allow room for diverse families, sexualities, and genders.

**Katherine R. Allen** is a Professor in the Department of Human Development and Family Science at Virginia Tech in Blacksburg, Virginia, USA. She received her DS in Child Development and Family Relations from the University of Connecticut and her MA and PhD from Syracuse University in Family Studies, with a Certificate in Gerontology. Her areas of expertise include family diversity over the life course, family gerontology, feminist family studies, LGBTQ families, and qualitative research methods.

# Contributors

**Katie L. Acosta** Georgia State University, Langdale Hall, Atlanta, GA, USA

**Katherine R. Allen** Department of Human Development and Family Science, Virginia Tech, Blacksburg, VA, USA

**M. V. Lee Badgett** Department of Economics, University of Massachusetts Amherst, Crotty Hall, Amherst, MA, USA

Williams Institute, UCLA, Los Angeles, CA, USA

**Pallavi Banerjee** Sociology, University of Calgary, Calgary, AB, Canada

**Katie M. Barrow** School of Human Ecology, Louisiana Tech University, Ruston, LA, USA

**Dana Berkowitz** Department of Sociology and Program in Women's and Gender Studies, Louisiana State University, Baton Rouge, LA, USA

**Meg D. Bishop** Population Research Center, Human Development and Family Sciences, University of Texas at Austin, Austin, TX, USA

**Henny Bos** Sexual and Gender Diversity in Families and Youth, Research Institute of Child Development and Education, Faculty of Social and Behavioural Sciences, University of Amsterdam, Amsterdam, The Netherlands

**Eric N. Boyum** Child and Adolescent Psychiatry, University of Iowa Hospitals & Clinics, Iowa City, IA, USA

**Amy Brainer** Womens and Gender Studies and Sociology, University of Michigan Dearborn, Dearborn, MI, USA

**Eliza Byard** GLSEN: The Gay, Lesbian & Straight Education Network, New York, NY, USA

**Megan Carroll** Department of Sociology, California State University – San Bernadino, CA, USA

**Pedro Alexandre Costa** William James Center for Research, ISPA – Instituto Universitário, Lisbon, Portugal

**Christa C. Craven** Anthropology and Women's, Gender, & Sexuality Studies, The College of Wooster, Wooster, OH, USA

**Peter T. Daniolos** Child and Adolescent Psychiatry, University of Iowa Hospitals & Clinics, Iowa City, IA, USA

**Laura E. Durso** Center for American Progress, Washington, DC, USA

**Rachel H. Farr** Department of Psychology, University of Kentucky, Lexington, KY, USA

**April L. Few-Demo** Department of Human Development and Family Science, Virginia Tech, Blacksburg, VA, USA

**Jacqui Gabb** Faculty of Arts and Social Sciences, The Open University, Milton Keynes, UK

**Randi L. Garcia** Department of Psychology, Smith College, Northampton, MA, USA

**Nanette Gartrell** Visiting Distinguished Scholar, The Williams Institute, U.C.L.A. School of Law, Los Angeles, CA, USA

Guest Appointee, Research Institute of Child Development and Education, Faculty of Social and Behavioural Sciences, University of Amsterdam, Amsterdam, Netherlands

**Valerie Q. Glass** Department of Marriage and Family Therapy, Northcentral University, San Diego, CA, USA

**Abbie E. Goldberg** Department of Psychology, Clark University, Worcester, MA, USA

**Naomi G. Goldberg** Movement Advancement Project, Boulder, CO, USA

**Elizabeth Grace Holman** Human Development and Family Studies Program, Bowling Green State University, Bowling Green, OH, USA

**Satoris S. Howes** College of Business, Oregon State University, Bend, OR, USA

**Ann Hergatt Huffman** Psychological Sciences and WA Franke College of Business, Northern Arizona University, Flagstaff, AZ, USA

**Kierra B. Jones** Department of Sociology, University of South Carolina, Columbia, SC, USA

**Katherine A. Kuvalanka** Department of Family Science and Social Work, Miami University, Oxford, OH, USA

**Erin S. Lavender-Stott** Department of Counseling & Human Development, South Dakota State University, Brookings, SD, USA

**Arlene Istar Lev** University at Albany, School of Social Welfare, and Choices Counseling and Consulting, Albany, NY, USA

**Allen B. Mallory** Population Research Center, Human Development and Family Sciences, University of Texas at Austin, Austin, TX, USA

**Melissa H. Manley** Department of Psychology, Clark University, Worcester, MA, USA

**Mignon R. Moore** Sociology, Barnard College, Columbia University, New York, NY, USA

**Ruby Mountford** Melbourne Bisexual Network, Melbourne, VIC, Australia

**Cat Munroe** University of California, San Francisco, San Francisco, CA, USA

**Joel A. Muraco** Student Engagement and Career Development, University of Arizona, Tucson, AZ, USA

**Nadine Nakamura** Department of Psychology, University of La Verne, La Verne, CA, USA

**Ramona Faith Oswald** Department of Human Development and Family Studies, University of Illinois at Urbana-Champaign, Urbana, IL, USA

**Maria Pallotta-Chiarolli** Deakin University, Melbourne, VIC, Australia

**Charlotte J. Patterson** Department of Psychology, University of Virginia, Charlottesville, VA, USA

**Carla A. Pfeffer** Department of Sociology, University of South Carolina, Columbia, SC, USA

**Amanda M. Pollitt** Population Research Center, University of Texas at Austin, Austin, TX, USA

**Daniel J. Potter** Houston Education Research Consortium, Rice University, Houston, TX, USA

**Emma C. Potter** Department of Psychology, University of Virginia, Charlottesville, VA, USA

**Corinne Reczek** Department of Sociology, The Ohio State University, Columbus, OH, USA

**Damien W. Riggs** College of Education, Psychology and Social Work, Flinders University, Adelaide, SA, Australia

**Lori E. Ross** Dalla Lana School of Public Health, University of Toronto, Toronto, ON, Canada

**Jasmine M. Routon** Department of Human Development and Family Studies, University of Illinois at Urbana-Champaign, Urbana, IL, USA

**Stephen T. Russell** Population Research Center, Human Development and Family Sciences, University of Texas at Austin, Austin, TX, USA

**Alyssa Schneebaum** Department of Economics, Vienna University of Economics and Business, Vienna, Austria

**Shannon L. Sennott** Smith College School for Social Work Translate Gender, Inc., The Center for Psychotherapy and Social Justice, Northampton, MA, USA

**Julie Shapiro** Seattle University School of Law, Faculty Fellow Fred T Korematsu Center for Law and Equality, Seattle, WA, USA

**Elisabeth Sheff** Sheff Consulting, Chattanooga, Tennessee, USA

**Geva Shenkman** Baruch Ivcher School of Psychology, Interdisciplinary Center (IDC) Herzliya, Herzliya, Israel

**Kyle A. Simon** Department of Psychology, University of Kentucky, Lexington, KY, USA

**JuliAnna Z. Smith** Independent Methodological Consultant, Amherst, MA, USA

**Nicholas A. Smith** Oregon Institute of Occupational Health Sciences, Oregon Health & Science University, Portland, OR, USA

**Fiona Tasker** Department of Psychological Sciences, Birkbeck University of London, London, UK
Bloomsbury, London, UK

**Cynthia J. Telingator** Harvard Medical School, Cambridge Health Alliance, Cambridge, MA, USA

**Debra Umberson** Department of Sociology, University of Texas at Austin, Austin, TX, USA

**Cassandra P. Vazquez** Department of Psychology, University of Kentucky, Lexington, KY, USA

# Part I

# Overview

# LGBTQ Parenting Post-Heterosexual Relationship Dissolution

Fiona Tasker and Erin S. Lavender-Stott

Various commentators have noted different sociohistorical trends in research on sexual and gender minority parenting and these trends contextualize the lives of lesbian, gay, bisexual, transgender, and queer (LGBTQ) people parenting a child or children from a post-heterosexual relationship dissolution (PHRD; Golombok, 2007; Johnson, 2012). For example, Johnson (2012) delineated three waves of research on lesbian parenting. The first wave consisted of lesbians who became parents while in heterosexual relationships who subsequently came out and decided to separate from their child's father. The second wave contained lesbians who then decide to have children (planned, primary, or "de novo" families). Johnson's third wave then saw research refocus away from negating deficit arguments (i.e., establishing no difference comparisons with heterosexual parent families) and turned attention to evaluate the unique challenges experienced within lesbian-headed families. Johnson acknowledged that parenting PHRD has contin-

ued beyond the crest of the first wave of research on lesbian parenting. Nonetheless, PHRD parenting has become a forgotten research backwater in recent decades (Tasker & Rensten, 2019).

In this chapter, we provide an updated version of what Tasker (2013) discussed, namely, what we currently know about LGBTQ-parenting PHRD. We begin by reviewing the key theoretical perspectives employed in the field. We then present the demographics and social trends currently known and understood in addition to examining how religion and race impact LGBTQ parenting PHRD. With the demographic context and intersectional identities in mind, we consider legislation and the well-being of LGBTQ parents PHRD. Next, we discuss the ongoing challenges of coming out PHRD, forming new partnerships, same-gender stepfamilies, and legal and policy impacts on well-being of LGBTQ parents PHRD. Finally, we discuss future research directions and implications for practice.

F. Tasker (✉)
Department of Psychological Sciences, Birkbeck University of London, London, UK

Bloomsbury, London, UK
e-mail: f.tasker@bbk.ac.uk;
http://www.bbk.ac.uk/psychology/our-staff/fiona-tasker

E. S. Lavender-Stott
Department of Counseling & Human Development, South Dakota State University, Brookings, SD, USA
e-mail: Erin.LavenderStott@sdstate.edu

## Theoretical Perspectives

Theoretical perspectives, and the sociohistorical trends that contextualize them, have influenced the waves of research on LGBT parenting PHRD. Against a background of contested custody cases, early quantitative research studies often derived hypotheses to test out developmental deficit approaches that the absence of two

© Springer Nature Switzerland AG 2020
A. E. Goldberg, K. R. Allen (eds.), *LGBTQ-Parent Families*,
https://doi.org/10.1007/978-3-030-35610-1_1

parents of different genders in the child's home would be detrimental to child well-being (Farr, Tasker, & Goldberg, 2017; Golombok & Tasker, 1994; see chapter "LGBTQ-Parent Families and Health"). More recently, some social scientists have employed deficit comparisons to mount a challenge to the "no differences" consensus reached in earlier studies (Allen, Pakaluk, & Price, 2013; Regnerus, 2012; Sullins, 2015) yet crucially failed to control for confounding factors accounting for disadvantage (Cenegy, Denney, & Kimbro, 2018; Gates et al., 2012; Potter & Potter, 2017; Rosenfeld, 2013).

Feminist theories also have influenced the research on LGBTQ parents PHRD from earlier studies (Ainslie & Feltey, 1991; Gabb, 2005) and in more recent years have emphasized the critical intersection of identities as the key factor contextualizing experience (Moore, 2008; Nixon, 2011). More recently, studies have begun to consider tenets from life course perspective (Bengtson & Allen, 1993; Elder, 1998), namely, cohort effects and linked lives (e.g., Berkowitz & Marsiglio, 2007; Delvoye & Tasker, 2016). Researchers also have begun to employ queer theory (Bermea, Eeden-Moorefield, Bible, & Petren, 2018; Carroll, 2018) and minority stress theory approaches to enlighten understanding of the unique context of parenting PHRD (Lassiter, Gutierrez, Dew, & Abrams, 2017). In addition, some pieces of work have assessed the relevance of specific models in relation to understanding LGBTQ parenting PHRD, for example, the concept of boundary ambiguity has been evaluated in relation to gay father stepfamilies (Jenkins, 2013).

## Demographics, Social Trends, and LGBTQ Parents PHRD

While scholars do not have exact numbers, it is agreed that the majority of children under the age of 18 who are in same-sex households entered them following a heterosexual relationship dissolution rather than through planned same-sex families using donor insemination, surrogates, or via foster care or adoption (Gates, 2015;

Goldberg, Gartrell, & Gates, 2014; Lynch & Murray, 2000; Potter & Potter, 2017; Robitaille & Saint-Jacques, 2009; Tasker, 2013). Approximately 28% of gay fathers and 37% of lesbian mothers with children became parents in the context of their current relationship (Henehan, Rothblum, Solomon, & Balsam, 2007); thus, roughly 60–70% of LG parents had children in a previous relationship. Additionally, using data from the National Survey of Family Growth, over 60% of lesbian mothers in the United States (US) report having been married (Brewster, Tillman, & Jokinen-Gordon, 2014). Data from the 2011 Canadian census indicated that one in eight stepfamilies headed by a same-gender couple contained residential children (Ferete, 2012). Within the Australian context, 40% of gay men became a parent while in a heterosexual relationship (Power et al., 2012). As societal acceptance leads to more people claiming a sexual minority identity at earlier ages and creating planned families using available medical technologies, it can be expected that fewer children in same-sex parent headed households will be entering this family structure following heterosexual relationship dissolution (Biblarz & Savci, 2010; Dunlap, 2016; Gates, 2015; Goldberg & Gartrell, 2014; Tasker, 2013; Tornello & Patterson, 2015).

As of yet there are minimal data on trans parents to know much about the demographics on the route to parenthood. Stotzer, Herman, and Hasenbush (2014) reviewed over 50 studies on trans parents to conclude that between one-quarter and one-half of trans people reported being parents. Using data from the Trans PULSE Project in Ontario, Canada, Pyne, Bauer, and Bradley (2015) found that trans parents were likely to be older rather than younger, were more likely to have had children prior to transitioning, and were more likely to be (or have been) married previously. Data from this Canadian survey also revealed that transgender individuals with children were more likely to be transwomen than transmen and were less likely to be engaging in medical transition (Pyne et al., 2015). Also, while *queer* is an identity for many, especially younger cohorts, and an umbrella term for sexual and gender minorities, there are minimal data specific to either queer or indeed bisexual identified parents, as many scholars refer to parents in same-sex- or same-gender-headed families as *lesbian* or *gay*.

## Intersections of Religion and Race and Doing LGBTQ Parenting PHRD

While rare, more research has begun to focus on exploring the intersection of identities in lived experience focusing on religion and race or ethnicity around LGBTQ parenting, including PHRD. Historically, religious groups, including Christianity, Judaism, and Islam, have not affirmed same-sex or same-gender attraction and relationships (Barnes & Meyer, 2012; Lytle, Foley, & Aster, 2013; see chapter "Religion in the Lives of LGBTQ-Parent Families"). Religious communities have barred LGB people from leadership positions and have not been willing to perform or sanction same-sex marriage ceremonies (Barnes & Meyer, 2012; Lytle et al., 2013; Woodell, Kazyak, & Compton, 2015). While some denominations and communities do affirm LGBTQ individuals and same-sex marriage, belonging to a non-affirming religious group or denomination can lead to additional stress and internal homophobia in LGBTQ persons (Barnes & Meyer, 2012). Being a member of a non-affirming religious group may be a challenge in disclosing an LGBTQ identity because heterosexual marriage feels like the only way to have children or indeed a recognized partnership (Tuthill, 2016).

Little is known about the experience of exiting a heterosexual relationship for LGBTQ parents who have different religious faiths. Lytle et al. (2013) studied 10 adult children's perceptions of growing up when one parent was LG and one parent was heterosexual and the family attended a Christian or Jewish place of worship. The adult children indicated that family breakup was the most difficult aspect of their experience, more so than the discovery that a parent was gay or lesbian or the process of redefining their relationship with religion. Positive aspects of having an LG parent also were identified, such as being more open-minded and accepting of people. A

rare example of the experience of being in a non-affirming religious atmosphere and parenting PHRD is outside the academic literature. In *Our Family Outing: A Memoir of Coming Out and Coming Through* (2011), Leigh Anne Taylor and Joe Cobb discuss their family's experience of Joe coming to terms of his sexuality as an ordained minister in the non-affirming United Methodist Church. Initially it was easier for Joe to keep the closet door closed when religious colleagues around Joe debated and cast doubt upon the existence of LGBTQ individuals in the faith. The memoir then covered their individual and joint crisis, their divorce and continued co-parenting, and the formation of their new families and ended with Reverend Cobb leading a Metropolitan Community Church congregation. Thus, through finding an affirming religious community, Reverend Cobb was able to hold the tension of various aspects of his identity together, as well as make family transitions.

For some LGBTQ people, their ethnicity or race may add additional challenges or pressures around sexual orientation identity disclosure (Aranda et al., 2015; Bowleg, Burkholder, Teti, & Craig, 2008; Greene, 1998; Moore, 2010). Racial and ethnic minority couples have higher rates of parenting than White same-sex couples, and as many mothers became parents while in a prior heterosexual relationship, scholars estimate that many PHRD parents are also parents of color (Goldberg et al., 2014). Racial integration within LGBTQ parenting community groups has been noted as a challenge. For example, gay fathers recruited for participant observation and interviews via gay parenting support groups in California, Texas, and Utah felt that gay parenting groups were gradually becoming more racially diverse but feelings of marginalization from the LGBTQ parenting community were prominent in the responses of the Black (11%) and Hispanic/Latino (9%) gay fathers interviewed (Carroll, 2018). In Carroll's study, single gay fathers, gay fathers of color, and PHRD gay fathers rarely attended gay father community events in any of the three states sampled due to feelings of being an "other" (p. 110).

Communities of color (particularly Black, African American, Hispanic, and Latinx) are put forward as less accepting of LGBTQ individuals, partly due to conservative Christian values (Barnes & Meyer, 2012; Greene, 1994; Morris, Balsam, & Rothblum, 2002; Tuthill, 2016). Lassiter et al. (2017) found that of 305 LG parents, parents of color ($n = 80$) were less out to faith communities and had higher identity confusion, but felt a lower need for privacy and tended to rely on their religious community for support. They also found that younger parents across race and ethnicity were less out than older parents to their religious communities (Lassiter et al., 2017). Carroll (2018) found that 90% of the PHRD gay fathers recruited to the study via a support group in Utah had belonged to the Jesus Christ of the Latter-Day Saints Church and some still felt depressed and guilty for breaking up the church expected family life.

In her groundbreaking work on lesbian mothers of color, Moore (2008, 2011) also found most had children within a prior heterosexual union. Lesbian mothers struggled to be seen as "good mothers" as shaped by gender, sexuality, and race specifically as defined within religious Black communities (Moore, 2011). Tuthill (2016) utilized the same framework as Moore (2011) to interview 15 Hispanic lesbian mothers living in Texas parenting biological, adopted, and step children. The lesbian mothers in Tuthill's sample found different solutions to their dilemma: retaining their spiritual beliefs while maintaining loose ties with Catholic traditions, redefining religious meanings such as the concept of sin and the authority of clergymen, or keeping their distance from formal religion by maintaining their Catholic identity without a church affiliation or developing beliefs that fit their lived experience and own understanding of faith.

## Legislation Rights and Well-Being of LGBTQ Parents

The legal rights of LGBTQ parents have been fraught for decades (see chapter "The Law Governing LGBTQ-Parent Families in the United States"). For many, the risk of losing their child by leaving a heterosexual relationship and coming out and/or entering a same-sex relationship influenced their decision on whether and how to disclose their sexuality. We first review the current legal situation for LGBTQ parents PHRD in the United States and other nations with more developed equal rights legislation. We then consider how social science research on lesbian parenting in particular has contributed to the equal rights debate in this regard.

In divorce settlements involving dependent children, the best interests of the child is seen as the paramount legal principle under which the court operates. Under the best interests principle, a key factor taken into consideration would be whether the child would be harmed or negatively impacted by being separated from a parent (Haney-Caron & Heilbrun, 2014; Holtzman, 2011). When there are custody and access disputes involving dissolution of a heterosexual relationship in which one partner has a new sexual identity, states that do take sexual orientation into account now note that sexual orientation cannot be the only factor considered (Haney-Caron & Heilbrun, 2014). This has led to courts scrutinizing the particular sexual activities of an LGBTQ parent and allowing this to influence legal decision-making (Haney-Caron & Heilbrun, 2014; Tasker & Rensten, 2019).

In addition to custody and access decisions, there are legal and social barriers restricting how people parent PHRD (Park, Kazyak, & Slauson-Blevins, 2016), such as legal challenges of adding parental figures when a child already has two parents. Thus, the LGBTQ stepparent who is not legally recognized as having a parenting role might face a lack of institutional support for their parenting (Moore, 2008; Park et al., 2016). For example, marriage alone does little to protect the rights of same-sex couples, leaving parent-child relationships legally vulnerable, especially in the case of a parent's death (Acosta, 2017). Acosta (2017) found that lesbian stepfamilies had three paths for planning to preserve stepparent-child relationships in the event of parent-of-origin death: relying on family members, using wills for extended family members to follow, and if the children were old enough that children would choose for themselves. All of the paths leave some ambiguity as to what will actually happen in the event of parent-of-origin death, especially if there is strain in the relationship with the co-parent or extended family (Acosta).

Historically, the newly identifying lesbian mother feared the loss of custody of her children (Tasker, 2013). In a number of high-profile legal cases in the United States, lesbian mothers lost custody, or had visitation restrictions imposed upon them; for example, in Bottoms v. Bottoms (1995), a child's grandmother was awarded custody because their mother's conduct was judged immoral. Seminal studies—such as those by Golombok, Spencer, and Rutter (1983) and Green, Mandel, Hotvedt, Gray, and Smith (1986)—found nothing to distinguish children raised by lesbian or heterosexual mothers PHRD and contributed to the "no difference" conclusion (Stacey & Biblarz, 2001). In an interview about her work, Golombok ascribed her initial research interest being kindled by reading about lesbian mothers in the United Kingdom losing custody upon exiting a relationship with their child's father (Florance, 2015). Subsequent reviews of research on the well-being of children in LGBTQ-parented families concluded that children in these families were not developmentally disadvantaged (LaSala, 2013; Manning, Fettro, & Lamidi, 2014; Patterson, 1992; Tasker, 2005) with only a minority of authors dissenting (American Psychological Association Amicus Brief, 2014).

Gradually through the work of legal activists and test cases, the "no difference" consensus began to hold sway in legal cases and precedents for custody and visitation were established (Tasker & Rensten, 2019). Further, the nexus principle governing admissible evidence—the direct association between the behavior in question and the likelihood of harm had to be clear—became a cornerstone of family law (Logue, 2002). Therefore, as long as the no difference conclusion remained, the nexus principle would ensure that sexual identity per se was not seen as grounds to discriminate against an LGBTQ parent PHRD.

Nonetheless, in recent years the "no difference" principle has come under challenge from reviews emphasizing the limited convenience sampling of LGBTQ parents conducted in many of the earlier studies (Amato, 2012; Marks, 2012). Linked to these critiques, new studies were generated that loosened sampling criteria to obtain larger samples (Allen et al., 2013; Regnerus, 2012; Sullins, 2015), crucially at the expense of accurately defining the groups of LGB parents purportedly studied, thus accentuating family type differences (Baiocco, Carone, Ioverno, & Lingiardi, 2018; Gates, 2015; Gates et al., 2012). Other studies have indicated that controlling for socioeconomic status and family instability—the history of exit and entry transitions surrounding the formation of single-parent or stepfamily forms—can nullify differences between young people from different family backgrounds that might otherwise be evident (Cenegy et al., 2018; Potter, 2012; Potter & Potter, 2017; Rosenfeld, 2013). Similarly, several major studies on the general effects of parental separation and divorce have implicated family instability as the major factor alongside socioeconomic disadvantage accounting for disparity in children's psychosocial adjustment and achievements not the family form itself (Fomby & Cherlin, 2007; Fomby & Osborne, 2017; Lansford, 2009). Notwithstanding the association of family instability and well-being, the combined vulnerability of being a newly out parent intersecting with class, race, religion, and cohort factors means that legal disputes involving LGBTQ parents do not happen within a neutral arena.

## The Ongoing Challenge of Coming Out PHRD and Forming New Partnerships

Despite the increased visibility of LGBTQ communities and equal rights legislation to acknowledge same-gender partnerships across much of the Western world, the psychosocial challenges of coming out as an LGBTQ parent with children from a prior heterosexual relationship are not to be underestimated. Single parenting, nonresidential parenting, and forming a new same-gender partnership all present complex challenges for the LGBTQ parent PHRD. First, we consider the LGBTQ parent's route into and out of heterosexual parenthood and then consider how this frames the LGBTQ parent's process of awareness and coming out later in life. Second, we consider how LGBTQ parents PHRD feel a powerful mix of stigma and pride in coming out with the complex intersections of class, race, religion, and cohort effects. Third, we review how disclosure is broached within their heterosexual relationship. Fourth, we examine how PHRD family relationships change and develop during this process. Lastly, we consider new same-gender partnerships and LGBTQ-parent stepfamily experiences PHRD.

## LGBTQ Parenting via Heterosexual Parenthood and Coming Out Later in Life

LGBTQ parents with children from a previous heterosexual relationship might encounter incredulity or suspicion from a variety of sources and feel called to account for their relationship history. Researchers have explored the varied reasons why an LGBTQ parent may have had children within a heterosexual partnership to reveal a mix of reasons. For example, in Figueroa's (2018) qualitative study of PHRD lesbian mothers in Chile, some had identified feelings for other women as teenagers. In a strongly conservative and predominantly Catholic milieu, Chilean lesbians assumed there was no option but to marry a man, especially if they wanted to have children.

In disentangling a complex mix of gender identity and sexual identity to understand relationship desires, many on the trans and gender nonconforming spectrum often identify later in life (Dierckx, Motmans, Mortelmans, & T'sjoen, 2015; Stotzer et al., 2014). Additionally, from clinical work and qualitative research, Mallon (2017) indicated that for many LGBTQ people, gender and sexual identity are not so clear-cut

when they embarked upon a heterosexual partnership. For instance, some of the other cisgender women in Figueroa's (2018) study of Chilean lesbian mothers described experiencing a change in their sexual identity from heterosexual to lesbian, not a rekindling of desire.

Using a life course perspective, qualitative research has begun to explore cisgender bisexual women's accounts of experiencing attractions to both women and men and how these intertwine with their perceptions of motherhood. The eight British and Irish bisexual mothers in Tasker and Delvoye's (2018) study had children through a relationship with a man in a variety of different family arrangements: some were now parenting PHRD while others were not. The mothers reported a complex mix of emotional and sexual attractions encountered as they self-defined their sexual identity across their life course (Delvoye & Tasker, 2016). Some of the cisgender women felt some degree of relief when they fell in love with a man because the normative pathway to marriage and having children then opened up. Participants felt perplexed, misunderstood, socially isolated, or invisible in their nascent bisexual identity until they made contact with the bisexual community (Tasker & Delvoye, 2015).

Life course and feminist approaches also have been useful in framing the reflections of lesbian and bisexual grandmother when reflecting upon their lives. For example, the US lesbian and bisexual grandmothers in Orel and Fruhauf's (2006) study said that when younger they saw their future only in terms of marriage to a man, even if they were aware at that time of something lacking in their lives. Lesbian grandmother's in Patterson's (2005a) study recalled three distinct time periods in their lives. Initially, when growing up as young women, if they had claimed a lesbian identity they could have been subjected to a criminal prosecution or labeled with a mental health problem. Consequently, most of Patterson's lesbian grandmothers had regarded a lesbian identity as simply taboo. Later in the 1970s and 1980s while lesbians were becoming steadily more visible, lesbian mothers were still seen only in the margins, including within the often child-free and separatist lesbian communities. Some of

Patterson's lesbian grandmothers did begin to come out during the 1970s and 1980s, but felt they risked their relationship with their children in doing so given the hostile judicial climate. Greater openness had only been feasible when equal rights legislation had lessened the possibility of experiencing discrimination and prejudice.

## Stigma and Pride in Coming Out: Experiencing the Intersection of Class, Race, Religion, and Cohort

Post *Obergefell* and equal rights legislation, we speculate that contemporary White middle-class LGBTQ parent PHRD may find coming out an easier prospect than did their counterparts in previous cohorts (Tasker & Rensten, 2019). Nevertheless, there are as yet few if any published studies that have investigated the polar experiences of stigma and pride and the intersection of LGBTQ parenting PHRD, social class, race, ethnicity, religion, and cohort.

Without formal educational and economic resources, working-class parents transitioning into a new sexual or gender identity are in a more vulnerable position in relation to disclosing their sexual identity and may not have the resources to fight any legal battles (Tasker & Rensten, 2019). In one study of White working-class mothers in the United Kingdom, even identifying as lesbian was a major challenge for some women who were in effect dependent upon their ex-husband for financial support for their children (Nixon, 2011). Furthermore, the women in Nixon's research recalled their own unhappy and marginalized experiences as young lesbians at school. These prior experiences, arising from the intersection of social class and sexual identity, spurred on the desires of these mothers to protect their children from being bullied by avoiding disclosure and fostering their child's ability to be independent.

Stigma is likely still a major part of the experience of LGBTQ parenthood in more socially conservative areas. One survey of over 60 mostly White and middle-class gay fathers compared respondents residing in California with those in Tennessee (Perrin, Pinderhughes, Mattern, Hurley, & Newman, 2016). Half of the gay men in the Tennessee group parented PHRD, whereas the large majority in California had planned fatherhood as gay men. Gay fathers in Tennessee were more likely to report worrying about stigma than were those in California. Surveying over 300 participants at a gay pride event in a city in a southern state in the United States, Lassiter et al. (2017) found intriguing differences in the responses of the lesbian and gay parents they surveyed. Older respondents were more likely to feel under pressure than were younger participants suggesting a cohort effect such that older generations were still more likely to feel vulnerable to sexual minority stress, despite a more accepting current zeitgeist. Plausibly older cohorts were more likely than younger cohorts to contain PHRD LG parents, although route to parenthood was not recorded in the survey. Compared to the lesbian parents surveyed, gay parents not only reported on the lack of social acceptance they experienced but also felt more directly threatened by their external environment. Gay parents additionally experienced more internalized homophobia than did lesbian parents. Both lesbian and gay parents of color (about 25% of the sample) reported more feelings of identity confusion than did White lesbian and gay parents (Lassiter et al., 2017). Carroll (2018) has drawn attention to the particular circumstances of PHRD gay fathers in Utah versus those attending community groups in California (predominantly fathers via surrogacy or adoption) and Texas where route to parenthood varied. Gay fathers PHRD felt marginalized in society and in relation to the LGBTQ communities in all three states, but gay fathers in California appeared to be particularly isolated from community assistance because of their minority within a minority status.

The negative effects of stigma and fear of stigmatization have been featured in the clinical case accounts of children of trans parents (Freedman, Tasker, & Di Ceglie, 2002; White & Ettner, 2004). Similarly, dealing with stigma, or the possibility of experiencing stigma, has been noted as a major aspect of life experience in survey research on transgender parents (Haines, Ajayi, & Boyd, 2014) and the adult children of transgender parents (Veldorale-Griffin, 2014).

The stark contrast between the socially privileged world of the parent who is read by others as heterosexual simply because they are in a different gender partnership and the parent who is read as lesbian or gay is crystalized in the difficulties bisexual parents have in achieving recognition both within their family of origin and in their friendship circles (Delvoye & Tasker, 2016). Bisexual mothers met separatist lesbian opposition and were rendered invisible as mothers overwhelmed by the presumptions of heteronormative motherhood (Tasker & Delvoye, 2015). Furthermore, the women in Tasker and Delvoye's study positioned themselves as mothers first and foremost as they recollected prioritizing the needs of their children over and above their own identification as a bisexual woman on various occasions. For example, some bisexual mothers avoided giving any clues as to their sexual identity while children were of school age and did not challenge others when they presumed heterosexuality (Tasker & Delvoye, 2015). Nonetheless, mothers took the opportunities they felt they could to raise the profile of LGBTQ equal rights issues within their local neighborhood.

One recurrent finding from earlier research on gay fathers and lesbian mothers exiting heterosexual relationships was that many expressed self-pride in their honesty and achievement in coming out, especially in the face of obstacles and opposition (Bigner & Bozett, 1990; Bozett, 1987; Coleman, 1990). A sense of achievement also featured in the early accounts of single Black lesbian mothers (Hill, 1987). As they reached young adulthood, some of the offspring of lesbian mothers also reported feeling proud of their mother and their family background (Tasker & Golombok, 1997). Nonetheless, expressing pride may have been more difficult for mothers, fathers, and children who came from PHRD backgrounds than for parents and children in planned LGB parent families (Goldberg, 2007; Perlesz et al., 2006; Van Dam, 2004). Nixon's (2011) research has indicated that pride is not just confined to middle-class samples as their children's displays

of tolerance and equality were qualities praised by working-class lesbian mothers too.

For older cohorts of PHRD lesbian and gay parents, continuing difficulties of feeling out of step with much younger LGBTQ parents also contribute to feelings of stigma and pride. Only with more recent cultural shifts marking the value of diversity have the Canadian lesbian grandmothers in Patterson's (2005b) study felt more valued and able to make a positive contribution towards political change. Reflections on pride in personal growth also were emphasized by the middle-aged and older Israeli PHRD gay fathers, who significantly differed from the comparison group of heterosexual fathers in this respect (Shenkman, Ifrah, & Shmotkin, 2018). Furthermore, Shenkman and colleagues noted that feelings of personal growth and purpose in life were rated more highly by gay fathers than by those in the comparison group of child-free gay men.

## Broaching Disclosure Within a Heterosexual Relationship

Speaking as a clinician, Mallon (2017) highlighted the emotional and social complexities for newly identifying LGBTQ parents in coming out within the context of an established heterosexual partnership in which children have been nurtured. The parent beginning their journey to self-actualization is faced with twin desires for authenticity and wanting to live a fuller life. Yet a painful sense of loss may ensue because they may feel deeply attached and committed to the children they share with their partner. Furthermore, emotional and/or sexual feelings for their partner may possibly linger after leaving the relationship. New excitement is thus tinged with sadness at the thought of what could be lost.

Diverse reflections over time upon the challenges and pleasures of coming out as an LGBTQ parent can be seen in the moving qualitative accounts of lesbian grandparents coming out to their adult children and grandchildren (Patterson, 2005b). Most of the women in Patterson's sample of Canadian lesbian grandmothers stressed the transformation of their lives through a late in life discovery of their feelings for another woman. Most did not manage or hide their feelings for women over a long period of time. Similarly, Orel and Fruhauf (2006) reported accounts by lesbian and bisexual grandmothers in a US sample of women who realized their own sexual identity later in life just prior to embarking on a relationship with another woman.

Leaving the security of a heterosexual future and coming out to their presumably heterosexual partner is often a tense process (Patterson, 2005a). On the one hand, the LGBTQ parent may have spent some time working out what their sexual feelings meant, or the realization may have suddenly dawned and helped to make sense of past experiences. On the other hand, their former partner is less likely to have been prepared, even if they had an inkling that something had changed in the relationship. Therefore, the reality of coming out will be linked into the reconfiguration of an existing family system formed around bringing up children. Sometimes the parenting couple may be able to reach a new accommodation in a mixed-orientation marriage and one or both of them may be keen to try this (Buxton, 2005, 2012). If a new accommodation within an existing parenting partnership is to work, then open communication is important (Mallon, 2017). If the partners are no longer prepared to be patient with or tolerate each other, then separation seems an inevitable consequence.

Being unfettered by a heterosexual partnership that is no longer sustainable, an LGBTQ parent has a chance to redefine both self and family relationships in a way that can be authentic and more meaningful (Benson, Silverstein, & Auerbach, 2005). Nevertheless, as with any relationship breakup and especially that of a partnership with children, the whole family system is challenged to redefine around a new reality. Mallon (2017) suggested that LGBTQ parents will likely experience challenges that are often more to do with solo parenting than with sexual identity. As a single parent, the LGBTQ parent will have the strain of sole day-to-day parental responsibility in the home and may experience multiple role strain if taking on additional respon-

sibilities for paid employment (Amato, 2014; Braver, Shapiro, & Goodman, 2006). The nonresidential LGBTQ parent PHRD has to face legal, financial, and/or psychological consequences as family relationships reconfigure around two separate residences (Amato & Dorius, 2010).

## PHRD Family Relationships: Conflict, Acceptance, and Building New Relationships

Earlier studies of lesbian or gay parents PHRD highlighted conflict with the child's other parent around the ending of the lesbian or gay parent's intimate heterosexual relationship as a critical influence on the LG parent's feelings about coming out (Bigner, 1996; Hare & Richards, 1993; Lott-Whitehead & Tully, 1992; Lynch & Murray, 2000; Morris et al., 2002). In the United States and elsewhere, the establishment of the nexus principle has meant that custody or visitation disputes are less likely to be enflamed by resentment over an ex-partner's sexual identity ostensibly lessening conflict between the LGBTQ parent and their ex-partner (Tasker & Rensten, 2019). Nonetheless, as Bermea et al.' (2018) in-depth case study of two nonresidential gay fathers parenting and stepparenting together revealed, ex-partners are in a legally powerful position to limit children's visits. In other countries where sexual identity is a more openly contested issue, conflict still features in accounts of PHRD lesbian mothers (Figueroa Guinez, 2018).

High levels of conflict between the trans parent and the child's other parent have been noted in survey research with transgender parents (Haines et al., 2014; White & Ettner, 2007). Parental conflict also featured in analyses of clinical accounts of children of transgender parents (Freedman et al., 2002; White & Ettner, 2004). In the 2015 US Transgender Survey, over 20% of trans parents reported that at least one of their children stopped seeing or speaking to them because of transition (James et al., 2016). Pyne et al. (2015) found that less than half of the transgender parents in the Canadian Trans PULSE survey reported receiving strong endorsement from their children regarding gender identity. Furthermore, 18% of trans parents surveyed had no legal access to their child and 18% reported having lost or reduced custody because they were transgender. Moreover, Green (2006) has pointed to parental alienation syndrome as a concern for trans parents (when a child's co-parent attempts to sever the child's connection with the child's transgender parent). Nonetheless, one in-depth UK-based case study found considerable variation in the partnership and parenting experiences reported by three transgender parents who transitioned post-parenthood (Hines, 2006). Hines indicated that family responses ranged from irreconcilable separation to a reconfiguration of family relationships around authenticity and celebration of gender nonconformity or romance.

In the United States and Canada, the continuing aftermath of relationship dissolution conflict between the LGBTQ parent and their former heterosexual partner is often associated with the ongoing quality of LGBTQ parent-child or LGBTQ grandparent-grandchild relationships. For example, Orel and Fruhauf (2006) reported that the lesbian and bisexual grandmothers they interviewed often attributed any ambivalence that adult children displayed to unresolved feelings about parental divorce or earlier difficulties in childhood. Analogous to this, studies with adult children of lesbian or gay parents have emphasized that feelings about their parent's sexual identity are complicated by their feelings about the ending of their parents' relationship (Daly, MacNeela, & Sarma, 2015; Lytle et al., 2013). The lesbian grandmothers in Patterson's (2005b) study also spoke of family members, particularly children, opportunistically using homophobia to keep themselves distant and create opposition. Clearly some grandmothers in Patterson's study had worked very hard to rebuild relationships with adult children. For some lesbian grandmothers, an ex-husband had given support to mediate family relationships (Orel & Fruhauf, 2006).

While most children of PHRD lesbian or gay parents seem to reach acceptance or at least tolerate to their parent's sexual identity over time, a few lesbian or bisexual grandmothers in both

Patterson's (2005a) and Orel and Fruhauf's (2006) studies reported that family gatherings were still difficult or that adult offspring had excluded them from their lives. An additional consequence was that the quality of participants' relationships with their adult children set the terms of engagement with grandchildren, for instance, in whether grandmothers could be open about their sexual identity (Orel & Fruhauf, 2006). Intergenerational family relationships that were accepting enabled lesbian and bisexual grandmothers to give their grandchildren unique insight into open-minded acceptance of diversity, on top of the usual support they would give their grandchildren (Whalen, Bigner, & Barber, 2000). In contrast, lesbian and bisexual grandmothers who could not be open with their grandchildren reported feeling distant from their grandchildren because of this lack of honesty (Patterson, 2005a).

The experiences of gay grandfathers in coming out to children and grandchildren appear to be similar to those described by lesbian and bisexual grandmothers. The 11 grandfathers in Fruhauf, Orel, and Jenkins' (2009) study all said they found it easier to come out to grandchildren compared to their children, partly because their adult children had helped to smooth the disclosure process (Fruhauf et al., 2009). Nevertheless, experiences varied. Some grandfathers said they feared disclosing, because they might lose their grandchildren's regard and affection. In other instances, grandfathers had at best minimal contact with their grandchildren because their adult offspring had blocked this. Other gay grandfathers described their relationship with their partner as part of the taken for granted everyday fabric of their grandchildren's lives.

Church, O'Shea, and Lucey (2014) reported that most of the 14 Irish trans parents they surveyed indicated good relationships with their children (i.e., for 25/28 children parented). Another study of seven Italian male-to-female trans parents indicated that they centered parenting not on gender but on affection for their child (Faccio, Bordin, & Cipolletta, 2013). One Australian survey of trans adults highlighted three components of hostility from different family members directed toward the trans person: refusal to use preferred pronouns, exclusion from family events, and pathologizing responses (Riggs, von Doussa, & Power, 2015). Other findings from the same survey indicated that trans parents' general perception of family support correlated with feeling specifically supported in their parenting (Riggs, Power, & von Doussa, 2016). In the United States, Tabor (2019) concluded that most of the 30 adult offspring interviewed were actively engaged in working to improve their relationship with their trans parent and only 10% described having disconnected from their trans parent. Over two-thirds of Tabor's participants spontaneously spoke about working on various ways to resolve role-relational ambiguity—that is, the disjuncture between gender role and designated relational status of their parent (as mom or dad). Reviewing the field of LGBTQ parenting from a clinical systemic perspective, Lev (2004) emphasized consideration of family relationships and adjustment to parental gender identity, which may include a medical or legal transition, as processes over time, in relation to the whole family.

## Same-Gender Partnership and Stepfamily Formation

While some LGBTQ parents remain single PHRD, many will re-partner at some point, either prior to the end of their heterosexual relationship, during the process of dissolving their heterosexual union, or subsequent to separation. Here we consider the limited research on same-gender dating relationships PHRD, before moving on to consider the couple relationship dynamics of PHRD re-partnerships, and then the quality of stepfamily relationships.

Early research on gay fathers emphasized the difficulties PHRD gay fathers faced in trying to find a new gay partner as they entered the gay arena at a later age than most (Bozett, 1987; Miller, 1978). However, recent research on Israeli middle-aged and older gay men has indicated that more PHRD gay fathers compared to child-free gay men reported being in a committed romantic relationship (Shenkman et al., 2018). While dating may be difficult PHRD, it seems that gay fathers PHRD look to form, and often find, a committed same-gender partnership as Bigner (1996) previously suggested. Nonetheless, in Shenkman et al.'s (2018) study, separated or divorced gay fathers were less likely than separated or divorced heterosexual fathers to be in an intimate partnership.

Dating was not the center of attention in research investigating the same-gender partnerships formed by lesbian, bisexual women, or trans parents PHRD. Instead, many of the early feminist studies on lesbian motherhood PHRD focused upon how PHRD lesbian mothers were attempting to put feminist principles into practice in their relationships (Tasker, 2013). Thus, many lesbians aspired to feminist principles of equality in their new relationship with another woman, yet those with children from a prior relationship often shouldered a disproportionate amount of child care labor compared to their partner (Rawsthorne & Costello, 2010). This seemed to apply to Black lesbian mothers in the United States (Moore, 2008) and also to White working-class lesbian mothers in the United Kingdom (Gabb, 2004).

Research on the division of child care and domestic labor has now explored how gay fathers with children from a previous heterosexual relationship divide up responsibilities in their new same-gender partnership. An online survey of gay couples with children less than 18 years old conducted by Tornello, Sonnenberg, and Patterson (2015) found that PHRD gay fathers with resident, or partially resident, children were less likely to share child care with a partner than were gay couples who became fathers in the context of the same-sex relationship. Nevertheless, household chores were likely to be divided equally in both types of partnership. Furthermore, just like the gay fathers in planned families, those parenting children PHRD found that their desire for a more equal division of labor was subject to other time constraints, namely, the number of hours each partner spent in paid employment (Tornello et al., 2015).

Not all new same-gender partners will want to become involved in their partner's children's lives. Similarly, some LGBTQ parents may want to keep partnership and parenting separate (Tasker & Delvoye, 2015). If partners do become involved, then there are challenges to be overcome in forming a new stepfamily (Ganong & Coleman, 2017). For example, partnered grandmothers in Orel and Fruhauf's (2006) study described the difficulties they and their same-gender partners experienced in gaining recognition of their partner's status in the family circle, initially as a parental figure and later as a co-grandmother. Sometimes partners felt painfully excluded. Similarly, in Patterson's (2005b) study, nonbiological grandmothers were often faced with the need to give an explanation of how they came to be a grandmother if they wanted recognition outside the home. Patterson considered how Canadian laws to permit same-sex marriage (Bill C-38) had impacted upon the lives of the lesbian grandmothers she interviewed (Hurley & Law and Government Division Canada, 2005). Most of Patterson's participants greeted the legislation as a positive step toward equal rights. Nevertheless, the partnered older women in Patterson's sample differed on whether they had married or not: some felt that marriage had helped others to recognize their relationship, while other women felt that they did not want their relationship constrained by heteronormative rules.

Earlier research often used Cherlin's (1978) incomplete institutionalization concept to research stepfamilies led by a lesbian or gay couple (e.g., Berger, 1998; Hequembourg, 2004). Building upon the idea of incomplete institutionalization, recent work has considered that LGBTQ-parent families may experience boundary ambiguity. Boundary ambiguity has been defined as the lack of common agreement on who is part of the new family and thus privy to stepfamily matters (Boss & Greenberg, 1984; Brown & Manning, 2009). In turn, greater boundary ambiguity may create conflict and stress leading to weakened family ties and access to family resources. For example, Jenkins (2013) interviewed and explored the experiences of nine gay

nonresidential fathers with children from a previous heterosexual union and nine gay stepfathers. Both gay fathers and stepfathers were proud and clear about who counted as family, but felt that they had struggled to blend their respective families together. Blending difficulties were encountered particularly when a child did not accept their father's gay identity, or saw his new same-gender partner as emblematic of this. Fathers in these situations mentioned that they had two equally close but distinct relationships: one with their child and one with their partner. Some gay fathers even described the stressful clash of preserving their relationship with their child at the expense of their relationship with their partner. Jenkins (2013) argued that members of gay-parent stepfamilies experienced more self-definitional challenges than did members of heterosexual stepparent families, because heterosexism and prejudice worked together to invalidate a same-gender partnership. Jenkins identified different pressures on gay father stepfamilies from both institutional sources, namely, legal obstacles or conservative religious beliefs, which operated often in conjunction with interpersonal challenges from children or ex-partners.

Writing from the perspective of a therapist who has counseled members of stepfamilies formed by a gay father, Gold (2017) suggested the couple must initially resolve how to address and delineate the role of the new gay stepparent and how he should interact with the children. As with any new parental relationship, Gold contended that the children involved may wonder whether their parent will be taken away from them by the presence of a new partner or how this will affect their own lives. In addition, older children might worry about the reaction of their peers if a parent's new relationship is disclosed (Papernow, 2018). Despite these challenges to stepfamily definition, the very lack of a role prescription for a new same-gender partner may also be an advantage in some instances as this can give stepfamily members the freedom to form relationships that suit them at the pace they want to do so (Tasker & Golombok, 1997). Gold also suggested that fostering a growing sense of appreciation of diversity within the LGBTQ community may assist in developing creativity and cooperation in new stepfamily relationships.

A further challenge for same-gender partnership stepfamilies is that the arrival of a same-gender partner may unsettle a previously cooperative relationship between ex-partners. For instance, it may only be when they hear about the LGBTQ-parent's new partnership that an ex-partner finally decides to let go of the relationship and comes to terms with the LGBTQ-parent's sexual identity (Gold, 2017). Gay fathers and stepfathers described how ongoing difficulties between the father and his ex-wife put pressure on the children's relationship with their father and simultaneously hindered the children from forming a relationship with their new stepparent (Jenkins, 2013). Indeed, continuing issues with an ex-partner can challenge relationships in any newly formed stepfamily (Ganong & Coleman, 2017). Nevertheless, LGBTQ-parent stepfamilies face the additional challenge of an ex-partner's indignation being endorsed by some parts of society and children internalizing the prejudice they have heard at home to feel embarrassed or ashamed of their father's relationship (Jenkins, 2013). For example, some of the gay fathers interviewed by Jenkins feared that their children would not be able to visit at all if they did not acquiesce to direct or indirect restrictions on their new partner's presence, such as not showing affection to each other in the children's presence. Thus, tensions arising from boundary ambiguity in the stepfamily, namely, the inability of being able to include the LGBTQ stepparent in the children's lives, can make stepfamily relationships fraught with problems. The strain of not being able to act as a couple may perhaps become too much for some same-gender partnerships. One study revealed that while gay fathers in stepfamilies reported having the highest level of couple relationship quality compared with other gay men, gay fathers in stepfamilies were generally less out and scored lower on cohesiveness than those in re-partnerships without children (van Eeden-Moorefield, Pasley, Crosbie-Burnett, & King, 2012).

Being able to act in concert as a same-gender couple depends in part upon others acknowledging the partnership, which in turn is facilitated by the disclosure of the relationship. Lynch (2000) discussed how differences in the level of comfort around disclosure of sexual identity could impact upon the couple relationship between the lesbian or gay parent and their new partner. The challenge for the lesbian or gay parent was to come to terms with coming out (Lynch, 2004). New partners, who often did not have children themselves, were often familiar with disclosure issues. However, new partners were unpracticed at how to disclose in a way that was appropriate both for a partner who might be hesitant and children who might be reticent (Lynch, 2005). Gold (2017) argued that this divergence in experience with disclosure is often a crucial issue faced by partners establishing a new same-gender partnership when one parent has children from a prior heterosexual relationship.

Research has begun to explore PHRD gay fathering as a site for queering family relationships, exploring how forming a new same-gender partnership can create and sustain a queer family against the pressures of heteronormativity. Bormea et al. (2018) explored the issues encountered by one family headed by two fathers who each had children from a previous relationship. Despite the relatively positive context of their extended family and local neighborhood, the fathers found that custody decisions went against them. Yet the fathers spoke warmly about the formation of family relationships created through performance, such as family mealtimes spent together when both sets of children visited.

## Directions for Future Research

Since the publication of Tasker's (2013) review of LG parenting post-heterosexual separation and divorce, data from large-scale surveys requesting information related to parental sexual orientation have become available for analyses. Yet, as we have detailed above, large data sets may be imprecise and thus problematic (Baumle & Compton, 2014; Gates et al., 2012). Nevertheless, new studies, such as those by Carroll (2018), Perrin et al. (2016), and van Eeden-Moorefield et al. (2012) in the United States and Shenkman et al. (2018) in Israel have increased our knowledge particularly of gay fathers parenting PHRD.

Much of the funding in the field has been for research related to the well-being of children in LGBTQ-parent households, and thus relatively few published studies directly address the concerns of LGBTQ parents PHRD or aim to hear their voices. Nevertheless, research studies have begun to consider wider concerns of PHRD parents and consider the intersection of sexual identity across class, race, ethnicity, religion, and cohort groups and to sample beyond the experience of lesbian or gay White, middle-class, urban parents.

Additionally, we challenge scholars to use queer theory in their research on PHRD families with one or more gender and sexual minority parent. Legal structures focus on two-parent families, which leaves out families with multiple parents with different identities. As scholars, we can challenge the assumptions of heteronormativity and, increasingly, homonormativity (Allen & Mendez, 2018). Queering families can include legal parents, biological parents, and social parents, creating a polyparenting situation (Park, 2013; Sheff, 2014; see chapter "Polyamorous Parenting in Contemporary Research: Developments and Future Directions"), which can also include grandparents. By taking a queer theoretical perspective, we can continue to acknowledge the lived experiences of malleable boundaries of sexual identity and of gender within families and be open to alternative relations (Halberstam, 2005; McGuire, Kuvalanka, Catalpa, & Toomey, 2016; Oswald, Blume, & Marks, 2005).

Many studies sampling LGBTQ parents do not clearly identify the route to parenthood in listing sampling criteria. Research focuses on LGBTQ parents as a whole (e.g., Lassiter et al., 2017) or focus specifically on LGBTQ parents who have adopted (e.g., Farr & Goldberg, 2015) or parents who used a donor or surrogate (e.g., Bos, Kuyper, & Gartrell, 2018). As in the research by Lassiter and colleagues, there are often underlying assumptions made by authors as to how same-sex-headed households are formed, but these are not always scrutinized within their research. We found that publications need careful reading to determine whether the LGBTQ-parent family formation investigated contained PHRD parents. More generally as researchers, we need to explore each participant's self-definition of not only sexual identity but also gender identity (Tasker, 2018). Many rich and meaningful self-definitions of gender and sexual identity exist; however, surveys often provide relatively few options for answer choices, even when allowing for self-definition (Galupo, Henise, & Mercer, 2016; Galupo, Ramirez, & Pulice-Farrow, 2017). Nevertheless, qualitative studies have begun to reveal the complex issues of identity definition and exploration for trans parents (Hines, 2006), and some studies have explored gender and sexual identity using a life course approach to consider how this intersects with defining family (Delvoye & Tasker, 2016).

Much of the data collected has been via cross-sectional surveys of self-identified LGBTQ parents, another limitation that again in part may be due to funding constraints or recruitment and access to members of the community. Most of our review has been pieced together from different publications detailing the reflections of LGBTQ parents given in a single research interview. Nonetheless, some studies have attempted to investigate family processes over time (Tasker & Golombok, 1997), collect multiple types of data (Gabb, 2005; Tasker & Delvoye, 2018), and consider multiple respondents (Bermea et al., 2018; Perlesz et al., 2006). Thus, while we urge researchers to continue to explore new research methods, our review has highlighted a myriad of processes that potentially influence the lived experiences of LGBTQ parents as they narrate their PHRD journey.

## Implications for Practice

When advocating for the best interests of the child and their LGBTQ parent, legal professionals need to be aware of the complexity of factors that need to be taken into account in social science research data (Baumle, 2018; Kazyak,

Woodell, Scherrer, & Finken, 2018). Early reviews of clinical practice concentrated on lesbian or gay parents coming out of previous heterosexual relationships (Bigner, 1996; Coleman, 1990). Little is known about the current issues facing lesbian or gay parents PHRD and even less about the issues facing bisexual and trans parents. Professionals assisting parents PHRD need to be aware that family composition and parental gender and/or sexual identity are projects under construction and may not align in a direct way at any one point in time (Tasker & Malley, 2012).

Professionals should be aware of the complexities facing individuals and families when a parent leaves a heterosexual relationship as a gender or sexual minority. Community members, teachers, therapists, judges, lawyers, legislators, and other professionals should be educated on the unique challenges facing LGBTQ parents and families. As family law and social conventions are predominantly based on heteronormative assumptions, it is especially important to acknowledge the various family structures and lived experiences among LGBTQ-parent families (Kim & Stein, 2019; Minter, 2019). This includes polyparenting families and single LGBTQ parent families.

## Conclusion

LGBTQ parents who have had children in a previous heterosexual relationship have a unique engagement with their sexual identity through changing their social and/or personal self-identification. Their journey to LGBTQ identification and beyond intersects with multiple identity issues concerning race and ethnicity, religion, and socioeconomic status. Instead of growing up contending with acceptance and integration into LGBTQ communities as self-maturation occurs, LGBTQ parents PHRD experience a late and often sudden entry into a marginalized group where they may feel disadvantaged not only by chronological age but also by feelings of responsibility for children and personal, social, and economic vulnerabilities from the ending of their previous relationship. The history of exit and entry transitions surrounding the formation of single-parent or stepfamily forms is critical to children's well-being too and appears to present more of a challenge in the long term than coming to terms with parental sexual identity. The challenges of leaving the social privileges that come with heterosexual identification, leaving a heterosexual relationship, and family instability should not be underestimated. Nonetheless, life course research on LGBTQ parents PHRD conveys a hopeful message of personal growth and meaning in life through authenticity and open-mindedness.

## References

Acosta, K. L. (2017). In the event of death: Lesbian families' plans to preserve stepparent-child relationships. *Family Relations, 66*, 244–257. https://doi.org/10.1111/fare.12243

Ainslie, J., & Feltey, K. M. (1991). Definitions and dynamics of motherhood and family in lesbian communities. *Marriage & Family Review, 17*, 63–85. https://doi.org/10.1300/J002v17n01_05

Allen, D. W., Pakaluk, C., & Price, J. (2013). Nontraditional families and childhood progress through school: A comment on Rosenfeld. *Demography, 50*, 955–961. https://doi.org/10.1007/s13524-012-0169-x

Allen, S. H., & Mendez, S. N. (2018). Hegemonic heteronormativity: Toward a new era of queer family theory. *Journal of Family Theory & Review, 10*, 70–86. https://doi.org/10.1111/jftr.12241

Amato, P. R. (2012). The well-being of children with gay and lesbian parents. *Social Science Research, 41*, 771–774. https://doi.org/10.1016/j.ssresearch.2012.04.007

Amato, P. R. (2014). The consequences of divorce for adults and children: An update. *Društvena IstraŽivanja (Social Research), 23*, 5–24. https://doi.org/10.5559/di.23.1.01

Amato, P. R., & Dorius, C. (2010). Fathers, children, & divorce. In M. E. Lamb (Ed.), *The role of the father in child development* (pp. 191–196). Chichester, UK: Wiley.

American Psychological Association. (2014). APA Amicus Brief Case Nos. 13-4178, 14-5003, and 14-5006, Tenth Circuit Court. Retrieved from https://www.apa.org/about/offices/ogc/amicus/kitchen.pdf

Aranda, F., Matthews, A. K., Hughes, T. L., Muramatsu, N., Wilsnack, S. C., Johnson, T. P., & Riley, B. B. (2015). Coming out in color: Racial/ethnic differences in the relationship between level of sexual identity disclosure and depression among lesbians. *Cultural Diversity and Ethnic Minority Psychology, 21*, 247–257. https://doi.org/10.1037/a0037644

Baiocco, R., Carone, N., Ioverno, S., & Lingiardi, V. (2018). Same-sex and different-sex parent families in Italy: Is parents' sexual orientation associated with child health outcomes and parental dimensions? *Journal of Developmental & Behavioral Pediatrics, 39*, 555–563. https://doi.org/10.1097/DBP.0000000000000583

Barnes, D. M., & Meyer, I. H. (2012). Religious affiliation, internalized homophobia, and mental health in lesbians, gay men, and bisexuals. *American Journal of Orthopsychiatry, 82*, 505–515. https://doi.org/10.1111/j.1939-0025.2012.01185.x

Baumle, A. K. (2018). Legal counselling and the marriage decision: The impact of same-sex marriage on family law practice. *Family Relations, 67*, 192–206. https://doi.org/10.1111/fare.12294

Baumle, A. K., & Compton, D. R. (2014). Identity versus identification: How LGBTQ parents identify their children on census surveys. *Journal of Marriage & Family, 76*, 94–104. https://doi.org/10.1111/jomf.12076

Bengtson, V. L., & Allen, K. R. (1993). The life course perspective applied to families over time. In P. G. Boss, W. J. Doherty, R. LaRossa, W. R. Schumm, & S. K. Steinmetz (Eds.), *Sourcebook of family theories and methods: A contextual approach* (pp. 469–499). New York, NY: Plenum Press.

Benson, A. L., Silverstein, L. B., & Auerbach, C. F. (2005). From the margins to the center: Gay fathers reconstruct the fathering role. *Journal of GLBT Family Studies, 1*, 1–29. https://doi.org/10.1300/J461v01n03_01

Berger, R. (1998). Gay stepfamilies: A triple-stigmatized group. *Families in Society, 81*, 504–516. https://doi.org/10.1300/J087v29n03_06

Berkowitz, D., & Marsiglio, W. (2007). Gay men: Negotiating procreative, father, and family identities. *Journal of Marriage & Family, 69*, 366–381. https://doi.org/10.1111/j.1741-3737.2007.00371.x

Bermea, A. M., van Eeden-Moorefield, B., Bible, J., & Petren, R. (2018). Undoing normativities and creating family: A queer stepfamily's experience. *Journal of GLBT Family Studies.*. Advance online publication. doi:https://doi.org/10.1080/1550428X.2018.1521760, 15, 357

Biblarz, T. J., & Savci, E. (2010). Lesbian, gay, bisexual, and transgender families. *Journal of Marriage and Family, 72*, 480–497. https://doi.org/10.1111/j.1741-3737.2010.00714.x

Bigner, J. J. (1996). Working with gay fathers: Developmental, post-divorce parenting, and therapeutic issues. In J. Laird & R. J. Green (Eds.), *Lesbians and gays in couples and families: A handbook for therapists* (pp. 370–403). San Francisco, CA: Jossey-Bass.

Bigner, J. J., & Bozett, F. W. (1990). Parenting by gay fathers. In F. W. Bozett & M. B. Sussman (Eds.), *Homosexuality and family relations* (pp. 155–176). New York, NY: Harrington Park Press.

Bos, H., Kuyper, L., & Gartrell, N. K. (2018). A population-based comparison of female and male same-sex parent and different-sex parent households. *Family Process, 57*, 148–164. https://doi.org/10.1111/famp.12278

Boss, P., & Greenberg, J. (1984). Family boundary ambiguity: A new variable in family stress theory. *Family Process, 23*, 535–546. https://doi.org/10.1111/j.1545-5300.1984.00535.x

Bottoms v Bottoms, (457 S.E. 2d 102 Va 1995).

Bowleg, L., Burkholder, G., Teti, M., & Craig, M. L. (2008). The complexities of outness: Psychosocial predictors of coming out to others among black lesbian and bisexual women. *Journal of LGBT Health Research, 4*, 153–166. https://doi.org/10.1080/15574090903167422

Bozett, F. W. (1987). Gay fathers. In F. W. Bozett (Ed.), *Gay and lesbian parents* (pp. 3–22). New York, NY: Praeger.

Braver, S. L., Shapiro, J. R., & Goodman, M. R. (2006). Consequences of divorce for parents. In M. A. Fine & J. H. Harvey (Eds.), *Handbook of divorce and relationship dissolution* (pp. 313–337). London, UK: Routledge.

Brewster, K. L., Tillman, K. H., & Jokinen-Gordon, H. (2014). Demographic characteristics of lesbian parents in the United States. *Population Research Policy Review, 33*, 503–526. https://doi.org/10.1007/s11113-013-9296-3

Brown, S. L., & Manning, W. D. (2009). Family boundary ambiguity and the measurement of family structure: The significance of cohabitation. *Demography, 46*, 85–101. https://doi.org/10.1353/dem.0.0043

Buxton, A. P. (2005). A family matter: When a spouse comes out as gay, lesbian, or bisexual. *Journal of GLBT Family Studies, 1*, 49–70. https://doi.org/10.1300/J461v01n02_04

Buxton, A. P. (2012). Straight husbands whose wives come out as lesbian or bisexual: Men's voices challenge the "masculinity myth". *Journal of GLBT Family Studies, 8*, 23–45. https://doi.org/10.1080/1550428X.2012.641369

Carroll, M. (2018). Gay fathers on the margins: Race, class, marital status, and pathway to parenthood. *Family Relations, 67*, 104–117. https://doi.org/10.1111/fare.12300

Cenegy, L. F., Denney, J. T., & Kimbro, R. T. (2018). Family diversity and child health: Where do same-sex couple families fit? *Journal of Marriage and Family, 80*, 198–218. https://doi.org/10.1111/jomf.12437

Cherlin, A. (1978). Remarriage as an incomplete institution. *American Journal of Sociology, 84*, 634–650. https://doi.org/10.1086/226830

Church, H. A., O'Shea, D., & Lucey, J. V. (2014). Parent-child relationships in gender identity disorder. *Irish Journal of Medical Science, 183*, 277–281. https://doi.org/10.1007/s11845-013-1003-1

Coleman, E. (1990). The married lesbian. In F. W. Bozett & M. B. Sussman (Eds.), *Homosexuality and family relations* (pp. 119–135). New York, NY: Harrington Park Press.

Daly, S. C., MacNeela, P., & Sarma, K. M. (2015). When parents separate and one parent "comes out" as lesbian, gay or bisexual: Sons and daughters engage with the tension that occurs when their family unit changes.

*PLoS One, 10*, e0145491. https://doi.org/10.1371/journal.pone.0145491

Delvoye, M., & Tasker, F. (2016). Narrating self-identity in bisexual motherhood. *Journal of GLBT Family Studies, 12*, 5–23. https://doi.org/10.1080/1550428X.2015.1038675

Dierckx, M., Motmans, J., Mortelmans, D., & T'sjoen, G. (2015). Families in transition: A literature review. *International Review of Psychiatry, 28*, 36–43. https://doi.org/10.3109/09540261.2015.1102716

Dunlap, A. (2016). Changes in coming out milestones across five age cohorts. *Journal of Gay & Lesbian Social Services, 28*, 20–38. https://doi.org/10.1080/10538720.2016.1124351

Elder, G. H., Jr. (1998). The life course as developmental theory. *Child Development, 69*, 1–12. https://doi.org/10.2307/1132065

Faccio, E., Bordin, E., & Cipolletta, S. (2013). Transsexual parenthood and new role assumptions. *Culture, Health & Sexuality, 15*, 1055–1070. https://doi.org/10.1080/13691058.2013.806676

Farr, R. H., & Goldberg, A. E. (2015). Contact between birth and adoptive families during the first year post-placement: Perspectives of lesbian, gay, and heterosexual parents. *Adoption Quarterly, 18*, 1–24. https://doi.org/10.1080/10926755.2014.895466

Farr, R. H., Tasker, F., & Goldberg, A. E. (2017). Theory in highly cited studies of sexual minority parent families: Variations and implications. *Journal of Homosexuality, 64*, 1143–1179. https://doi.org/10.1080/00918369.2016.1242336

Ferete, J. (2012, January 25). Step-families becoming the new normal in Canada. Retrieved from http://news.nationalpost.com/news/canda/step-families-becoming-the-new-normalin-Canada

Figueroa Guinez, V. M. (2018). *Lesbian motherhood in a Chilean cultural context* (Doctoral thesis). Birkbeck University, London, UK.

Florance, I. (2015). Ian Florance talks to Susan Golombok: "we need to link our research to the real world". *The Psychologist, 28*, 586–587.

Fomby, P., & Cherlin, A. J. (2007). Family instability and child well-being. *American Sociological Review, 72*, 181–204. https://doi.org/10.1177/000312240707200203

Fomby, P., & Osborne, C. (2017). Family instability, multipartner fertility, and behavior in middle childhood. *Journal of Marriage & Family, 79*, 75–93. https://doi.org/10.1111/jomf.12349

Freedman, D., Tasker, F., & Di Ceglie, D. (2002). Children and adolescents with transsexual parents referred to a specialist gender identity development service: A brief report of key developmental features. *Clinical Child Psychology & Psychiatry, 7*, 423–432. https://doi.org/10.1177/1359104502007003009

Fruhauf, C. A., Orel, N. A., & Jenkins, D. A. (2009). The coming-out process of gay grandfathers: Perceptions of their adult children's influence. *Journal of GLBT Family Studies, 5*, 99–118. https://doi.org/10.1080/15504280802595402

Gabb, J. (2004). Critical differentials: Querying the incongruities within research on lesbian parent families. *Sexualities, 7*, 167–182. https://doi.org/10.1177/1363460704042162

Gabb, J. (2005). Lesbian M/Otherhood: Strategies of familial-linguistic management in lesbian parent families. *Sociology, 39*, 585–603. https://doi.org/10.1177/0038038505056025

Galupo, M. P., Henise, S. B., & Mercer, N. L. (2016). "The labels don't work very well": Transgender individuals' conceptualizations of sexual orientation and sexual identity. *International Journal of Transgenderism, 17*, 93–104. https://doi.org/10.1080/15532739.2016.1189373

Galupo, M. P., Ramirez, J. L., & Pulice-Farrow, L. (2017). "Regardless of their gender": Descriptions of sexual identity among bisexual, pansexual, and queer identified individuals. *Journal of Bisexuality, 17*, 108–124. https://doi.org/10.1080/15299716.2016.1228491

Ganong, L., & Coleman, M. (2017). *Stepfamily relationships: Development, dynamics, and interventions* (2nd ed.). New York, NY: Springer.

Gates, G. J. (2015). Marriage and family: LGBT individuals and same-sex couples. *The Future of Children, 25*, 67–89. https://doi.org/10.1353/foc.2015.0013

Gates, G. J., et al. (2012). Letter to the editors and advisory editors of Social Science Research. *Social Science Research, 41*, 1350–1351. https://doi.org/10.1016/j.ssresearch.2012.08.008

Gold, J. M. (2017). Honoring the experiences of gay stepfamilies: An unnoticed population. *Journal of Divorce & Remarriage, 58*, 126–133. https://doi.org/10.1080/10502556.2016.1268020

Goldberg, A. E. (2007). (How) does it make a difference? Perspectives of adults with lesbian, gay, and bisexual parents. *American Journal of Orthopsychiatry, 77*, 550–562. https://doi.org/10.1037/0002-9432.77.4.550

Goldberg, A. E., & Gartrell, N. K. (2014). LGB-parent families: The current state of the research and directions for the future. *Advances in Child Development and Behavior, 46*, 57–88. https://doi.org/10.1016/B978-0-12-800285-8.00003-0

Goldberg, A. E., Gartrell, N. K., & Gates, G. (2014). *Research report on LGB-parent families*. The Williams Institute. Retrieved from http://williamsinstitute.law.ucla.edu/research/parenting/lgb-parent-families-jul-2014/

Golombok, S. (2007). Foreword. *Journal GLBT Family Studies, 3*, xxi–xxvii. https://doi.org/10.1300/J461v03n02_a

Golombok, S., Spencer, A., & Rutter, M. (1983). Children in lesbian and single-parent households: Psychosexual and psychiatric appraisal. *Journal of Child Psychology and Psychiatry, 24*, 551–572. https://doi.org/10.1111/j.1469-7610.1983.tb00132.x

Golombok, S., & Tasker, F. (1994). Children in lesbian and gay families: Theories and evidence. *Annual Review of Sex Research, 5*, 73–100. https://doi.org/10.1080/10532528.1994.10559893

Green, R. (2006). Parental alienation syndrome and the transsexual parent. *International Journal of Transgenderism, 9*, 9–13. https://doi.org/10.1300/1485v09n01.02

Green, R., Mandel, J. B., Hotvedt, M. E., Gray, J., & Smith, L. (1986). Lesbian mothers and their children: A comparison with solo parent heterosexual mothers and their children. *Archives of Sexual Behavior, 7*, 175–181. https://doi.org/10.1007/BF01542224

Greene, B. (1994). Ethnic-minority lesbians and gay men: Mental health and treatment issues. *Journal of Consulting and Clinical Psychology, 62*, 243–251. https://doi.org/10.1037/0022-006X.62.2.243

Greene, B. (1998). Family, ethnic identity, and sexual orientation: African-American lesbians and gay men. In C. Patterson & A. R. D'Augelli (Eds.), *Lesbian, gay, and bisexual identities in families: Psychological perspectives* (pp. 40–52). New York, NY: Oxford University Press.

Haines, B. A., Ajayi, A. A., & Boyd, H. (2014). Making trans parents visible: Intersectionality of trans and parenting identities. *Feminism & Psychology, 24*, 238–247. https://doi.org/10.1177/0959353514526219

Halberstam, J. (2005). *In a queer time and place: Transgender bodies, subcultural lives.* New York, NY: NYU Press.

Haney-Caron, E., & Heilbrun, K. (2014). Lesbian and gay parents and determination of child custody: The changing legal landscape and implications for policy and practice. *Psychology of Sexual Orientation and Gender Diversity, 1*, 19–29. https://doi.org/10.1037/sgd0000020

Hare, J., & Richards, L. (1993). Children raised by lesbian couples: Does context of birth affect father and partner involvement? *Family Relations, 42*, 249–255. https://doi.org/10.2307/585553

Henehan, D., Rothblum, E. D., Solomon, S. E., & Balsam, K. F. (2007). Social and demographic characteristics of gay, lesbian, and heterosexual adults with and without children. *Journal of GLBT Family Studies, 3*, 35–79. https://doi.org/10.1300/J461v03n02_03

Hequembourg, A. (2004). Unscripted motherhood: Lesbian mothers negotiating incompletely institutionalized family relationships. *Journal of Social & Personal Relationships, 21*, 739–762. https://doi.org/10.1177/0265407504047834

Hill, M. (1987). Child rearing attitudes of black lesbian mothers. In the Boston Lesbian Psychologies Collective (Eds.), *Lesbian psychologies: Explorations and challenges* (pp. 215–226). Chicago, IL: University of Illinois Press.

Hines, S. (2006). Intimate transitions: Transgender practices of partnering and parenting. *Sociology, 40*, 353–371. https://doi.org/10.1177/0038038506062037

Holtzman, M. (2011). Nonmarital unions, family definitions, and custody decision making. *Family Relations, 60*, 617–632. https://doi.org/10.1111/j.1741-3729.2011.00670.x

Hurley, M. C. & Law and Government Division Canada (2005). Bill C-38: The civil marriage act (Legislative Summary LS-502E). Retrieved from https://lop.parl.ca/sites/PublicWebsite/default/en_CA/ResearchPublications/LegislativeSummaries/381LS502E

James, S., Herman, J., Rankin, S., Keisling, M., Mottet, L., & Anafi, M. (2016). *The Report of the 2015 U.S. Transgender Survey.* National Center for Transgender Equality. Retrieved from https://transequality.org/sites/default/files/docs/usts/USTS-Full-Report-Dec17.pdf

Jenkins, D. A. (2013). Boundary ambiguity in gay stepfamilies: Perspectives of gay biological fathers and their same-sex partners. *Journal of Divorce & Remarriage, 54*, 329–348. https://doi.org/10.1080/10502556.2013.780501

Johnson, S. M. (2012). Lesbian mothers and their children: The third wave. *Journal of Lesbian Studies, 16*, 45–53. https://doi.org/10.1080/10894160.2011.557642

Kazyak, E., Woodell, B., Scherrer, K., & Finken, E. (2018). Law and family formation among LGBQ-parent families. *Family Court Review, 56*, 364–373. https://doi.org/10.1111/fcre.12353

Kim, S. A., & Stein, E. (2019). The role of gender and gender dynamics in same-sex divorce and dissolution. In A. E. Goldberg & A. P. Romero (Eds.), *LGBTQ divorce and relationship dissolution: Psychological and legal perspectives and implications for practice* (pp. 353–382). New York, NY: Oxford University Press.

Lansford, J. E. (2009). Parental divorce and children's adjustment. *Perspectives in Psychological Science, 4*, 140–152. https://doi.org/10.1111/j.1745-6924.2009.01114.x

LaSala, M. C. (2013). Out of the darkness: Three waves of family research and the emergence of family therapy for lesbian and gay people. *Clinical Social Work Journal, 41*, 267–276. https://doi.org/10.1007/s10615-012-0434-x

Lassiter, P. S., Gutierrez, D., Dew, B. J., & Abrams, L. P. (2017). Gay and lesbian parents: An exploration of wellness, sexual orientation identity, and level of outness. *The Family Journal: Counseling and Therapy for Couples and Families, 25*, 327–335. https://doi.org/10.1177/1066480717731204

Lev, A. I. (2004). *Transgender emergence: Therapeutic guidelines for working with gender-variant people and their families.* New York, NY: Routledge.

Logue, P. M. (2002). The rights of lesbian and gay parents and their children. *Journal of the American Academy of Matrimonial Lawyers, 18*, 95–129.

Lott-Whitehead, L., & Tully, C. (1992). The family of lesbian mothers. *Smith College Studies in Social Work, 63*, 265–280.

Lynch, J. M. (2000). Considerations of family structure and gender composition: The lesbian and gay stepfamily. *Journal of Homosexuality, 40*, 81–95. https://doi.org/10.1300/J082v40n02_06

Lynch, J. M. (2004). The identity transformation of biological parents in lesbian/gay stepfamilies. *Journal of*

*Homosexuality, 47*, 91–107. https://doi.org/10.1300/ J082v47n02_06

Lynch, J. M. (2005). Becoming a stepparent in gay/lesbian stepfamilies: Integrating identities. *Journal of Homosexuality, 48*, 45–60. https://doi.org/10.1300/ J082v48n02_03

Lynch, J. M., & Murray, K. (2000). For the love of the children: The coming out process for lesbian and gay parents and stepparents. *Journal of Homosexuality, 39*, 1–24. https://doi.org/10.1300/J082v39n01_01

Lytle, M. C., Foley, P. F., & Aster, A. M. (2013). Adult children of gay and lesbian parents: Religion and the parent-child relationship. *The Counseling Psychologist, 41*, 530–567. https://doi. org/10.1177/0011000012449658

Mallon, G. P. (2017). Practice with LGBT parents. In G. P. Mallon (Ed.), *Social work practice with lesbian, gay, bisexual, and transgender people* (pp. 165–197). London, UK: Routledge.

Manning, W. D., Fettro, M. N., & Lamidi, E. (2014). Child well-being in same-sex parent families: Review of research prepared for American Sociological Association amicus brief. *Population Research and Policy Review, 33*, 485–502. https://doi.org/10.1007/ s11113-014-9329-6

Marks, L. (2012). Same-sex parenting and children's outcomes: A closer examination of the American Psychological Association's Brief on lesbian and gay parenting. *Social Science Research, 41*, 735–751. https://doi.org/10.1016/j.ssresearch.2012.03.006

McGuire, J. K., Kuvalanka, K. A., Catalpa, J. M., & Toomey, R. B. (2016). Transfamily theory: How the presence of trans* family members informs gender development in families. *Journal of Family Theory & Review, 8*, 60–73. https://doi.org/10.1111/jftr.12125

Miller, B. (1978). Adult sexual resocialization: Adjustments toward a stigmatized identity. *Alternative Lifestyles, 1*, 207–234. https://doi.org/10.1007/ BF01082077

Minter, S. P. (2019). Legal issue in divorce for transgender individuals. In A. E. Goldberg & A. P. Romero (Eds.), *LGBTQ divorce and relationship dissolution: Psychological and legal perspectives and implications for practice* (pp. 312–326). New York, NY: Oxford University Press.

Moore, M. R. (2008). Gendered power relations among women: A study of household decision making in Black, lesbian stepfamilies. *American Sociological Review, 73*, 335–356. https://doi. org/10.1177/000312240807300208

Moore, M. R. (2010). Articulating a politics of (multiple) identities: LGBT sexuality and inclusion in Black community life. *Du Bois Review, 7*, 315–334. https:// doi.org/10.1017/S1742058X10000275

Moore, M. R. (2011). *Invisible families: Gay identities, relationships, and motherhood among black women*. Berkeley, CA: University of California.

Morris, J. F., Balsam, K. F., & Rothblum, E. D. (2002). Lesbian and bisexual mothers and nonmothers: Demographics and the coming-out process. *Journal*

*of Family Psychology, 16*, 144–156. https://doi. org/10.1037/0893-3200.16.2.144

Nixon, C. A. (2011). Working-class lesbian parents' emotional engagement with their children's education: Intersections of class and sexuality. *Sexualities, 14*, 79–99. https://doi.org/10.1177/1363460710390564

Orel, N. A., & Fruhauf, C. (2006). Lesbian and bisexual grandmothers' perceptions of the grandparent-grandchild relationship. *Journal of GLBT Family Studies, 2*, 43–70. https://doi.org/10.1300/ J461v02n01_03

Oswald, R. F., Blume, L. B., & Marks, S. R. (2005). Decentering heteronormativity: A model for family studies. In V. L. Bengtson, A. C. Acock, K. R. Allen, P. Dilworth-Anderson, & D. M. Klein (Eds.), *Sourcebook of family theory and research* (pp. 143– 165). Thousand Oaks, CA: Sage.

Papernow, P. L. (2018). Clinical guidelines for working with stepfamilies: What family, couple, individual, and child therapists need to know. *Family Process, 57*, 25–51. https://doi.org/10.1111/famp.12321

Park, N. K., Kazyak, E., & Slauson-Blevins, K. (2016). How law shapes experiences of parenthood for same-sex couples. *Journal of GLBT Family Studies, 12*, 115–137. https://doi.org/10.1080/15504 28X.2015.1011818

Park, S. M. (2013). *Mothering queerly, queering motherhood: Resisting monomaternalism in adoptive, lesbian, blended, and polygamous families*. Albany, NY: SUNY Press.

Patterson, C. J. (1992). Children of lesbian and gay parents. *Child Development, 63*, 1025–1042. https://doi. org/10.2307/1131517

Patterson, S. (2005a). Better one's own path: The experience of lesbian grandmothers in Canada. *Canadian Women's Studies, 24*, 118–122.

Patterson, S. (2005b). "This is so you know you have options": Lesbian grandmothers and the mixed legacies of nonconformity. *Journal of the Association for Research on Mothering, 7*, 38–48.

Perlesz, A., Brown, R., McNair, R., Lindsay, J., Pitts, M., & de Vaus, D. (2006). Lesbian family disclosure: Authenticity and safety within private and public domains. Lesbian and Gay Psychology Review, 7, 54–65.

Perrin, E. C., Pinderhughes, E. E., Mattern, K., Hurley, S. M., & Newman, R. A. (2016). Experiences of children with gay fathers. *Clinical Pediatrics, 55*, 1305– 1317. https://doi.org/10.1177/0009922816632346

Potter, D. (2012). Same-sex parent families and children's academic achievement. *Journal of Marriage & Family, 74*, 556–571. https://doi. org/10.1111/j.1741-3737.2012.00966.x

Potter, D., & Potter, E. C. (2017). Psychosocial well-being in children of same-sex parents: A longitudinal analysis of familial transitions. *Journal of Family Issues, 38*, 2303–2328. https://doi.org/10.1177/01925 13X16646338

Power, J., Perlesz, A., McNair, R., Schofield, M., Pitts, M., Brown, R., et al. (2012). Gay and bisexual dads and diversity: Fathers in the work, love, play study. *Journal of Family Studies, 18*, 143–154. https://doi.org/10.5172/jfs.2012.18.2-3.143

Pyne, J., Bauer, G., & Bradley, K. (2015). Transphobia and other stressors impacting trans parents. *Journal of GLBT Family Studies, 11*, 107–126. https://doi.org/10.1080/1550428X.2014.941127

Rawsthorne, M., & Costello, M. (2010). Cleaning the sink: Exploring the experiences of Australian lesbian parents reconciling work/family responsibilities. *Community, Work, & Family, 13*, 189–204. https://doi.org/10.1080/13668800903259777

Regnerus, M. (2012). How different are the adult children of parents who have had same-sex relationships? Findings from the New Family Structures Study. *Social Science Research, 41*, 752–770. https://doi.org/10.1016/j.ssresearch.2012.03.009

Riggs, D. W., Power, J., & von Doussa, H. (2016). Parenting and Australian trans and gender diverse people: An exploratory survey. *International Journal of Transgenderism, 17*, 59–65. https://doi.org/10.1080/15532739.2016.1149539

Riggs, D. W., von Doussa, H., & Power, J. (2015). The family and romantic relationships of trans and gender diverse Australians: An exploratory survey. *Sexual and Relationship Therapy, 30*, 243–255. https://doi.org/10.1080/14681994.2014.992409

Robitaille, C., & Saint-Jacques, M. C. (2009). Social stigma and the situation of young people in lesbian and gay stepfamilies. *Journal of Homosexuality, 56*, 421–442. https://doi.org/10.1080/00918360902821429

Rosenfeld, M. J. (2013). Reply to Allen et al. *Demography, 50*, 963–969. https://doi.org/10.1007/s13524-012-0170-4

Sheff, E. (2014). *The polyamorists next door*. Lanham, MD: Rowman & Littlefield.

Shenkman, G., Ifrah, K., & Shmotkin, D. (2018). Meaning in life among middle-aged and older gay and heterosexual fathers. *Journal of Family Issues, 39*, 2155–2173. https://doi.org/10.1177/0192513X17741922

Stacey, J., & Biblarz, T. J. (2001). (How) does the sexual orientation of parents matter? *American Sociological Review, 66*, 159–183. https://doi.org/10.2307/2657413

Stotzer, R. L., Herman, J. L., & Hasenbush, A. (2014). Transgender parenting: A review of existing research. Williams Institute. Retrieved from https://williamsinstitute.law.ucla.edu/research/parenting/transgender-parenting-oct-2014/

Sullins, P. D. (2015). Emotional problems among children with same-sex parents: Difference by definition. *British Journal of Education, Society & Behavioural Science, 7*, 99–120. https://doi.org/10.9734/BJESBS/2015/15823

Tabor, J. (2019). Mom, dad, or somewhere in between: Role-relational ambiguity and children of transgender parents. *Journal of Marriage & Family, 81*, 506–519. https://doi.org/10.1111/jomf.12537

Tasker, F. (2005). Lesbian mothers, gay fathers and their children: A review. *Journal of Developmental & Behavioral Pediatrics, 26*, 224–240. https://doi.org/10.1097/00004703-200506000-00012

Tasker, F. (2013). Lesbian and gay parenting post-heterosexual divorce and separation. In A. E. Goldberg & K. R. Allen (Eds.), *LGBT-parent families: Innovations in research and implications for practice* (pp. 3–20). New York, NY: Springer.

Tasker, F. (2018, September). *Today's family maps & tomorrow's possibilities: Family formations and LGBTQ parenting*. Keynote address at the Ninth European Society on Family Relations Congress, Porto, Portugal.

Tasker, F., & Delvoye, M. (2015). Moving out of the shadows: Accomplishing bisexual motherhood. *Sex Roles, 73*, 125–140. https://doi.org/10.1007/s11199-015-0503-z

Tasker, F., & Delvoye, M. (2018). Maps of family relationships drawn by women engaged in bisexual motherhood: Defining family membership. *Journal of Family Issues, 39*, 4248–4274. https://doi.org/10.1177/0192513X18810958

Tasker, F., & Malley, M. (2012). Working with LGBT parents. In J. J. Bigner & J. L. Wetchler (Eds.), *Handbook of LGBT-affirmative couple and family therapy* (pp. 149–165). New York, NY: Routledge.

Tasker, F., & Rensten, K. (2019). Social science research on heterosexual relationship dissolution and divorce where one parent comes out as LGB. In A. E. Goldberg & A. P. Romero (Eds.), *LGBTQ divorce and relationship dissolution: Psychological and legal perspectives and implications for practice* (pp. 173–194). New York, NY: Oxford University Press.

Tasker, F. L., & Golombok, S. (1997). *Growing up in a lesbian family: Effects on child development*. New York, NY: Guilford Press.

Taylor, L. A., & Cobb, J. (2011). *Our family outing: A memoir of coming out and coming through*. Tusla, OK: Total Publishing and Media.

Tornello, S., & Patterson, C. (2015). Timing of parenthood and experiences of gay fathers: A life course perspective. *Journal of GLBT Family Studies, 11*, 35–56. https://doi.org/10.1080/1550428X.2013.878681

Tornello, S. L., Sonnenberg, B. N., & Patterson, C. J. (2015). Division of labor among gay fathers: Associations with parent, couple, and child adjustment. *Psychology of Sexual Orientation and Gender Diversity, 2*, 365–375. https://doi.org/10.1037/sgd0000109

Tuthill, Z. (2016). Negotiating religiosity and sexual identity among Hispanic lesbian mothers. *Journal of Homosexuality, 63*, 1194–1210. https://doi.org/10.1080/00918369.2016.1151691

Van Dam, M. A. A. (2004). Mothers in two types of lesbian families: Stigma experiences, supports, and burdens. *Journal of Family Nursing, 10*, 450–484. https://doi.org/10.1177/1074840704270120

van Eeden-Moorefield, B., Pasley, K., Crosbie-Burnett, M., & King, E. (2012). Explaining couple cohesion in different types of gay families. *Journal of Family Issues, 33*, 182–201. https://doi.org/10.1177/0192513X11418180

Veldorale-Griffin, A. (2014). Transgender parents and their adult children's experiences of disclosure and transition. *Journal of GLBT Family Studies, 10,* 475–501. https://doi.org/10.1080/1550428X.2013.866063

Whalen, D. M., Bigner, J. J., & Barber, C. E. (2000). The grandmother role as experienced by lesbian women. *Journal of Women & Aging, 12*(3–4), 39–58. https://doi.org/10.1300/J074v12n03_04

White, T., & Ettner, R. (2004). Children of parents who make a gender transition: Disclosure, risks, and protective factors. *Journal of Gay & Lesbian Psychotherapy, 8,* 129–145. https://doi.org/10.1300/J236v08n01_10

White, T., & Ettner, R. (2007). Adaptation and adjustment in children of transsexual parents. *European Child & Adolescent Psychiatry, 16,* 215–221. https://doi.org/10.1007/s00787-006-0591-y

Woodell, B., Kazyak, E., & Compton, D. (2015). Reconciling LGB and Christian identities in the rural south. *Social Sciences, 4,* 859–878. https://doi.org/10.3390/socsci4030859

# Lesbian-Mother Families Formed Through Donor Insemination

Henny Bos and Nanette Gartrell

For decades, theory and research on family functioning focused on two-parent families consisting of a father and a mother. Over the past 30 years, however, the concept of what makes a family has changed. Some children now grow up in patchwork or blended families, namely, families headed by two parents, one of whom has a child or children from a previous relationship. Other children grow up in planned lesbian-parent families, that is, those headed by lesbians who decide to have children through adoption, foster care, or donor insemination. These lesbian mothers and their children differ from lesbian mothers whose children were born into a previous heterosexual relationship. Such children typically experience their mother's coming out and her separation or divorce from the children's father. This type of transition could potentially influence the child's psychological well-being. Many other variations in family structures, or combinations of the abovementioned family types, are possible (e.g., a child is born after two lesbian women form a relationship, and both mothers also have a child or children from a previous heterosexual relationship or marriage; see chapter "LGBTQ Parenting Post-Heterosexual Relationship Dissolution"). The present chapter focuses specifically on lesbian-mother families in which the children were conceived through donor insemination (i.e., planned lesbian-mother families).

Since the 1980s, assisted reproductive technologies (ART) have made it possible for lesbians to become parents through sperm banks (if they have the economic means) or private arrangements with known donors. As a result, planned lesbian-mother families are now an integral part of the social structure of many economically developed countries (Parke, 2004). According to data compiled in a 2018 report from the Williams Institute, approximately 114,000 same-sex couples in the USA are raising children; these include 86,000 female couples and 28,000 male couples (Goldberg & Conron, 2018). Most of these couples are raising biological children. It is unclear, however, whether those raised by female couples were born into lesbian relationships or to lesbian-identified mothers.

It is expected that the number of children born into planned lesbian-parent families and raised

H. Bos (✉)
Sexual and Gender Diversity in Families and Youth,
Research Institute of Child Development and
Education, Faculty of Social and Behavioural
Sciences, University of Amsterdam,
Amsterdam, Netherlands
e-mail: h.m.w.bos@uva.nl

N. Gartrell
Visiting Distinguished Scholar, The Williams
Institute, U.C.L.A. School of Law,
Los Angeles, CA, USA

Guest Appointee, Research Institute of Child
Development and Education, Faculty of Social and
Behavioural Sciences, University of Amsterdam,
Amsterdam, Netherlands
e-mail: ngartrell@nllfs.org

© Springer Nature Switzerland AG 2020
A. E. Goldberg, K. R. Allen (eds.), *LGBTQ-Parent Families*,
https://doi.org/10.1007/978-3-030-35610-1_2

by lesbian mothers will continue to increase. Based on data from the 2011–2013 US National Survey of Family Growth (a nationally representative probability sample of 15–44-year-olds), Riskind and Tornello (2017) found that 78% of childless women identifying as lesbian ($n = 39$) answered "yes" to the question, "Looking to the future, if it were possible, would you, yourself, want to have a baby at some time in the future?" Similar results were reported in the Netherlands where 63% of 464 females between 12 and 24 years of age who identified as lesbian or bisexual wanted to become parents in the future, and 22% indicated that they did not yet know (Nikkelen & Vermey, 2018).

Attitudes toward lesbian parenting have improved during the past 30 years. In 1992, 29% of participants in a US population-based study reported that same-sex couples should have the legal right to adopt a child, and by 2014, 63% of participants agreed (Gallup, 2014). A 2006/2007 report from the Netherlands found that 54% of respondents supported adoption by same-sex couples; this increased to 73% in 2016/2017 (Kuyper, 2018).

These changing attitudes towards same-sex parenting also have meant that ART has become more accessible to lesbian women. For example, in 2008, the statement that a "child needs a father" was removed from the UK Human Fertilization and Embryology Act (see: http://www.dh.gov.uk/en/Publicationsandstatistics/Legislation/Actsandbills/DH_080211), and between 2013 and 2015, the Ethics Committee of the American Society for Reproductive Medicine concluded that denying access to fertility services for lesbian, gay, transgender, and unmarried people is not justified (Ethics Committee of the American Society for Reproductive Medicine, 2013, 2015).

Nevertheless, the right and fitness of sexual minorities to parent is still widely disputed in the media and in the legal and policy arenas. Opponents of sexual minority parenting claim that the children are at risk of developing a variety of behavior problems. It is assumed that children of lesbians who are raised in fatherless households might be teased by peers because of their mothers' sexual orientation (for analyses of opponents' arguments, see Clarke, 2001; Gabb, 2018). To address these concerns, proponents of marriage equality and lesbian parenthood rely on studies that have been conducted on planned lesbian-mother families. These studies found no evidence to support claims that the traditional mother–father family is the ideal environment in which to raise children (Rosky, 2009).

## Research Approaches and Theoretical Perspectives

In general, the studies cited in this chapter can be divided in two groups: those conducted from a between-difference approach (in which planned lesbian families with donor-conceived offspring are compared with different-sex parent families) and a within-difference approach (focusing on diversity within planned lesbian families; Bos, 2019). Studies based on both approaches represent a variety of disciplines, varying from psychology, medicine, and public health to social work and sociology (Farr, Tasker, & Goldberg, 2017). Between-difference studies are often driven by the public debate over whether the two types of families differ in parenting capabilities and child outcomes. The backdrop of this debate includes questions about whether: (a) lesbian mothers should be allowed to parent, (b) lesbian mothers can be appropriate socialization agents, and (c) children need both a mother and a father for a healthy development (Biblarz & Stacey, 2010; Farr et al., 2017; Lamb, 2012). Several of these studies are simultaneously driven by public debate and based on theory. In addition, research question(s) are often derived from a combination of theories (i.e., eclectic paradigm; Eldredge et al., 2016), such as Bronfenbrenner's (2001) ecological theory, family systems theory (Boss, 2001), and gender and queer theory (Butler, 1990) (for overview, see Farr et al., 2017).

Within-difference investigations focus more on nuanced family dynamics and unique family processes that are specific to lesbian mothers and children conceived through ART (e.g., relationships with donors, parenting with different biological relationships to the child). An important topic in within-difference investigations is the role of stigmatization on parenting and child development in planned lesbian families with donor-conceived offspring. The frameworks used for these studies are based mainly on theories of stigmatization (Goffman, 1963) and minority stress (Meyer, 2003). Recent studies based on the within-difference approach have focused on resilience within lesbian-parent families. Although grounded in minority stress theory, these investigations not only examined minority stressors as risk factors, but also explored influences that protect families against the impact of these stressors on well-being and development. Resilience studies in lesbian-parent families have been underutilized. However, they offer research opportunities for the future since the outcomes may facilitate the development of clinical and educational programs to promote key family strengths (Prendergast & MacPhee, 2018).

## Planned Lesbian-Mother Families Compared with Different-Sex Parent Families

Early studies on planned lesbian-mother families were often aimed at establishing whether lesbians can be good parents, whether they should be granted legal parenthood, and whether they should have access to assisted reproductive technologies (e.g., Kirkpatrick, Smith, & Roy, 1981; Mucklow & Phelan, 1979). The emphasis was originally on proving the normality of planned lesbian-mother families and the children who grow up in them (for overviews, see Clarke, 2008; Sandfort, 2000; Stacey & Biblarz, 2001). In order to inform family policy and regulations on assisted reproduction, it continues to be important to compare parents and children in planned lesbian-mother and different-sex parent families. It is also important to continue this research focus in order to further theoretical understanding of the influence of family structure (same-sex vs. different-sex parents) and family processes (parent-child relationships, relationships between parents) on child development.

The association between family structure and outcomes for children can be complex, with family structure often playing a less important role in children's psychological development than the quality of the family relationships (Golombok, 2015).

The results of studies that compare planned lesbian-mother and different-sex parent families are presented below. These studies focused on three main areas: (a) family characteristics, (b) parenting, and (c) the development of offspring.

## Family Characteristics

**Age of Mother and Motivation to Have Children** In a Dutch study of 100 planned lesbian-mother families and 100 heterosexual two-parent families (with children between 4 and 8 years old), Bos, van Balen, and van den Boom (2003) found that both biological and co-mothers in planned lesbian-mother families were, on average, older than heterosexual parents. At that time, the age difference may have been related to several issues: (a) lesbian women may have begun to think about having children later than heterosexual women; (b) lesbians have to make several decisions regarding the conception (e.g., deciding on donors), which takes time; and (c) it takes longer to achieve pregnancy through donor insemination than by natural conception (Botchan et al., 2001). Now that sexual minority parent families are more visible and accepted in society, it is conceivable that lesbian family planning will start at an earlier age.

In Bos et al.'s (2003) study, participants were also asked about their motives for parenthood. The lesbian biological mothers and co-mothers differed from heterosexual mothers and fathers in that they spent more time thinking about their motives for having children. Because lesbians carefully weigh the pros and cons of having children, their process to parenthood may be comparable to that of infertile heterosexual couples, with an enhanced awareness of the importance of parenthood in their lives. However, Bos et al. (2003) found that lesbian and heterosexual parents ranked their parenthood motives similarly. Both types of parents reported that their most important motives were feelings of affection toward children and an expectation that parenthood would provide life fulfillment (Bos et al., 2003).

**Division of Family Tasks** How parents in lesbian-mother families and heterosexual two-parent families divide their time between family tasks (unpaid work such as household tasks and childcare) and paid work tends to be measured in two ways: via questionnaire (e.g., the "Who Does What?" measure [Chan, Brooks, Raboy, & Patterson, 1998; Cowan & Cowan, 1988] or via a structured diary record of daily activities [e.g., Bos, van Balen, & van den Boom, 2007]). Overall these studies found that lesbian-parent families with young children were more likely to share family tasks to a greater degree than mothers and fathers in heterosexual two-parent families. It is possible that the absence of gender polarization and having more flexible gender identities in lesbian-mother families led to more equal burden-sharing (Goldberg, 2013), which might explain findings that lesbian mothers were more satisfied with their partners as co-parents than heterosexual parents (Bos et al., 2007). Analysis of diary data also revealed that lesbian biological mothers and co-mothers spent similar amounts of time on employment outside the home, in contrast to heterosexual two-parent families in which the fathers spent much more time at their work outside the home than their partners did (Bos et al., 2007). It is also possible that lesbian partners may be more attentive and sensitive to issues of (in)equality in their relationships (Goldberg, 2013) and understand each other's career opportunities and challenges better than do heterosexual partners (see Dunne, 1998).

**Parental Justification and Self-Efficacy** Parental justification or the feeling that one has to demonstrate to people that one is a good parent has been an important concept to examine because it is potentially related to parenting stress. Bos et al.

(2007) found that Dutch lesbian co-mothers felt more pressured to justify the quality of their parenting than heterosexual fathers. An explanation for this finding might be that, in the absence of a biological tie to the children, co-mothers do their utmost to be "good moms."

Feeling obligated to demonstrate their competence as parents could influence the parental self-efficacy of lesbian mothers. However, a nationally representative Dutch survey on parenting and child development found that the birth mothers in two-mother families felt more competent than mothers in different-sex parent households (Bos, Kuyper, & Gartrell, 2017). The unequal division of labor within mother–father families may provide a possible explanation for this finding. Mothers in different-sex parent households carry a greater burden of household responsibilities, which may contribute to their feeling they have less time to devote to competent parenting.

## Parenting

**Parental Stress** In their study of Dutch lesbian-mother families with young children, Bos, Van Balen, and Van Den Boom (2004a) found that parental stress among lesbian mothers was comparable to that of heterosexual parents. These data are congruent with reports from other countries. Shechner, Slone, Meir, and Kalish (2010) examined maternal stress in 30 Israeli lesbian two-mother families, 30 heterosexual two-parent families, and 30 single-mother families (all with children between 4 and 8 years old). Single heterosexual mothers reported higher levels of stress than lesbian or heterosexual mothers; lesbian mothers' stress scores did not differ from those of the heterosexual mothers. Similar findings were found in a Dutch study of first-time parents whose children were 4 months old. There were no significant differences between lesbian mothers with donor-conceived infants, heterosexual parents with in vitro fertilization (IVF)-conceived infants (who did not use gamete donation), and gay fathers who became parents through surrogacy (van Rijn-van Gelderen et al., 2017). In contrast, a US population-based study drawn from the National Survey of Children's Health found that female same-sex parents of children and adolescents experienced more parenting stress than different-sex parents to whom they were demographically matched (Bos, Knox, van Rijn-van Gelderen, & Gartrell, 2016). A similarly designed population-based study in the Netherlands reported no differences in parenting stress when same- and different-sex parents were compared, but fathers in same-sex couples and mothers in different-sex couples felt less parental competence than their counterparts (Bos et al., 2017).

**Parenting Styles** Studies based on parental self-report data in the UK, the USA, the Netherlands, and Belgium found that lesbian co-mothers of young children had higher levels of emotional involvement, parental concern, and parenting awareness skills than fathers in heterosexual two-parent families (Bos et al., 2004a; Bos et al., 2007; Brewaeys, Ponjaert, van Hall, & Golombok, 1997; Flaks, Ficher, Masterpasqua, & Joseph, 1995; Golombok, Tasker, & Murray, 1997). In the Bos et al. (2007) Dutch study comparing lesbian and heterosexual two-parent families, data were also gathered through observations of the parent relationship during a home visit in which the parent and child were videotaped performing two instructional tasks, which were later scored by two different trained raters. Co-mothers differed from fathers in that they showed lower levels of limit-setting during the parent–child interaction (Bos et al., 2007). These differences were not found between lesbian biological mothers and heterosexual mothers. Explanations offered for these findings focused on gender: Women are expected to be more expressive, nurturant, and sensitive, while men more often exhibit instrumental competence, such as disciplining (Lamb, 1999).

In a follow-up of the aforementioned Dutch 2007 study, when the offspring reached adolescence (average age 16 years), they were asked about parental monitoring of their behavior, disclosure about their personal lives to their parents, and the quality of the relationship with their parents (Bos, van Gelderen, & Gartrell, 2014). The adolescents' scores on these variables (measured with standardized instruments) were compared with a matched group of adolescents in different-sex parent families; no significant differences were found. Of note is the offspring were asked about their parents in general, and no distinction was made between parents.

Golombok et al. (2003) used standardized interviews to assess the quality of parent–child relationships in a community sample of 7-year-old children from 39 lesbian-mother families (20 headed by a single mother and 19 by a lesbian couple), 74 heterosexual two-parent families, and 60 families headed by single heterosexual mothers. In this study a significant difference was found for emotional involvement, with fathers scoring higher than co-mothers. However, it should be noted that a substantial number of the lesbian co-mothers were stepmothers who had not been involved in the decision to have the child and did not raise the child from birth.

In their longitudinal study in the UK, Golombok and Badger (2010) compared 20 families headed by lesbian mothers, 27 families headed by single heterosexual mothers, and 36 two-parent heterosexual families, at the time their offspring reached early adulthood. Lesbian and single heterosexual mothers were more emotionally involved with their offspring than heterosexual mothers in two-parent families. Lesbian and single heterosexual mothers also showed lower levels of separation anxiety than mothers in the heterosexual two-parent families. Single mothers reported less conflict and less severe disputes with their adult offspring than did the lesbian mothers.

In sum, empirical studies reveal some differences between lesbian and heterosexual parents. Lesbian mothers are more committed as parents, spend more time caring for their children, and show higher levels of emotional involvement with their children.

## Child and Adolescent Development

**Psychosocial Development** Research on the children raised in planned lesbian-mother families has mainly focused on their psychological adjustment and peer relationships. Most studies found no significant differences between children raised in lesbian-parent and heterosexual two-parent families with regard to problem behavior, well-being, and emotion regulation (Baiocco et al., 2015; Bos et al., 2007; Bos & van Balen, 2008; Brewaeys, Ponjaert-Kristoffersen, van Steirteghem, & Devroey, 1993; Crouch, Waters, McNair, Power, & Davis, 2014; Flaks et al., 1995; Patterson, 1994; Steckel, 1987). There are, however, some exceptions to the abovementioned findings. In the US National Longitudinal Lesbian Family Study (NLLFS), for example, the 38 10-year-old daughters of lesbian parents had significantly lower mean scores on externalizing problem behavior (as measured by the Child Behavior Checklist, or CBCL; Achenbach, 1991; Achenbach & Rescorla, 2001) than the Achenbach age-matched normative sample of girls (Gartrell, Deck, Rodas, Peyser, & Banks, 2005). Golombok et al. (1997) found that when the offspring from planned lesbian-mother families in the UK were 6 years old, they rated themselves less cognitively and physically competent than did their counterparts in father-present families. At the age of 9, however, there were no significant differences on psychological adjustment between the two groups (MacCallum & Golombok, 2004). In Belgium, Vanfraussen, Ponjaert-Kristoffersen, and Brewaeys (2002) reported that although the 24 children in lesbian-parent families were not more frequently teased than the 24 children in heterosexual two-parent families about such matters as clothes or physical appearance, family-related incidents of teasing were mentioned only by children from lesbian-parent families. Vanfraussen et al. also gathered data on the children's well-being through reports from teachers, parents, and children. Teachers reported more attention problem behavior in children from lesbian-mother families than in children from mother–father families. However, based on reports from mothers and the children

themselves, no significant differences in the children's problem behavior were found. An explanation for this discrepancy could be that the teachers' evaluations were influenced by their own negative attitudes towards lesbianism. A US study revealed that preservice teacher attitudes toward gay and lesbian parents were more negative than their attitudes towards heterosexual parents (Herbstrith, Tobin, Hesson-McInnis, & Joel Schneider, 2013).

In the earlier mentioned Dutch follow-up study, it was found that the adolescents raised in lesbian two-mother families had higher scores on self-esteem and lower scores on conduct problems than their counterparts raised in mother–father families (Bos et al., 2014). However, it should be mentioned that like many other investigations on adolescents with lesbian mothers, this study did not use a multi-informant approach; the findings were based only on the information provided by the adolescents. As a consequence, the results could be influenced by reporter bias as adolescents in same-sex parent families develop a keener awareness of their minority status (Rivers, Poteat, & Noret, 2008).

The abovementioned studies on the psychological development of children were all based on convenience samples: The planned lesbian-mother families were recruited with the help of gay and lesbian organizations, through friendship networks or hospital fertility departments, or sometimes through a combination of these methods. However, other studies used a different recruitment strategy. Golombok et al. (2003) extracted household composition data from the UK Avon Longitudinal Study of Parents and Children dataset. They used this information to identify households headed by two women and compared them with different-sex parent families. They found no differences in the psychological well-being of young children in the two types of households.

A similar strategy was used by Wainright and colleagues (Wainright & Patterson, 2006, 2008; Wainright, Russell, & Patterson, 2004), who used the US National Longitudinal Study of Adolescent Health (Add Health) dataset to identify households headed by two mothers. They identified 44 families headed by two mothers, and each of them was matched with an adolescent of the Add Health dataset who was reared in a different-sex parent family. They found no differences in substance use, relationships with peers, and progress through school between adolescents in households headed by two women and those in different-sex parent families.

Because of their strong associations with child and adolescent health outcomes, parental relationship (in)stability or (dis)continuity, and family transitions (e.g., fostering or adopting) have been considered in some population-based comparative studies. Using aggregate 1997 to 2013 data from the National Health Interview Survey, Sullins (2015a, 2015b) found higher rates of emotional problems in children with same-sex parents. However, the Sullins studies did not account for family stability and transitions (e.g., separation/divorce, foster care, adoption) in comparing the different types of families, which may have influenced the outcomes (American Sociological Association, 2015). In a comparison of 6- to 17-year-olds with same- and different-sex parents drawn from the US National Survey of Children's Health, Bos et al. (2016) focused only on families in which neither the parents (i.e., through divorce or separation) nor the children (i.e., through adoption or foster care) had experienced a major instability or transition. The 95 children and adolescents with female same-sex parents did not differ in general health, emotional difficulties, coping behavior, or learning behavior from a demographically matched sample of 95 children and adolescents with different-sex parents. Likewise, using data from the Dutch Youth and Development Survey, 43 female and 52 male same-sex couple families were demographically matched with 95 different-sex parent families (Bos et al., 2017). None of the 5- to 18-year-olds in either type of family had experienced major instability or transition, and no differences associated with family type were found in their psychological well-being.

Among other studies on adolescents, Golombok & Badger's, 2010 longitudinal study in the UK found that at the age of 19, adolescents born into lesbian-mother families showed lower levels of anxiety, depression, hostility, and problematic alcohol use, and higher levels of self-esteem, than adolescents in father–mother families. Likewise, Gartrell and Bos (2010) found that at the age of 17 years, the US NLLFS offspring (39 boys and 39 girls) demonstrated higher levels of social, school/academic, and total competence than gender-matched normative samples of American teenagers (49 girls and 44 boys). Although the US NLLFS sample and the comparison sample were similar in socioeconomic status, they were not matched on, nor did the authors control for, race/ethnicity or region of residence. This type of matching was done in another US NLLFS publication about substance use (Goldberg, Bos, & Gartrell, 2011). The researchers used the Monitoring the Future (MTF) data as a comparison group, and by using a 1:1 matching procedure on gender, age, race/ethnicity, and parental education, they randomly selected 78 17-year-old adolescents from the MTF dataset. There were no differences in the two groups on the likelihood of reporting heavy substance use (Goldberg et al., 2011). On a standardized assessment of quality of life, the US NLLFS adolescents scored comparably to their matched counterparts, who were drawn from a representative sample and raised by different-sex parents (van Gelderen, Bos, Gartrell, Hermanns, & Perrin, 2012).

When the US NLLFS offspring reached the age of 25, they completed the Achenbach Adult Self-Report, which assesses mental health through a series of questions about relationships and school/job performance and a checklist about behavior (Gartrell, Bos, & Koh, 2018). The scores of these adults raised in two-mother households were compared to a demographically matched group from the population-based Achenbach normative sample (Gartrell et al., 2018). No significant differences were found in the two groups with respect to family, friends, spouse/partner relationships, school/college or job performance, behavioral/emotional problems, or the mental health diagnostic scales. These positive findings regarding individuals raised in planned lesbian-parent families may be partly explained by the mothers' commitment to and involvement in the rearing of their children, or by other aspects regarding the quality of the relationships within the family (e.g., sharing parental responsibilities).

**Gender Role, Sexual Questioning, and Sexual Behavior** Other frequently studied aspects of the development of children in planned lesbian-parent families are the children's gender roles and sexual behavior. MacCallum and Golombok (2004) studied 25 lesbian-mother families, 38 families headed by a single heterosexual mother, and 38 two-parent heterosexual families in the UK and found that boys in lesbian- or single-mother families showed more feminine personality traits than boys in two-parent heterosexual families. However, other studies that focused on children's aspirations to traditionally masculine or feminine occupations and activities did not find differences between children in lesbian-parent families and those in two-parent heterosexual families (Brewaeys et al., 1997; Fulcher, Sutfin, & Patterson, 2008; Golombok et al., 2003).

In the Netherlands, Bos and Sandfort (2010) studied the gender development of 63 children with lesbian mothers and 68 children with heterosexual parents from a multidimensional perspective by focusing on five issues: (a) gender typicality (the degree to which the children felt that they were typical members of their gender category), (b) gender contentedness (the degree to which the children felt happy with their assigned gender), (c) pressure to conform (the degree to which the children felt pressure from parents and peers to conform to gender stereotypes), (d) intergroup bias (the degree to which the children felt that their gender was superior to the other gender), and (e) children's anticipation of future heterosexual romantic involvement. The authors found that when the children were between 8 and 12 years old, those in lesbian-parent families felt less parental pressure to conform to gender stereotypes, were less likely to experience their own gender as superior (intergroup bias), and were more likely to question

future heterosexual romantic involvement than those in heterosexual two-parent families. An explanation for these findings might be that lesbian mothers have more liberal attitudes than heterosexual parents toward their children's gender-related behavior (Fulcher et al., 2008). That children in lesbian-mother families are less certain about future heterosexual romantic involvement might also be a result of growing up in a family environment that is more accepting of homoerotic relationships.

The abovementioned findings are all based on studies of children. Three studies on adolescents also included questions about sexual and romantic behavior and sexual orientation. The Wainright et al. (2004) study using Add Health data revealed no significant differences in heterosexual intercourse or romantic relationships between young adults with female same-sex parents and young adults with different-sex parents. The 2010 longitudinal UK study by Golombok and Badger found that as young adults (mean age 19), individuals with lesbian mothers were more likely to have started dating than young adults from heterosexual-parent families. However, the US NLLFS found that the 17-year-old female offspring of lesbian mothers were significantly older at the time of their first heterosexual contact compared to an age- and gender-matched comparison group from the National Survey of Family Growth (Gartrell, Bos, & Goldberg, 2012). The daughters of US NLLFS lesbian mothers were also significantly less likely to have been pregnant and more likely to have used emergency contraception than their peers (Gartrell et al., 2012). In both the UK and the US studies, most offspring of lesbian mothers identified as heterosexual. However, nearly one in five of the US NLLFS girls identified in the bisexual spectrum, which is consistent with the theory that an accepting family environment makes it more comfortable for adolescent girls with same-sex attractions to explore intimate relationships with their peers (Biblarz & Stacey, 2010; Stacey & Biblarz, 2001). At the age of 25, although most NLLFS offspring identified as "heterosexual or straight," compared to their counterparts in a population-based survey, the adult offspring were significantly more to likely to report same-sex attraction, sexual minority identity, and same-sex sexual experience (Gartrell, Bos, & Koh, 2019).

## Comparison Between Biological Mothers and Nonbiological Mothers in Planned Lesbian-Mother Families

In studies that compare biological and nonbiological mothers in planned lesbian- parent families, there are three main topics of interest: (a) the pregnancy decision-making process and the desire and motivation to have children, (b) the division of tasks (household and childrearing), and (c) parenting. Interest in the differences and similarities between biological and nonbiological mothers is linked to the role and position of the mothers who did not bear the child, especially because these mothers are living in a societal context in which the biological relatedness of the parents is often perceived as important.

## Pregnancy Decision-Making Process and Desire and Motivation to Have Children

Several studies have examined the decision-making process concerning which of the partners in lesbian couples will conceive and bear the children. Goldberg (2006) interviewed 29 American lesbian couples about their decision regarding who would try to become pregnant and the reasons behind this decision. The most frequently mentioned reason was the biological mother's desire to experience pregnancy and childbirth; for some, it was also important to have a genetic connection with the child (Goldberg, 2006). However, many couples had other reasons, such as age: The older partner was chosen because it could have been her last chance to become pregnant, or the younger partner was chosen because they both thought that the age of the older partner might make it difficult for her to conceive. Additionally, some couples invoked their employment situation, such that the partner with the

most flexible job was chosen to conceive. Chabot and Ames (2004) interviewed 10 American lesbian couples (with children between 3 months and 8 years old) and observed these couples during support group meetings for lesbian parents. Similar results were found to Goldberg's, 2006 study on how the couples decided who would carry the child.

Each partner in a lesbian couple can theoretically carry a child. Studies have shown, however, that few couples make the decision to do this. For example, a study of 95 lesbian couples who were undergoing donor insemination at a clinic in Belgium found that only 14% wanted both partners to become pregnant; these couples wanted first the older and then the younger partner to do so (Baetens, Camus, & Devroey, 2002). A study of 100 Dutch lesbian couples with one or more children (the oldest between 4 and 8 years old) found that in only a minority (33%) of cases had both mothers given birth to a child (Bos et al., 2003). While in Baetens et al.'s (2002) study it was the older partner who had been the first to attempt pregnancy, in Bos et al.'s (2003) study there was no significant age difference between the two would-be parents.

Bos et al. (2003) also compared mothers who became pregnant with those who did not. They found that the former group had spent more time thinking about why they wanted to become mothers, stated more frequently that they had had to "give up almost everything" to become pregnant, and more frequently described "parenthood as a life fulfillment." Indeed, it would be interesting to examine the extent to which gender identity (i.e., whether women use stereotypic feminine or masculine personality traits to describe themselves) is a predictor of the desire to experience pregnancy and childbirth. For heterosexual women in economically developed cultures, being a mother is considered evidence of femininity (Ulrich & Weatherall, 2000).

In 2010, shared IVF motherhood began to receive more attention in the literature about lesbian-mother families (Marina et al., 2010). This practice, also called "reception of oocyte from partner" (ROPA), involves one partner in a lesbian couple providing the ovum and the other carrying the fetus to term. ROPA reflects the wish of a lesbian couple to conceive a child together (although they still need the contribution of a sperm donor) through a combined genetic and biological link (Pennings, 2016). ROPA is also consistent with egalitarianism in lesbian relationships (Pelka, 2009), because it avoids the biological versus nonbiological asymmetry (Raes et al., 2014) and diminishes feelings of envy (Pelka, 2009). ROPA is an acceptable, successful, and safe treatment option for lesbian couples with financial means (e.g., Bodri et al., 2018). The number of ROPA pregnancies seems to be growing (Machin, 2014), although in 2017, ROPA was only allowed in a few countries (i.e., in countries where same-sex marriage is allowed, lesbian women are eligible for all forms of ART, and known egg donation is legally authorized; Bodri et al., 2018). ROPA is still an understudied topic in research on lesbian-mother families.

## Division of Tasks

There is a great deal of variability in the labor arrangements (paid and unpaid work) within lesbian parenting relationships (Goldberg, 2010, 2013). Several studies found an equal division of both child-rearing tasks and paid work between the partners in planned lesbian-mother families (Chan et al., 1998; Gartrell et al., 1999; Gartrell et al., 2000). However, other research found that biological lesbian mothers were more involved in childcare than their partners and that the nonbiological lesbian mothers spent more time working outside the home (Bos et al., 2007; Downing & Goldberg, 2011; Goldberg & Perry-Jenkins, 2007; Patterson, 2002; Short, 2007). In interviews with biological and nonbiological mothers about differences in their contribution to paid and unpaid (childcare) work, they rarely mentioned the biological link as an explanation of the division of their roles in family tasks (Downing & Goldberg, 2011). There is evidence that when differences in the division of

family tasks occur in lesbian-mother families, the partner with less job prestige, less income, and/or less formal education typically does more of the unpaid work (Sutphin, 2013).

## Parenting

Relatively few studies have examined whether there are differences in parenting styles and parenting behavior between partners in planned lesbian-mother families. When such a comparison is made, the unit of analyses is the biological tie (or its absence) with the child(ren). Goldberg, Downing, and Sauck (2008) asked the lesbian mothers whom they interviewed whether they observed in their children a preference for the biological or the nonbiological mother. Many of the women mentioned that as infants their children had preferred the birth mother, but that over the years this preference had faded such that at the time of the interviews, the children (who were then 3.5 years old) had no preference. According to the mothers, the initial preference of the child was related to the pregnancy and breastfeeding. Notably, some nonbiological mothers were jealous of these experiences of their partners. Gartrell et al. (1999) found that lesbian co-mothers of 2-year-old children reported feelings of jealousy related to their partners' bonding with the child during breastfeeding (see Gartrell, Peyser, & Bos, 2011).

Bos et al. (2007) compared Dutch biological and nonbiological mothers in 100 planned lesbian-mother families with respect to parenting styles and parental behavior. No differences were found between the partners on most of the variables: They did not differ significantly on emotional involvement, parental concern, power assertion, induction (all measured with questionnaires), supportive presence, or respect for the child's autonomy (all measured through observations of child–parent interactions). However, lesbian biological mothers scored higher on limit-setting the child's behavior during the observed parent–child interactions.

## Diversity Within Planned Lesbian-Mother Families

The third set of studies focused on diversity among planned lesbian-mother families and the potential effects of such diversity on child-rearing and children. Three aspects of diversity within planned lesbian-mother studies that have been investigated are: (a) donor status (known or as-yet-unknown donor), (b) absence of male role models, and (c) parent and offspring experiences of stigmatization. The focus on diversity within lesbian-parent families represents a relatively new type of inquiry in studies of lesbian-mother families.

Questions regarding why mothers use known or as-yet-unknown donors, and what the choice means for the mothers and their offspring, should be placed in a broader discussion about how the absence of information about their donors may affect offspring identity and psychological development, especially during the vulnerable period of adolescence. Interest in the role of male involvement in these families is based on theories and ideas about gender identification and how the absence of a traditional father or father figure may affect children. The experience of stigmatization in lesbian-mother families should be understood in terms of the role of personal, family, and community resources in reducing the negative impact of homophobia on the offspring's psychological development (van Gelderen, Gartrell, Bos, & Hermanns, 2009).

## Donor Status

Many fertility clinics in the USA offer couples a double-track option of using either the sperm of a donor who will remain permanently anonymous (unknown donor) or that of a donor who may be met by the offspring when she or he reaches the age of 18 (identity-release donor) (Scheib, Riordan, & Rubin, 2005). It is increasingly being argued that gamete donor offspring have a fundamental right to know the identity of their sperm donor (see Ravelingien & Pennings, 2013 for analyses of the arguments).

The right to know the sperm donor is based on the proceedings from the United Nations Convention on the Rights of the Child (1989) which state that children have the right to preserve their identity and know/be cared for by their parents (McWhinnie, 2001). As a result of these proceedings, several countries (e.g., the Netherlands) implemented legal and policy changes such that sperm donation from a permanently anonymous donor is no longer allowed. However, in her US study of 29 pregnant lesbians and their partners, Goldberg (2006) found that 59% of the women preferred an unknown donor, because they wanted to raise their children without interference from a third party. Touroni and Coyle (2002), who interviewed nine lesbian couples in the UK, found that six had chosen a known donor because they believed that children have the right to know their genetic origins and/or to form relationships with their donors early in life. Gartrell et al. (1996) found that among the lesbian women in the US NLLFS who preferred a known donor were many who worried that children conceived by unknown donors might experience psychological and identity problems during adolescence or later in life.

Few studies have assessed the impact on offspring to have known or unknown donors. In Belgium, Vanfraussen, Pontjaert-Kristoffersen, and Brewaeys (2003a, 2003b) asked 24 children (mean age = 10 years old) with lesbian mothers whether, if it were possible, they would want to have more information about their donors. Nearly 50% of the children answered "yes"; they were especially curious about their donors' physical features and personalities. Scheib et al. (2005) found that for adolescents conceived by identity-release donors and raised in lesbian-mother families, the most frequently mentioned questions were, "What's he like?", "What does he look like?", "What's his family like?", and "Is he like me?" The Belgian study also assessed whether the children who wanted to know more about their donors differed in self-esteem or emotional and behavioral functioning from their counterparts who did not share this curiosity, and no significant differences were found (Vanfraussen et al., 2003a, 2003b).

At the time of the first US NLLFS data collection, the mothers-to-be were either pregnant or inseminating, and the donor preferences were almost equally divided between permanently anonymous and identity-release donors (Gartrell et al., 1996). In the fifth wave of the US NLLFS, nearly 23% of the adolescents with unknown donors stated that they wished they knew their donors, while 67% of those who would have the option to meet their donors when they turned 18 planned to do so (Bos & Gartrell, 2010).

Analysis of the data collected by the Donor Sibling Registry (i.e., the largest US web-based registry) revealed that of the 133 individuals (age range: 13–41+) conceived in the context of two-parent planned lesbian families, 8% reported that they had met the donor (Nelson, Hertz, & Kramer, 2013). Of those who had not yet met their donor, three-quarters mentioned that they hoped to contact the donor; the most frequently mentioned reason was curiosity about his physical appearance. Some individuals reported that they already had contact in some way (e.g., by email or in person) with one or more half-siblings (Nelson et al., 2013; Persaud et al., 2017).

The US NLLFS (Bos & Gartrell, 2010) assessed the associations between donor status and problem behavior among youth over time through parental responses to the Child Behavior Checklist (CBCL; Achenbach & Rescorla, 2001). This data collection was done in the fourth and fifth waves (when the children were 10 and 17 years old, respectively). The analyses revealed that donor type (known and as-yet-unknown donors) had no bearing on the development of the psychological well-being of youth over a 7-year period from childhood through adolescence. These results are important, because lesbian prospective parents are often uncertain about the long-term effects of donor selection on the well-being of their children.

Also, when their offspring were 17 years old, the NLLFS mothers were asked about their retrospective feelings concerning the types of sperm donors they selected. More than three-quarters (77.5%) indicated that they would make the same choice if they had it do over again, regardless of the type of donor chosen (Gartrell, Bos, Goldberg,

Deck, & van Rijn-van Gelderen, 2015). Of those who were satisfied with their choice of a known donor, nearly all mentioned reasons that were related to the relationship between the donor and the offspring and/or the mother(s). That their 17-year-old offspring would soon have the option to meet their donors and learn more about them was the most frequently mentioned reason for being satisfied among mothers who chose an open-identity donor. Among the mothers who used an unknown donor, most were satisfied because they had avoided legal conflicts and/or parenting involvement by a third person. In addition, these mothers were pleased with the overall outcome that having an unknown donor did not negatively affect their children's life and well-being.

Some studies investigated the narratives that were used to describe the donor. Goldberg and Allen (2013) reported that adolescent and adults raised by lesbian mothers used a variety of terms to refer to their donors: (a) strictly donors and not members of their family, (b) extended family members but not parents, and (c) fathers. Other studies document similar narratives (Mahlstedt, Labounty, & Kennedy, 2010; Raes et al., 2015). The data from the earlier mentioned Donor Sibling Registry showed that most individuals raised in lesbian-parent families used the terms "donor" or "sperm donor" (Nelson et al., 2013).

## Male Role Models

Little research has focused on lesbian mothers' ideas about male involvement in the lives of their offspring, and only one study has examined the effects on adolescents of growing up in lesbian-mother families with or without male role models. Goldberg and Allen (2007) interviewed 30 lesbian couples in the USA during pregnancy and when their children were 3 months old. More than two-thirds of the mothers were highly conscious of the fact that their children would grow up in the absence of a male figure, and these mothers believed that this could negatively impact their children's psychological well-being. Many of these parents, in turn, had already made plans to find such men. According to the authors, as well as Clarke and Kitzinger (2005), this concern may be a response to cultural anxieties about the necessity for male role models in the development of children.

The US NLLFS found that when the mothers were inseminating or pregnant, 76% stated that they hoped to provide their children with positive male role models (often described as "good, loving men"; Gartrell et al., 1996), and by the time the children were 10 years old, half of the families had incorporated male role models into these children's lives (Gartrell et al., 2005). During wave 5, the 17-year-old US NLLFS adolescents with and without male role models were compared on the feminine and masculine scales of the Bem Sex-Role Inventory and on psychological adjustment (Bos, Goldberg, van Gelderen, & Gartrell, 2012). No differences were found on any of these comparisons based on the presence or absence of male role models.

## Stigmatization

**Mothers' Experiences of Stigmatization** The US NLLFS found that most prospective lesbian mothers viewed raising a child in a heterosexist and homophobic society as potentially challenging (Gartrell et al., 1996). Experiences of stigmatization and rejection were assessed in the Dutch longitudinal study by Bos, Van Balen, Van den Boom, and Sandfort (2004b). The 200 mothers (100 couples) were asked about such experiences when the children were between 4 and 8 years old. The authors developed a scale to measure the mothers' perceived experiences of rejection. This instrument included 7 forms of rejection related to being a lesbian mother. Lesbian mothers were asked to indicate how frequently each form of rejection had occurred in the previous year (Bos et al., 2004). The forms of rejection that were most frequently reported were "Other people asking me annoying questions related to my lifestyle" (reported by 68% and 72% of the biological mothers and the co-mothers, respectively) and "Other people gossiping about me" (27.3% and 32.7% of the biological and the co-mothers,

respectively). Less frequently reported experiences were disapproving comments (13% and 12.1% of the biological and the co-mothers, respectively) and being excluded (12% and 9.1% of the biological and the co-mothers, respectively). These 7 items formed a reliable scale, and higher levels of rejection were found to be associated with more experiences of parenting stress, feeling a greater need to justify the quality of the parent–child relationship, and feeling less competent as a parent (Bos et al., 2004). The study from which these data were drawn was conducted in the Netherlands, which is relatively accepting of lesbian and gay people and same-sex marriage (Sandfort, McGaskey, & Bos, 2008). Shapiro, Peterson, and Stewart (2009) found that living in a country with same-sex marriage had a positive effect on lesbian parents.

Lesbian-parent families also experience homophobic stigmatization and heteronormativity in the child healthcare system. In the UK, USA, Canada, Australia, and New Zealand, same-sex couples have reported anxiety about prejudicial treatment by child health professionals (e.g., Chapman, Watkins, Zappia, Combs, & Shields, 2012; Cherguit, Burns, Pettle, & Tasker, 2013; Hayman, Wilkes, Halcomb, & Jackson, 2013). Fearing judgment, some female same-sex parents were reluctant to seek professional support (Alang & Fomotar, 2015). Wells and Lang (2016) reviewed the literature on lesbian parents' experiences with child healthcare in Nordic countries (e.g., Sweden, Norway, Denmark, Finland, and Iceland). Even though these countries rank as the most gender-equal countries in the world, lesbian parents still faced discriminatory practices and procedures. For example, co-mothers felt that they were inappropriately treated like fathers (Wells & Lang, 2016).

**Offspring Experiences of Stigmatization** In the follow-up of the longitudinal Dutch study, the children (aged 8–12 years) were asked about their experiences of rejection (Bos & van Balen, 2008). Sixty percent of the children in the lesbian-mother families reported that peers made jokes about them because of their mothers' lesbianism. Other frequently reported forms of rejection were: annoying questions (56.7%) and abusive language (45.2%) related to the mothers' sexual orientation, gossip about their lesbian mothers (30.6%), and exclusion because of their family type (26.2%).

Here, differences in sociolegal context between countries are also important. In the fourth wave of the US NLLFS, Gartrell et al. (2005) assessed experiences of homophobia by asking the children: "Do other kids ever say mean things to you about your mom(s) being lesbian?" Nearly 38% of the 41 boys and 46% of the 38 girls responded affirmatively. In Dutch planned lesbian families (Bos & van Balen, 2008), 14.7% of the 36 boys and 22.2% of the 38 girls answered "yes" to the same question. When the NLLFS offspring were 25 years old, the most frequently cited experiences of homophobia were (a) asking annoying questions about the mother(s)' sexual orientation and (b) making jokes about the mother(s)' sexual orientation (Koh, Bos, & Gartrell, 2019).

Although studies comparing children of lesbian and heterosexual parents (or comparing the former group with nationally representative samples) have found that having sexual minority parents is not in itself a risk factor for developing psychological problems (e.g., Bos et al., 2007; Carone, Lingiardi, Chirumbolo, & Baiocco, 2018; Golombok et al., 2003), children who were stigmatized because of their mothers' lesbianism had lower scores on self-confidence and exhibited more behavioral problems (Bos et al., 2004b; Bos & van Balen, 2008; Gartrell et al., 2005). This association between homophobic stigmatization and behavioral problems was also found in emerging adults with lesbian parents (Koh et al., 2019). Attending schools with LGBTQ curricula, their mothers' participation in the lesbian community, and having frequent contact with other offspring of sexual minority parents protected children against the negative influences of stigmatization on their well-being (Bos & van Balen, 2008).

## Future Directions for Research

Most studies described in this chapter were based on data from parents (semistructured interviews with parents, or self-administered questionnaires completed by them). Parental reports could be biased if the mothers are motivated to impress the researchers with their parenting skills. To limit self-report bias, future research should utilize other sources such as teacher reports or researcher observations of parent–child interactions (which some studies already have).

Another issue for future research concerns the representativeness of the study samples and the generalizability of the findings. Most studies on planned lesbian-mother families used comparatively small samples, and respondents were recruited via such sources as organizations of lesbian and gay parents. As a consequence, they are not representative, which limits the generalizability of the findings (Tasker, 2010). Large general population studies with an intersectional focus offer an opportunity to conduct analyses based on family type and structure, genetic and nongenetic relationships between parents and children, parental gender identity and sexual orientation, race/ethnicity, and socioeconomic status. These studies will be an important contribution to the literature, because the parents in a majority of planned lesbian-mother families studied to date have been White, middle to upper middle class, highly educated, and urban-dwelling (see chapter "Race and Ethnicity in the Lives of LGBTQ Parents and Their Children: Perspectives from and Beyond North America").

In general, previous studies on planned lesbian-mother families used a cross-sectional design; thus, causal directions cannot be determined for the associations that were found (e.g., between experiences of stigmatization and a child's psychological adjustment). There are several studies in which data are gathered over multiple waves (e.g., Bos et al., 2007; Bos & Sandfort, 2010; Gartrell et al., 1996, 2018; Goldberg, 2006; Golombok et al., 1997; Golombok & Badger, 2010). However, the instruments that were used were sometimes different across phases, and as a consequence it was not possible to examine children's psychological well-being longitudinally. More longitudinal studies focusing on the long-term consequences of stigmatization and resilience are needed.

Finally, studies based on the within-difference approach that focused on the role of stigmatization underscore the importance of conducting research on lesbian-parent families with a goal of understanding resilience and protective factors— that is, the ability of the parents and children to function well despite challenging circumstances (Prendergast & MacPhee, 2018). A theoretical model of family resilience may facilitate our understanding of factors on the parental, family, and child levels that buffer youth from the effects of stigmatization and discrimination (Masten, 2018; Prendergast & MacPhee, 2018).

## Practical Implications

The overall finding that lesbian-mother families formed through donor insemination are functioning well has implications for the clinical care of lesbian-parent families, for the expert testimony on lesbian-mother custody, and for public policies concerning sexual minority parenting. Overall, the data provide no justification for restricting access to reproductive technologies or child custody on the basis of the sexual orientation of the parents. Pediatricians and other health care professionals should provide the findings of the studies mentioned in this review to prospective lesbian parents. It would also be useful to review information provided at clinics to assess whether all types of families are represented, including lesbian-parent families with children born through sperm donation. Making these families more visible enhances their feelings of inclusion and legitimacy.

Clinicians and educators working with planned lesbian-parent families should be prepared to counsel them about the direct and indirect effects of heterosexism and homophobia and provide resources to those who have been stigmatized. Clinicians and educators should be aware of possible difficulties that children of sexual minorities may face as a result of discrimi-

nation, and they should be able to discuss how protective factors, such as socializing with or attending school with other children with lesbian and gay parents, affect children's well-being (see chapter "Clinical Work with Children and Adolescents Growing Up with LGBTQ Parents"). Clinicians and educators should also reflect on their own views on and behavior toward sexual minority parent families. If aware of inherent bias, it is incumbent that the clinician or educator receive training on confronting and unlearning homophobia.

All types of families face challenges, some of which are unique to members of minority groups. Although they show more similarities to than differences from heterosexual-parent families, lesbian families formed through donor insemination still struggle with societal acceptance even though their egalitarian parenting style serves as a model for co-parents everywhere.

## References

Achenbach, T. M. (1991). *Manual for the child behavior checklist/4–18 and 1991 profile*. Burlington, VT: University of Vermont, Department of Psychiatry.

Achenbach, T. M., & Rescorla, L. A. (2001). *Manual for ASEBA school-age forms and profiles*. Burlington, VT: University of Vermont, Research Center for Children Youth and Families.

Alang, S. M., & Fomotar, M. (2015). Postpartum depression in an online community of lesbian mothers: Implications for clinical practice. *Journal of Gay & Lesbian Mental Health, 19*, 21–39. https://doi.org/10.1080/19359705.2014.910853

American Sociological Association. (2015). Brief of amicus curiae American Sociological Association in support of petitioners. *Obergefell v. Hodges, 576*. Retrieved from http://www.asanet.org/sites/default/files/savvy/documents/ASA/pdfs/ASA_March_2015_Supreme_Court_Marriage_Equality_Amicus_Brief.pdf on 18 March 2019.

Baetens, P., Camus, M., & Devroey, P. (2002). Counseling lesbian couples: Request for donor insemination on social grounds. *Reproductive Biomedicine Online, 6*, 75–83. https://doi.org/10.1016/S1472-6483(10)62059-7

Baiocco, R., Santamaria, F., Ioverno, S., Fontanesi, L., Baumgartner, E., Laghi, F., & Lingiardi, V. (2015). Lesbian mother families and gay father families in Italy: Family functioning, dyadic satisfaction, and child well-being. *Sexuality Research and Social Policy, 12*, 202–212. https://doi.org/10.1007/s13178-015-0185-x

Biblarz, T. J., & Stacey, J. (2010). How does the gender of the parents matter? *Journal of Marriage and Family, 72*, 3–22. https://doi.org/10.1111/j.1741-3737.2009.00678.x

Bodri, D., Nair, S., Gill, A., Lamanna, G., Rahmati, M., Arian-Schad, M., … Ahuja, K. K. (2018). Shared motherhood IVF: High delivery rates in a large study of treatments for lesbian couples using partner-donated eggs. *Reproductive Biomedicine Online, 36*, 130–136. https://doi.org/10.1016/j.rbmo.2017.11.006

Bos, H. M. W. (2019). Oratie: "Somewhere over the rainbow". Werkelijkheid, nog steeds een droom, of iets ter tussen in? [Somewhere over the rainbow: Reality, still a dream, or something between?] *Tijdschrift Pedagogiek, 39*, 5–27.

Bos, H., Goldberg, N., Van Gelderen, L., & Gartrell, N. (2012). Adolescents of the US National Longitudinal Lesbian Family Study: Male role models, gender role traits, and psychological adjustment. *Gender & Society, 26*, 603–638. https://doi.org/10.1177/0891243212445465

Bos, H., van Gelderen, L., & Gartrell, N. (2014). Lesbian and heterosexual two-parent families: Adolescent–parent relationship quality and adolescent well-being. *Journal of Child and Family Studies, 24*, 1031–1046. https://doi.org/10.1007/s10826-014-9913-8

Bos, H. M., & Gartrell, N. K. (2010). Adolescents of the US National Longitudinal Lesbian Family Study: The impact of having a known or an unknown donor on the stability of psychological adjustment. *Human Reproduction, 26*, 630–637. https://doi.org/10.1093/humrep/deq359

Bos, H. M., Kuyper, L., & Gartrell, N. K. (2017). A population-based comparison of female and male same-sex parent and different-sex parent households. *Family Process, 57*, 148–164. https://doi.org/10.1111/famp.12278

Bos, H. M. W., Knox, J. R., van Rijn-van Gelderen, L., & Gartrell, N. K. (2016). Same-sex and different-sex parent households and child health outcomes: Findings from the National Survey of Children's Health. *Journal of Developmental and Behavioral Pediatrics, 37*, 1–9. https://doi.org/10.1097/DBP.0000000000000288

Bos, H. M. W., & Sandfort, T. (2010). Children's gender identity in lesbian and heterosexual two-parent families. *Sex Roles, 62*, 114–126. https://doi.org/10.1007/s11199-009-9704-7

Bos, H.M.W., & Van Balen, F. (2008). Children in planned lesbian families: stigmatisation, psychological adjustment and protective factors. *Culture, Health, & Sexualities, 10*, 221–236.

Bos, H. M. W., van Balen, F., & van den Boom, D. C. (2003). Planned lesbian families: Their desire and motivation to have a child. *Human Reproduction, 18*, 2216–2224. https://doi.org/10.1093/humrep/deg427

Bos, H. M. W., van Balen, F., & van den Boom, D. C. (2004a). Experience of parenthood, couple relationship, social support, and child rearing goals in planned lesbian families. *Journal of Child*

*Psychology and Psychiatry, 45*, 755–764. https://doi.org/10.1111/j.1469-610.2004.00269.x

Bos, H. M., Van Balen, F., Van Den Boom, D. C., & Sandfort, T. G. (2004b). Minority stress, experience of parenthood and child adjustment in lesbian families. *Journal of Reproductive and Infant Psychology, 22*(4), 291–304.

Bos, H. M. W., van Balen, F., & van den Boom, D. C. (2007). Child adjustment and parenting in planned lesbian-parent families. *American Journal of Orthopsychiatry, 77*, 38–48. https://doi.org/10.1037/0002-9432.77.1.38

Boss, P. (2001). *Family stress management*. Newbury Park, CA: Sage.

Botchan, A., Hauser, R., Gamzu, R., Yogev, L., Paz, G., & Yavetz, H. (2001). Results of 6139 artificial insemination cycles with donor spermatozoa. *Human Reproduction, 16*, 2298–2304. https://doi.org/10.1093/humrep/16.11.2298

Brewaeys, A., Ponjaert, I., van Hall, E. V., & Golombok, S. (1997). Donor insemination: Child development & family functioning in lesbian mother families. *Human Reproduction, 12*, 1349–1359. https://doi.org/10.1093/humrep/deh581

Brewaeys, A., Ponjaert-Kristoffersen, I., van Steirteghem, A. C., & Devroey, P. (1993). Children from anonymous donors: An inquiry into homosexual and heterosexual parents' attitudes. *Journal of Psychosomatic Obstetrics and Gynaecology, 14*, 23–35. https://europepmc.org/abstract/med/8142986

Bronfenbrenner, U. (Ed.). (2001). *Making human beings human: Bioecological perspectives on human development*. Thousand Oaks, CA: Sage.

Butler, J. (1990). *Gender trouble*. New York, NY: Routledge.

Carone, N., Lingiardi, V., Chirumbolo, A., & Baiocco, R. (2018). Italian gay father families formed by surrogacy: Parenting, stigmatization, and children's psychological adjustment. *Developmental Psychology, 54*, 1904–1916. https://doi.org/10.1037/dev0000571

Chabot, J. M., & Ames, B. D. (2004). "It wasn't 'let's get pregnant and go do it':" decision-making in lesbian couples planning motherhood via donor insemination. *Family Relations, 53*, 348–356. https://doi.org/10.1111/j.0197-6664.2004.00041.x

Chan, R. W., Brooks, R. C., Raboy, B., & Patterson, C. J. (1998). Division of labor among lesbian and heterosexual parents: Associations with children's adjustment. *Journal of Family Psychology, 12*, 402–419. https://doi.org/10.1037/0893-3200.12.3.402

Chapman, R., Watkins, R., Zappia, T., Combs, S., & Shields, L. (2012). Second-level hospital health professionals' attitudes to lesbian, gay, bisexual and transgender parents seeking health for their children. *Journal of Clinical Nursing, 21*, 880–887. https://doi.org/10.1111/j.1365-2702.2011.03938.x

Cherguit, J., Burns, J., Pettle, S., & Tasker, F. (2013). Lesbian co-mothers' experiences of maternity healthcare services. *Journal of Advanced Nursing, 69*, 1269–1278. https://doi.org/10.1111/j.1365-2648.2012.06115.x

Clarke, V. (2001). What about the children? Arguments against lesbian and gay parenting. *Women's Studies International Forum, 24*, 555–570. https://doi.org/10.1016/S0277-5395(01)00193-5

Clarke, V. (2008). From outsiders to motherhood to reinventing the family: Constructions of lesbian parenting in the psychological literature – 1886–2006. *Women's Studies International Forum, 31*, 118–128. https://doi.org/10.1016/j.wsif.2008.03.004

Clarke, V., & Kitzinger, C. (2005). 'We're not living on planet lesbian': Constructions of male role models in debates about lesbian families. *Sexualities, 8*, 137–152. https://doi.org/10.1177/1363460705050851

Cowan, C. P., & Cowan, P. A. (1988). Who does what when partners become parents: Implications for men, women and marriage. *Marriage and Family Review, 12*, 105–131. https://doi.org/10.1300/J002v12n03_07

Crouch, S. R., Waters, E., McNair, R., Power, J., & Davis, E. (2014). Parent-reported measures of child health and wellbeing in same-sex parent families: A cross-sectional survey. *BMC Public Health, 14*, 635. https://doi.org/10.1186/1471-2458-14-635

Downing, J. B., & Goldberg, A. E. (2011). Lesbian mothers' constructions of the division of paid and unpaid labor. *Feminism & Psychology, 21*, 100–120. https://doi.org/10.1177/0959353510375869

Dunne, G. A. (1998). Pioneers behind our own front doors: New models for the organization of work in domestic partnerships. *Work, Employment, and Society, 12*, 273–296. https://doi.org/10.1177/0950017098122004

Eldredge, L. K. B., Markham, C. M., Ruiter, R. A., Kok, G., Fernandez, M. E., & Parcel, G. S. (2016). *Planning health promotion programs: An intervention mapping approach*. Hoboken, NJ: John Wiley & Sons.

Ethics Committee of the American Society for Reproductive Medicine. (2013). Access to fertility treatment by gays, lesbians, and unmarried persons: A committee opinion. *Fertility and Sterility, 100*, 1524–1527. https://doi.org/10.1016/j.fertnstert.2013.08.042

Ethics Committee of the American Society for Reproductive Medicine. (2015). Access to fertility services by transgender persons: An Ethics Committee opinion. *Fertility and Sterility, 104*, 1111–1115. https://doi.org/10.1016/j.fertnstert.2015.08.021

Farr, R. H., Tasker, F., & Goldberg, A. E. (2017). Theory in highly cited studies of sexual minority parent families: Variations and implications. *Journal of Homosexuality, 64*, 1143–1179. https://doi.org/10.1080/00918369.2016.1242336

Flaks, D. K., Ficher, I., Masterpasqua, F., & Joseph, G. (1995). Lesbian choosing motherhood: A comparative study of lesbian and heterosexual parents and their children. *Developmental Psychology, 31*, 105–114. https://doi.org/10.1037/0012-1649.31.1.105

Fulcher, M., Sutfin, E. L., & Patterson, C. (2008). Individual differences in gender development: Associations with parental sexual orientation, attitudes, and division of labor. *Sex Roles, 58*, 330–341. https://doi.org/10.1007/s11199-007-9348-4

Gabb, J. (2018). Unsettling lesbian motherhood: Critical reflections over a generation (1990–2015). *Sexualities, 21*, 1002–1020. https://doi.org/10.1177/1363460717718510

Gallup. (2014). *Most American say same-sex couples entitled to adopt. Right to adopt children outpaces Americans' acceptance of same-sex marriage*. Retrieved from https://news.gallup.com/poll/170801/americans-say-sex-couples-entitled-adopt.aspx on 18 March 2019.

Gartrell, N., Banks, A., Hamilton, J., Reed, N., Bishop, H., & Rodas, C. (1999). The National Lesbian Family Study: 2. Interviews with mothers of toddlers. *American Journal of Orthopsychiatry, 69*, 362–369. https://doi.org/10.1037/h0080410

Gartrell, N., Banks, A., Reed, N., Hamilton, J., Rodas, C., & Deck, A. (2000). The National Lesbian Family Study: 3. Interviews with mothers of five-year-olds. *American Journal of Orthopsychiatry, 70*, 542–548. https://doi.org/10.1037/h0087823

Gartrell, N., Bos, H., & Koh, A. (2018). National Longitudinal Lesbian Family Study—Mental health of adult offspring. *New England Journal of Medicine, 379*, 297–299. https://doi.org/10.1056/NEJMc1804810

Gartrell, N., Bos, H., & Koh, A. (2019). Sexual attraction, sexual identity, and same-sex sexual experiences of adult offspring in the US National Longitudinal Lesbian Family Study. *Archives of Sexual Behavior.* Advance online publication, 48, 1495. https://doi.org/10.1007/s10508-019-1434-5

Gartrell, N., & Bos, H. M. W. (2010). The US National Longitudinal Lesbian Family Study: Psychological adjustment of 17-year-old adolescents. *Pediatrics, 126*, 1–9. https://doi.org/10.1542/peds.2010-1807

Gartrell, N., Bos, H. M. W., & Goldberg, N. (2012). New trends in same-sex sexual contact for American adolescents? *Archives of Sexual Behavior, 41*, 5–7. https://doi.org/10.1007/s10508-011-9883-5

Gartrell, N., Deck, A., Rodas, C., Peyser, H., & Banks, A. (2005). The National Lesbian Family Study: 4. Interviews with the 10-year-old children. *American Journal of Orthopsychiatry, 75*, 518–524. https://doi.org/10.1037/0002-9432.75.4.518

Gartrell, N., Hamilton, J., Banks, A., Mosbacher, D., Reed, N., Sparks, C. H., & Bishop, H. (1996). The National Lesbian Family Study: 1. Interviews with prospective mothers. *American Journal of Orthopsychiatry, 66*, 272–281. https://doi.org/10.1037/h0080178

Gartrell, N., Peyser, H., & Bos, H. (2011). Planned lesbian families: A review of the U.S. National Longitudinal Lesbian Family Study. In D. M. Brodzinsky & A. Pertman (Eds.), *Adoption by lesbian and gay men* (pp. 112–129). Oxford, NY: Oxford University Press.

Gartrell, N. K., Bos, H., Goldberg, N. G., Deck, A., & van Rijn-van Gelderen, L. (2015). Satisfaction with known, open-identity, or unknown sperm donors: Reports from lesbian mothers of 17-year-old adolescents. *Fertility and Sterility, 103*, 242–248. https://doi.org/10.1016/j.fertnstert.2014.09.019

Goffman, E. (1963). *Stigma: Notes on the management of spoiled identity*. New York, NY: Prentice-Hall.

Goldberg, A. E. (2006). The transition to parenthood for lesbian couples. *Journal of GLBT Family Studies, 2*, 13–42. https://doi.org/10.1300/J461v02n01_02

Goldberg, A. E. (2010). *Lesbian and gay parents and their children: Research on the family life cycle*. Washington, DC: American Psychological Association.

Goldberg, A. E. (2013). "Doing" and "undoing" gender: The meaning and division of housework in same-sex couples. *Journal of Family Theory & Review, 5*, 85–104. https://doi.org/10.1111/jftr.12009

Goldberg, A. E., & Allen, K. R. (2007). Lesbian mothers' ideas and intentions about male involvement across the transition to parenthood. *Journal of Marriage and Family, 69*, 352–365. https://doi.org/10.1111/j.1741-3737.2007.00370.x

Goldberg, A. E., & Allen, K. R. (2013). Donor, dad, or…? Young adults with lesbian parents' experiences with known donors. *Family Process, 52*, 338–350. https://doi.org/10.1111/famp.12029

Goldberg, A. E., Downing, J. B., & Sauck, C. C. (2008). Perceptions of children's parental preferences in lesbian two-mother households. *Journal of Marriage and Family, 70*, 419–434. https://doi.org/10.1111/j.1741-3737.2008.00491.x

Goldberg, A. E., & Perry-Jenkins, M. (2007). The division of labor and perceptions of parental roles: Lesbian couples across the transition to parenthood. *Journal of Social and Personal Relationships, 24*, 297–318. https://doi.org/10.1177/0265407507075415

Goldberg, N., Bos, H. M. W., & Gartrell, N. (2011). Substance use by adolescents of the US National Longitudinal Lesbian Family Study. *Journal of Health Psychology, 16*, 1231–1240. https://doi.org/10.1177/1359105311403522

Goldberg, S. K., & Conron, K. J., & The Williams Institute UCLA School of Law. (2018). *How many same-sex couples in the U.S. are raising children?* Retrieved from https://williamsinstitute.law.ucla.edu/wp-content/uploads/Parenting-Among-Same-Sex-Couples.pdf

Golombok, S. (2015). *Modern families: Parents and children in new family forms*. Cambridge, UK: Cambridge University Press.

Golombok, S., & Badger, S. (2010). Children raised in mother-headed families from infancy: A follow-up of children of lesbian and heterosexual mothers, at early adulthood. *Human Reproduction, 25*, 150–157. https://doi.org/10.1093/humrep/dep345

Golombok, S., Perry, B., Burston, A., Murray, C., Mooney-Somers, J., Stevens, M., & Golding, J. (2003). Children with lesbian parents: A community study. *Developmental Psychology, 39*, 20–33. https://doi.org/10.1037/0012-1649.39.1.20

Golombok, S., Tasker, F. L., & Murray, C. (1997). Children raised in fatherless families from infancy: Family relationships and the socio-emotional development of children of lesbian and single heterosexual mothers. *Journal of Child Psychology and Psychiatry, 38*, 783–791. https://doi.org/10.1111/j.1469-7610.1997.tb01596.x

Hayman, B., Wilkes, L., Halcomb, E., & Jackson, D. (2013). Marginalised mothers: Lesbian women negotiating heteronormative healthcare services. *Contemporary Nurse, 44*, 120–127. https://doi.org/10.5172/conu.2013.44.1.120

Herbstrith, J. C., Tobin, R. M., Hesson-McInnis, M. S., & Joel Schneider, W. (2013). Preservice teacher attitudes toward gay and lesbian parents. *School Psychology Quarterly, 28*, 183. https://doi.org/10.1037/spq0000022

Kirkpatrick, M., Smith, C., & Roy, P. (1981). Lesbian mothers and their children: A comparative survey. *American Journal of Orthopsychiatry, 51*, 545–551. https://doi.org/10.1111/j.1939-0025.1981.tb01403.x

Koh, A. S., Bos, H. M., & Gartrell, N. K. (2019). Predictors of mental health in emerging adult offspring of lesbian-parent families. *Journal of Lesbian Studies*. Advance online publication, *23*, 257. https://doi.org/10.1080/10894160.2018.1555694

Kuyper, L. (2018). *Opvattingen over seksuele en genderdiversiteit in Nederland en Europa*. Den Haag, Netherlands: Sociaal en Cultureel Planbureau.

Lamb, M. E. (1999). Parental behavior, family processes, and child development in non-traditional and traditionally understudied families. In M. E. Lamb (Ed.), *Parenting and child development in 'non-traditional families'* (pp. 1–14). Mahwah, NJ: Lawrence Erlbaum Associates.

Lamb, M. E. (2012). Infant–father attachments and their impact on child development. In N. J. Cabrera & C. S. Tamis-LeMonda (Eds.), *Handbook of father involvement* (pp. 109–133). New York, NY: Routledge Academic.

MacCallum, F., & Golombok, S. (2004). Children raised in fatherless families from infancy: A follow-up of children of lesbian and single heterosexual mothers at early adolescence. *Journal of Child Psychology and Psychiatry, 45*, 1407–1419. https://doi.org/10.1111/j.1469-7610.2004.00324.x

Machin, R. (2014). Sharing motherhood in lesbian reproductive practices. *BioSocieties, 9*, 42–59. https://doi.org/10.1057/biosoc.2013.40

Mahlstedt, P. P., LaBounty, K., & Kennedy, W. T. (2010). The views of adult offspring of sperm donation: Essential feedback for the development of ethical guidelines within the practice of assisted reproductive technology in the United States. *Fertility and Sterility, 93*, 2236–2246. https://doi.org/10.1016/j.fertnstert.2008.12.119

Marina, S., Marina, D., Marina, F., Fosas, N., Galiana, N., & Jové, I. (2010). Sharing motherhood: Biological lesbian co-mothers, a new IVF indication. *Human Reproduction, 25*, 938–941. https://doi.org/10.1093/humrep/deq008

Masten, A. S. (2018). Resilience theory and research on children and families: Past, present, and promise. *Journal of Family Theory & Review, 10*, 12–31. https://doi.org/10.1111/jftr.12255

McWhinnie, A. (2001). Gamete donation and anonymity: Should offspring from donated gametes continue to be denied knowledge of their origins and antecedents? *Human Reproduction, 16*, 807–817. https://doi.org/10.1093/humrep/16.5.807

Meyer, I. H. (2003). Prejudice, social stress, and mental health in lesbian, gay, and bisexual populations: Conceptual issues and research evidence. *Psychological Bulletin, 129*(5), 674–697. https://psycnet.apa.org/buy/2003-99991-002

Mucklow, J. F., & Phelan, G. (1979). Lesbian and traditional mother's responses to child behavior and self-concept. *Psychological Report, 44*, 880–882. https://doi.org/10.2466/pr0.1979.44.3.880

Nelson, M. K., Hertz, R., & Kramer, W. (2013). Making sense of donors and donor siblings: A comparison of the perceptions of donor-conceived offspring in lesbian-parent and heterosexual-parent families. *Contemporary Perspectives in Research, 7*, 1–42. https://www.emeraldinsight.com/doi/abs/10.1108/S1530-3535(2013)0000007004

Nikkelen, S., & Vermey, K. (2018). Seksuele orientatie en gender identiteit [Sexual orientation and gender identity]. In H. de Graaf, M. van den Borne, S. Nikkelen, D. Twisk, & S. Meijer (Eds), *Seks onder je 25ste. Seksuele gezondheid van jongeren in Nederland anno 2017* [Sex below the age of 25. Sexual health among youth in the Netherlands anno 2017] (pp. 37–60). Delft, Netherlands: Eburon.

Parke, R. D. (2004). Development in the family. *Annual Review of Psychology, 55,* 365–399. https://doi.org/10.1146/annurev.psych.55.090902.141528

Patterson, C. J. (1994). Children of the lesbian baby boom: Behavioral adjustment, self-concepts, and sex-role identity. In B. Greene & G. Herek (Eds.), *Psychological perspectives on lesbian and gay issues: Vol. 1. Lesbian and gay psychology: Theory, research, and clinical applications* (pp. 156–175). Thousand Oaks, CA: Sage.

Patterson, C. J. (2002). Children of lesbian and gay parents: Research, law, and policy. In B. L. Bottoms, M. Bull Kovera, & B. D. McAuliff (Eds.), *Children, social science, and the law* (pp. 176–199). Cambridge, MA: Cambridge University Press.

Pelka, S. (2009). Sharing motherhood: Maternal jealousy among lesbian co-mothers. *Journal of Homosexuality, 56*, 195–217. https://doi.org/10.1080/00918360802623164

Pennings, G. (2016). Having a child together in lesbian families: Combining gestation and genetics. *Journal of Medical Ethics, 42*, 253–255. https://doi.org/10.1136/medethics-2015-102948

Persaud, S., Freeman, T., Jadva, V., Slutsky, J., Kramer, W., Steele, M., … Golombok, S. (2017). Adolescents conceived through donor insemination in mother-headed families: A qualitative study of motivations and experiences of contacting and meeting same-donor offspring. *Children & Society, 31*, 13–22. https://doi.org/10.1111/chso.12158

Prendergast, S., & MacPhee, D. (2018). Family resilience amid stigma and discrimination: A conceptual model for families headed by same-sex parents. *Family Relations, 67*, 26–40. https://doi.org/10.1111/fare.12296

Raes, I., Van Parys, H., Provoost, V., Buysse, A., De Sutter, P., & Pennings, G. (2014). Parental (in) equality and the genetic link in lesbian families. *Journal of Reproductive and Infant Psychology, 32*, 457–468. https://doi.org/10.1080/02646838.2014.947473

Raes, I., Van Parys, H., Provoost, V., Buysse, A., De Sutter, P., & Pennings, G. (2015). Two mothers and a donor: Exploration of children's family concepts in lesbian households. *Facts, Views & Vision in ObGyn, 7*, 83–90. https://www.ncbi.nlm.nih.gov/pmc/articles/PMC4498173/

Ravelingien, A., & Pennings, G. (2013). The right to know your genetic parents: From open-identity gamete donation to routine paternity testing. *The American Journal of Bioethics, 13*, 33–41. https://doi.org/10.1080/15265161.2013.776128

Riskind, R. G., & Tornello, S. L. (2017). Sexual orientation and future parenthood in a 2011–2013 nationally representative United States sample. *Journal of Family Psychology, 31*, 792–297. https://doi.org/10.1037/fam0000316

Rivers, I., Poteat, V. P., & Noret, N. (2008). Victimization, social support, and psychosocial functioning among children of same-sex and opposite-sex couples in the United Kingdom. *Developmental Psychology, 44*, 127–134. https://doi.org/10.1037/0012-1649.44.1.127

Rosky, C. J. (2009). Like father, like son: Homosexuality, parenthood, and the gender of homophobia. *Yale Journal of Law and Feminism, 20*, 256–355.

Sandfort, T. G. M. (2000). Homosexuality, psychology, and gay and lesbian studies. In T. G. M. Sandfort, J. Schuyf, J. W. Duyvendak, & J. Weeks (Eds.), *Lesbian and gay studies. An introductory, interdisciplinary approach* (pp. 14–45). London, UK: Sage.

Sandfort, Th. G. M., McGaskey, J & Bos, H. M. W. (2008, July). Cultural and structural determinants of acceptance of homosexuality: A cross-national comparison. *Paper presented at the International Congress of Psychology*, Berlin, Germany.

Scheib, J. E., Riordan, M., & Rubin, S. (2005). Adolescents with open-identity sperm donors: Reports from 12-17 year olds. *Human Reproduction, 20*, 239–252. https://doi.org/10.1093/humrep/deh581

Shapiro, D. N., Peterson, C., & Stewart, A. J. (2009). Legal and social contexts and mental health among lesbian and heterosexual mothers. *Journal of Family Psychology, 23*, 255–262. https://doi.org/10.1037/a0014973

Shechner, T., Slone, M., Meir, Y., & Kalish, Y. (2010). Relations between social support and psychological and parental distress for lesbian, single heterosexual by choice, and two-parent heterosexual mothers. *American Journal of Orthopsychiatry, 80*, 283–292. https://doi.org/10.1111/j.1939-0025.2010.01031.x

Short, L. (2007). Lesbian mothers living well in the context of heterosexism and discrimination: Resources, strategies, and legislative changes. *Feminism & Psychology, 13*, 106–126. https://doi.org/10.1177/0959353507072912

Stacey, J., & Biblarz, T. (2001). (How) does the sexual orientation of parents matter? *American Sociological Review, 66*, 159–183. https://doi.org/10.1111/j.1741-3737.2009.00678.x

Steckel, A. (1987). Psychosocial development of children of lesbian mothers. Gay and lesbian parents. In F. Bozett (Ed.), *Homosexuality and family relations* (pp. 23–36). New York, NY: Harrington Park Press.

Sullins, D. (2015a). Emotional problems among children with same-sex parents: Difference by definition. *British Journal of Education, Society and Behavioural Science, 7*, 99–120. https://doi.org/10.9734/BJESBS/2015/15823

Sullins, D. (2015b). Child attention-deficit hyperactivity disorder (ADHD) in same-sex parent families in the United States: Prevalence and comorbidities. *British Journal of Medicine & Medical Research, 6*, 987–998. https://doi.org/10.9734/BJMMR/2015/15897

Sutphin, S. (2013). The division of child care tasks in same-sex couples. *Journal of GLBT Family Studies, 9*, 474–491. https://doi.org/10.1080/1550428X.2013.826043

Tasker, F. (2010). Same-sex parenting and child development: Reviewing the contribution of parental gender. *Journal of Marriage and Family, 72*, 35–40. https://doi.org/10.1111/j.1741-3737.2009.00681.x

Touroni, E., & Coyle, A. (2002). Decision-making in planned lesbian parenting: An interpretative phenomenological analysis. *Journal of Community & Applied Social Psychology, 12*, 194–209. https://doi.org/10.1002/casp.672

Ulrich, M., & Weatherall, A. (2000). Motherhood and infertility. Viewing motherhood through the lens of infertility. *Feminism and Psychology, 10*, 323–336. https://doi.org/10.1177/0959353500010003003

United Nations Convention on the Rights of the Child. (1989). Retrieved from http://wunrn.org/reference/pdf/Convention_Rights_Child.PDF on 18 March 2019.

van Gelderen, L., Bos, H., Gartrell, N., Hermanns, J., & Perrin, E. C. (2012). Quality of life of adolescents raised from birth by lesbian mothers. *Journal of Developmental and Behavioral Pediatrics, 33*, 1–7. https://doi.org/10.1097/DBP.0b013e31823b62af

van Gelderen, L., Gartrell, N., Bos, H. M. W., & Hermanns, J. (2009). Stigmatization and resilience in adolescent children of lesbian mothers. *Journal of GLBT Family Studies, 5*, 268–279. https://doi.org/10.1080/15504280903035761

van Rijn-van Gelderen, L., Bos, H. W. M., Jorgensen, T. D., Ellis-Davies, K., Winstanley, A., Golombok, S., … Lamb, M. E. (2017). Wellbeing of gay fathers with children born through surrogacy: A comparison with lesbian-mother families and heterosexual IVF parent families. *Human Reproduction, 33*, 101–108. https://doi.org/10.1093/humrep/dex339

Vanfraussen, K., Ponjaert-Kristoffersen, I., & Brewaeys, A. (2002). What does it mean for youngsters to grow up in a lesbian family created by means of donor insemination? *Journal of Reproductive and Infant Psychology, 20*, 237–252. https://doi.org/10.1080/0264683021000033165

Vanfraussen, K., Pontjaert-Kristoffersen, I., & Brewaeys, A. (2003a). Family functioning in lesbian families created by donor insemination. *American Journal of Orthopsychiatry, 73*, 78–90. https://doi.org/10.1037/0002-9432.73.1.78

Vanfraussen, K., Pontjaert-Kristoffersen, I., & Brewaeys, A. (2003b). Why do children want to know more about the donor? The experience of youngsters raised in lesbian families. *Journal of Psychosomatic Obstetrics and Gynecology, 24*, 31–38. https://doi.org/10.3109/01674820309042798

Wainright, J. L., & Patterson, C. J. (2006). Delinquency, victimization, and substance use among adolescents with female same-sex parents. *Journal of Family Psychology, 20*, 526–530. https://doi.org/10.1037/0893-3200.20.3.526

Wainright, J. L., & Patterson, C. J. (2008). Peer relations among adolescents with female same-sex parents. *Developmental Psychology, 44*, 117–126. https://doi.org/10.1037/0012-1649.44.1.117

Wainright, J. L., Russell, S. T., & Patterson, C. J. (2004). Psychosocial adjustment, school outcomes, and romantic relationships of adolescents with same-sex parents. *Child Development, 75*, 1886–1898. https://doi.org/10.1111/j.1467-8624.2004.00823.x

Wells, M. B., & Lang, S. N. (2016). Supporting same-sex mothers in the Nordic child health field: A systematic literature review and meta-synthesis of the most gender equal countries. *Journal of Clinical Nursing, 25*, 3469–3483. https://doi.org/10.1111/jocn.13340

# LGBTQ Adoptive Parents and Their Children

Rachel H. Farr, Cassandra P. Vázquez, and Charlotte J. Patterson

Many lesbian, gay, bisexual, transgender, and queer (LGBTQ) adults express a desire to become parents (Riskind & Tornello, 2017; Simon, Tornello, Farr, & Bos, 2018; Stotzer, Herman, & Hasenbush, 2014) and often report adoption as a preferred pathway to parenthood (dickey, Ducheny, & Ehrbar, 2016; Farr & Patterson, 2009). In the USA and other parts of the world, many LG adults have adopted children (Gates, 2013; Patterson & Tornello, 2011). (Please note, we use acronyms that best describe the reprosented identities from the research we describe, such as LG for lesbian/gay.) According to data from national surveys in the USA, the numbers of adoptive families headed by LG parents have doubled in recent years (Gates, 2011), and same-sex couples are much more likely than other-sex couples to have adopted children (Goldberg & Conron, 2018). There is continued controversy, however, surrounding the adoption of children by LGBTQ adults (Farr & Goldberg, 2018a). Although LG adults may jointly adopt as same-sex couples across the USA, adoption laws remain regulated on the state level (Farr & Goldberg, 2018a). As a result of different state-level laws and policies that govern adoption (e.g., religious freedom bills; Movement Advancement Project, 2018a), there are variations in the experiences of sexual and gender minority adults seeking to adopt. Over the last two decades, a growing body of research on the adoption of children by LGBTQ parents has emerged and rapidly expanded that helps to address questions that continue to be at the center of public controversies.

In the context of research on adoption and controversies about LGBTQ adoptive parents, we provide an overview of recent research in this area. We include discussions of work that is inclusive of understudied (e.g., BTQ) identities wherever possible. Much of the literature addressing sexual and gender minority parent adoptive families has, however, focused on LG parents— to the exclusion of other sexual and gender minority identities (Goldberg, Gartrell, & Gates, 2014; Moore & Stambolis-Ruhstorfer, 2013; Patterson, 2017).

In this chapter, we review research on LGBTQ adoptive parents and their children in the context of an interdisciplinary, international, and intersectional framework. Studies of LGBTQ adoptive parenting have emerged primarily from developmental and clinical psychology, but research from social work, family science, demography, sociology, public policy, law, and economics is also relevant. Here, we consider the

R. H. Farr (✉) · C. P. Vázquez
Department of Psychology, University of Kentucky, Lexington, KY, USA
e-mail: rachel.farr@uky.edu; casey.vazquez@uky.edu

C. J. Patterson
Department of Psychology, University of Virginia, Charlottesville, VA, USA
e-mail: cjp@virginia.edu

© Springer Nature Switzerland AG 2020
A. E. Goldberg, K. R. Allen (eds.), *LGBTQ-Parent Families*, https://doi.org/10.1007/978-3-030-35610-1_3

theoretical framings (or lack thereof) that have characterized this body of work emerging from these disparate fields. In addition, most research on LGBTQ parenting has focused on the roles of sexual and gender identity (Fish & Russell, 2018)—in our review, where possible, we evaluate how other intersecting identities (e.g., race, class), geographic location (e.g., US South, Western Europe), and historical-sociopolitical context (e.g., marriage equality) relate to the experiences of LGBTQ-parent adoptive families. Within these frameworks then, we consider work in this chapter describing the pathways to adoption for LGBTQ adults, and we summarize findings on the experiences of LGBTQ individuals and couples during the adoption process. We also review research on psychosocial and adjustment outcomes for children, parents, and families when LGBTQ adults adopt children. Throughout the chapter, similarities among LGBTQ and cisgender heterosexual adoptive parent families are discussed, such as those regarding outcomes for children adopted by LGBTQ and cisgender heterosexual parents. The ways in which LGBTQ adoptive parents may differ from cisgender heterosexual adoptive parents are also noted, such as in their reasons for adopting children. We describe findings that are specific to processes among LGBTQ adoptive parent families, such as talking to children about having LGBTQ parents. Finally, we offer recommendations for future research and practice.

## Research on Adoptive Families

One context for understanding issues facing LGBTQ adoptive parents and their children is the body of research on adoption. A large literature explores adoptive family dynamics and psychosocial outcomes of adopted children, with samples predominantly comprised of cisgender heterosexual couples and parents and their adopted children (Brodzinsky, 2015; Davis, 2013; Palacios & Brodzinsky, 2010). Research regarding outcomes of children who have been adopted has indicated that, relative to their non-adopted peers (i.e., children remaining with

their biologically related families), adopted children are at risk for some negative outcomes such as behavior problems (Palacios & Brodzinsky, 2010). The contexts in which adoptive placements occur are, however, paramount to consider in understanding the outcomes of adopted children.

In a literature review examining research about adopted children's social and behavioral outcomes, Julian (2013) uncovered greater social and behavioral problems (and a higher risk of these problems being long-lasting) among children who had been placed in an institution at older (versus younger) ages prior to adoption, as well as among children who were adopted at older (versus younger) ages postinstitutionalization. Research has also indicated that compared with children adopted through private domestic or international agencies, children adopted through foster care (who generally have experienced various forms of abuse and neglect) often fare worse in terms of behavioral and adjustment outcomes, experience lower-quality peer relationships, and are at risk for heightened mental health challenges (DeLuca, Claxton, & van Dulmen, 2018; Tan & Marn, 2013; Vandivere & McKlindon, 2010). Jiménez-Morago, León, and Román (2015) assessed early adversity and psychological adjustment among 230 Spanish children in various placement settings. Although children generally displayed positive levels of adjustment, they found that children in institutional care ($n = 50$) experienced the greatest adjustment issues, followed by children in nonrelative foster placements ($n = 28$), as compared to internationally adopted children ($n = 40$) and to children in a control group ($n = 58$). Thus, children who experience adversity (e.g., institutionalization, abuse, neglect) before being adopted appear to be particularly at risk for later difficulties.

Negative outcomes do not, however, characterize adopted children across the board. For instance, in a longitudinal study examining developmental outcomes among a sample of 872 adopted Chinese girls in the USA, Tan and Carmas (2011) found that adopted children demonstrated greater social skills, as reported by their teachers ($n = 611$) and parents ($n = 869$), when compared with published normative scores of nonadopted children. Teachers also reported that adopted children had higher than average academic performance as compared to the US normative range. Consistent with Julian's (2013) review, girls had better social and academic outcomes when they had been adopted at younger ages. Overall, adoption appears to be an effective intervention for children who face adversity in various forms (e.g., removal from families and/or cultures of origin, institutionalization, abuse, or neglect) early in life and particularly when adoptive placements occur at younger ages.

In an effort to reconcile variations in results among studies of adopted children's outcomes, cross-cultural research, generally conducted among cisgender heterosexual parent families, has also expanded to include consideration of many different adoption-related issues in examining associations with behavioral adjustment, self-worth, and other developmental health outcomes. These topics include a number of factors like preadoptive life circumstances and adoptive family environments (Balenzano, Coppola, Cassibba, & Moro, 2018; Crea, Chan, & Barth, 2013; del Pozo de Bolger, Dunstan, & Kaltner, 2018; Harwood, Feng, & Yu, 2013; Ji, Brooks, Barth, & Kim, 2010; Kendler, Turkheimer, Ohlsson, Sundquist, & Sundquist, 2015; Rosnati, Ranieri, & Barni, 2013; Rueter, Keyes, Iacono, & McGue, 2009; Rushton, 2014), communication about adoption (Brodzinsky, 2015; del Pozo de Bolger et al., 2018; Grotevant, McRoy, Wrobel, & Ayers-Lopez, 2013; Le Mare & Audet, 2011; Reinoso, Juffer, & Tieman, 2013), awareness of adoption and adoptive identity (Brodzinsky, 2011a; Grotevant et al., 2013), openness arrangements and contact with birth family (del Pozo de Bolger et al., 2018; Grotevant et al., 2013; Siegel & Smith, 2012), transracial adoption and racial/ethnic socialization (Brodzinsky, 2015; Hrapczynski & Leslie, 2018) and the role of adoptees' appraisal about their adoption (i.e., thoughts and attitudes related to the transitions, separations, and losses involved in adoption; Storsbergen, Juffer, van Son, & Hart, 2010). As in

other types of families, the qualities of parenting and family interactions have been found to be significantly associated with child outcomes and family functioning (Lamb, 2012; Rueter et al., 2009).

Most of the research on adoptive families to date has focused on families with cisgender heterosexual parents. More recently, research including LGBTQ adoptive parents (and prospective adoptive parents) has been conducted; however, this research has primarily focused on cisgender LG parents. In this chapter, research findings about LGBTQ adoptive parents and their children are compared with the broader literature about adoptive families wherever possible. We address dominant theories applied to this work and also use developmental, family systems, and ecological perspectives in considering the experiences of LGBTQ-parent adoptive families in the context of broader social structure issues such as the intersection of multiple minority identities (e.g., race, class), geographic region, and associated cultural context in which the research was conducted. The emergence of studies about adoptive families with LGBTQ parents seems to have been motivated, in part, by controversy surrounding the adoption of children by LGBTQ parents, and it is to this topic that we turn next.

## Controversy Surrounding LGBTQ-Parent Adoption

The adoption of children by LGBTQ adults has been a controversial issue in the USA and around the world (Davis, 2013; Farr & Goldberg, 2018a; Patterson & Goldberg, 2016). Questions have been raised about the suitability of LGBTQ parents as role models for children, with contentions that a heterosexual mother and father are necessary for children's optimal development. Such concerns have affected policy and law regarding adoption by LGBTQ adults. As a result, the adoption of children by LGBTQ adults is permitted by law in some parts of the world, but not in others (International Lesbian, Gay, Bisexual, Trans and Intersex Association, 2019; U.S. Department of State, 2019).

In the USA, the Supreme Court's 2015 ruling on marriage equality (*Obergefell v. Hodges*, 2015) paved the way for many LG couples to marry and become adoptive parents. All 50 states and the District of Columbia permit married couples to petition for joint adoption (e.g., both petitioners are recognized as legal parents; Movement Advancement Project, 2018b). Stepparent adoptions by LG adults are also permitted across the USA, and 15 states (e.g., Illinois, California, Colorado) and the District of Columbia permit second-parent adoptions by LG adults[1] (Movement Advancement Project, 2018b). There are no specific legal barriers in the USA at this time to gender minority adults wishing to adopt (dickey et al., 2016; Farr & Goldberg, 2018a). And yet, three states (Kansas, Georgia, Oklahoma) have recently passed bills that allow state-licensed child welfare agencies to refuse services to LGBTQ foster and adoptive parents based on religious belief. Seven other states have passed discriminatory "religious freedom" legislation (Movement Advancement Project, 2018a). In 2018, the US House of Representatives considered the so-called Aderholt Amendment to a federal appropriations bill; if it had been enacted, it would have allowed state-funded agencies across the USA to reject otherwise qualified LGBTQ adoptive parent applicants based on religious belief and would have limited federal funding to states that currently enforce antidiscrimination laws and policies (Movement Advancement Project, 2018a). At this time, only seven states (e.g., California, Massachusetts, New York) prohibit discrimination on the basis of sexual orientation in matters of adoption (Movement Advancement Project, 2018b), and only three states (California, New Jersey, Rhode Island) and the District of Columbia also prohibit discrimination based on gender identity.

Around the world, there is also considerable variation in law and policy relevant to adoption. In the USA and in other countries, religious and political leaders have clashed repeatedly about whether the law should allow LGBTQ adults to adopt minor children (American Psychological Association, 2015; Davis, 2013; Webb & Chonody, 2014). Information on adoption policy and law is generally available for sexual minority (i.e., LGBQ) adults; however, sparse information exists regarding adoption by gender minority adults (i.e., transgender and gender diverse individuals; Farr & Goldberg, 2018a). Thus, with regard to joint adoption by same-sex couples, this practice is currently permitted in 26 countries (17 of which are located in Europe); many countries, however, still do not permit adoption by LG adults (Carroll & Mendos, 2017). Controversy surrounding the adoption of children by LGBTQ persons has contributed, in part, to research addressing questions about outcomes for children adopted by LGBTQ parents, about the capabilities of LGBTQ adults as parents, and about overall family processes in adoptive families with LGBTQ parents. We next turn to discussing this research.

## Research on LGBTQ-Parent Adoptive Families

In this section, we discuss the findings of research on how LGBTQ adults become adoptive parents, their strengths and challenges, their transition to adoptive parenthood, and outcomes for children, parents, and parenting couples. As is true of much work on LGBTQ-parent families specifically, research examining adoption by LGBTQ adults has often seemed to be driven more by matters of public debate and policy than by theoretical concerns (Farr, Tasker, & Goldberg, 2017; van Eeden-Moorefield, Few-Demo, Benson, Bible, & Lummer, 2018). When theories have been applied to studies of LGBTQ-parent adoptive families, these often have included ecological, feminist, queer, and minority stress theories (Farr et al., 2017; van Eeden-Moorefield et al., 2018). In addition, much of the research conducted on the

---

[1] In stepparent and second-parent adoptions, legal parenting status is created for an additional parent without terminating the rights or responsibilities of another legal parent (Patterson, 2013). Stepparent adoption requires parents to be in a legally recognized relationship (e.g., marriage); second-parent adoption does not (Movement Advancement Project, 2018a).

topic of LGBTQ-parent adoptive families has occurred in the USA or UK. Regardless, many LGBTQ adults do become parents through adoption around the world. In some respects, LGBTQ adoptive parents have experiences like those of other adoptive parents, but they also face some issues that are specific to their circumstances.

## Adoption as a Pathway to Parenthood

National survey data from the USA, together with findings from other research, suggest that LG and heterosexual adoptive parents share a number of demographic characteristics (Gates, 2011). Like heterosexual adoptive parents, LG adoptive parents are often older, well-educated, affluent, and predominantly white (Brewster, Tillman, & Jokinen-Gordon, 2014; Davis, 2013; Farr, Forssell, & Patterson, 2010a; Gates, 2011; Goldberg, 2009a, 2009b). These demographic factors are generally characteristic of known cases of legally recognized adoption or census data recorded from householders in the USA (Davis, 2013). Census data reflect information about female and male same-sex couple households and do not include direct information about sexual orientation or gender identity (Gates, 2013)—rendering many bisexual, transgender, and queer adoptive parent families invisible. Thus, the demographic profile of families formed through second-parent adoptions by unmarried same-sex partners or through informal methods, such as kinship adoption, may be different in the USA and elsewhere (Brewster et al., 2014; Davis, 2013).

LGBTQ adults may adopt children for reasons that are both similar to, and distinct from, those of cisgender heterosexual adults (Goldberg, 2012; Goldberg, Gartrell, & Gates, 2014; Mallon, 2011; Tornello & Bos, 2017). In Farr and Patterson's (2009) study of 106 adoptive families (29 lesbian, 27 gay, and 50 heterosexual couples) in the USA, virtually all couples gave "wanted to have children" as a reason for pursuing adoption, regardless of parental sexual orientation. The majority of heterosexual couples reported "challenges with infertility" as another motivation for adopting children, but fewer than half of same-

sex couples reported this. Many more same-sex than other-sex couples reported that they "did not have a strong desire for biological children." Similarly, in other studies with US samples of lesbian ($n = 30, 36$) and heterosexual ($n = 30, 39$) adoptive couples, respectively, lesbian couples have less often reported a commitment to biological parenthood, attempts to conceive, or pursuit of fertility treatments as compared to heterosexual couples (Goldberg, Downing, & Richardson, 2009; Goldberg & Smith, 2008).

Many gay men in the USA have also been found to pursue adoption rather than other pathways to parenthood (Goldberg, 2012); however, gay men oftentimes experience particular difficulties in achieving biological parenthood (e.g., inability to conceive; cost of surrogacy) and therefore may not even consider other pathways as feasible options (Goldberg, Gartrell, & Gates, 2014). Many investigators have reported that heterosexual adoptive parents often described adoption as a "second choice" pathway to parenthood, chosen only after struggles with infertility convinced them that biological parenthood was not a realistic option (e.g., Mallon, 2011). Similar findings have been reported in a sample of lesbian ($n = 40$), gay ($n = 41$) and heterosexual ($n = 49$) adoptive parent couples in the UK, such that same-sex adoptive parents were less likely than heterosexual adoptive parents to desire, value, or attempt to have a biologically related child (Jennings, Mellish, Tasker, Lamb, & Golombok, 2014). Many transgender adults also report adoption as their preferred pathway to parenthood (dickey et al., 2016; Farr & Goldberg, 2018a; Tornello & Bos, 2017). Thus, when compared to cisgender heterosexual parents, LGBTQ adoptive parents are more likely to have chosen adoption as a "first choice" route to parenthood (Mallon, 2011).

Another way that LGBTQ adoptive parents may differ from cisgender heterosexual adoptive parents, at least among studies conducted in the USA, is in their willingness to adopt a child from a racial/ethnic background different than their own. Among preadoptive couples, lesbian couples have been found to be more open than heterosexual couples to transracial adoption (Goldberg, 2009a). Some studies have found LG adoptive couples to be more likely than heterosexual adoptive couples to have completed a transracial adoption (Farr & Patterson, 2009; Lavner, Waterman, & Peplau, 2012; Raleigh, 2012). Conversely, in a sample of lesbian ($n = 111$), gay ($n = 98$), and heterosexual ($n = 671$) adoptive parents, no significant differences were found between parental sexual orientation and likelihood of completing a transracial adoption (Brodzinsky & Goldberg, 2016). Discrepancies in completion rates for transracial adoptions by LG and heterosexual couples warrant further review.

One reason that LGBTQ couples in the USA may be more willing to adopt transracially is that same-sex couples are more likely than heterosexual couples to be interracial, and, in turn, interracial couples are more likely than same-race couples to complete transracial adoptions (Farr & Patterson, 2009; Raleigh, 2012). Indeed, LGBTQ parents tend to live in communities with greater racial diversity within the USA (Gates, 2013), which may increase levels of comfort in interracial interactions and could relate to greater openness to transracial adoption. Because they are often less committed than heterosexual couples to achieving biological parenthood, LGBTQ couples in the USA and UK may also be more open than cisgender heterosexual couples to transracial adoptions (dickey et al., 2016; Farr & Patterson, 2009; Goldberg et al., 2009; Jennings et al., 2014).

Another way that LGBTQ adoptive couples may be different than cisgender heterosexual adoptive couples is in terms of child gender preferences in adoption. Goldberg (2009b) studied 47 lesbian, 31 gay, and 56 heterosexual couples in the USA who were actively seeking to adopt and reported that, while heterosexual men were unlikely to express a gender preference, gay men often preferred to adopt boys. Lesbian participants who expressed a preference, however, generally preferred to adopt girls, as did the heterosexual women in the sample. Thus, only about half of participants overall expressed gender preferences. These findings are consistent with research conducted in the USA and in Europe regarding preferences for child gender among other lesbian, gay, and heterosexual adoptive couples, as well as lesbian couples using

donor insemination (Baccara, Collard-Wexler, Felli, & Yariv, 2014; Gumus & Lee, 2012; Herrmann-Green & Gehring, 2007).

What might account for these gender preferences? LG adoptive parents in Goldberg's (2009b) study often explained their preferences for child gender by referring to concerns about gender socialization and heterosexism. For example, some participants felt uncertain about parenting a child of a gender different than their own. It is possible that LG couples, being made up of two parents of the same gender, may feel inadequate to parent a child of a different gender. Heterosexual couples, on the other hand, may not question their ability to parent a child of either gender since one parent of each gender is represented in the parenting couple. In this case, at least one partner in the couple may feel prepared for and knowledgeable about gender-specific socialization issues. Overall, however, little is known about why LG preadoptive parents expressed this feeling more often than did heterosexual preadoptive parents.

Research has also begun to explore dynamics among LG adoptive families in the USA related to openness arrangements (e.g., contact between adoptive and birth families; Farr & Goldberg, 2015). Preliminary research suggests that as compared to heterosexual adoptive parents, same-sex adoptive parents may be more open to contact with birth relatives (Goldberg, Kinkler, Richardson, & Downing, 2011) and report more positive relationships with birth relatives in certain adoption types (Brodzinsky & Goldberg, 2016). Consistent with the research described above (e.g., transracial adoption), these findings may be attributed to LG adults placing less emphasis on heteronormative nuclear family ideals (Farr, Ravvina, & Grotevant, 2018). In choosing adoption as a route to parenthood, LGBTQ adults may have preferences for the child's race, gender, and openness arrangement, but there are many other issues to consider as well. Indeed, gay men have described consideration of children's age, race, health, and other factors in selecting their particular routes to adoption (Downing, Richardson, Kinkler, & Goldberg, 2009).

Adoptions may be domestic or international; may be accomplished through public or private agencies; may involve adoption of infants, children, or adolescents; and may involve open as well as closed arrangements. Much remains to be learned about varied pathways to adoptive parenthood among LGBTQ adults and about factors related to these variations. Each variation comes with its own challenges, and with adoption policy and law in constant flux, research is in the early stages of examining the relevant issues (Farr & Goldberg, 2018a; Goldberg, Gartrell, & Gates, 2014). For example, now that LG married couples can jointly adopt across the USA, how will this affect choices related to adoption, individual outcomes, or family dynamics? Future research should explore how changes in adoption law influence LGBTQ adults' decision-making about family formation, as well as overall family dynamics and individual adjustment.

## Challenges and Strengths of Adoptive LGBTQ Parents

Although all prospective adoptive parents progress through a series of steps in adopting their child (e.g., an application process, training and workshops, a home study[2]; Mallon, 2011), LGBTQ parents often face additional challenges. In addition to variations in the legal and policy landscape for LGBTQ adoptive parents in the USA (Farr & Goldberg, 2018a), not all adoption agencies and/or adoption workers openly work with LGBTQ prospective parents. Brodzinsky (2011b) found that, among 307 public and private adoption agencies throughout the USA, 60% of reporting agencies had accepted applications from LG prospective adoptive parents, and 39% had placed children with LG parents. The acceptance of applications from LG parents, number of children placed with LG parents, interest in training geared toward working with LG parents, and active recruitment of LG adoptive parents varied as a function of agencies' religious affiliations

and adoption program focus. Jewish, Lutheran, and private nonreligious agencies, as well as public agencies or those with a focus on special needs adoptions, were most willing to work with LG parents. Conservative religiously affiliated agencies (e.g., Baptist, Mormon, fundamentalist Christian churches) were among the least likely to work with LG parents. Brodzinsky (2011b) also found that some agency workers lacked knowledge of adoption law pertaining to LG adults, which has been echoed in subsequent work examining agency workers' perceptions of LGBTQ adoption laws (Farr & Goldberg, 2018a). Thus, LGBTQ adults face a number of institutional and attitudinal barriers in the adoption process.

Societal resistance to LGBTQ parenting and adoption is commonplace around the world in the forms of homophobia, stereotyping, and discrimination, particularly among religious and politically conservative groups (Brodzinsky, 2011b; Perry, 2017; Takács, Szalma, & Bartus, 2016; Vecho, Poteat, & Schneider, 2016). In reports of the adoption journeys of LGBTQ adults, discrimination from adoption agencies and workers is a recurring theme (Brodzinsky, 2015; Goldberg, Moyer, Kinkler, & Richardson, 2012; Kinkler & Goldberg, 2011; Mallon, 2011; Stotzer et al., 2014). LGBTQ parents have reported experiencing discrimination and significant barriers to becoming adoptive parents not only in the USA, but also in Canada and Europe (Messina & D'Amore, 2018; Ross, Epstein, Anderson, & Eady, 2009). For example, in a study of 96 Swedish mothers who completed a second-parent adoption with a same-sex partner, Malmquist (2015) found that many mothers reported that social workers asked inappropriate questions about sexual orientation and displayed bias toward heteronormative family ideals (e.g., expressed the belief that a child must have one mother and one father). In addition to facing discrimination during all phases of the adoption process, Brown, Smalling, Groza, and Ryan (2009) found that LG adoptive parents ($N = 182$) in the USA saw themselves as having few role models to guide them through this process. Transgender parents in the USA and Canada have reported similar experiences of discrimination and fear of

---

[2] A home study is the in-depth evaluation that any prospective adoptive parent must complete in the USA as a requirement of the adoption process. It is intended as a way to educate and support parents throughout the adoption process and also to evaluate their fitness as potential parents (Mallon, 2011).

bias during the adoption process, such as concerns about whether to "come out" as transgender; limited research, however, is available in this area (Farr & Goldberg, 2018a ; Pyne, 2012; Stotzer et al., 2014; see chapter "Transgender-Parent Families").

At the same time, LGBTQ individuals and couples may offer special strengths as adoptive parents. Indeed, overall, LGBTQ adoptive parents have been found to display some positive characteristics that may benefit their children (Golombok et al., 2014; Perry, 2017). For example, Farr and Patterson (2013) found that, among 104 adoptive couples from their study in the USA (i.e., Farr et al., 2010a), LG couples were more likely than heterosexual couples to report sharing the duties of parenthood in an equal fashion. Moreover, among same-sex couples, shared parenting was associated with greater couple relationship adjustment and greater perceived parenting competence. With regard to family interaction, lesbian mothers were more supportive of one another in observations of triadic (i.e., parent/parent/child) interaction than were heterosexual or gay parents. Among all family types, more supportive interaction was associated with positive adjustment for young adopted children in this sample.

Likewise, a study by Goldberg, Kinkler, and Hines (2011) reported that among couples who had recently adopted a child in the USA, lesbian ($n = 45$) and gay adoptive couples ($n = 30$) were less likely to internalize adoption stigma (e.g., feeling that being an adoptive parent is inferior to being a biological parent) than were heterosexual adoptive couples ($n = 51$). Those parents who reported lower internalization of stigma also reported fewer depressive symptoms.

Many LG adoptive and foster parents report satisfaction in being a parent. For example, in a sample of 60 heterosexual, 15 gay, and 7 lesbian parents of children adopted from foster care in the USA, Lavner, Waterman, and Peplau (2014) found that parents generally reported being satisfied with their adoption, reported few depressive symptoms, and low levels of parental stress across three time points (2, 12, and 24 months postplacement). Indeed, many adoptive parents

report enjoying being a role model for other LG and/or adoptive parents, receiving more support than expected from families of origin after adopting, and feeling satisfied with their adoption experience (Brown et al., 2009; Goldberg & Smith, 2014; Wells, 2011). Thus, not only do LGBTQ adults who adopt children appear to be generally equipped as effective parents, but they also demonstrate a variety of distinct and unique strengths in these roles.

## The Transition to Adoptive Parenthood Among LGBTQ Adults

The transition to adoptive parenthood has been studied most carefully among heterosexual couples, but several studies have also examined this life transition among LG adoptive couples. Regardless of parents' gender or sexual identity, the transition to parenthood brings both joys and challenges. The broader literature indicates that after the adoption of a first child, there is a period of adjustment that can be marked by stress and compromised mental and physical health as well as by happiness and excitement (McKay, Ross, & Goldberg, 2010). For those adopting children, the transition to parenthood involves a rigorous screening process by adoption professionals and a variable waiting time for placement of a child (Mallon, 2011). In a systematic review of the literature, McKay et al. (2010) reported that rates of distress appear to be lower among adoptive parents as compared with biological parents, but post-adoption depressive symptoms are not uncommon. Post-adoption services appear to be helpful for some families (McKay et al., 2010). Consistent with the general literature on the transition to adoptive parenthood, Goldberg, Smith, and Kashy (2010) found that, among 44 lesbian, 30 gay, and 51 heterosexual adoptive couples in the USA, relationship quality declined across the transition to parenthood for all types of couples. Women reported the greatest declines in love and those in relationships with women (i.e., both heterosexual and lesbian partners) reported the greatest ambivalence. In another study of the same sample, Goldberg and Smith (2009) found that all parents reported increases in perceived parenting skill across the transition to parenthood. Relational conflict and expectations of completing more childcare were related to smaller increases in perceived parenting skill.

In a longitudinal study examining factors affecting LG adoptive couples across the transition to parenthood in the USA, Goldberg and Smith (2008, 2011) found that greater perceived social support and better relationship quality were associated with more favorable mental health, as would be expected from the general adoption literature. Sexual minority parents who had higher levels of internalized homophobia and who lived in areas with unfavorable legal climates with regard to adoption by LG parents experienced the greatest increases in anxiety and depression across the transition to parenthood. Indeed, it appears that the factors that contribute most to parental well-being and couple dynamics within LG adoptive families (at least within the USA) during their transition to parenthood are related to the age of a child, presence of social support, and family processes broadly, rather than parents' sexual or gender identity (Goldberg, Kinkler, Moyer, & Weber, 2014; Lavner et al., 2014; Sumontha, Farr, & Patterson, 2016).

LGBTQ adults who adopt may benefit from fewer "prescribed" cultural scripts to follow in parenting their children due to their "deviation" from heteronormative and cisnormative family structures that are based on biological parent-child relationships and headed by one mother and one father (who are both cisgender and heterosexual). For example, during the transition to parenthood, one important set of decisions that parents must make involves the choice of children's names. Interesting differences may emerge in this area, as a function of parental sexual orientation. In their study of 27 lesbian, 29 gay, and 50 heterosexual adoptive parents in the USA, Patterson and Farr (2017) found that heterosexual couples were more likely than LG couples to follow patronymic conventions. Thus, whereas children of heterosexual parents were most likely to have been given the last names of their fathers, children of LG parents were more often given hyphenated last names that had been created by combining the last names of both parents. Thus, same- and other-sex couples in this study took different approaches to naming their children (Patterson & Farr, 2017). A related study in the USA by Frank, Manley, and Goldberg (2019) involved an examination of how children referred to their parents (e.g., "Mommy," "Daddy") among sexual minority parent families, uncovering that many lesbian and gay parents often experience potential creativity as well as tension in considering what their children will call them. Little additional information is available about naming of adopted children by sexual and gender minority parents, and this is a topic that would benefit from further study, particularly given the implications related to family dynamics in the absence of felt pressure about heteronormative cultural values.

## Child Development and Outcomes for Parents, Couples, and Families

In controversies surrounding the adoption of children by LGBTQ parents, debate has often centered on children's development. Questions have been raised about whether LGBTQ adults can provide children with adequate parenting, appropriate role models, and effective socialization, particularly in the areas of gender development and sexual identity. The overall research on sexual orientation and parenting has been informative here; children of LGBTQ parents in general appear to develop in similar ways to their peers with cisgender heterosexual parents (Biblarz & Stacey, 2010; Moore & Stambolis-Ruhstorfer, 2013; Patterson, 2013, 2017). Until recently, however, this research rarely focused specifically on outcomes among adoptive families. Consistent with findings from the broader literature, we review existing studies about LGBTQ adoptive parent families, focusing on children's behavioral adjustment, gender development, and lived experiences related to adoptive and racial/ethnic identities. We also summarize results of research on parenting, couple relationships, parent-child relationships, and adoptive family systems. Considered as a group, these studies indicate that parental sexual orientation is not a strong predictor of individual or family outcomes. Rather, other factors, such as the qualities of parenting and family relationships, as well as prevailing laws and policies in a family's environment, may be more important.

Behavioral adjustment has been a topic of great interest in studies of child outcomes in adoptive families with LG parents. Early studies reported that assessments of adopted children's behavior problems were unrelated to parental sexual orientation, even after controlling for child age, child sex, and family income (Averett, Nalavany, & Ryan, 2009; Farr et al., 2010a; Farr & Patterson, 2009; Tan & Baggerly, 2009). A subsequent study by Goldberg and Smith (2013) also reported no significant differences in young children's internalizing or externalizing behavior problems as a function of parental sexual orientation. Similarly, Farr (2017) reported no differences in behavior problems among elementary school-aged children as a function of parental sexual orientation. Golombok and her colleagues (2014) studied lesbian, gay, and heterosexual parent families in the UK and reported that young children of heterosexual parents were more likely than those of LG parents to show externalizing behavior problems. Thus, it appears that adopted children with LG parents develop well, with behavioral outcomes that are at least on par with those with heterosexual parents.

A few longitudinal studies have examined children's gender development over time in families headed by LG and heterosexual adoptive parents. Among 106 adoptive families with lesbian, gay, and heterosexual parents, no significant differences were found in parents' reports or observational data of preschoolers' gender development, as a function of parental sexual orientation; across family types, children showed preferences for toys and activities typical of their gender (Farr et al., 2010a; Farr, Bruun, Doss, & Patterson, 2018). Moreover, these findings were consistent over time—child and parent reports, in addition to observational data from early to middle childhood, revealed that children were generally gender-typical and that gender development was similar across family types (Farr, Bruun, et al., 2018). In another study, Goldberg and

Garcia (2016) examined lesbian, gay, and heterosexual adoptive parents' reports of their children's gender-typed play behavior across early childhood. Children with lesbian mothers were less likely to demonstrate gender-typical play behavior compared to children with gay and heterosexual parents across multiple time points. This could be attributed to sexual minorities being more likely to display gender-flexible attitudes (Biblarz & Stacey, 2010). Relatedly, in a study of the within-family processes that shape children's gender attitudes, Sumontha, Farr, and Patterson (2017) found that school-age children adopted by LG parents had more flexible gender attitudes when parents also had more flexible attitudes and when they divided childcare labor more evenly. Future research using multiple methods of data collection over time could illuminate possible associations between adoptive parents' sexual orientation and their children's gender development. Overall, it seems that parental sexual orientation is not a strong predictor of gender identity and development among adopted children; rather, factors such as parents' attitudes and behaviors (e.g., divisions of labor) may be more relevant.

How do children who are adopted by LG parents actually describe their experiences? In one study, adolescents' practices surrounding disclosure about family were examined, with particular attention to issues related to having been adopted by LG parents. Using qualitative interview data from 14 racially diverse adopted children ranging in age from 13 to 20 years old, Gianino, Goldberg, and Lewis (2009) explored how adolescents disclose their adoptive status and parental sexual orientation within friendship networks and school environments. Adolescents reported using a wide variety of strategies, ranging from not disclosing to anyone to telling others openly. Several participants noted that they had felt "forced" to disclose by virtue of their visibility as a transracial adoptive family with same-sex parents, and many indicated their apprehension in "coming out" about their families. Overall, adolescents indicated that they had received positive reactions and responses from others about their adoptive status. In another study of adolescents adopted through foster care by LG parents, participants reported feeling more open-minded and tolerant of others based on their adoptive parents' sexual orientation (Cody, Farr, McRoy, Ayers-Lopez, & Ledesma, 2017). Among school-age children adopted by LG parents, despite reports of experiencing some bullying related to their parents' sexual orientation, participants described positive feelings about their family and did not usually fear disclosing about them (Farr, Crain, Oakley, Cashen, & Garber, 2016; Farr, Oakley, & Ollen, 2016).

Gianino et al. (2009) suggested that parental preparation for dealing with issues surrounding their child's adoption, racism, and heterosexism and homophobia may have helped children in negotiating the disclosure process. Sparse research exists examining how LGBTQ adoptive parents socialize their children around minority statuses they may hold (e.g., race, adoption), but existing evidence suggests that LG adoptive parents value these practices (Wyman Battalen, Farr, Brodzinsky, & McRoy, 2018) and that parents often engage in processes of adoptive, racial/ethnic, and sexual minority parent family socialization with their young children (Goldberg & Smith, 2016; Oakley, Farr, & Scherer, 2017). Future research should explore how such socialization shapes children's experiences.

A handful of studies of adoptive families with LG parents have examined mental health or relationship outcomes for parents and for couples in the USA, as well as for parent-child relationships and overall family functioning. Goldberg and Smith (2011) reported relatively few depressive symptoms overall among a sample of 52 lesbian and 38 gay adoptive couples. An earlier report based on the same sample had also revealed that, among lesbian and heterosexual couples waiting to adopt children, there were no differences in overall well-being as a function of parental sexual orientation (Goldberg & Smith, 2008). In a study of gay adoptive fathers, Tornello, Farr, and Patterson (2011) found that participants ($N = 231$) reported levels of parenting stress that were well within the normative range. Farr and her colleagues (2010a) found that lesbian, gay, and heterosexual adoptive parents in their sample of 106 adoptive families reported relatively little parenting stress, with no significant differences as a function of family type. Moreover, studies examining parenting stress over time among samples of

lesbian, gay, and heterosexual adoptive parents have demonstrated that parenting stress is not a function of sexual orientation (Farr, 2017; Goldberg & Smith, 2014; Lavner et al., 2014). Similarly, lesbian, gay, and heterosexual adoptive parents in Farr et al.'s (2010a) study reported using effective parenting techniques, with no significant differences in effectiveness as a function of parental sexual orientation. In observational data on family interaction in this same sample, lesbian, gay, and heterosexual adoptive parents were found to be relatively warm and accepting with their children overall; regardless of sexual orientation, mothers tended to be warmer with their children than did fathers (Farr & Patterson, 2013).

In terms of couple relationships among LG adoptive parents in the USA, Goldberg and Smith (2009) found that lesbian ($n = 47$) and gay adoptive couples ($n = 56$) in their sample reported relatively low levels of relationship conflict. Interestingly, Goldberg, Garcia, and Manley (2018) also found that sexual identity was relevant to levels of couple relationship among members of female adoptive same-sex couples, with higher conflict among individuals who had plurisexual identities (e.g., bisexual, queer) as compared to those with monosexual identities (e.g., lesbian, gay). In terms of additional couple relationship dynamics, Farr et al. (2010a) also found that among their sample of 106 adoptive couples, adoptive parents reported high average levels of couple relationship adjustment with no significant differences across family type. A majority of couples reported long-term relationships with their partners or spouses, in which they reported feeling secure and satisfied (Farr, Forssell, & Patterson, 2010b). LG parents in this sample also reported overall satisfaction with current divisions of childcare labor, which participants generally described as being shared by both parents in the couple—both when children were in early childhood and in middle childhood (Farr & Patterson, 2013; Sumontha et al., 2017). Interestingly, in both Goldberg and Garcia's (2015) and Farr's (2017) samples, rates of couple dissolution over time were higher among lesbian than gay or heterosexual adoptive parents. As these are among the first studies to examine couple dynamics over time among LGBTQ adoptive parent couples, continued research in this area is warranted (Farr & Goldberg, 2018b).

Consistent with findings from the broader literature, quality of parenting and of parent-child relationships appear to be more influential than parental sexual orientation to individual outcomes. In their study of 106 families headed by lesbian, gay, and heterosexual adoptive couples in the USA, Farr et al. (2010a) found that qualities of family interactions were more strongly associated with child outcomes than was family structure. Across all families, positive parenting, harmonious couple relationships, and healthy family functioning were associated with parents' reports of fewer child behavior problems when children were in early and middle childhood (Farr, 2017; Farr et al., 2010a). Drawing on data from the same sample, Farr and Patterson (2013) found that quality of co-parenting interaction was related to children's behavioral adjustment, such that more supportive and less undermining behavior between parents was associated with fewer child behavior problems. Erich, Kanenberg, Case, Allen, and Bogdanos (2009), in their study of 210 adopted adolescents and 154 parents in the USA, also reported that qualities of adolescents' relationships with their lesbian, gay, or heterosexual adoptive parents were associated with adolescents' reported life satisfaction, parents' satisfaction with their child, and the number of prior placements the adolescent had experienced, but were unrelated to parental sexual orientation. In Golombok et al.'s (2014) study of lesbian, gay, and heterosexual adoptive families in the UK, gay fathers reported significantly greater parental well-being and more positive relationships with their children than did heterosexual parents. Thus, associations between parental sexual orientation and family relationships have generally not been discovered, and when they have been identified, the results have favored families with LGBTQ parents.

## Summary, Conclusions, and Future Directions

In this final section, we summarize the overall findings of research to date and consider what conclusions may be justified. We also suggest directions for further research and practice.

## Summary of the Research Findings

Research on LGBTQ adoptive parents and their children has grown markedly in the last several years. In the USA, many LGBTQ adults are adoptive parents, and many more wish to adopt children. Some of the reasons that LGBTQ adults adopt children, as well as some of the experiences of LGBTQ adoptive parents, are similar to, and some are different from, those of cisgender heterosexual adoptive parents. In recent studies, LGBTQ adults have reported experiencing discrimination and facing many obstacles in becoming adoptive parents. At the same time, having overcome obstacles to parenthood, LGBTQ adoptive parents appear to be as capable and effective as are cisgender heterosexual adults in their roles as adoptive parents. Children adopted by LGBTQ parents have been found to develop in ways that are similar to development among children adopted by cisgender heterosexual parents. Regardless of parental sexual orientation and gender identity and expression, quality of parenting and quality of family relationships are significantly associated with adopted children's adjustment. Thus, as in other types of families, it is family processes, rather than family structure, that matter more to child outcomes and to overall family functioning among adoptive families.

## Directions for Future Research

Although existing research on adoption by LGBTQ parents is informative, work in this area has only recently begun, and there are many directions for further study in terms of research design, conceptual frameworks, and legal and policy implications. From a methodological standpoint, use of more diverse research strategies seems likely to be fruitful (Fish & Russell, 2018). Much of the empirical work to date has relied on cross-sectional and self-report data, yet utilizing longitudinal designs, multiple informants from sources outside the family (e.g., teachers, peers), and observations of actual behavior have the potential to make strong contributions to this literature. Much existing work has used either quantitative or qualitative approaches to research, but mixed-methods approaches that embrace both quantitative and qualitative approaches to data collection could enrich our understanding.

In terms of sampling, many studies in this area have included predominantly white, well-educated samples of LG adoptive parents. More diverse samples could make valuable contributions, as the experiences of racial minority adoptive parents likely differ from those of white adoptive parents. Low-income adoptive parents, who may be likely to adopt children through public versus private agencies (or to foster children for long periods of time without legally adopting them) would also be expected to differ in their experiences from the more affluent adoptive parents who have been included in most studies to date. Furthermore, research has generally not included bisexual or transgender adoptive parents, although work in this area has begun to emerge. Greater integration across fields of adoption study would also be beneficial in providing a more comprehensive understanding of adoptive families with LGBTQ parents. Scholarship in fields as diverse as law, economics, demography, family science, social work, sociology, and psychology is already contributing to understanding in this area. Further integration of work in these diverse fields might contribute to a more comprehensive understanding of the social, psychological, and economic aspects of LGBTQ adoptive parent family life experiences. Relatedly, recent literature reviews have underscored the dearth in published studies on LGBTQ-parent families that explicitly use theoretical frames within their research; rather, the majority of studies reviewed focused on public policy debate (Farr et al., 2017; van Eeden-Moorefield et al., 2018). More inclusive samples of sexual and gender minority adoptive parents, as well as more strongly integrated theoretical frameworks in conjunction with rigorous methodological designs, would contribute to our more comprehensive understanding of the experiences of diverse adoptive family systems.

Adoption is a complex topic, and different issues arise in public versus private adoptions, domestic versus international adoptions, and adoptions of infants versus adoptions of children or adolescents. Similarly, transracial adoptions bring with them issues that are not always posed by same-race adoptions, such as considerations of racial and ethnic socialization, identity, and diversity in one's community. Little is known about how the intersections of race, class, and parents' sexual minority status affect adoptive families and children, especially in the context of child welfare adoptions (Goldberg, Gartrell, & Gates, 2014). Future research could be strengthened by consideration of the variations among adoption pathways.

Another valuable direction for future research would be more attention to family processes and dynamics, as well as to family outcomes. What are the special family dynamics, if any, that are associated with LGBTQ adoptive parent families, and how do these affect children, for better or for worse? What are the important ways in which LGBTQ adoptive parents may be similar to and different from one another, and what does this mean for children? How, in short, are changing family configurations related to family interactions and relationships?

The voices of adopted children themselves also need to be heard. How do children and youth understand the difficulties and the opportunities of their lives as adopted offspring of LGBTQ parents? How do children and youth see their experiences as having been linked with (or unaffected by) the contextual factors and varied family configurations discussed above? Preliminary work has demonstrated that although children of LG adoptive parents may face adversity related to their parents' sexual orientation, a number of factors contribute to resilience and positive child outcomes (Cody et al., 2017; Farr, Crain, et al., 2016; Farr, Oakley, & Ollen, 2016). Greater attention to the views of individuals adopted by LGBTQ parents seems likely to broaden understanding in this area.

Future research on adoptive LGBTQ-parent families would also benefit from fuller consideration of the contexts of adoptive family life. These might include social, economic, and legal aspects of family environments. Research might consider the importance of proximal (e.g., social contacts for families in their daily lives) and distal aspects of family environments (e.g., regional, state, and national laws and policies). Federal, state, and local laws may affect the choices that adoptive LGBTQ parents make for their families, and daily interactions with neighbors, coworkers, and friends are also likely to exert important influences on their experiences. Indeed, research has demonstrated that policy and law shape how LG parents perceive and experience parenthood, through their influence on choices among pathways to adoption and among residential neighborhoods (Farr & Goldberg, 2018a). Inasmuch as laws, policies, and attitudes vary considerably across jurisdictions, in the USA and elsewhere, and inasmuch as change in this area is more the rule than the exception today, the impact of broader social contexts on adoptive LGBTQ-parent families is a rich and important topic for further study.

## Directions for Policy and Practice

With regard to policy implications of research on LGBTQ-parent adoptive families, a number of directions can be identified. First and foremost, the results of research in this area should be used to inform law, policy, and practice. If the Aderholt Amendment had become law in the USA, it would have allowed discrimination against otherwise qualified LG prospective adoptive parents (Movement Advancement Project, 2018a). Currently, however, there are 10 states in the USA with religious exemption laws that allow for discrimination against qualified LGBTQ adults when they apply to adopt children through state-funded child welfare agencies (Movement Advancement Project, 2018a). Research findings to date clearly demonstrate the parenting proficiency of LGBTQ adults and thus do not support such policies as being beneficial to children.

More than 440,000 children are in the child welfare system in the USA and more than 120,000 children are currently waiting to be adopted (U.S. Department of Health & Human Services, 2018). Existing evidence suggests that discriminatory policies related to parental sexual and gender identity are detrimental to the welfare of children awaiting adoptive placement. Kaye and Kuvalanka (2006) compared placement rates of children from foster care in states with laws that prohibit adoptions by openly LG adults with placement rates in states that permit such adoptions. They found that, in states where adoption laws prohibit adoptions by openly LG adults, proportionately more children remained in foster care. In contrast, states that permitted LG adults to adopt children had proportionately fewer children in foster care. Indeed, if LG adults had been permitted to adopt children in every jurisdiction within the USA and if discrimination against them was forbidden, Gates, Badgett, Macomber, and Chambers (2007) estimated that between 9,000 and 14,000 children could be removed from foster care and placed in permanent homes each year. Moreover, in a study examining the development of high-risk children adopted from foster care in the USA, it was found that child development did not differ between lesbian, gay, and heterosexual adoptive parent families—despite LG parents having children with significantly higher levels of biological and environmental risks (e.g., prenatal substance exposure, birth complications, neglect and abuse) typical of children with special needs (Lavner et al., 2012). Compounding the challenge of finding permanent families for waiting children is a perceived dearth of prospective parents. If adoption agencies were to recruit more prospective LGBTQ parents, many additional children might find permanent homes (Brodzinsky, 2011a).

To support LGBTQ adults seeking to adopt children, a number of organizations have begun programs related to adoption issues. For example, the Human Rights Campaign (HRC) has an initiative called the "All Children – All Families" program (HRC, 2017) that seeks to assist adoption agencies and child welfare professionals in their efforts to recruit prospective adoptive parents from LGBTQ communities, work successfully with them, and in so doing, place more children into permanent homes. In addition, agencies can complete the HRC's training program and become recognized as organizations that are affirming to LGBTQ adults seeking adoption services (Farr & Goldberg, 2018a; HRC, 2017).

## Conclusion

In conclusion, the adoption of children by LGBTQ parents is a growing reality in the USA and in at least some other parts of the world. Empirical research on adoptive families with LGBTQ parents has begun to address some questions about how children adopted by LGBTQ parents fare. While LGBTQ individuals may face a number of challenges in becoming adoptive parents, LGBTQ-parent families formed through adoption appear to experience generally positive outcomes. Much remains to be learned, however, especially about diversity among LGBTQ adoptive parents and their children and about the ways in which their lives are shaped by characteristics of the environments in which they live.

## References

American Psychological Association. (2015). *Amicus brief in Obergefell v. Hodges*. Washington, DC: American Psychological Association. Retrieved from http://www.apa.org/about/offices/ogc/amicus/obergefell-supreme court.pdf

Averett, P., Nalavany, B., & Ryan, S. (2009). An evaluation of gay/lesbian and heterosexual adoption. *Adoption Quarterly, 12*, 129–151. https://doi.org/10.1080/10926750903313278

Baccara, M., Collard-Wexler, A., Felli, L., & Yariv, L. (2014). Child-adoption matching: Preferences for gender and race. *American Economic Journal: Applied Economics, 6*(3), 133–158. https://doi.org/10.1257/app.6.3.133

Balenzano, C., Coppola, G., Cassibba, R., & Moro, G. (2018). Pre-adoption adversities and adoptees' outcomes: The protective role of post-adoption variables in an Italian experience of domestic open adoption. *Children and Youth Services Review, 85*, 307–318. https://doi.org/10.1016/j.childyouth.2018.01.012

Biblarz, T. J., & Stacey, J. (2010). How does the gender of parents matter? *Journal of Marriage and Family, 72*, 3–22. https://doi.org/10.1111/j.1741-3737.2009.00678.x

Brewster, K. L., Tillman, K. H., & Jokinen-Gordon, H. (2014). Demographic characteristics of lesbian parents in the United States. *Population Research and Policy Review, 33*, 503–526. https://doi.org/10.1007/s11113-013-9296-3

Brodzinsky, D. M. (2011a). Children's understanding of adoption: Developmental and clinical implications. *Professional Psychology, 42*, 200–207. https://doi.org/10.1037/a022415

Brodzinsky, D. M. (2011b). Adoption by lesbians and gay men: A national survey of adoption agency policies and practices. In D. Brodzinsky & A. Pertman (Eds.), *Adoption by lesbians and gay men: A new dimension in family diversity* (pp. 62–84). New York, NY: Oxford University Press.

Brodzinsky, D. M. (2015). *The modern adoptive families study: An introduction*. New York, NY: Evan B. Donaldson Adoption Institute. Retrieved from https://www.adoptioninstitute.org/wp-content/uploads/2015/09/DAI_MAF_Report_090115_R7_Edit.pdf

Brodzinsky, D. M., & Goldberg, A. E. (2016). Contact with birth family in adoptive families headed by lesbian, gay male, and heterosexual parents. *Children and Youth Services Review, 62*, 9–17. https://doi.org/10.1016/j.childyouth.2016.01.014

Brown, S., Smalling, S., Groza, V., & Ryan, S. (2009). The experiences of gay men and lesbians in becoming and being adoptive parents. *Adoption Quarterly, 12*, 226–246. https://doi.org/10.1080/10926750903313294

Carroll, A. & Mendos, L. R. (2017). *State-Sponsored Homophobia 2017: A world survey of sexual orientation laws: Criminalisation, protection and recognition*. International Lesbian, Gay, Bisexual, Trans and Intersex Association. Retrieved from https://ilga.org/downloads/2017/ILGA_State_Sponsored_Homophobia_2017_WEB.pdf

Cody, P. A., Farr, R. H., McRoy, R. G., Ayers-Lopez, S. J., & Ledesma, K. J. (2017). Youth perspectives on being adopted from foster care by lesbian and gay parents: Implications for families and adoption professionals. *Adoption Quarterly, 20*, 98–118. https://doi.org/10.1080/10926755.2016.1200702

Crea, T. M., Chan, K., & Barth, R. P. (2013). Family environment and attention-deficit/hyperactivity disorder in adopted children: Associations with family cohesion and adaptability. *Child: Care, Health and Development, 40*, 853–862. https://doi.org/10.1111/cch.12112

Davis, M. A. (2013). Demographics of gay and lesbian adoption and family policies. In A. K. Baumle (Ed.), *International handbook on the demography of sexuality* (pp. 383–401). Dordrecht, The Netherlands: Springer. https://doi.org/10.1007/978-94-007-5512-3_19

del Pozo de Bolger, A., Dunstan, D., & Kaltner, M. (2018). A conceptual model of psychosocial adjustment of foster care adoptees based on a scoping review of contributing factors. *Clinical Psychologist, 22*, 3–15. https://doi.org/10.1111/cp.12090

DeLuca, H. K., Claxton, S. E., & van Dulmen, M. H. (2018). The peer relationships of those who have experienced adoption or foster care: A meta-analysis. *Journal of Research on Adolescence*. Advance online publication. https://doi.org/10.1111/jora.12421

dickey, L. M., Ducheny, K. M., & Ehrbar, R. D. (2016). Family creation options for transgender and gender nonconforming people. *Psychology of Sexual Orientation and Gender Diversity, 3*, 173–179. https://doi.org/10.1037/sgd0000178

Downing, J., Richardson, H., Kinkler, L., & Goldberg, A. (2009). Making the decision: Factors influencing gay men's choice of an adoption path. *Adoption Quarterly, 12*, 247–271. https://doi.org/10.1080/10926750903313310

Erich, S., Kanenberg, H., Case, K., Allen, T., & Bogdanos, T. (2009). An empirical analysis of factors affecting adolescent attachment in adoptive families with homosexual and straight parents. *Children & Youth Services Review, 31*, 398–404. https://doi.org/10.1016/j.childyouth.2008.09.004

Farr, R. H. (2017). Does parental sexual orientation matter? A longitudinal follow-up of adoptive families with school-age children. *Developmental Psychology, 53*, 252–264. https://doi.org/10.1037/dev0000228

Farr, R. H., Bruun, S. T., Doss, K. M., & Patterson, C. J. (2018). Children's gender-typed behavior from early to middle childhood in adoptive families with lesbian, gay, and heterosexual parents. *Sex Roles, 78*, 528–541. https://doi.org/10.1007/s11199-017-0812-5

Farr, R. H., Crain, E. E., Oakley, M. K., Cashen, K. K., & Garber, K. J. (2016). Microaggressions, feelings of difference, and resilience among adopted children with sexual minority parents. *Journal of Youth and Adolescence, 45*, 85–104. https://doi.org/10.1007/s10964-015-0353-6

Farr, R. H., Forssell, S. L., & Patterson, C. J. (2010a). Parenting and child development in adoptive families: Does parental sexual orientation matter? *Applied Developmental Science, 14*, 164–178. https://doi.org/10.1080/10888691.2010.500958

Farr, R. H., Forssell, S. L., & Patterson, C. J. (2010b). Lesbian, gay, and heterosexual adoptive parents: Couple and relationship issues. *Journal of GLBT Family Studies, 6*, 199–213. https://doi.org/10.1080/15504281003705436

Farr, R. H., & Goldberg, A. E. (2015). Contact between birth and adoptive families during the first year postplacement: Perspectives of lesbian, gay, and heterosexual parents. *Adoption Quarterly, 18*, 1–24. https://doi.org/10.1080/10926755.2014.895466

Farr, R. H., & Goldberg, A. E. (2018a). Same-sex relationship dissolution and divorce: How will children be affected? In A. E. Goldberg & A. Romero (Eds.), *LGBTQ divorce and relationship dissolution: Psychological and legal perspectives and implications for practice* (pp. 151–172). New York, NY: Oxford University Press.

Farr, R. H., & Goldberg, A. E. (2018b). Sexual orientation, gender identity, and adoption law. *Family Court Review, 56*, 374–383. https://doi.org/10.1111/fcre.12354

Farr, R. H., Oakley, M. K., & Ollen, E. W. (2016). School experiences of young children and their lesbian and gay adoptive parents. *Psychology of Sexual Orientation and Gender Diversity, 3*, 442–447. https://doi.org/10.1037/sgd0000187

Farr, R. H., & Patterson, C. J. (2009). Transracial adoption by lesbian, gay, and heterosexual parents: Who completes transracial adoptions and with what results? *Adoption Quarterly, 12*, 187–204. https://doi.org/10.1080/10926750903313328

Farr, R. H., & Patterson, C. J. (2013). Coparenting among lesbian, gay, and heterosexual couples: Associations with adopted children's outcomes. *Child Development, 84*, 1226–1240. https://doi.org/10.1111/cdev.12046

Farr, R. H., Ravvina, Y., & Grotevant, H. (2018). Birth family contact experiences among lesbian, gay, and heterosexual adoptive parents with school-age children. *Family Relations, 67*, 132–146. https://doi.org/10.1111/fare.12295

Farr, R. H., Tasker, F., & Goldberg, A. E. (2017). Theory in highly cited studies of sexual minority parent families: Variations and implications. *Journal of Homosexuality, 64*, 1143–1179. https://doi.org/10.1080/00918369.2016.1242336

Fish, J. N., & Russell, S. T. (2018). Queering methodologies to understand queer families. *Family Relations, 67*, 12–25. https://doi.org/10.1111/fare.12297

Frank, E., Manley, M., & Goldberg, A. E. (2019). Parental naming practices in same-sex adoptive families. *Family Relations*. Advance online publication. https://doi.org/10.1111/fare.12390

Gates, G. J. (2011). *Family formation and raising children among same-sex couples*. National Council of Family Relations. Retrieved from https://escholarship.org/uc/item/5pq1q8d7

Gates, G. J. (2013). *LGBT parenting in the United States*. The Williams Institute. Retrieved from http://williamsinstitute.law.ucla.edu/wp-content/uploads/LGBT-Parenting.pdf

Gates, G. J., Badgett, M. V. L., Macomber, J. E., & Chambers, K. (2007). *Adoption and foster care by gay and lesbian parents in the United States*. The Williams Institute. Retrieved from https://escholarship.org/uc/item/2v4528cx

Gianino, M., Goldberg, A., & Lewis, T. (2009). Disclosure practices among adopted youth with gay and lesbian parents. *Adoption Quarterly, 12*, 205–228. https://doi.org/10.1080/10926750903313344

Goldberg, A. E. (2009a). Lesbian and heterosexual preadoptive couples' openness to transracial adoption. *American Journal of Orthopsychiatry, 79*, 103–117. https://doi.org/10.1037/a0015354

Goldberg, A. E. (2009b). Heterosexual, lesbian, and gay preadoptive parents' preferences about child gender. *Sex Roles, 61*, 55–71. https://doi.org/10.1007/s11199-009-9598-4

Goldberg, A. E. (2012). *Gay dads: Transitions to adoptive fatherhood*. New York, NY: NYU Press.

Goldberg, A. E., Downing, J. B., & Richardson, H. B. (2009). The transition from infertility to adoption: Perceptions of lesbian and heterosexual preadoptive couples. *Journal of Social & Personal Relationships, 26*, 938–963. https://doi.org/10.1177/0265407509345652

Goldberg, A. E., & Garcia, R. (2015). Predictors of relationship dissolution in lesbian, gay, and heterosexual adoptive parents. *Journal of Family Psychology, 29*, 394–404. https://doi.org/10.1037/fam0000095

Goldberg, A. E., & Garcia, R. L. (2016). Gender-typed behavior over time in children with lesbian, gay, and heterosexual parents. *Journal of Family Psychology, 30*, 854–865. https://doi.org/10.1037/fam0000226

Goldberg, A. E., Garcia, R., & Manley, M. H. (2018). Monosexual and nonmonosexual women in same-sex couples' relationship quality during the first five years of parenthood. *Sexual and Relationship Therapy, 33*, 190–212. https://doi.org/10.1080/14681994.2017.1419561

Goldberg, A. E., Gartrell, N. K., & Gates, G. J. (2014). *Research report on LGB-parent families*. The Williams Institute. Retrieved from https://escholarship.org/uc/item/7gr4970w

Goldberg, A. E., Kinkler, L. A., & Hines, D. A. (2011). Perception and internalization of adoption stigma among gay, lesbian, and heterosexual adoptive parents. *Journal of GLBT Family Studies, 7*, 132–154. https://doi.org/10.1080/1550428X.2011.537554

Goldberg, A. E., Kinkler, L. A., Moyer, A. M., & Weber, E. (2014). Intimate relationship challenges in early parenthood among lesbian, gay, and heterosexual couples adopting via the child welfare system. *Professional Psychology, 45*, 221–230. https://doi.org/10.1037/a0037443

Goldberg, A. E., Kinkler, L. A., Richardson, H. B., & Downing, J. B. (2011). Lesbian, gay, and heterosexual couples in open adoption arrangements: A qualitative study. *Journal of Marriage and Family, 73*, 502–518. https://doi.org/10.1111/j.1741-3737.2010.00821.x

Goldberg, A. E., Moyer, A. M., Kinkler, L. A., & Richardson, H. B. (2012). "When you're sitting on the fence, hope's the hardest part": Challenges and experiences of heterosexual and same-sex couples adopting through the child welfare system. *Adoption Quarterly, 15*, 288–315. https://doi.org/10.1080/10926755.2012.731032

Goldberg, A. E., & Smith, J. Z. (2008). Social support and psychological well-being in lesbian and heterosexual preadoptive couples. *Family Relations, 57*, 281–294. https://doi.org/10.1111/j.1741-3729.2008.00500.x

Goldberg, A. E., & Smith, J. Z. (2009). Perceived parenting skill across the transition to adoptive parenthood among lesbian, gay, and heterosexual couples. *Journal of Family Psychology, 23*, 861–870. https://doi.org/10.1037/a0017009

Goldberg, A. E., & Smith, J. Z. (2011). Stigma, social context, and mental health: Lesbian and gay couples across the transition to adoptive parenthood. *Journal of Counseling Psychology, 58*, 139–150. https://doi.org/10.1037/a0021684

Goldberg, A. E., & Smith, J. Z. (2013). Predictors of psychological adjustment in early placed adopted children with lesbian, gay, and heterosexual parents. *Journal of Family Psychology, 27*, 431–442. https://doi.org/10.1037/a0032911

Goldberg, A. E., & Smith, J. Z. (2014). Predictors of parenting stress in lesbian, gay, and heterosexual adoptive parents during early parenthood. *Journal of Family Psychology, 28*, 125–137. https://doi.org/10.1037/a0036007

Goldberg, A. E., & Smith, J. Z. (2016). Predictors of race, adoption, and sexual orientation related socializa-tion of adoptive parents of young children. *Journal of Family Psychology, 30*, 397–408. https://doi.org/10.1037/fam0000149

Goldberg, A. E., Smith, J. Z., & Kashy, D. A. (2010). Preadoptive factors predicting lesbian, gay, and heterosexual couples' relationship quality across the transition to adoptive parenthood. *Journal of Family Psychology, 24*, 221–232. https://doi.org/10.1037/a0019615

Goldberg, S. K., & Conron, K. J. (2018). *How many same-sex couples in the U.S. are raising children?* The Williams Institute. Retrieved from https://williamsinstitute.law.ucla.edu/research/parenting/how-many-same-sex-parents-in-us/

Golombok, S., Mellish, L., Jennings, S., Casey, P., Tasker, F., & Lamb, M. E. (2014). Adoptive gay father families: Parent-child relationships and children's psychological adjustment. *Child Development, 85*, 456–468. https://doi.org/10.1111/cdev.12155

Grotevant, H. D., McRoy, R. G., Wrobel, G. M., & Ayers-Lopez, S. (2013). Contact between adoptive and birth families: Perspectives from the Minnesota/Texas Adoption Research Project. *Child Development Perspectives, 7*, 193–198. https://doi.org/10.1111/cdep.12039

Gumus, G., & Lee, J. (2012). Alternative paths to parenthood: IVF or child adoption? *Economic Inquiry, 50*, 802–820. https://doi.org/10.1111/j.1465-7295.2011.00401.x

Harwood, R., Feng, X., & Yu, S. (2013). Preadoption adversities and postadoption mediators of mental health and school outcomes among international, foster, and private adoptees in the United States. *Journal of Family Psychology, 27*, 409–420. https://doi.org/10.1037/a0032908

Herrmann-Green, L. K., & Gehring, T. M. (2007). The German lesbian family study: Planning for parenthood via donor insemination. *Journal of GLBT Family Studies, 3*, 351–395. https://doi.org/10.1300/J461v03n04_02

Hrapczynski, K. M., & Leslie, L. A. (2018). Engagement in racial socialization among transracial adoptive families with white parents. *Family Relations, 67*, 354–367. https://doi.org/10.1111/fare.12316

Human Rights Campaign. (2017). *All children—all families: List of participating agencies*. Retrieved from http://www.hrc.org/resources/all-children-all-families-list-of-participating-agencies

International Lesbian, Gay, Bisexual, Trans and Intersex Association. (2019). *Sexual orientation laws in the world – 2019*. Retrieved from https://ilga.org/downloads/ILGA_Sexual_Orientation_Laws_Map_2019.pdf

Jennings, S., Mellish, L., Tasker, F., Lamb, M., & Golombok, S. (2014). Why adoption? Gay, lesbian, and heterosexual adoptive parents' reproductive experiences and reasons for adoption. *Adoption Quarterly, 17*, 205–226. https://doi.org/10.1080/10926755.2014.891549

Ji, J., Brooks, D., Barth, R. P., & Kim, H. (2010). Beyond preadoptive risk: The impact of adoptive family environment on adopted youth's psychosocial adjustment. *American Journal of Orthopsychiatry, 80*, 432–442. https://doi.org/10.1111/j.1939-0025.2010.01046.x

Jiménez-Morago, J. M., León, E., & Román, M. (2015). Adversity and adjustment in children in institutions, family foster care, and adoption. *The Spanish Journal of Psychology, 18*, E45. https://doi.org/10.1017/sjp.2015.49

Julian, M. M. (2013). Age at adoption from institutional care as a window into the lasting effects of early experiences. *Clinical Child and Family Psychology Review, 16*, 101–145. https://doi.org/10.1007/s10567-013-0130-6

Kaye, S., & Kuvalanka, K. (2006). *State gay adoption laws and permanency for foster youth.* Maryland Family Policy Impact Seminar. Retrieved http://www.hhp.umd.edu/FMST/_docsContribute/GayadoptionbriefFINAL0806.pdf

Kendler, K. S., Turkheimer, E., Ohlsson, H., Sundquist, J., & Sundquist, K. (2015). Family environment and the malleability of cognitive ability: A Swedish national home-reared and adopted-away cosibling control study. *Proceedings of the National Academy of Sciences, 112*, 4612–4617. https://doi.org/10.1073/pnas.1417106112

Kinkler, L. A., & Goldberg, A. E. (2011). Working with what we've got: Perceptions of barriers and supports among small-metropolitan-area same-sex adopting couples. *Family Relations, 60*, 387–403. https://doi.org/10.1111/j.1741-3729.2011.00654.x

Lamb, M. E. (2012). Mothers, fathers, families, and circumstances: Factors affecting children's adjustment. *Applied Developmental Science, 16*, 98–111. https://doi.org/10.1080/10888691.2012.667344

Lavner, J. A., Waterman, J., & Peplau, L. A. (2012). Can gay and lesbian parents promote healthy development in high-risk children adopted from foster care? *American Journal of Orthopsychiatry, 82*, 465–472. https://doi.org/10.1111/j.1939-0025.2012.01176.x

Lavner, J. A., Waterman, J., & Peplau, L. A. (2014). Parent adjustment over time in gay, lesbian, and heterosexual parent families adopting from foster care. *American Journal of Orthopsychiatry, 84*, 46–53. https://doi.org/10.1037/h0098853

Le Mare, L., & Audet, K. (2011). Communicative openness in adoption, knowledge of culture of origin, and adoption identity in adolescents adopted from Romania. *Adoption Quarterly, 14*, 199–217. https://doi.org/10.1080/10926755.2011.608031

Mallon, G. P. (2011). The home study assessment process for gay, lesbian, bisexual, and transgender prospective foster and adoptive families. *Journal of GLBT Family Studies, 7*, 9–29. https://doi.org/10.1080/1550428X.2011.537229

Malmquist, A. (2015). A crucial but strenuous process: Female same-sex couples' reflections on second-parent adoption. *Journal of GLBT Family Studies, 11*, 351–374. https://doi.org/10.1080/15504 28X.2015.1019169

McKay, K., Ross, L. E., & Goldberg, A. E. (2010). Adaptation to parenthood during the post-adoption period: A review of the literature. *Adoption Quarterly, 13*, 125–144. https://doi.org/10.1080/10926755.2010.481040

Messina, R., & D'Amore, S. (2018). Adoption by lesbians and gay men in Europe: Challenges and barriers on the journey to adoption. *Adoption Quarterly, 21*, 59–81. https://doi.org/10.1080/10926755.2018.1427641

Moore, M. R., & Stambolis-Ruhstorfer, M. (2013). LGBT sexuality and families at the start of the twenty-first century. *Annual Review of Sociology, 39*, 491–507. https://doi.org/10.1146/annurev-soc-071312-145643

Movement Advancement Project. (2018a, July). *Creating a license to discriminate: 2018 Federal Child Welfare Amendment.* (Issue Brief). Retrieved from http://www.lgbtmap.org/2018-child-welfare-amendment

Movement Advancement Project. (2018b, August). *Foster and adoption laws* [Map illustration of U.S. foster and adoption laws August, 2018]. Retrieved from http://www.lgbtmap.org/equality-maps/foster_and_adoption_laws/

Oakley, M. K., Farr, R. H., & Scherer, D. G. (2017). Same-sex parent socialization: Understanding gay and lesbian parenting practices as cultural socialization. *Journal of GLBT Family Studies, 13*, 56–75. https://doi.org/10.1080/1550428X.2016.1158685

*Obergefell v. Hodges*, 135 S. Ct. 2584 (2015).

Palacios, J., & Brodzinsky, D. (2010). Review: Adoption research: Trends, topics, outcomes. *International Journal of Behavioral Development, 34*, 270–284. https://doi.org/10.1177/0165025410362837

Patterson, C. J. (2013). Children of lesbian and gay parents: Psychology, law, and policy. *Psychology of Sexual Orientation and Gender Diversity, 1*, 27–34. https://doi.org/10.1037/2329-0382.1.S.27

Patterson, C. J. (2017). Parents' sexual orientation and children's development. *Child Development Perspectives, 11*, 45–49. https://doi.org/10.1111/cdep.12207

Patterson, C. J., & Farr, R. H. (2017). What shall we call ourselves? Last names among lesbian, gay, and heterosexual couples and their adopted children. *Journal of GLBT Family Studies, 13*, 97–113. https://doi.org/10.1080/1550428X.2016.1169239

Patterson, C. J., & Goldberg, A. E. (2016). *Lesbian and gay parents and their children.* National Council on Family Relations Policy Brief. Minneapolis, MN: Author.

Patterson, C. J., & Tornello, S. L. (2011). Gay fathers' pathways to parenthood: International perspectives. *Zeitschrift für Familienforschung (Journal of Family Research), 7*, 103–116.

Perry, J. R. (2017). *Promising practices for serving transgender & non-binary foster & adoptive parents.* Washington, DC: The Human Rights Campaign Foundation.

Pyne, J. (2012). *Transforming family: Trans parents and their struggles, strategies, and strengths.* Toronto,

ON: LGBTQ Parenting Network, Sherbourne Health Clinic. Retrieved from http://lgbtqpn.ca/wp-content/uploads/2014/10/Transforming-Family-Report-Final-Version-updated-Sept-30-2014-reduced.pdf

Raleigh, E. (2012). Are same-sex and single adoptive parents more likely to adopt transracially? A national analysis of race, family structure, and the adoption marketplace. *Sociological Perspectives, 55*, 449–471. https://doi.org/10.1525/sop.2012.55.3.449

Reinoso, M., Juffer, F., & Tieman, W. (2013). Children's and parents' thoughts and feelings about adoption, birth culture identity and discrimination in families with internationally adopted children. *Child and Family Social Work, 18*, 264–274. https://doi.org/10.1111/j.1365-2206.2012.00841.x

Riskind, R. G., & Tornello, S. L. (2017). Sexual orientation and future parenthood in a 2011–2013 nationally representative United States sample. *Journal of Family Psychology, 31*, 792–798. https://doi.org/10.1037/fam0000316

Rosnati, R., Ranieri, S., & Barni, D. (2013). Family and social relationships and psychosocial well-being in Italian families with internationally adopted and non-adopted children. *Adoption Quarterly, 16*, 1–16. https://doi.org/10.1080/10926755.2012.731030

Ross, L. E., Epstein, R., Anderson, S., & Eady, A. (2009). Policy, practice, and personal narratives: Experiences of LGBTQ people with adoption in Ontario, Canada. *Adoption Quarterly, 12*, 272–293. https://doi.org/10.1080/10926750903313302

Rueter, M., Keyes, M., Iacono, W. G., & McGue, M. (2009). Family interactions in adoptive compared to nonadoptive families. *Journal of Family Psychology, 23*, 58–66. https://doi.org/10.1037/a0014091

Rushton, A. (2014). Early years adversity, adoption and adulthood: Conceptualising long-term outcomes. *Adoption and Fostering, 38*, 374–385. https://doi.org/10.1177/0308575914553363

Siegel, D. H., & Smith, S. L. (2012). *Openness in adoption: From secrecy and stigma to knowledge and connections.* New York, NY: Evan B. Donaldson Adoption Institute. Retrieved from https://www.adoptioninstitute.org/wp-content/uploads/2013/12/2012_03_OpennessInAdoption.pdf

Simon, K. A., Tornello, S. L., Farr, R. H., & Bos, H. M. (2018). Envisioning future parenthood among bisexual, lesbian, and heterosexual women. *Psychology of Sexual Orientation and Gender Diversity, 5*, 253–259. https://doi.org/10.1037/sgd0000267

Storsbergen, H. E., Juffer, F., van Son, M. J. M., & Hart, H. (2010). Internationally adopted adults who did not suffer severe early deprivation: The role of appraisal of adoption. *Children and Youth Services Review, 32*, 191–197. https://doi.org/10.1016/j.childyouth.2009.08.015

Stotzer, R. L., Herman, J. L., & Hasenbush, A. (2014). *Transgender parenting: A review of existing literature.* The Williams Institute. Retrieved from https://escholarship.org/uc/item/3rp0v7qv

Sumontha, J., Farr, R. H., & Patterson, C. J. (2016). Social support and coparenting among lesbian, gay, and heterosexual adoptive parents. *Journal of Family Psychology, 30*, 987–996. https://doi.org/10.1037/fam0000253

Sumontha, J., Farr, R. H., & Patterson, C. J. (2017). Children's gender development: Associations with parental sexual orientation, division of labor, and gender ideology. *Psychology of Sexual Orientation and Gender Diversity, 4*, 438–450. https://doi.org/10.1037/sgd0000242

Takács, J., Szalma, I., & Bartus, T. (2016). Social attitudes toward adoption by same-sex couples in Europe. *Archives of Sexual Behavior, 45*, 1787–1798. https://doi.org/10.1007/s10508-016-0691-9

Tan, T. X., & Baggerly, J. (2009). Behavioral adjustment of adopted Chinese girls in single-mother, lesbian-couple, and heterosexual-couple households. *Adoption Quarterly, 12*, 171–186. https://doi.org/10.1080/10926750903313336

Tan, T. X., & Marn, T. (2013). Mental health service utilization in children adopted from U.S. foster care, U.S. private agencies and foreign countries: Data from the 2007 National Survey of Adoption Parents (NSAP). *Children and Youth Services Review, 35*, 1050–1054. https://doi.org/10.1016/j.childyouth.2013.04.020

Tornello, S. L., & Bos, H. (2017). Parenting intentions among transgender individuals. *LGBT Health, 4*, 115–120. https://doi.org/10.1089/lgbt.2016.0153

Tornello, S. L., Farr, R. H., & Patterson, C. J. (2011). Predictors of parenting stress among gay adoptive fathers in the United States. *Journal of Family Psychology, 25*, 591–600. https://doi.org/10.1037/a0024480

U.S. Department of Health & Human Services. (2018). *Trends in foster care and adoption, FY 2008–FY 2017.* Retrieved from https://www.acf.hhs.gov/cb/resource/trends-in-foster-care-and-adoption

U.S. Department of State. (2019). *Resources for LGBTI adoptions.* Retrieved from https://travel.state.gov/content/travel/en/Intercountry-Adoption/Adoption-Process/before-you-adopt/LGBTI-adoption-resources.html

Vandivere, S., & McKlindon, A. (2010). The well-being of U.S. children adopted from foster care, privately from the United States and internationally. *Adoption Quarterly, 13*, 157–184. https://doi.org/10.1080/10926755.2010.524871

van Eeden-Moorefield, B., Few-Demo, A. L., Benson, K., Bible, J., & Lummer, S. (2018). A content analysis of LGBT research in top family journals 2000-2015. *Journal of Family Issues, 39*, 1374–1395. https://doi.org/10.1177/0192513X17710284

Vecho, O., Poteat, V. P., & Schneider, B. (2016). Adolescents' attitudes toward same-sex marriage and adoption in France. *Journal of GLBT Family Studies, 12*, 24–45. https://doi.org/10.1080/1550428X.2015.1040530

Webb, S. N., & Chonody, J. (2014). Heterosexual attitudes toward same-sex marriage: The influence of attitudes toward same-sex parenting. *Journal of GLBT Family Studies, 10*, 404–421. https://doi.org/10.1080/15504 28X.2013.832644

Wells, G. (2011). Making room for daddies: Male couples creating families through adoption. *Journal of GLBT Family Studies, 7*, 155–181. https://doi.org/10.1080/1 550428X.2011.537242

Wyman Battalen, A., Farr, R. H., Brodzinsky, D. M., & McRoy, R. G. (2018). Socializing children about family structure: Perspectives of lesbian and gay adoptive parents. *Journal of GLBT Family Studies, 15*, 235. https://doi.org/10.1080/1550428X.2018.1465875

# What Do We Now Know About Bisexual Parenting? A Continuing Call for Research

Melissa H. Manley and Lori E. Ross

In the context of a now robust body of scholarship examining LGBTQ parenting and families, remarkably little research has focused on the specific experiences of bisexual and other plurisexual [e.g., pansexual, omnisexual, two-spirit; see Galupo, Mitchell, & Davis, 2015] parents. In her landmark book on lesbian and gay (L/G) parenting, Goldberg (2010) noted that bisexual parenting experiences and perspectives had been rarely acknowledged and explored and, further, that in most cases, inclusion of "bisexual" within the acronym "LGBTQ" was misleading, given that most studies simply pooled bisexual and L/G parents, or included only bisexual people with same-sex partners. In the first edition of this chapter, Ross and Dobinson (2013) conducted a systematic review of the research literature and identified only seven academic articles that reported any findings particular to bisexual parents. Now, 5 years later, the revised edition of this book provides the opportunity to revisit the state of the literature, to determine whether in the intervening years, it

has become more appropriate to speak of the field of "LGBTQ parenting."

Bisexuality has been defined and operationalized in research in many ways, including self-identification as bisexual or another plurisexual identity label, attractions to multiple genders, and engaging in sexual or romantic relationships with partners of more than one gender (Flanders, 2017). In addition, the range of plurisexual identity labels in use has been increasingly documented, with many individuals identifying as pansexual, queer, fluid, or a combination of terms (Galupo et al., 2015). Such variation reflects increased awareness of and opportunities to capture nuances of bisexual experience, including parenting experiences. Given these variations in definition, we take care to identify the definitions utilized in each study discussed in this chapter.

The range of bisexual parenting experiences matches this diversity in definitions of bisexuality. That is, bisexual people may be parents through a variety of routes and raise children in any of myriad possible relationship configurations. This chapter includes bisexual parents in monogamous relationships with same-gender partners and different-gender partners, bisexual parents who have separated from their partners or who are raising children as single parents, and bisexual parents in a variety of consensually nonmonogamous relationships. These individuals often become parents through biological

M. H. Manley (✉)
Department of Psychology, Clark University, Worcester, MA, USA
e-mail: memanley@clarku.edu

L. E. Ross
Dalla Lana School of Public Health, University of Toronto, Toronto, ON, Canada
e-mail: l.ross@utoronto.ca

© Springer Nature Switzerland AG 2020
A. E. Goldberg, K. R. Allen (eds.), *LGBTQ-Parent Families*,
https://doi.org/10.1007/978-3-030-35610-1_4

means, yet they may also be nonbiological (social) parents, adoptive parents, stepparents, or foster parents. Additionally, social contexts and partner gender may impact bisexual people's paths to parenthood.

Biphobia (i.e., prejudice or discrimination directed toward bisexual individuals) and bisexual erasure represent considerable challenges for bisexual parents. That is, bisexual individuals encounter stereotypes and stigma such as beliefs that bisexual people are indecisive, promiscuous, or unfaithful, and people's bisexual identities are often erased based on the gender of their partner(s) (Klesse, 2011). Additionally, bisexual parents are typically assumed to be heterosexual (given the heteronormativity of parenthood) unless they have a same-sex partner, in which case they are assumed to be gay or lesbian. This societal context of bisexual negativity and invisibility has relevance for bisexual identity development, disclosure decisions, relationship and parenting experiences, and other social and legal repercussions.

The relative growth in scholarship on bisexual parents reflects an increasing awareness and interest in the unique issues and experiences bisexual parents may navigate. Although the research discussed here is still in its infancy (with many publications derived from the same larger projects), it represents a significant foundation for a more nuanced and comprehensive understanding of the diverse experiences of bisexual parents. This chapter aims to summarize the existing literature to orient readers toward what is most meaningful in examining experiences of bisexuality and parenting.

We begin the chapter with a brief overview of the key themes identified in the early literature reviewed in the first edition of this chapter (Ross & Dobinson, 2013). Then, we outline the methods and findings of our current literature search. Finally, we close with a discussion of the contemporary state of the literature in this field and highlight some important remaining gaps. We hope that this chapter will serve to further encourage meaningful inclusion of bisexual and other plurisexual parents in future research in the field of LGBTQ family science.

## In Search of the "B": Early Bisexual Parenting Research

In this first edition of this chapter, Ross and Dobinson's (2013) systematic search of the peer-reviewed research literature identified only seven articles that reported any findings specific to bisexual parents. These were supplemented with two papers that had been published subsequent to the original literature search and several other (largely non-peer-reviewed) sources identified though expert consultation and a broader Internet search. On the basis of these sources, Ross and Dobinson (2013) summarized six primary themes in the literature available at that time. For the first theme, Ross and Dobinson (2013) highlighted research reporting *statistics regarding the number of bisexual parents*, revealing that at least as many, and perhaps more, bisexual people than L/G people desire to be and are actually parents (Gates, Badgett, Macomber, & Chambers, 2007; Paiva, Filipe, Santos, Lima, & Segurado, 2003). The second theme summarized research addressing *outcomes in children of bisexual parents*, revealing that insufficient research had been conducted treating bisexual parents as an analytic category to draw any conclusions about outcomes specific to bisexual parents, but like the children of L/G parents, there are likely both challenges (e.g., exposure to stigma and discrimination; see Snow, 2004) and advantages (e.g., open-mindedness; see Jones & Jones, 1991) of being parented by bisexual people. Third, Ross and Dobinson (2013) summarized research focusing on *disclosure of sexual identity* as an issue that can often be more challenging for bisexual parents than for L/G parents, given that one's bisexual identity cannot be inferred on the basis of one's primary (and often, parenting) partner. As a result, bisexual parents must consider whether, how, and when to disclose their sexual identity to their partners (McClellan, 2006; Ross, Dobinson, & Eady, 2010) and children (Anders, 2005); however, almost no literature had addressed these experiences among bisexual parents (Ross & Dobinson, 2013). Similarly, for the fourth theme, Ross and Dobinson (2013) reviewed research reporting on the *experiences of bisexual people with systems and supports* and particularly social services. Some writers suggested that bisexual parents fare better in custody decisions than do L/G parents (Lahey, 1999) while others described specific forms of discrimination encountered by bisexual people in custody cases and the process of adoption (Cahill, Mitra, & Tobias, 2003; Eady, Ross, Epstein, & Anderson, 2009). Given that social attitudes toward bisexuality are changing at a much slower rate than those toward L/G identities (Dodge et al., 2016), it will be important to determine the contemporary state of bisexual individuals' experiences interacting with a variety of structures and systems, including the legal system and children's schools. Fifth, with respect to *health and well-being* of bisexual parents, Ross and Dobinson (2013) drew attention to the very limited literature available suggesting that bisexual parents may fare worse than those of other sexual identities on various indicators of mental health (Ross et al., 2010; Ross, Siegel, Dobinson, Epstein, & Steele, 2012) and access to mental health services (Steele, Ross, Epstein, Strike, & Goldfinger, 2008), and these disparities are in turn linked with experiences of invisibility and exclusion (Ross et al., 2012). Finally, Ross and Dobinson (2013) identified limited evidence that parenting and parenting desires shaped *bisexual identity development* among bisexual women. Namely, two papers reported on cisgender bisexual women who reported that parenting desires shifted their attractions more toward men (Ross et al., 2012; Wells, 2011), and a first person narrative from a cisgender bisexual woman described how becoming a parent increased her commitment to political activism (Blanco, 2009). In summary, Ross and Dobinson's (2013) review of this nascent field of scholarship concluded that more research was needed in virtually every domain of study.

## A Review of Contemporary Research on Bisexual Parenting

To determine if the state of the literature had improved in the intervening years, we conducted a systematic search of the peer-reviewed litera-ture published in social, health, and psychological sciences between 2010 and June 2018. We used various combinations of keywords related to bisexuality (e.g., bisexual, plurisexual, "men who have sex with men and women") and parenting (e.g., parent, mother, father—full list of keywords available from the authors upon request) in the databases Medline (OVID—including Epub ahead of print, in process, and other non-indexed citations), PsycINFO (EBSCOhost), and Sociological Abstracts (Proquest). We screened in review papers identified in the search that included bisexual-specific findings that were not captured in the original studies also identified in the review. Excluding duplicates, our search identified 674 citations for screening, of which we determined 582 studies to be irrelevant based on titles and abstracts. Of the 92 full-text studies screened for eligibility, we excluded 66; notably, 58 (88%) of these were excluded either because bisexual people were not disaggregated in the reporting of data (e.g., they were simply lumped in with L/G people) or because bisexual people were not treated as an analytical category in the analysis (that is, no findings particular to bisexual people could be extracted from the article given that the qualitative or quantitative analysis did not explore the possibility that experiences of bisexual parents could differ from those of L/G parents).

In total, the search yielded 26 studies reporting on parenting-related issues among bisexual people; we supplemented these studies with a further 10 studies conducted by our author team that were published or accepted for publication between the end date of our search and the writing of this chapter (September 2018). Thus, our review below is based on a total of 36 peer-reviewed papers published or accepted for publication between January 2010 and September 2018 (Table 1).

In order to compile this narrative review, both authors reviewed the full text of the included papers to identify findings that explicitly linked bisexuality with some aspect of parenting. Then, through a process of consensus, we organized these findings into seven key themes: identity management, paths to parenthood, relationship

**Table 1** Summary of included studies

| Article | Data source and country of study | Areas of focus |
| --- | --- | --- |
| Bartelt et al. (2017) | Qualitative study of 33 adult bisexual parents (USA) | Parenting issues<br>Identity management<br>Intersections |
| Eong (2011) | Qualitative case study of a bisexual mother (Malaysia) | Intersections |
| Bowling et al. (2017) | Qualitative study of 33 adult bisexual parents (USA) | Parenting issues |
| Bowling, Dodge, and Bartelt (2018) | Qualitative study of 33 adult bisexual parents (USA) | Relationship issues |
| Bowling, Dodge, Bartelt, Simmons, and Fortenberry (2019) | Qualitative study of 33 adult bisexual parents (USA) | Paths to parenthood |
| Brewster et al. (2014) | 2002 and 2006–2010 National Survey of family growth (USA) | Paths to parenthood<br>Intersections |
| Budnick (2016) | Qualitative study of 35 women reporting same-sex attraction, sexual behavior, and/or nonheterosexual identity; recruited through their participation in the relationship dynamics and social life study (USA) | Parenting issues<br>Identity management<br>Intersections |
| Calzo et al. (2017) | 2013–2015 National Health Interview Survey (USA) | Health outcomes |
| Costa and Bidell (2017) | Survey of 568 LGB individuals ($n = 89$ bisexual) (Portugal) | Paths to parenthood |
| Delvoye and Tasker (2016) | Qualitative interviews with 8 bisexual mothers (UK) | Identity management |
| DeVault and Miller (2017) | Survey of 515 MTurk workers and 539 students asked to rate vignettes of couples wishing to adopt a child | Social stigma |
| Flanders et al. (2016) | Survey of 107 pregnant women of any sexual orientation, including 5 bisexual-identified (Canada) | Health outcomes |
| Flanders, Legge, Plante, Goldberg, and Ross (2019) | Analysis of qualitative data from 25 nonmonosexual women in different gender partnerships interviewed over the course of 1 year who participated in the postpartum wellbeing study (USA and Canada) | Parenting issues |
| Gibson (2018) | Qualitative study of 15 LGBT parents of children with disabilities ($n = 3$ identified as bisexual or bisexual in combination with another identity) | Social stigma |
| Goldberg, Ross, et al. (2017) | Analysis of qualitative data from 28 male-partnered sexual minority women interviewed in late pregnancy or early postpartum who participated in the postpartum wellbeing study (USA and Canada) | Identity management |
| Goldberg, Allen, et al. (2018) | Analysis of qualitative data from 22 male-partnered bisexual women interviewed during the perinatal period and at 1 year postpartum who participated in the postpartum wellbeing study (USA and Canada) | Identity management |
| Goldberg, Garcia, and Manley (2017) | Survey of same-sex female couples (including 50 nonmonosexual participants) who adopted children 5 years prior (USA) | Relationship issues |
| Goldberg, Manley, et al. (2019) | Analysis of qualitative data from 28 plurisexual, male-partnered women interviewed 4 times during pregnancy and the first postpartum year who participated in the postpartum wellbeing study (USA and Canada) | Parenting issues<br>Identity management |
| Hardesty et al. (2011) | Qualitative study of 24 "lesbian/bisexual" mothers who were in or had left abusive same-sex relationships | Social stigma |
| Hartnett et al. (2017) | 2006–2015 National Survey of family growth (USA) | Health outcomes |
| Hodson et al. (2017) | Systematic review of 30 papers comparing pregnancy rates across sexual orientation groups | Paths to parenthood |

| Source | Description | Themes |
|---|---|---|
| Januwalla, Goldberg, Flanders, Yudin, and Ross (2019) | Analysis of quantitative data from 30 male-partnered sexual minority women and 32 female-partnered sexual minority women who participated in the postpartum wellbeing study (USA and Canada) | Health outcomes |
| Kangasvuo (2011) | Qualitative study of 11 bisexual adults (Finland) | Identity management |
| Mallon (2011) | Commentary on state of the knowledge regarding adoption home study processes for LGBT people | Social stigma |
| Manley, Goldberg, and Ross (2018) | Analysis of qualitative data from 29 plurisexual women with different-gender partners interviewed 4 times during pregnancy and the first postpartum year who participated in the postpartum wellbeing study (USA and Canada) | Parenting issues; Identity management; Social stigma |
| Manley, Legge, et al. (2018) | Analysis of qualitative data from 21 bisexual and plurisexual women interviewed 4 times during pregnancy and the first postpartum year who participated in the postpartum wellbeing study (USA and Canada) | Relationship issues |
| McCabe and Sumerau (2018) | Qualitative study of 20 women in college (n = 5 bisexual) (USA) | Paths to parenthood |
| Power et al. (2012) | Analysis of data from the work, love, play study of 455 LGBT parents (n = 48 bisexual) (Australia and New Zealand) | Paths to parenthood; Relationship issues; Parenting issues |
| Riskind and Tornello (2017) | 2011–2013 National Survey of family growth (USA) | Paths to parenthood |
| Ross et al. (2018) | Analysis of qualitative data from 29 plurisexual women with different-gender partners interviewed during pregnancy who participated in the postpartum wellbeing study (USA and Canada) | Relationship issues |
| Ross, Manley, et al. (2017) | Mixed-methods analysis of data from 39 pregnant nonmonosexual women who participated in the postpartum wellbeing study (USA and Canada) | Health outcomes |
| Ross et al. (2012) | Mixed methods study of 64 sexual minority women (n = 14 bisexual) who were currently pregnant, parenting, or trying to conceive (Canada) | Identity management; Social stigma; Health outcomes |
| Ross, Tarasoff, et al. (2017) | Analysis of qualitative data from 29 plurisexual women with different-gender partners interviewed during pregnancy who participated in the postpartum wellbeing study (USA and Canada) | Relationship issues |
| Simon et al. (2018) | Online survey of 196 bisexual (n = 35), lesbian, and heterosexual women (USA) | Paths to parenthood |
| Tasker and Delvoye (2015) | Qualitative interviews with 7 bisexual mothers (UK) | Relationship issues; Parenting issues; Identity management |
| Tasker and Delvoye (2018) | Qualitative study including interviews and drawing of family maps with 8 cisgender bisexual mothers (UK) | Relationship issues |

factors, social stigma, parenting issues, health outcomes, and intersections between bisexuality and other socially significant identities. Below, we discuss each of the themes in turn, organized by prevalence in the literature reviewed, before discussing directions for future research and clinical practice in the final section.

## What Do We Now Know About Bisexual Parenting?

### Identity Management

Research on trajectories of bisexual and parental identities suggests that the salience of bisexual identity may decline in the context of long-term relationships with a partner of one gender (Budnick, 2016; Goldberg, Manley, Ellawala, & Ross, 2019; Kangasvuo, 2011; Tasker & Delvoye, 2015). This may be related to the invisibility of individuals' bisexual identities in the context of a mixed-gender relationship, or to the increased prioritization of children during the transition to parenthood (Budnick, 2016; Goldberg, Manley, et al., 2019; Kangasvuo, 2011; Tasker & Delvoye, 2015). Eleven qualitative or mixed-methods papers (most of which focused on bisexual mothers partnered with men) discussed identity management, including developing a bisexual identity and making decisions about disclosure.

Goldberg et al. (2019) and Tasker and Delvoye (2015) documented how bisexual women in relationships with men may place their sexuality "on the backburner" after giving birth. Additionally, women—particularly women with less social privilege—may view bisexuality as conflicting with ideas of "good motherhood" and intentionally distance themselves from bisexual identity, attractions, or personal histories (Budnick, 2016; Goldberg, Manley, et al., 2019). Nevertheless, many bisexual parents maintained their sexual identities (Bartelt, Bowling, Dodge, & Bostwick, 2017; Goldberg, Manley, et al., 2019; Tasker & Delvoye, 2015). Bisexual mothers described various ways that they maintained connections with their bisexual identities, including engaging in consensual nonmonogamy such as sexual friend-

ships or threesomes with women, engaging in sexual fantasy, disclosing their sexual identities to others, becoming involved or maintaining involvement in the LGBTQ community, and teaching children that different kinds of gender expression and relationships are valid (Budnick, 2016; Goldberg, Manley, et al., 2019; Manley, Legge, Flanders, Goldberg, & Ross, 2018). Some research even suggests that having children may motivate some bisexual parents to raise their children with LGBTQ role models or bring their children to LGBTQ community events, to foster their children's awareness and acceptance of sexual and gender diversity (Manley, Goldberg, & Ross, 2018). Furthermore, bisexual parents' sexual identities may become more salient again as children grow up and parents have more time to focus on their own identities (Tasker & Delvoye, 2015), or during children's puberty or adolescence (Bartelt et al., 2017). Specifically, in Bartelt et al. (2017), parents discussed bisexuality as an asset in relating to teenage children who were beginning to date, or parents found that their bisexuality became salient when discussing sexuality with their children in the context of sexual education or children's own coming out.

Activism, the LGBTQ community, and community biphobia were regularly invoked as influential to bisexual parents' identity development. Bisexual stereotypes, the absence of bisexual role models, and lack of knowledge about bisexuality can make it more difficult for individuals to identify as bisexual, leading some parents to adopt other identities or question their sexuality (Delvoye & Tasker, 2016). Across studies, bisexual parents described appreciating opportunities to connect with similar others or engage in some forms of community or activism (Bartelt et al., 2017; Manley, Goldberg, & Ross, 2018; Ross et al., 2012; Tasker & Delvoye, 2015). However, invalidating and biphobic reactions from others were common, and bisexual mothers in particular often felt that lesbian communities were exclusive or unwelcoming to them (Bartelt et al., 2017; Kangasvuo, 2011; Manley, Goldberg, & Ross, 2018 ; Ross et al., 2012). Indeed, bisexual parents may desire bi-affirming family-friendly spaces and groups, but feel that they must choose between heteronormative parenting communities and nonparent or bi-exclusive L/G communities (Manley, Goldberg, & Ross, 2018; Ross et al., 2012).

Studies have begun to explore how bisexual parents experience disclosure to family, children, and health care providers. Common themes include bisexuality "not coming up" and invisibility and concerns about negative reactions—particularly how others' negative reactions could impact children. Experiences of biphobia such as others questioning the authenticity of their sexuality or challenging parents' commitments to their partners may discourage bisexual parents from future disclosure, leading some parents to engage in LGBTQ activism or advocacy work without being out (Bartelt et al., 2017; Tasker & Delvoye, 2015). Because others assumed that bisexual parents are heterosexual or L/G based on partner gender (and sometimes gender expression), opportunities to disclose were not readily available (Goldberg, Ross, Manley, & Mohr, 2017; Ross et al., 2012). Bisexual parents in some studies have feared that correcting others' assumptions about their identities would have negative repercussions or upset others (Goldberg, Allen, Ellawala, & Ross, 2018; Goldberg, Ross, et al., 2017; Tasker & Delvoye, 2015). However, allowing others to assume that they are heterosexual or not bisexual can be uncomfortable for many, and bisexual parents have also voiced discomfort or guilt because they are able to pass as heterosexual (Manley, Goldberg, & Ross, 2018; Ross et al., 2012).

Overall, it appears that the salience of one's bisexual identity and sexuality more generally may decrease during the transition to parenthood, although bisexual parents may engage in efforts to maintain connections with or distance oneself from bisexuality depending on their social locations, exposure to bi-negative contexts and ideas, and parenting goals. Bisexuality may also reemerge as a salient identity when discussing dating or sexuality during children's adolescence. Biphobia may influence parents' feelings about their bisexuality and decisions about disclosure, especially given parental concerns that biphobia could negatively impact children. Bisexual par-

ents may draw support from LGBTQ communities or activism, but many communities are not inclusive to bisexual parents. Because bisexuality is such an invisible identity, these parents often must make difficult trade-offs in deciding whether to disclose their identities to others, including children. However, many parents who have disclosed have reported positive experiences. Next, we consider the transition to parenthood for bisexual parents more closely by examining the literature on how bisexual individuals become parents.

## Paths to Parenthood

The second theme addresses bisexual individuals' aspirations for and paths to parenthood. First, we explore nonparents' plans, desires, and perceptions of parenthood, with research suggesting relatively high parenting desire among bisexual individuals (which differed by partner gender). We then discuss the pathways bisexual people take to achieve parenthood.

Riskind and Tornello (2017) examined parenting desires (i.e., wishing to parent) and intentions (i.e., planning to parent or viewing it as feasible) using data from the 2011–2013 National Survey of Family Growth in the USA. They found that the vast majority (75%) of self-identified bisexual men ($n = 48$) reported both desire and intention for parenthood, similar to heterosexual men (85% of $n = 2211$) but not gay men (47% of $n = 89$). Similarly, 69% of self-identified bisexual women ($n = 120$) reported both desire and intention for parenthood, and their parenting desires did not differ from those of heterosexual women ($n = 1434$) but were higher than those of lesbian women ($n = 39$) (Riskind & Tornello, 2017). Notably, partner gender played an important role in predicting parenting desires and intentions. Women whose most recent sexual partner was male were 3.29 times more likely to report parenting desires than those with a same-gender partner, and men with a most recent same-gender partner were also less likely to express parenting desire or the ability to fulfill parenting desires. Thus, bisexual women and men were similar to their heterosexual counterparts in desire to have a child, and desires for children tended to be higher for individuals with a recent different-gender partner. However, a study of Portuguese individuals including bisexual men and women did not find differences in parenting intention by sexual orientation (Costa & Bidell, 2017). Yet it should be noted that this study included only 89 bisexual participants (relative to 479 L/G participants) and thus may have lacked statistical power to detect differences for this group.

Other research on parenting expectations and desires adds to this picture, though all other studies we found on this topic examined predominantly White bisexual women. One study of currently childless, partnered women with intention to become a parent in the future (including 35 bisexual women) found that bisexual women reported lower partner expectations (i.e., anticipated less involvement and support from their partner after becoming parents) compared to heterosexual women, but not compared to lesbian women (Simon, Tornello, Farr, & Bos, 2018). The authors suggest that bisexual women's uniquely invisible status and the pressure to adopt a monosexual identity may in part account for lower partner expectations. Additionally, McCabe and Sumerau (2018) included five middle−/ upper-class bisexual undergraduate women in a qualitative study on reasons to have or not have children and noted that all of the bisexual respondents spoke about desire to have children in terms of a search for fulfilment, rather than to conform to societal expectations or to replicate positive experiences—reasons endorsed by heterosexual participants. These studies begin to suggest that bisexual women may have expectations of parenthood that are distinct from heterosexual and lesbian women's and that they may be likely to view parenthood through a lens of personal fulfilment and lower partner expectations. It is important to note, however, that the papers which have drawn these conclusions are based on small samples of mostly White bisexual women and thus likely miss many bisexual parents' perspectives and experiences.

Turning to how bisexual individuals actually become parents, research suggests that a variety

of family-building strategies may be used, but biological parenthood is most common (Bowling et al., 2019; Brewster, Tillman, & Jokinen-Gordon, 2014; Power et al., 2012). Using nationally representative data from the 2002 and 2006–2010 in the USA, Brewster et al. (2014) compared heterosexual ($n$ = 14,981), bisexual ($n$ = 593), and lesbian women's ($n$ = 210) parenthood. A majority (56%) of self-identified bisexual women aged 20–44 were parents—50.2% of bisexual women had only biological children, 1.1% only adoptive, 1.6% both biological and adoptive, 0.9% social (i.e., no legal ties), and 2.3% combined legal and social parenthood. Additionally, there is some evidence that the high proportion of bisexual women who are biological parents in their adult years may be in part accounted for by higher rates of adolescent pregnancy among these mothers. Specifically, a meta-analysis found that bisexual adolescent girls are more likely than their heterosexual counterparts to become pregnant, whereas bisexual adult women were less likely to be pregnant than heterosexual counterparts (Hodson, Meads, & Bewley, 2017). Additionally, the average age of bisexual mothers in Brewster et al.' (2014) analysis of data from the US National Survey of Family Growth was 30.6, as compared to 34.5 for heterosexual mothers and 36.1 for lesbian mothers, suggesting bisexual women may become parents at an earlier age, or that younger mothers may be more likely than older mothers to identify as bisexual (Brewster et al., 2014). Thus, bisexual women are relatively likely to become parents by giving birth, yet their trajectories to biological parenthood may be shaped by unique social or relational factors at different developmental timepoints. A dearth of research has explored women's experiences of becoming pregnant, such as the context of their relationships with co-parents or intimate partners.

Very limited research has examined paths to parenthood among bisexual men and/or transgender people. However, two qualitative studies documented experiences of bisexual parents of multiple genders. Bowling et al. (2019) interviewed 33 bisexual parents (15 women, 15 men, three genderqueer or nonconforming) in the

USA, and Power et al. (2012) interviewed 48 bisexual parents (42 women, four men, two "other") in Australia and New Zealand. Most of these parents had biological children, though other legal and social parent-child relationships were also represented. While many parents had children in a different-gender partnership (particularly in Bowling et al.'s study), separations and new relationships were not uncommon. Bowling et al. (2019) also found that several participants had children at a young age, and participants did not make a clear or simple delineation between intended and unintended pregnancies. A minority of parents viewed their bisexuality as significant in becoming a parent (Bowling et al., 2019).

## Relationship Histories, Structures, and Dynamics

This theme explores what is known about bisexual parents' relationship histories, relationship configurations including consensual nonmonogamy and co-parenting after separation, and relationship maintenance and quality. The research discussed here illuminates the diverse structures of bisexual parents' relationships and factors that may be important to the relationship health of bisexual parents.

In one sample of 29 pregnant plurisexual women with different-gender partners, the majority had predominantly partnered with men across their lifetimes (Ross, Tarasoff, Goldberg, & Flanders, 2017). For some, this pattern related to heterosexist bias (i.e., experiencing or internalizing pressure to be in relationships with men) and/or limited opportunity to date women, whereas others conceptualized their relationships with women as casual, short term, and/or sexual in nature. A smaller number had partnerships with men and women that were equal in number or significance, and this group of women were likely to state that if their current relationship ended, they would be open to partnering with women in the future. The smallest group consisted of those who had predominantly partnered with women, and they were likely to indicate that

their current relationship was their only significant relationship with a man. For some of these women, being partnered with a man and pregnant led others to assume they were heterosexual, which participants experienced as uncomfortable. Some similar themes were endorsed in a study of 33 bisexual parents, none of whom were in committed relationships with same-gender partners at the time of interviews or at the time that their children were born (Bowling, Dodge, & Bartelt, 2018). In their sample, several fathers expressed short-term or casual interest in men, yet wanting more long-term or committed relationships with women. Additionally, some mothers and nonbinary parents in that study stated that they avoided partnering with men, or at least heterosexual men.

Turning to current partnerships and relationship configurations, studies have documented bisexual parents who are single, dating, in committed relationships with same-gender or different-gender partners, co-parenting with former partners, and/or engaging in consensually nonmonogamous relationships (Bowling, Dodge, & Bartelt, 2018; Power et al., 2012). Despite these varied family forms, a study of eight bisexual mothers found that most participants conceptualized family according to a heteronormative model including themselves, their children, and one partner/co-parent—however, some participants did expand their definitions to include additional partners or chosen family (Tasker & Delvoye, 2018).

One relationship configuration that appeared in several studies was consensual nonmonogamy (CNM). For example, eight of 33 bisexual parents in one sample were currently in consensually nonmonogamous relationships, and 22 had previously engaged in CNM or were currently seeking a nonexclusive relationship (Bowling, Dodge, & Bartelt, 2018). In another study, 21 of 29 plurisexual mothers had considered or engaged in CNM (Manley, Legge, et al., 2018). Finally, three of eight bisexual mothers interviewed by Tasker and Delvoye (2015) were currently engaged in CNM while another three had questioned monogamy. Thus, CNM emerged as a common topic of discussion and as a not uncommon practice across interviews with bisexual and plurisexual parents. Participants who engaged in CNM endorsed a variety of relationship agreements, including polyamory, casually dating other partners, swinging, and threesomes (Bowling, Dodge, & Bartelt, 2018; Manley, Legge, et al., 2018). Yet parents with young children often closed the relationship, at least temporarily, due to limited time and energy and their prioritization of children (Bowling, Dodge, & Bartelt, 2018; Manley, Legge, et al., 2018). Despite its association with some challenges, including stigma, CNM sometimes facilitated intimacy or fostered feelings of support between partners (Ross, Goldberg, Tarasoff, & Guo, 2018).

Relationship dissolution was another relationship experience that some bisexual parents encountered, similar to parents in general. Several studies discussed experiences with separation and divorce, as well as co-parenting with former partners (Bowling, Dodge, & Bartelt, 2018; Power et al., 2012; Tasker & Delvoye, 2018). Among 33 parents in one study, 12 were divorced (Bowling, Dodge, & Bartelt, 2018). These participants reported a mix of positive co-parenting experiences and negative, conflictual situations. Negative experiences sometimes related to biphobia or discrimination from ex-partners, such as the cases of two bisexual fathers whose ex-partners outed them to their families and friends after relationship dissolution. Similarly, 17 of 48 bisexual parents in another study reported they were co-parenting with ex-partners (Power et al., 2012). Again, many parents reported both positive aspects and challenges, only one of which related to biphobia (i.e., an ex-partner disapproved of a new same-sex partner and communicated this disapproval to their children). Overall then, the dynamics of relationship dissolution among bisexual parents were similar in many ways to those of parents in general, except biphobia could be mobilized in conflicts before or after separation.

Finally, several studies discussed relationship maintenance, partner support, and relationship satisfaction (Bowling, Dodge, & Bartelt, 2018; Goldberg, Garcia, & Manley, 2017; Manley,

Legge, et al., 2018; Ross et al., 2018). Research has suggested that parents, particularly women, often prioritize children over their own relationship desires, such as dating relationships or CNM engagement (Bowling, Dodge, & Bartelt, 2018; Manley, Legge, et al., 2018; Tasker & Delvoye, 2015). Given that most time and internal resources are directed to children during their early years, relationship satisfaction is likely to decrease, and relationship maintenance (e.g., talking about or "working on" the relationship) may become more important (Goldberg, Garcia, & Manley, 2017). Some studies have identified maintenance strategies used by bisexual parents; these include open communication, negotiating boundaries, prioritizing physical intimacy between partners, sharing social networks such as LGBTQ communities or activist circles, and utilizing therapy resources (Bowling, Dodge, & Bartelt, 2018; Manley, Legge, et al., 2018; Ross et al., 2018). Less is known about how the relative levels of maintenance or strategies may differ by parents' sexual identity, gender, or partner gender. However, one study including 50 plurisexual adoptive mothers in same-sex relationships found that, regardless of the partner's sexual identity, plurisexual women reported significantly higher levels of relationship maintenance and conflict (Goldberg, Garcia, & Manley, 2017). The authors hypothesized the difference could relate to high levels of openness about needs and desires in the relationship, or due to awareness of stereotypes and partners' potential insecurities— suggesting that the partner's acceptance of bisexuality may be an important variable in relationship satisfaction. Indeed, qualitative studies corroborate the key role of acceptance from partners, suggesting that partner attitudes of ambivalence, insecurity, or disapproval may undermine relationship health (Bowling, Dodge, & Bartelt, 2018; Ross et al., 2018).

In sum, the available literature suggests that the relationship structures of bisexual parents take many forms, with diversity in gender of partners, number of partners, and types of relationships. Existing studies have sampled mostly bisexual parents in different-gender relationships and found a considerable proportion have engaged in or considered CNM. Transition to parenthood and parenting experiences have been associated with relationship challenges (such as deprioritizing sexuality and difficulty finding time for intimacy), and emerging evidence suggests that bisexual parents may engage in more relationship maintenance than monosexual parents.

## Social Stigma

Assumptions that bisexual parents are monosexual can lead to feelings of invisibility and difficulty accessing supportive communities (Manley, Goldberg, & Ross, 2018; Ross et al., 2012). In addition, bisexual parents who are perceived to be heterosexual tend to be highly cognizant of the privilege of not experiencing overt discrimination and having their relationship with a different-gender partner recognized and respected (Gibson, 2018; Manley, Goldberg, & Ross, 2018; Ross et al., 2012), and they also know that if they openly disclose their bisexuality, they will be vulnerable to discrimination (Gibson, 2018). This anticipated stigma and the need to consider the trade-offs of disclosure (e.g., disclosing identity to access LGBTQ community support but contending with negative reactions, versus avoiding overt discrimination but feeling inauthentic or invisible) is experienced as stressful by many bisexual parents (Ross et al., 2012). Further, bisexual parents have reported a range of concerns about disclosing their sexuality (e.g., fearing loss of employment, worry that children will be teased or rejected; Bartelt et al., 2017). They have also documented negative experiences, including: being outed to family by partners or ex-partners, being expected to engage in threesomes or to be incapable of monogamy, being told their identity does not exist, and facing rejection from valued communities or their own families (Bartelt et al., 2017; Bowling, Dodge, Bartelt, Simmons, & Fortenberry, 2019; Goldberg, Allen, et al., 2018; Hardesty, Oswald, Khaw, & Fonseca, 2011; Manley, Goldberg, & Ross, 2018; Manley, Legge, et al., 2018). Indeed, one study of intimate partner violence among same-sex female couples

included a small number of bisexual participants and found that, unlike lesbian participants who were more often willing to seek formal or informal help in leaving violent partnerships, bisexual women in the sample exclusively attempted to solve the situation alone. These women tended to have fewer social supports, feel less protected by legal policies, and fear more negative repercussions such as job loss if their sexual orientation was disclosed, relative to the lesbian-identified participants in the sample (Hardesty et al., 2011).

Despite this evidence of stigma against bisexual parents, one study using an MTurk and college student sample found that participants perceived a same-sex male couple consisting of one bisexual parent as *more* committed potential adoptive parents than a heterosexual or lesbian couple (DeVault & Miller, 2017). The authors suggested that participants may have been overcompensating based on their awareness of anti-bisexual stereotypes. Broadly, institutional discrimination against bisexual people (e.g., in adoption applications, reproductive rights, and child custody) and the effects of that discrimination on bisexual parents have been understudied (Mallon, 2011). However, many of the health disparities seen among bisexual parents (discussed later) are believed to result from minority stress and stigma experienced by bisexual people.

## Parenting Issues

Like parents of other sexual identities, bisexual parents reported issues related to child discipline, negotiating quality time with children and partner(s), financial concerns, and managing co-parenting and custody after separation. Here we explore findings related to parents' attitudes, behaviors, and experiences raising children.

Although most of the parenting issues faced by bisexual people appear to be common among parents of other sexual identities, one parenting issue that appears to be uniquely influenced by bisexual identity is attitudes and decisions related to gender and sexuality. Specifically, recent research suggests that bisexual peoples' parenting strategies may be informed by openness and egalitarian values, knowledge of diverse genders, sexualities, and relationship types, partner gender and life contexts, and experiences of gendered and/or sexual stigma (Bowling, Dodge, & Bartelt, 2017). For example, Flanders and colleagues (2019) examined gender socialization practices among 25 new mothers with bisexual attractions in mixed-gender relationships. They found that these women tended to provide both stereotypically same-gender and cross-gender opportunities for their children, and some explicitly expressed openness to the possibility that their children could identify as trans or nonbinary. Even participants who self-identified as heterosexual (while acknowledging a bisexual relationship history) expressed flexibility in their gender socialization practices, and participants' cisgender male partners were not perceived to encourage gender-normative behaviors (perhaps reflecting women's choice of partners). Still, many of these women felt they could not or should not engage in feminine gender socialization with their sons due to anticipated social stigma for their children.

Similarly, Bowling et al. (2017) studied family sexuality-related communications discussed by 33 bisexual parents and found that parents emphasized talking to their children about sexual and gender diversity, hoping to promote open and accepting attitudes toward others and children's own selves. Other studies have also suggested that bisexual parents may work to create inclusive environments for children through conversations about sexuality or gender, advocacy work, or LGBTQ community involvement (Bartelt et al., 2017; Manley, Goldberg, & Ross, 2018; Tasker & Delvoye, 2015). Thus, the limited research on bisexual parenting suggests that parents effortfully try to practice and pass on knowledge and acceptance of gender and sexual diversity.

With respect to parenting challenges, the research again suggests that these are predominantly not specific to bisexual identity (Power et al., 2012). However, some studies suggest that bisexual parents may worry that their bisexual identity will in some way be challenging for children. They may fear their children will hold neg-

ative ideas about bisexuality and be embarrassed or ashamed of them (Bartelt et al., 2017), that others' biphobia will negatively impact their children's lives (Bartelt et al., 2017), or, particularly for religious parents, that bisexuality or LGBTQ sexualities will conflict with their parenting goals (Budnick, 2016; Goldberg, Manley, et al., 2019). Some parents have reported hesitating to disclose their bisexual attractions or identities to children because they felt their children were too young, or because they worried biphobia would negatively impact their children (Bartelt et al., 2017; Bowling et al., 2017; Tasker & Delvoye, 2015). Those who did disclose to children were often met with positive or supportive reactions (Bowling et al., 2017; Tasker & Delvoye, 2015). Taken together, the available research suggests that bisexuality can be conceptualized both as a potential parenting challenge (e.g., in the form of conflicts with religious or cultural beliefs or via the impact of anti-bisexual stereotypes) and a parenting strength (i.e., in that some parents viewed themselves as more open-minded or better equipped to talk about sexuality with their children).

## Health Outcomes

This theme relates to the limited research on health outcomes and disparities among bisexual parents and their children. Of particular note is an analysis of a nationally representative sample (the US National Health Interview Survey), which found that bisexual parents reported significantly higher levels of psychological distress than did lesbian, gay, or heterosexual parents; more than one in five bisexual parents reported distress levels indicative of a probable psychological disorder (Calzo et al., 2017). Further, unlike the children of L/G parents, children of bisexual parents had higher levels of emotional and mental health difficulties compared to children of heterosexual parents (as rated by a parent or other family member). This difference was no longer statistically significant after controlling for the higher levels of distress among bisexual parents. Significantly, 61% of bisexual parents were the single parent in the household, 36% were in different-gender parent households, and only 3% were in same-gender parent households.

Smaller samples of sexual minority women have found similar patterns. For example, studies have suggested that bisexual-identified women, sexual minority women who reported sex with men during the past 5 years, and sexual minority men with a current male partner may have higher levels of anxiety and depression compared to lesbian women during the perinatal period (Flanders, Gibson, Goldberg, & Ross, 2016; Ross et al., 2012). Among bisexual mothers, those who are currently partnered with men or who have been partnered with men during the past 5 years reported higher rates of perinatal anxiety in one study (Ross et al., 2017). Additionally, one study found that sexual minority women (including bisexual, lesbian, and same-sex-attracted heterosexual-identified women) generally reported less happiness about being pregnant than did heterosexual women with no same-sex attractions. This was accounted for by whether the pregnancy was intended or desired at that time for the lesbian and bisexual-identified women in the sample (Hartnett, Lindley, Walsemann, & Negraia, 2017). However, pregnancy intention only partially accounted for the lower happiness reported by same-sex-attracted women who identified as heterosexual. The authors suggest several possible explanations for this finding, including the possibility of feeling "stuck" with a male partner when women may feel ambivalent or conflicted about their heterosexuality. Additionally, heterosexual-identified women with same-sex attractions may feel more beholden to expectations that they "should" feel happy.

We only identified one paper that explored bisexual parents' physical or reproductive health. This analysis compared reproductive history and pregnancy information among pregnant heterosexual women, female-partnered sexual minority (e.g., lesbian and bisexual) women, and male-partnered sexual minority women (Januwalla et al., 2019). The three groups did not differ significantly in their reports of reproductive history

variables, but trends were identified wherein a higher proportion of male-partnered sexual minority women indicated experiences of miscarriage, terminated pregnancies, and fertility problems compared to female-partnered women. Given the small sample size for these comparisons, these trends require further investigation in a larger study of male- and female-partnered sexual minority women.

Studies have begun to explore the mental health outcomes of bisexual parents and their children. This work suggests that bisexual mothers, particularly single parents and those partnered with men, may be at higher risk for poor mental health outcomes. More research is needed with bisexual fathers and transgender parents, as well as research examining physical health outcomes for bisexual parents and their children.

## Intersecting Identities

Recognition of the need for awareness of how individuals' multiple intersecting identities shape experiences and outcomes has been growing, yet much of the research on bisexual parents has focused on White women in Western countries. To address this gap, we attended to studies that reported on more diverse samples of bisexual people, in order to characterize the state of existing knowledge on important intersections of bisexuality with other identities and experiences. Given the prominence of experiences of discrimination in the previous themes reviewed in this chapter, intersectionality is a helpful framework through which to interpret our findings. The term intersectionality was first coined by legal scholar Kimberlé Crenshaw (1989), building on the ideas of Black and Indigenous scholars and activists (Clark, 2016; Davis, 1981). Intersectionality attends to the unique experiences that are produced at the intersection of socially significant identities, experiences that must be understood as more than simply the sum of experiences associated with each identity alone (Crenshaw, 1991). Patricia Hill Collins (2000) has highlighted the ways in which identities associated with privilege or marginalization together produce a mutually reinforcing matrix of domination, which profoundly determines the everyday experiences of the individuals who embody these intersecting identities. Intersectionality has been useful in understanding the experiences of bisexual people, including bisexual people of color (Ghabrial & Ross, 2018) and bisexual people living in poverty (Ross et al., 2016). Thus, in this section, we draw upon an intersectional lens to first highlight the demographic features of bisexual mothers (as demographics of other bisexual parents were not available) in a representative sample of the USA in order to examine which important intersections may be understudied in the existing literature. We then review research identified that has included more intersectional perspectives.

Using nationally representative data from 2002 and 2006–2010 in the USA, Brewster et al. (2014) found that bisexual-identified mothers ($n = 593$) appeared to be younger than heterosexual- ($n = 14,981$) or lesbian-identified mothers ($n = 210$) with an average age of 30.6 years. These mothers tended to have lower levels of educational attainment than mothers of other sexual identities, as more than one-quarter did not complete high school and less than 8% attained a college degree. Bisexual mothers appeared to live in metropolitan areas at a similar distribution as heterosexual mothers, and they were less likely to live in central cities and more likely to live in nonmetropolitan areas than lesbian mothers. Bisexual mothers in this sample appeared less likely than heterosexual mothers to be currently married and more likely to be separated or never married. Finally, 73% of bisexual mothers were White non-Hispanic, as compared to 36% of lesbian mothers and 62% of heterosexual mothers.

A possible explanation for the overrepresentation of White women in the Brewster et al. (2014) national sample of bisexual-identified mothers may be related to how women in different social locations identify their sexuality. When studying racially and socioeconomically diverse women, Budnick (2016) found that many young mothers did not perceive bisexual identity as a viable option and instead referred to themselves as heterosexual. These data suggest bisexuality is more accessible to some parents than others. Thus,

recruitment based on self-identification only may exclude individuals with bisexual patterns of attractions or behavior who do not identify as sexual minorities—individuals who may be systematically underrepresented in existing research.

Little research discusses the specific intersection of being a bisexual parent of color in a US or Western context. Some research has described specific themes brought up by bisexual parents of color. For example, some of the eight parents of color interviewed by Bartelt et al. (2017) mentioned their children's understanding of their multiple identities and the multiple types of stigma children may encounter. Even less published research explores experiences of parents outside of Western contexts. Indeed, only one article, a case study of a Malaysian bisexual mother (Bong, 2011), sampled from outside of the USA, Canada, Western Europe, Australia, or New Zealand. Among other topics, Bong (2011) discussed how the participant's Tibetan faith allowed more flexibility and openness than the Christianity and Islam practiced in Malaysia, which largely condemned same-sex sexuality. Much of the participant's story addressed different ways of managing disclosure and concealment, which was situated in the national context (e.g., institutional and legal discrimination against sexual and gender minorities). Clearly, much remains to be learned about the experiences of bisexual parents with different matrices of identities.

In addition to being limited in terms of racial representation, the research on bisexual parents has also tended to be limited in terms of gender representation. Much of the published research on bisexual parents focuses on mothers. In the current literature, there is a paucity of knowledge about bisexual fathers and transgender and nonbinary parents. Inclusion of these parents is important, as one would anticipate that gendered norms associated with parenting would intersect with bisexual identity to produce unique experiences and concerns. For example, Bartelt et al. (2017) included three parents with nonbinary gender identities and noted that all three mentioned the importance of activism or being out when discussing their parenting experiences (whereas these findings were relatively less common among cisgender parents in the sample). More research is thus needed to further understand intersections between gender and bisexuality as they pertain to parenting experiences.

## Where Do We Go from Here? Future Research Directions

The recent research reviewed here on bisexual parenting include both extensions of earlier research and new directions. For example, the first theme of identity management builds upon earlier work on identity disclosure, and the theme of health outcomes extends prior work related to health and well-being. In other areas, recent research appears to have narrowed the focus of broader themes identified earlier, such that experiences with systems and supports are now summarized within the theme of social stigma. Still other themes represent new directions in the field, such as the emerging focus on bisexual parents' paths to parenthood. In this section, we review the implications of this proliferation of studies on bisexual parenting and the possibilities for future work.

This review documents significant growth in the research literature on bisexual parents that has helped to identify several key areas of interest and concern. We have included 36 articles published in the last 6 years with relevance for bisexual parents. However, 10 of these papers derived from one longitudinal data set sampling just under 100 women in the perinatal period (Goldberg, Ross, et al., 2017; Ross, Manley, et al., 2017), four from another sample of 33 bisexual parents (Bowling et al., 2017), and three from a smaller sample of bisexual mothers (Tasker & Delvoye, 2015); thus the existing scholarship remains limited and somewhat homogenous in the perspectives it represents. Considering the number of articles excluded because authors did not report analyses specific to bisexual orientation, we encourage researchers to include sufficient numbers of bisexual parents in their studies to permit for stratified analyses, in order to identify both issues that are unique to

bisexual parents, as well as potentially interesting and important differences between bisexual parents and other sexual minority parents. The articles utilizing nationally representative data sets by Brewster et al. (2014) and Calzo et al. (2017) also highlight the potential for secondary data analysis to reveal novel and important findings specific to bisexual parents. These variable sampling strategies (i.e., bisexual-specific samples, broader LGBTQ samples with stratified analyses, and secondary analysis of larger data sets) each offer important contributions to understanding the unique concerns and experiences of bisexual parents. In addition, the variety of methodological approaches included in the existing body of research constitute a significant strength in building our knowledge of bisexual parents, and we encourage researchers to continue utilizing qualitative, quantitative, and meta-analytic strategies, among other approaches.

We have identified several promising areas for future research on bisexual parenting and family issues, including mental health disparities, experiences of stigma, identity development and disclosure, and parenting decisions and communications related to sexuality and gender socialization. However, the existing literature has focused very predominantly on White cisgender bisexual women, most of whom gave birth to children with male partners, located in the USA, Canada, Western Europe, and Australia. Moving forward, it will be necessary to carefully consider the diversity of experiences encapsulated within the umbrella of bisexual identity or experience. For example, some bisexual people—like some heterosexual, lesbian, and gay people—may conceptualize family in ways that run counter to the socially constructed nuclear family model. In other words, some bisexual people may choose not to marry or have children, may raise children to whom they are not biologically related, or may raise children in the context of alternative family forms, such as polyamorous families (see chapter "Polyamorous Parenting in Contemporary Research: Developments and Future Directions"). The extent to which choices in this regard are related to personal constructions of bisexual identity is worthy of study. This means that examination of the ways in which bisexual identity informs beliefs and decisions about family and parenting is an important area of study, including among those bisexual people who are not parenting, or not parenting in the traditional contexts typically captured in parenting and family studies research.

Also critical in future research will be consideration of the diversity within the broad category of bisexual parents and careful definition/description of who is included within the category of bisexual. For example, we have defined bisexuality very broadly to include those who self-identify as bisexual, as well as those who report attraction to and/or sexual activity with both men and women (sometimes in addition to people of other genders); the experiences of individuals who do endorse a bisexual identity vs. those who do not may differ. Experiences of male, female, transgender, and nonbinary bisexual people are similarly likely to differ significantly based on socially constructed ideas about gender and parenting, as well as gendered notions of sexuality. As evidenced in the literature, partner status of bisexual parents may also determine their experiences in important ways. That is, partner status (single vs. partnered), gender of partner(s), and number of partners are important factors in shaping bisexual parents' visibility, self-definition, and parenting experience, and in contrast to the traditional notion of nuclear family, a significant proportion of bisexual parents may be single and/ or consensually nonmonogamous. Furthermore, intersections with other important identities, including race, class and ability, among others, will shape the ways in which bisexuality affects parenting and family experiences; despite its strengths, the existing body of literature is currently very limited in its capacity to take up these intersections.

## Implications for Practice

The findings of this review suggest several practice implications for providers who deliver services to bisexual parents and their families. Perhaps most critical, the broad array of unique issues and outcomes for bisexual parents identi-

fied in this review clearly indicate the importance for providers of asking their clients about sexual identity and sexual history. Given that those bisexual parents who are in different gender partnerships may have particularly unique parenting-related needs associated with their experiences of invisibility, it is especially important that these questions be asked of clients who present in different-gender partnerships. Resources such as the Asking the Right Questions 2 (ARQ2) assessment tool are available to assist providers in asking questions about sexual identity, sexual behavior, and sexual history in sensitive and appropriate ways (Barbara, Chaim, & Doctor, 2007). Our review suggests that bisexual identity may increase in salience during key periods, including the transition to parenthood, children's adolescence, and relationship transitions, including dissolution; thus, these may be particularly important opportunities to inquire about sexual identity and history.

Given that relationship dynamics were an important theme in this review, our findings suggest particular implications for sexual and relationship therapists. These providers may invite couples to talk about their sexual identities, including individual's perceptions of their partner's identities. In this way, sexual and relationship therapists can encourage support and acceptance of individuals' bisexual identities, counter negative stereotypes or stigmas about bisexuality, open up conversations about monogamy and nonmonogamy, and highlight the potential importance of accepting social networks such as LGBTQ communities.

Many providers will find that they lack knowledge about bisexuality and related issues (such as consensual nonmonogamy), given the invisibility of bisexuality and lack of related content in most training curricula. Thus, we invite providers to make efforts to educate themselves on these topics.

Experiences with anticipated and enacted stigma associated with bisexuality were prominent in our review; as such, providers should be prepared to work with bisexual parents and their children around these issues. In parallel, providers can help families find or create bisexual-friendly and affirming parenting or family spaces, whether they be formal (e.g., through LGBTQ2 parenting organizations) or informal (e.g., through connecting with other bisexual families in their community). Such spaces may serve to reduce bisexual parents' experiences of invisibility and isolation and buffer potential experiences of discrimination through community support.

Finally, providers can help bisexual parents to recognize the strengths or benefits that bisexuality may bring to their parenting. As noted in this review, these may include open-mindedness and comfort with sexuality-related issues and communication, which could support their children's healthy sexual and relational development. Bisexual parents can be encouraged to reenvision their identities through a strength-based model and to celebrate the positive impacts on their parenting experiences.

In conclusion, this review illuminates both the important issues for bisexual parents that are beginning to receive scholarly attention and important questions that remain, such as bisexual parents' physical health outcomes and experiences with institutional stigma. Consideration of these complex and rich intersections and persisting questions will help to illuminate the breadth of parenting and family experiences within the bisexual community.

**Acknowledgments** The authors wish to acknowledge the contributions of Cheryl Dobinson to the earlier edition of this chapter.

# References

Anders, M. (2005). Miniature golf. *Journal of Bisexuality, 5*, 111–117. https://doi.org/10.1300/J159v05n02_13

Barbara, A. M., Chaim, G., & Doctor, F. (2007). *Asking the right questions 2: Talking with clients about sexual orientation and gender identity in mental health, counselling, and addiction settings*. Toronto, CA: Centre for Addiction and Mental Health.

Bartelt, E., Bowling, J., Dodge, B., & Bostwick, W. (2017). Bisexual identity in the context of parenthood: An exploratory qualitative study of self-identified bisexual parents in the United States. *Journal of Bisexuality, 17*, 378–399. https://doi.org/10.1080/15299716.2017.1384947

Blanco, M. C. (2009). What I did on my ten-year vacation. *Bi Women, 27*(1), 1–6. Retrieved from http://www.robynochs.com/Bi_Women/Bi_Women_V27-1_DJF_09_web.pdf

Bong, S. A. (2011). Beyond queer: An epistemology of bi choice. *Journal of Bisexuality, 11*, 39–63. https://doi.org/10.1080/15299716.2011.545304

Bowling, J., Dodge, B., & Bartelt, E. (2017). Sexuality-related communication within the family context: Experiences of bisexual parents with their children in the United States of America. *Sex Education, 17*, 86–102. https://doi.org/10.1080/14681811.2016.1238821

Bowling, J., Dodge, B., & Bartelt, E. (2018). Diversity and commonalities in relationship experiences among self-identified bisexual parents in the United States. *Sexual and Relationship Therapy, 33*, 169–189. https://doi.org/10.1080/14681994.2017.1419565

Bowling, J., Dodge, B., Bartelt, E., Simmons, M., & Fortenberry, J. D. (2019). Paths to parenthood among self-identified bisexual individuals in the United States. *Archives of Sexual Behavior, 48*, 277–289. https://doi.org/10.1007/s10508-017-1090-6

Brewster, K. L., Tillman, K. H., & Jokinen-Gordon, H. (2014). Demographic characteristics of lesbian parents in the United States. *Population Research and Policy Review, 33*, 503–526. https://doi.org/10.1007/s11113-013-9296-3

Budnick, J. (2016). "Straight girls kissing"? Understanding same-gender sexuality beyond the elite college campus. *Gender & Society, 30*, 745–768. https://doi.org/10.1177/0891243216657511

Cahill, S., Mitra, E., & Tobias, S. (2003). *Family policy: Issues affecting gay, lesbian, bisexual, and transgender families*. New York, NY: National Gay and Lesbian Task Force Policy Institute.

Calzo, J. P., Mays, V. M., Bjorkenstam, C., Bjorkenstam, E., Kosidou, K., & Cochran, S. D. (2017). Parental sexual orientation and children's psychological well-being: 2013–2015 National Health Interview Survey. *Child Development*. Advance online publication, *90*, 1097. https://doi.org/10.1111/cdev.12989

Clark, N. (2016). Red intersectionality and violence-informed witnessing praxis with indigenous girls. *Girlhood Studies, 9*, 46–64. https://doi.org/10.3167/ghs.2016.090205

Collins, P. H. (2000). *Black feminist thought: Knowledge, consciousness, and the politics of empowerment*. New York, NY: Routledge.

Costa, P. A., & Bidell, M. (2017). Modern families: Parenting desire, intention, and experience among Portuguese lesbian, gay, and bisexual individuals. *Journal of Family Issues, 38*, 500–521. https://doi.org/10.1177/0192513X16683985

Crenshaw, K. (1989). Demarginalizing the intersection of race and sex: A black feminist critique of antidiscrimination doctrine, feminist theory and antiracist politics. *The University of Chicago Legal Forum, 140*, 139–167.

Crenshaw, K. (1991). Mapping the margins: Intersectionality, identity politics, and violence against women of color. *Stanford Law Review, 43*, 1241–1299.

Davis, A. Y. (1981). *Women, race, and class*. New York, NY: Random House.

Delvoye, M., & Tasker, F. (2016). Narrating self-identity in bisexual motherhood. *Journal of GLBT Family Studies, 12*, 5–23. https://doi.org/10.1080/15504 28X.2015.1038675

DeVault, A., & Miller, M. K. (2017). Justification-suppression and normative window of prejudice as determinants of bias toward lesbians, gays, and bisexual adoption applicants. *Journal of Homosexuality, 66*, 465–486. https://doi.org/10.1080/00918369.2017.14 14497

Dodge, B., Herbenick, D., Friedman, M. R., Schick, V., Fu, T. C. J., Bostwick, W., ... Sandfort, T. G. (2016). Attitudes toward bisexual men and women among a nationally representative probability sample of adults in the United States. *PLoS One, 11*(10), e0164430. https://doi.org/10.1371/journal.pone.0164430

Eady, A., Ross, L. E., Epstein, R., & Anderson, S. (2009). To bi or not to bi: Bisexuality and disclosure in the adoption system. In R. Epstein (Ed.), *Who's your daddy? And other writings on queer parenting* (pp. 124–132). Toronto, ON: Sumach Press.

Flanders, C. E. (2017). Under the bisexual umbrella: Diversity of identity and experience. *Journal of Bisexuality, 17*, 1–6. https://doi.org/10.1080/1529971 6.2017.1297145

Flanders, C. E., Gibson, M. F., Goldberg, A. E., & Ross, L. E. (2016). Postpartum depression among visible and invisible sexual minority women: A pilot study. *Archives of Women's Mental Health, 19*, 299–305. https://doi.org/10.1007/s00737-015-0566-4

Flanders, C. E., Legge, M. M., Plante, I., Goldberg, A. E., & Ross, L. E. (2019). Gender socialization practices among bisexual and other nonmonosexual mothers: A longitudinal qualitative examination. *Journal of GLBT Family Studies, 15*, 105–126. https://doi.org/10.1080/ 1550428X.2018.1461583

Galupo, M. P., Mitchell, R. C., & Davis, K. S. (2015). Sexual minority self-identification: Multiple identities and complexity. *Psychology of Sexual Orientation and Gender Diversity, 2*, 355–364. https://doi.org/10.1037/ sgd0000131

Gates, G. J., Badgett, M. V. L., Macomber, J. E., & Chambers, K. (2007). *Adoption and foster care by gay and lesbian parents in the United States*. Los Angeles, CA: The Williams Institute.

Ghabrial, M., & Ross, L. E. (2018). Representation and erasure of bisexual people of color in mental health research. *Psychology of Sexual Orientation and Gender Diversity, 5*, 132–142. https://doi.org/10.1037/ sgd0000286

Gibson, M. F. (2018). Predator, pet lesbian, or just the nanny? LGBTQ parents of children with disabilities describe categorization. *Journal of Homosexuality, 65*, 860–883. https://doi.org/10.1080/00918369.2017.13 64565

Goldberg, A. E. (2010). *Lesbian and gay parents and their children: Research on the family life cycle*. Washington, DC: American Psychological Association.

Goldberg, A. E., Allen, K. R., Ellawala, T., & Ross, L. E. (2018). Male-partnered bisexual women's perceptions of disclosing sexual orientation to family across the transition to parenthood: Intensifying heteronormativity or queering family? *Journal of Marital and Family Therapy, 44*, 150–164. https://doi.org/10.1111/ jmft.12242

Goldberg, A. E., Garcia, R., & Manley, M. H. (2017). Monosexual and nonmonosexual women in same-sex couples' relationship quality during the first five years of parenthood. *Sexual and Relationship Therapy, 33*, 190–212. https://doi.org/10.1080/14681994.2017.14 19561

Goldberg, A. E., Manley, M. H., Ellawala, T., & Ross, L. E. (2019). Sexuality and sexual identity across the first year of parenthood among male-partnered plurisexual women. *Psychology of Sexual Orientation and Gender Diversity, 6*, 75–87. https://doi.org/10.1037/ sgd0000307

Goldberg, A. E., Ross, L. E., Manley, M. H., & Mohr, J. J. (2017). Male-partnered sexual minority women: Sexual identity disclosure to health care providers during the perinatal period. *Psychology of Sexual Orientation and Gender Diversity, 4*, 105–114. https:// doi.org/10.1037/sgd0000215

Hardesty, J. L., Oswald, R. F., Khaw, L., & Fonseca, C. (2011). Lesbian/bisexual mothers and intimate partner violence: Help seeking in the context of social and legal vulnerability. *Violence Against Women, 17*, 28–46. https://doi.org/10.1177/1077801209347636

Hartnett, C. S., Lindley, L., Walsemann, K. M., & Negraia, D. V. (2017). Sexual orientation concordance and (un)happiness about births. *Perspectives on Sexual and Reproductive Health, 49*, 213–221. https://doi. org/10.1363/psrh.12043

Hodson, K., Meads, C., & Bewley, S. (2017). Lesbian and bisexual women's likelihood of becoming pregnant: A systematic review and meta-analysis. *BJOG: An International Journal of Obstetrics and Gynaecology, 124*, 393–402. https://doi. org/10.1111/1471-0528.14449

Januwalla, A., Goldberg, A. E., Flanders, C. E., Yudin, M. H., & Ross, L. E. (2019). Reproductive and pregnancy experiences of diverse sexual minority women: A descriptive exploratory study. *Maternal and Child Health Journal*. Advance online publication, *23*, 1071. https://doi.org/10.1007/ s10995-019-02741-4

Jones, B., & Jones, P. (1991). Growing up with a bisexual dad. In L. Hutchins & L. Kaahumanu (Eds.), *Bi any other name: Bisexual people speak out* (pp. 159–166). Boston, MA: Alyson.

Kangasvuo, J. (2011). "There has been no phase in my life when I wasn't somehow bisexual": Comparing the experiences of Finnish bisexuals in 1999 and 2010. *Journal of Bisexuality, 11*, 271–289. https://doi.org/1 0.1080/15299716.2011.571989

Klesse, C. (2011). Shady characters, untrustworthy partners, and promiscuous sluts: Creating bisexual intimacies in the face of heteronormativity and biphobia. *Journal of Bisexuality, 11*, 227–244. https://doi.org/10.1080/15299716.2011.571987

Lahey, K. A. (1999). *Are we 'persons' yet?: Law and sexuality in Canada*. Toronto, ON: University of Toronto Press.

Mallon, G. P. (2011). The home study assessment process for gay, lesbian, bisexual, and transgender prospective foster and adoptive families. *Journal of GLBT Family Studies, 7*, 9–21. https://doi.org/10.1080/1550428X.2011.537229

Manley, M. H., Goldberg, A. E., & Ross, L. E. (2018). Invisibility and involvement: LGBTQ community connections among plurisexual women during pregnancy and postpartum. *Psychology of Sexual Orientation and Gender Diversity, 5*, 169–181. https://doi.org/10.1037/sgd0000285

Manley, M. H., Legge, M. M., Flanders, C. E., Goldberg, A. E., & Ross, L. E. (2018). Consensual nonmonogamy in pregnancy and parenthood: Experiences of bisexual and plurisexual women with different-gender partners. *Journal of Sex & Marital Therapy, 44*, 721–736. https://doi.org/10.1080/0092623X.2018.1462277

McCabe, K., & Sumerau, J. E. (2018). Reproductive vocabularies: Interrogating intersections of reproduction, sexualities, and religion among U.S. cisgender college women. *Sex Roles, 78*, 352–366. https://doi.org/10.1007/s11199-017-0795-2

McClellan, D. L. (2006). Bisexual relationships and families. In D. F. Morrow & L. Messinger (Eds.), *Sexual orientation & gender expression in social work practice: Working with gay, lesbian, bisexual, & transgender people* (pp. 243–262). New York, NY: Columbia University Press.

Paiva, V., Filipe, E. V., Santos, N., Lima, T. N., & Segurado, A. (2003). The right to love: The desire for parenthood among men living with HIV. *Reproductive Health Matters, 11*, 91–100. https://doi.org/10.1016/S0968-8080(03)02293-6

Power, J. J., Perlesz, A., Brown, R., Schofield, M. J., Pitts, M. K., McNair, R., & Bickerdike, A. (2012). Bisexual parents and family diversity: Findings from the Work, Love, Play study. *Journal of Bisexuality, 12*, 519–538. https://doi.org/10.1080/15299716.2012.729432

Riskind, R. G., & Tornello, S. L. (2017). Sexual orientation and future parenthood in a 2011–2013 nationally representative United States sample. *Journal of Family Psychology, 31*, 792–798. https://doi.org/10.1037/fam0000316

Ross, L. E., & Dobinson, C. (2013). Where is the "B" in LGBT parenting? A call for research on bisexual parenting. In A. E. Goldberg & K. R. Allen (Eds.), *LGBT-parent families: Innovations in research and implications for practice* (pp. 87–103). New York, NY: Springer.

Ross, L. E., Dobinson, C., & Eady, A. (2010). Perceived determinants of mental health for bisexual people: A qualitative examination. *American Journal of Public Health, 100*, 496–502. https://doi.org/10.2105/AJPH.2008.156307

Ross, L. E., Goldberg, A. E., Tarasoff, L. A., & Guo, C. (2018). Perceptions of partner support among plurisexual women: A qualitative study. *Sexual and Relationship Therapy, 33*, 59–78. https://doi.org/10.1080/14681994.2017.1419562

Ross, L. E., Manley, M. H., Goldberg, A. E., Januwalla, A., Williams, K., & Flanders, C. E. (2017). Characterizing non-monosexual women at risk for poor mental health outcomes: A mixed methods study. *Canadian Journal of Public Health, 108*, e296–e305. https://doi.org/10.17269/CJPH.108.5884

Ross, L. E., O'Gorman, L., MacLeod, M. A., Bauer, G. R., MacKay, J., & Robinson, M. (2016). Bisexuality, poverty and mental health: A mixed methods analysis. *Social Science & Medicine, 156*, 64–72. https://doi.org/10.1016/j.socscimed.2016.03.009

Ross, L. E., Siegel, A., Dobinson, C., Epstein, R., & Steele, L. S. (2012). "I don't want to turn totally invisible": Mental health, stressors, and supports among bisexual women during the perinatal period. *Journal of GLBT Family Studies, 8*, 137–154. https://doi.org/10.1080/1550428X.2012.660791

Ross, L. E., Tarasoff, L. A., Goldberg, A. E., & Flanders, C. E. (2017). Pregnant plurisexual women's sexual and relationship histories across the life span: A qualitative study. *Journal of Bisexuality, 17*, 257–276. https://doi.org/10.1080/15299716.2017.1311177

Simon, K. A., Tornello, S. L., Farr, R. H., & Bos, H. M. W. (2018). Envisioning future parenthood among bisexual, lesbian, and heterosexual women. *Psychology of Sexual Orientation and Gender Diversity, 5*, 253–259. https://doi.org/10.1037/sgd0000267

Snow, J. (2004). *How it feels to have a gay or lesbian parent: A book by kids for kids of all ages*. New York, NY: Harrington Park Press.

Steele, L. S., Ross, L. E., Epstein, R., Strike, C., & Goldfinger, C. (2008). Correlates of mental health service use among lesbian, gay, and bisexual mothers and prospective mothers. *Women & Health, 47*(3), 95–112. https://doi.org/10.1080/03630240802134225

Tasker, F., & Delvoye, M. (2015). Moving out of the shadows: Accomplishing bisexual motherhood. *Sex Roles, 73*, 125–140. https://doi.org/10.1007/s11199-015-0503-z

Tasker, F., & Delvoye, M. (2018). Maps of family relationships drawn by women engaged in bisexual motherhood: Defining family membership. *Journal of Family Issues, 39*, 4248–4274. https://doi.org/10.1177/0192513X18810958

Wells, J. (2011). Tuxedo shirts. *Bi Women, 29*, 8. Retrieved from http://biwomenboston.org/2010/12/01/tuxedo-shirts/

# Race and Ethnicity in the Lives of LGBTQ Parents and Their Children: Perspectives from and Beyond North America

Amy Brainer, Mignon R. Moore,
and Pallavi Banerjee

In 2016, Black Lives Matter Toronto (BLM-TO) immobilized the Toronto Pride Parade to protest anti-Black racism in pride organizing and other LGBTQ spaces. Protestors presented pride organizers with a list of demands that centered queer and trans communities of color, including specific needs of Black, indigenous, and South Asian queer groups.[1] The BLM-TO action and similar actions at pride parades in other Canadian and US cities are part of a legacy of protest and dialogue around issues of racial exclusion within LGBTQ communities. From the inception of LGBTQ movements in North America as well as in many European nations, activists of color have critiqued, disrupted, and at times successfully dismantled unjust structures and practices in society and within the movements themselves (see, for example, Alimahomed, 2010; Boston & Duyvendak, 2015; Chambers-Letson, 2018; Stormhøj, 2018). The BLM-TO protest was responsive as well to a contemporary climate in which White supremacy, nationalism, homonationalism, and a variety of anti-Black and anti-immigrant measures structure people's daily lives. It is in this climate that queer and trans people form and sustain their families. Thus, as the BLM-TO protestors stressed, in order to adequately understand, represent, and support LGBTQ communities, it is necessary to see race and address racial oppression.

In the USA today, Black, indigenous, and Latinx[2] LGBTQ people are the most likely among all LGBTQ people to be raising children (Kastanis & Wilson, 2014). Johnson (2018) writes that when he began conducting interviews with Black queer southern women, he had no idea how powerful a role motherhood would play in their lives or how deeply the desire to have children would run for many of his interviewees. A growing number of scholars focus on LGBTQ parents of color and push queer theories and methodologies to be more responsive to issues of race, class, citizenship, and colonialism (e.g., Acosta, 2013, 2018; Battle, Pastrana, &

---

[1] For a complete list of demands and record of achievements, see: https://blacklivesmatter.ca/demands/ (retrieved September 5, 2018).

A. Brainer (✉)
Womens and Gender Studies and Sociology, University of Michigan Dearborn, Dearborn, MI, USA
e-mail: brainer@umich.edu

M. R. Moore
Sociology, Barnard College, Columbia University, New York, NY, USA
e-mail: mmoore@barnard.edu

P. Banerjee
Sociology, University of Calgary, Calgary, AB, Canada
e-mail: pallavi.banerjee@ucalgary.ca

[2] See Salvador Vidal Ortiz and Juliana Martínez, "Latinx Thoughts: Latinidad with an X" (2018) for a discussion of contestations around Latinx and its connections to other forms of linguistic resistance.

© Springer Nature Switzerland AG 2020
A. E. Goldberg, K. R. Allen (eds.), *LGBTQ-Parent Families*,
https://doi.org/10.1007/978-3-030-35610-1_5

Harris, 2017a, 2017b; Glass, 2014; Karpman, Ruppel, & Torres, 2018; Leibetseder, 2018; Moore, 2011a, 2011b; Pastrana, Battle, & Harris, 2017; Rodriguez, 2014). At the same time, White lesbian and gay parents remain overrepresented in the literature on LGBTQ-parent families as well as in popular culture (see Bible, Bermea, van Eeden-Moorefield, Benson, & Few-Demo, 2018; Huang et al., 2010; Singh & Shelton, 2011; van Eeden-Moorefield, Few-Demo, Benson, Bible, & Lummer, 2018). As one Black gay father put it,

> We're in the gay community, and the gay community itself is segregated. So we're the Black guys, you know, the Black section of the gay community. And then we're in a smaller—we're in the Black section with children in the gay community. We don't see our image around anywhere. (Carroll, 2018a, p. 111)

The invisibility articulated by this father goes beyond a politics of representation to reveal the interlocking systems of power that shape the lives of LGBTQ parents and their children. In this chapter, we highlight work by scholars who make the intersections of race, ethnicity, gender, and sexuality more central to the production of knowledge about LGBTQ-parent families.

## Theoretical Frameworks

In the second edition of *Black Feminist Thought: Knowledge, Consciousness and the Politics of Empowerment*, Collins (2000) conceptualizes sexuality in three ways: as a freestanding system of oppression similar to oppressions of race, class, nation, and gender, as an entity that is manipulated within each of these distinctive systems of oppression, and as a social location or conceptual glue that binds intersecting oppressions together and shows how oppressions converge. In her later work, Collins (2004) theorizes sexuality through the lens of heterosexism, which she identifies as a system of power similar to racism, sexism, and class oppression that suppresses heterosexual and homosexual African Americans in ways that foster Black subordination. As we demonstrate in this chapter, Collins' (2004)

application of the intersectionality paradigm to the study of Black women's sexuality is also a useful way to conceptualize sexuality as one of several social locations that LGBTQ parents inhabit.

LGBTQ group interests are often analyzed and advocated for in ways that privilege the interests of higher-income White individuals within those groups (DeFilippis, 2018). When these interests are constructed as separate from and even oppositional to the interests of (presumably heterosexual) racial communities, it is queer people of color and their families who are especially harmed (Cahill, 2010; Romero, 2005). Cahill (2010) argues that while antigay groups have constructed LGBTQ rights as "special rights" that threaten the civil liberties of people of color, antigay policies in fact have a disproportionate impact on Black and Latinx same-sex couple families who are more likely to be raising children and to have economic challenges—points we return to later in this chapter.

The study of race is also important within the larger discourses of diversity politics. For example, Hicks (2011) argues that White LGBTQ parents have the privilege to ignore inequalities around race and racism in a way that people of color do not. In his analysis of in-depth interviews with lesbian, gay, and queer parents, Hicks describes one White gay father who claimed that race was a "nonissue" for him and his two adopted Vietnamese sons. However, Hicks notes that this White father could not possibly know all the ways his sons will be positioned racially by others. The literature we review rejects a color-blind view of race as a "nonissue" for parents and families and instead acknowledges the significance of race, ethnicity, citizenship, and colonial legacies in queer family formation.

Conversations about how best to integrate intersectionality frameworks with queer theory have also come to bear on family studies (see Few-Demo, Humble, Curran, & Llyod, 2016). Allen and Mendez (2018) find that efforts to decenter heteronormativity in family studies often do not address the racialized contexts in which families are situated. Acosta (2018) argues that a "queerer" family scholarship is possible when we theorize in the flesh and from the borderlands, connecting with material realities and attending to race in our work. Allen and Mendez, Acosta, and other scholars working at the intersections of race and sexuality hold that queer theories will be strongest when they are race-conscious and mindful of how these constructs shape people's real lives.

The chapter begins with demographic characteristics of racially and ethnically diverse LGBTQ parents in North America and structural inequalities that emerge as salient for these groups. We next examine racial variation in how LGBTQ people become parents and navigate the gendered institutions of motherhood and fatherhood. While our focus is on families of color, we include studies of race and ethnicity in the lives of White lesbians and gay men who become parents through transracial adoption or surrogacy. The global reach of the surrogacy industry (see chapter "Gay Men and Surrogacy") underscores the need for studies that do not conceptualize the intersections of race and sexuality solely through the lens of US history and culture. As Purkayastha (2012) argues, a more robust intersectionality theory is possible when we look beyond Euro-American societies and attend to axes such as race within, between, and across nation-states. We offer a small step in this direction by engaging with studies of LGBTQ-parent families in geographic and cultural contexts that have received less scholarly attention. Throughout the chapter, we discuss ways to decenter assumptions about LGBTQ parenthood and approaches to this field of study that implicitly privilege White, North American families.

## Portrait of LGBTQ Parents of Color: Demographic Characteristics and Structural Inequalities

Census and other survey data point to consistently high rates of parenting among queer and trans people of color. Among the 6450 trans and gender nonconforming people who took part in the National Transgender Discrimination Survey (NTDS), American Indian respondents were the most likely to have children (45%) followed by respondents who are Latinx (40%), White (40%), Black (36%), multiracial (29%), and Asian (18%) (Stotzer, Herman, & Hasenbush, 2014). Among same-sex couples (and same-sex couples may include trans and gender nonconforming people), 41% of women of color and 20% of men of color have children under 18 in the home; for White women and men, these estimates are 23% and 8%, respectively (Gates, 2013b). As of the 2010 US census (the most recent census data available as of this review), 34% of African American, 29% of Latinx, and 26% of Asian American same-sex couples report that they are raising children (Kastanis & Gates, 2013a, 2013b, 2013c). These families tend not to be clustered in areas with proportionately large numbers of LGBTQ residents. Instead, they are most likely to reside in cities, towns, and rural areas with other members of their racial and ethnic communities (Kastanis & Gates, 2013a, 2013b, 2013c; see Battle et al., 2017a, 2017b; Pastrana et al., 2017). Efforts to support LGBTQ parents and their children must be attentive to the broader racial and ethnic communities of which they are a part.

Racially unjust systems—including economic, social, legal, healthcare, and immigration systems—shape LGBTQ parenting possibilities and practices for people of color as well as for Whites who are racially privileged within these systems. Numerous studies show that among same-sex couples, those who are Black, Latinx, Native American, and/or recent immigrants are more likely to be poor, less likely to own their homes, and more likely to lack health insurance compared to those who are White and native born (DeFilippis, 2016). Thirty-eight percent of Black children in households headed by two women and 52% in households headed by two men are living in poverty, the highest poverty rate of any group (Badgett, Durso, & Schneebaum, 2017). The 2015 US Transgender Survey reveals greater vulnerability among trans people of color to housing insecurity and homelessness, job loss, unemployment, police harassment, and imprisonment (James, Brown, & Wilson, 2017; James, Jackson, & Jim, 2017; James & Magpantay, 2017; James & Salcedo, 2017). Among families that include children, each of these vulnerabilities has lasting implications for the adult's ability to parent effectively and for the children witnessing the unequal treatment of their parents. Similarly, in a statewide needs assessment of LGBTQI (lesbian, gay, bisexual, transgender, queer, and intersex) people in Hawai'i, Native Hawaiians reported more discrimination based on gender identity/expression and sexual orientation compared to other groups (Stotzer, 2013). While not disaggregated by parental status, many of the areas where this discrimination and poor treatment occurred, such as in social service settings, are relevant to parents and children who are disproportionately likely to need such services.

The racism that is prevalent at all levels of the criminal legal system in the USA has direct and deleterious effects on LGBTQ parents of color who come into contact with the courts and the law. For example, among trans people who have separated from a partner or spouse, 29% of Black parents report that courts or judges have limited or terminated their relationships with their children on the basis of their transgender identity or gender nonconformity; the same is true for 20% of multiracial, 17% of American Indian, 12% of White, and 9% of Latinx NTDS respondents (Grant et al., 2011; of note is that the Asian sample size for this question was too low to report). Such decisions unjustly sever parent-child bonds, with lasting consequences for these children and families (see Lens, 2019; Roberts, 2009).

The healthcare system is another site of struggle for many trans parents and prospective parents, with implications for parent and child wellness and for trans people's pathways to parenthood. Nixon (2013) argues that sterilization requirements for sex reassignment and discrimination at multiple levels of the healthcare system—from insurance to fertility preservation and other reproductive options—result in passive eugenics for trans populations. She notes that in the USA, eugenics ideologies have historically taken three forms: immigration restrictions that target specific racial groups, anti-miscegenation laws, and coercive sterilization of "people deemed unfit to reproduce," overwhelmingly people with disabilities and women of color

(Nixon, 2013, p. 81). This legacy of racialized eugenics practices informs and intersects with trans-specific eugenics discourses to impinge on the reproductive autonomy of trans people of color.

Immigration policies and practices matter to LGBTQ-parent families as well. Researchers estimate that LGBTQ people comprise 2.4% of adult immigrants who are documented and 2.7% of adult immigrants who are undocumented in the USA, and parenthood is prevalent among these groups (Gates, 2013a). Twenty-five percent of binational same-sex couples and 58% of same-sex couples that include two noncitizen partners have children under 18. Among all Latinx same-sex couples raising children, 1 in 3 include at least one noncitizen partner (Kastanis & Gates, 2013b). The same is true for 1 in 4 Asian and Pacific Islander same-sex couples raising children (Kastanis & Gates, 2013a). Approximately 75,000 LGBTQ people qualify for the Development, Relief, and Education for Alien Minors (DREAM) Act and 36,000 have participated in Deferred Action for Child Arrivals (DACA) (Conran & Brown, 2017). We do not currently have data on how many DREAMers and DACA recipients have children, but we do know that immigration policies have a significant impact on parent and child well-being (Androff, Ayon, Becerra, Gurrola, & Salas, 2011; Dreby, 2015), and this is certainly true for LGBTQ parents and children in these communities. In a nationwide survey of Asian and Pacific Islander (API) LGBT Americans, respondents ranked immigration as the number one issue facing all APIs in the USA and one of the top four issues facing API LGBT Americans (Dang & Vianney, 2007).

Prior to 2013, same-sex couples were excluded from family unification under federal law (Cianciotto, 2005; Romero, 2005). US Supreme Court decisions to strike down the Defense of Marriage Act (DOMA) and to legalize same-sex marriage nationwide have since opened pathways to citizenship and increased security for some binational couples and their children. However, it is important to recognize that the US immigration system remains oppressive to many and that in an era of heightened White nationalism, LGBTQ parents and children of color who immigrate to the USA, or arrive seeking refugee or asylee status, continue to face exclusion, forced separation, and other forms of violence that are not remedied by legal same-sex marriage (Brandzel, 2016; Chávez, 2013).

## Gaps in Our Knowledge and Areas for Future Research

### Family Resilience

Amid pervasive discrimination in social institutions and interactions, LGBTQ people of color also exhibit unique parenting strengths. For example, Asian, Black, and Latinx trans people report greater improvement in parent-child relationships after coming out and lower rates of rejection by their children than do White trans people (Grant et al., 2011). This points to the quality of parental bonds between trans parents of color and their children as an important area for researchers to explore. LGBTQ parents of color are more likely to report that they are supported by their extended families, while rejection by blood relatives after coming out is more common among White LGBTQ parents (National Black Justice Coalition, 2012). Such findings challenge the assumption that LGBTQ people of color are more likely to be rejected by their families due to intersections of race and religiosity and related culturalist and often racist assumptions that communities of color are "more homophobic" (see Han, 2015, 2017). Increased focus on community strengths and assets will help to counter the deficit model that persists in research on LGBTQ families and families of color (Akerlund & Cheung, 2000; Prendergast & MacPhee, 2018).

### Gaps in Census and Other Survey Data

North American census data remain limited in ways that are directly linked to issues of race, ethnicity, and sexuality. Most of the demographic data

on LGBTQ families of color in Canada are found in the context of health (Balsam, Molina, Beadnell, Simoni, & Walters, 2011; Ross, Epstein, Goldfinger, Steele, Anderson, & Strike, 2014). Little is available on parenting, parenthood, or even family structures and compositions. One of the reasons for the paucity of data on race and LGBTQ families in Canada may be the abolition of the long-form census by the conservative government between 2010 and 2015. Justin Trudeau reintroduced the long-form in the 2016 census, but the data from the long-form are still being collated. In the USA, we lack information about Middle Eastern and North African LGBTQ people, who are racialized in US society (Hakim, Molina, & Branscombe, 2017; Strmic-Pawl, Jackson, & Garner, 2018). Data on American Indian and Alaskan Native (AIAN) populations remain slim (see Goldberg & Conron, 2018 for preliminary estimates of LGBTQ AIAN adults by region). In addition, counting only same-sex couple-headed households excludes single LGBTQ parents and other family arrangements (Battle et al., 2017a; Compton & Baumle, 2018). Efforts are underway to "queer the census," to include a Middle Eastern and North African (MENA) option, and to further refine the census around issues of race, ethnicity, and sexuality in ways that may expand research possibilities.[3] At the same time, some scholars have drawn attention to the White supremacist and eugenicist roots of counting populations and have raised questions about the implications of doing so in this political moment (Spade & Rohlfs, 2016; Strmic-Pawl et al., 2018). Our calls for better census and survey data must be carefully balanced with a critical eye toward how and by whom these data are used.

### Multiracial Families

Compared to different-sex couples, same-sex couples are more likely to be interracial or interethnic and more likely to create families that

---

[3] See examples of these campaigns here http://www.thetaskforce.org/thanks-for-keeping-the-census-queer/ (retrieved September 8, 2018) and here http://www.aaiusa.org/2020census (retrieved September 8, 2018).

include parents and children from different racial and ethnic backgrounds (Kastanis & Wilson, 2014). Eighty percent of Asian and Pacific Islander, 63% of Latinx, and 47% of African American individuals who are part of a same-sex couple have a partner of a different race or ethnicity (Kastanis & Gates, 2013a, 2013b, 2013c). Yet even discourses at the intersections of race and sexuality often fail to acknowledge these families. For example, many analyses of same-sex couples raising children follow the census approach of categorizing families by the race of the head of household. Multiracial households are not visible in this framework.

In recent years, qualitative researchers have brought multiracial families into focus. Acosta (2013) analyzed the ways that sexually nonconforming Latinas navigate their interracial and interethnic relationships, including relationships with other women of color who share a *mestiza* consciousness but are differentially positioned within US racial hierarchies. Although her 42 study participants did not automatically experience power imbalances based on gender, they did have to navigate imbalances based on race, language, and citizenship status. Some participants experienced conflict with families of origin over their partners' race and culture—an important reminder that LGBTQ family issues do not concern gender and sexuality only. These negotiations inform many dimensions of family life, including parenting practices and experiences. Karpman et al. (2018) found that lesbian, bisexual, and queer women of color who became parents in the context of an interracial partnership ($n = 11$ of 13 couples interviewed) were thoughtful about the racial characteristics the child would share with each mother. LBQ women of color in this study were attuned to issues surrounding transracial adoption and parenting—which is discussed in a later section of this chapter—and they brought this into their decision-making about donor selection and adoption.

In an interview with psychologist Sekneh Beckett, Alyena Mohummadally discussed her experiences as a Pakistani, Australian, queer Muslim who is also a mother (Beckett, Mohummadally, & Pallotta-Chiarolli, 2014).

Mohummadally has chosen to raise her child as a Muslim in the context of her interethnic and interfaith relationship. Her partner, a White Australian woman, had initial concerns about this decision but became supportive after learning more about Islam and about Mohummadally's family life; both women agree that raising their son as a Muslim "just feels right" (Beckett et al., 2014; Mohummadally, 2012, p. 1). Such negotiations are not unique to same-sex couples but may be uniquely inflected by intersections of sexuality and gender with ethnicity, faith, and culture. Same-sex couples may, for instance, have additional obstacles to overcome in finding a faith community that welcomes their family as one that is both interethnic and queer. As we learn more about multiracial families in general, it is important that we include LGBTQ parents and their children, who are disproportionately likely to be a part of such families.

## Pathways to Parenting

### Parenting Children from a Prior Heterosexual Relationship

The best available data suggest that a large percentage of queer parents had their children in the context of a prior heterosexual relationship and that this pathway to parenting is most common among queer people of color (Tasker & Rensten, 2019). Many researchers have framed their studies of lesbian and gay parenthood to make their results comparable to those of other empirical studies of family structure and family process in heterosexual two-parent families. Such an analogous research design makes it easier to test central assumptions in the literature regarding the division of household labor and the distribution of childcare and childrearing tasks, for example (Compton & Baumle, 2018). Research on lesbian-headed families also tends to be framed around long held assumptions about lesbian identity, particularly the idea that lesbians as a group are egalitarian in their distribution of paid work, housework, and childcare and that they organize their households and interact with each other in ways that support this principle (Dunne, 2000; Sullivan, 2004). Unfortunately, restricting samples so that they only include women who take on a lesbian identity before becoming parents over-represents White middle- and upper-income lesbians, who are more likely to support the ideological principles of feminism and who are better able to afford costly insemination procedures (Moore, 2011a).

In her three-year, mixed-methods study of African American lesbian families, Moore (2011a) found that many lesbian women who had become mothers in the context of a prior heterosexual union continued to make a concentrated effort to satisfy the societal definition of a "good mother" that is implicitly linked to heterosexuality. This expectation produced a conflict for lesbian mothers, who had to contend not only with the construction of lesbian identity as deviant, but also with negative stereotypes around race and Black women's sexuality. Their sexual orientation forced a sexual self into visibility in the context of motherhood, which frightened some and went against a politics of silence in this arena.[4] While lesbian mothers across racial groups may struggle to be viewed as "good mothers," the standards to which they are held are shaped not only by constructions of gender and sexuality, but also by constructions of race, racism, and intraracial group dynamics.

Gay and bisexual men who become fathers through their heterosexual relationships face similar pressures. In the largest qualitative study to date of sexuality and migration, comprising in-depth interviews with 150 Mexican-origin and Latinx gay and bisexual men and their partners, Carrillo (2018) identifies fatherhood as one of many factors shaping the men's immigration trajectories. This is evident in the life story of a study participant, Cuauhtémoc, who became a father through heterosexual marriage and migrated to the USA primarily to provide for his wife and children financially. He maintained this role as a provider to his family at the same time that he formed sexual and romantic relationships

with men in San Diego and gradually developed a bisexual identity. Contrary to normative expectations about "coming out," Cuauhtémoc continued to value his life as a straight-identified husband and father in Mexico, keeping his family circle carefully separated from his gay, bisexual, and transgender friendships and relationships in San Diego. Carrillo notes that men in the study were able to craft new lives in the USA while also maintaining what they liked about their lives in Mexico. Their journeys were not from "traditional" to "modern" modes of sexuality; Mexico has its own versions of sexual modernity and the men in the study are participants, not objects, in processes of sexual globalization. A simplistic reading of Cuauhtémoc's life might cast him as a "closeted" bisexual man. However, the portrait that emerges from Carrillo's research is far more complex. Such critical and compassionate research is needed to bring light to the largely invisible experiences of men who balance the expectations of heterosexual fatherhood with their bisexual and gay identities and lives.

## Parenting in Extended Families and Communities

In many racial and ethnic communities, family responsibilities, including the provision of financial and emotional support, elder and child care-taking, and other household duties are shared throughout social networks that may involve extended family and friends' participation in a variety of familial roles (Cross, 2018). Research on Black families has shown that kinship arrangements commonly include multigenerational family structures as well as other types of extended family households (Moras, Shehan, & Berardo, 2007). Several researchers have found that Latinx, Asian, and Caribbean immigrant families sustain complex networks that join households and communities, even across geographic borders, to provide assistance and support after immigration (e.g., Menjívar, Abrego, & Schmalzbauer, 2016; Taylor, Forsythe-Brown, Lincoln, & Chatters, 2015). LGBTQ people are also a part of these multigenerational and extended family networks.

---

[4]For more information on the politics of silence, see Hammonds, 1997.

In addition to parenting their own biological, foster, and adopted children, many queer people provide financial and emotional support to siblings, nieces and nephews, and grandchildren and to other children within their racial and ethnic communities (Mays, Chatters, Cochran, & Mackness, 1998; Moore, 2011a). Black same-sex couples are more than twice as likely as White same-sex couples to be parenting at least one nonbiological child, including children of relatives (Moore & Stambolis-Ruhstorfer, 2013). These parenting and family arrangements often do not show up in research studies that define same-sex parenting more narrowly.

Gilley (2006) spent 6 years living and working with members of two southwestern organizations for Native people who identify themselves as Two-Spirit. His work explores many dimensions of what it means for contemporary Indian people to "become" Two-Spirit through a synthesis of male and female qualities and gay and Native identities. Gilley's informants explained that Two-Spirit people have historically had caregiving roles, teaching children (especially girls) about Indian ceremonies and other cultural practices and caring for children when their parents are unable to do so. Two-Spirit men in the study cared for nieces, nephews, and other family members, supervised organizations for local teens, and reached out in formal and informal ways to support gay Indian youth. In keeping with their Two-Spirit identity, the men were called upon to stand in as both male and female role models for young people. The men did not describe their parenting activities in terms of a personal desire to have children or form a nuclear family together with a same-sex partner. Instead, their parenting roles were largely indistinguishable from their obligations to the larger family, community, and tribe. By teaching children and youth about Indian culture, Two-Spirit people positioned themselves as integral to Indian life (Gilley, 2006). Other researchers working with Two-Spirit populations that are diverse in terms of tribe, culture, and region have reported similar findings regarding caregiving roles (Evans-Campbell, Fredriksen-Goldsen, Walters, & Stately, 2007).

A second example of parenting to sustain the community emerges from Lewin's (2009) research on gay fathers. Drawing from interviews with 95 gay fathers in four metropolitan areas, Lewin analyzes the meanings gay men attach to their parenting roles and aspirations as they move across spaces defined as "gay" and those related to family and thus "not gay" by conventional standards. Among other meaning-making strategies, gay men in this research constructed fatherhood as the right thing to do in moral terms, often in response to stereotypes of gay men as morally deficient. For Black gay men, the moral impetus for fatherhood took on a special urgency, framed as a responsibility that extended beyond their immediate circle of kin. Non-Black men also described fatherhood as "doing the right thing," but for Black fathers this included doing the right thing for the racial community by caring for Black children who might otherwise languish in the foster care system. Lewin's research shows the salience of race even in patterns that occur across racial groups. While racially and ethnically diverse gay men used similar narrative constructs to describe their parenting, these took on different contours for Black gay fathers, who were most likely to connect their parenting narratives to larger issues of systemic racism and the survival of Black children.

## Transracial Adoption and Surrogacy

As the numbers of LGBTQ-parent families increase, so do the numbers of White LGBTQ parents raising children of color (Farr & Patterson, 2009; Goldberg, 2019). Lesbian and gay people are more likely than heterosexual people to adopt a child of a different race or ethnicity (Brooks, Whitsett, & Goldbach, 2016; Goldberg, Sweeney, Black, & Moyer, 2016). Substantial research makes it clear that race and color consciousness, not "color blindness," is the best practice approach to transracial adoption (e.g., Fong & McRoy, 2016; Quiroz, 2007; Wyman-Battalen, Dow-Fleisner, Brodzinsky, & McRoy, 2019). Thus, White LGBTQ parents who adopt children of color need to be prepared to engage with issues of race and racial inequality.

Goldberg et al. (2016) examined approaches to racial socialization among 82 lesbian, gay, and heterosexual adoptive parents, a majority of whom were White and raising children of color. Consistent with prior research, about one-half of these parents engaged actively in racial socialization, about one-third did so but more cautiously, and a smaller group of parents avoided addressing race in their families. Lesbian and gay adoptive parents were less likely to use an avoidant approach, more likely to engage in "positive race talk," and more likely to prioritize ties with communities of color compared to heterosexual parents in the study. The authors connect these qualities to parents' own experiences of difference as a source of pride, identity, and community (Goldberg et al., 2016; see Goldberg & Smith, 2016). In a later analysis of school decision-making among lesbian and gay adoptive parents, Goldberg and colleagues (2018) find that while all parents juggled children's intersecting identities, lesbian mothers placed greater emphasis on a racially diverse school environment to enhance their child's racial identity and sense of self. This work highlights additional dimensions of gender and class in racial socialization and race consciousness among adoptive parents.

Hicks (2011) argues that transracial adoption by lesbian, gay, and queer parents forces scholars to consider how race is related to ideas about resemblance and belonging—what it means to "look like" family. In interviews with lesbian adoptive couples creating multiracial families, Hicks analyzes the importance to many of these mothers of "looking like" a family with regard to skin color, often in anticipation of how their family will be perceived by others. While lesbian and gay parenting may destabilize notions of racial inheritance and biological bonds and while some parents explicitly challenge these ideals, they should also be aware of ways that racism may be expressed through insistence upon likeness as a criterion for family formation. Researchers have made similar observations in studies of sperm donor selection among lesbian couples (Andreassen, 2019; Ryan & Moras, 2017) and

surrogacy arrangements among gay men (Berkowitz, 2013; Ryan & Berkowitz, 2009). Such desires and demands among White lesbian and gay prospective parents show the hegemonic power of fitting into what Pyke (2000) calls the normal American family and Smith (1993) calls the standard North American family—a heteronormative, classed, and racialized ideology of what a family ought to be.

There is a paucity of statistical data on the numbers of LGBTQ-parent families who use surrogacy as way to have children. A small but growing number of research studies suggest that surrogacy has become a particularly popular pathway to parenthood for cisgender gay men (Patterson & Tornello, 2010) and that most of the gay men who access surrogacy are White and wealthy (see chapter "Gay Men and Surrogacy"). Surrogacy has produced a new layer of racialized, gendered, classed, and colonial stratification on a global level (DasGupta & DasGupta, 2010; Gondouin, 2012; Nebeling Petersen, 2018; Pande, 2015; Rudrappa & Collins, 2015; Vora, 2012). While many gay men work with altruistic surrogates (i.e., surrogates who do not receive monetary compensation), commercial surrogacy is fast becoming a common feminized vocation (Jacobson, 2016). Given the high cost of surrogacy in the West, many people, including gay men who want to pursue surrogacy, are turning to the Global South due to its lax laws and large supply of what Pande (2015) calls the "perfect surrogate—cheap, docile, selfless, and nurturing" (p. 970).

In their interviews with gay men from the USA and Australia who had availed commercial surrogacy services in India, Rudrappa and Collins (2015) found that men used "strategic moral frames" of surrogates' financial empowerment, access to reproductive rights, and liberation from patriarchy as justification for surrogacy. But the authors' interviews with the surrogates reveal how these moral frames were systematically created by the multimillion-dollar surrogacy industry by maintaining a commercial distance between the surrogate mothers and their Western clients. This distance maintained the surrogate mothers as singular monolithic "third-world" subjects (Mohanty, 1984), who are poor, shy but loving, ready to serve and fulfill the dreams of childless parents, and in need of rescue from their impoverished conditions by White men. The binaries created between the clients and the surrogates produced a classed and racialized image of the surrogate and a benevolent and wealthy image of Western clients who needed the surrogates to fulfill a familial dream. These images made the commercial exchange of intimate reproductive labor seamless while maintaining power hierarchies and keeping global inequalities intact.

## LGBTQ-Parent Families Beyond North America

We have noted in several places that global exchanges and inequities matter for LGBTQ parents and their children. Euro-American perspectives, while important, do not represent the experiences and interests of a majority of the world's families. In this final section, we turn our attention to studies of sexually nonconforming parents and prospective parents in Suriname, urban China, Tunisia, Chile, rural India, South Africa, Taiwan, and New Zealand indigenous communities. We present these eight cases (illustrative of a much larger body of international work) to highlight the rich variation in ways that heteronormative definitions of family are constructed and contested and theoretical implications that emerge from this variation.

## Rethinking the Distinction Between "Heterosexual" and "Same-Sex" Parent Families

It is common within family scholarship to classify couples and households as *either* "heterosexual" *or* "same-sex." Such a typology enables researchers to compare outcomes for children raised in these households and to make arguments about the unique strengths or deficits of same-sex-parent families. However, this is often an artificial distinction and one that has limited

the scope of LGBTQ family research in many parts of the world.

Wekker's (2006) ethnographic research on women engaged in "the *mati* work" in Paramaribo, Suriname, is instructive with regard to the limits of the heterosexual/same-sex-parent typology. Mati refers to love and sexual intimacy between women, conceived of as a pleasing behavior rather than as the basis of an individual or collective identity. Wekker found that women who mati usually have children by men and maintain sexual relationships with the fathers of their children, often in exchange for men's financial contributions to their households. Their primary emotional and romantic attachments, however, are to other women and most rely on the help of other women to bring up their children. Wekker uses the case of Afro-Surinamese women who mati to expose the limits of the Western concept of homosexual identity. We use it here to show the limits of the concept of same-sex parenting. Women who mati actively parent with other women and find sexual and romantic fulfillment in these relationships. However, they do not adopt a lesbian identity or see themselves as belonging to a community based on their sexual object choice, nor do they necessarily discontinue all sexual relations with men. Wekker's findings are consistent with reports that in African and other non-Western societies, women who are engaged in same-sex relationships may have men to fulfill certain functions, one of them being to reproduce (Aarmo, 1999; Potgieter, 2003). Conventional definitions of lesbian parenting that focus on the same-sex couple do not account for these kinds of arrangements.

Throughout the world, many people who have same-sex relationships enter or remain in concurrent heterosexual marriages (recall Cuauhtémoc, the father in Carrillo's, 2018 study discussed earlier in this chapter, as another illustration of this practice carried out across borders). Engebretsen (2009) presents three case studies to highlight a range of *lala* (lesbian) family arrangements in Beijing, China. One woman remained heterosexually married and mothered a child in the context of this marriage while also dating her lala partner. Two other lalas created a marriage-like relationship with one another and merged families, sharing care work for elderly parents. In the third case, a self-identified *chunde T* (pure T; similar, though not equivalent, to stone butch) chose to marry a gay male friend to satisfy her parents. Those who married men were able to maintain what Engebretsen calls "hetero-marital face," but found it difficult to form and keep lasting same-sex relationships because of the demands their marital and family arrangements placed on them. The women who formed a marriage-like relationship with one another found more lasting satisfaction in that relationship but expressed deep regret at their inability to have a child together. Engebretsen does not conclude that any one of these family arrangements is superior to or ultimately more satisfying than the others. Instead, she critiques Western discourses that prioritize certain marital ideologies and relationship strategies, without fully recognizing the diversity of nonnormative sexualities globally.

In contexts where gay sexuality is prohibited and/or where assisted reproductive technologies and adoption services are only available to heterosexually married couples, heterosexual marriage remains the planned pathway to parenthood for many LGBTQ people. Hamdi, Lachheb, and Anderson (2018) conducted cyber interviews with 28 gay Muslim men living in Tunisia; while the interviews focus on the integration of religion and sexuality, plans for marriage and fatherhood also surface in the men's narratives. Those who hope or plan to become fathers expect to do so through marriage to a woman. As one interviewee shared: "I did not choose homosexuality, and I would like to get married [to a woman] one day and have children, even though I cannot imagine myself with a woman on a bed" (Hamdi, Lachheb, & Anderson, 2018, p. 1301). Another man compromised by looking for a lesbian to marry, not unlike the *chunde T* interviewed by Engebretsen (2009); for other examples of gay-lesbian marriages in Taiwan, Korea, and China, see Brainer, 2019; Cho, 2009; and Huang & Brouwer, 2018, respectively).

Rearing a child conceived within a heterosexual marriage can carry some unique challenges and costs. Child custody is a particularly high stakes area for LGBTQ people who became parents in this way and whose marriages later end. Herrera (2009) identified this issue in her fieldwork and interviews with 29 Chilean lesbian women. Many of the women hid their sexual orientation from their families and especially from their ex-husbands because they feared losing custody of their children. These women saw their motherhood and their lesbian identities and relationships as compatible, yet recognized that they would be viewed and treated as "bad mothers" within the court system because of their sexuality. Herrera noted that a legitimate fear of having one's children taken away "profoundly marks the way [Chilean lesbians] experience motherhood" (p. 50).

By classifying households as *either* heterosexual *or* same-sex, researchers exclude those households where parenting arrangements are shared among multiple adults who may be romantically and/or sexually connected to one another. This classification does not prepare us to recognize and support LGBTQ parents who are balancing more traditional or traditional-seeming marriages with their nonnormative identities and relationships and who may face particularly difficult custody battles if and when those marriages dissolve. Studies by Wekker (2006), Carrillo (2018), Engebretsen (2009), Hamdi, Lachheb, and Anderson (2018), Herrera (2009), and other scholars working in diverse geographic and social locations require family scholars to think more broadly about what queer parenting might look like and the issues that these families face.

## Alternatives to a Politics of "Sameness"

A central feature of the same-sex/heterosexual parent typology is the ability to compare and contrast these households, often to counter (or in some cases, bolster) political claims that heterosexual parenting is superior and should be uniquely protected. Several scholars have pointed out that basing LGBTQ parents' rights on claims that they are *the same as* heterosexual parents is methodologically and epistemologically flawed (e.g., Berkowitz, 2009; Carroll, 2018b; Dozier, 2015). Moreover, queer and trans people do not necessarily see heterosexuals raising children as the model or gold standard for parenting. Many LGBTQ parents make conscious choices to parent in ways that differ from other members of their communities and to pursue countercultural goals for their children's futures.

One such example is offered by Swarr and Nagar (2003) in their case analysis of a masculine-feminine female couple raising two daughters in rural India. The couple chose not to arrange marriages for their daughters despite family and community pressure to do so. These mothers explained that they wanted their daughters to receive an inheritance so that they would have the option not to marry. For a similar reason, they chose not to follow social convention by adopting a son, as the son would then have rights to all they owned. The mothers connected their vision for their daughters' inheritance rights and future independence to their own struggles for independence from compulsory heterosexual marriage. In doing so, they voiced a desire to make the institutions of marriage and family fairer for sexually nonconforming people and for women.

Another pointed critique of family as a heteronormative institution appears in Lynch and Morison's (2016) analysis of media discourses about gay fathers and their children in South Africa. The range of discourses Lynch and Morison describe make it clear that normalizing strategies, including efforts to downplay or deny differences between gay and heterosexual parents, remain quite common in South African media. But more resistant talk is also present, constructing queer parents as different in positive and desirable ways and challenging the heteronormative "gold standard." For example, in response to a government document that presented the heterosexual nuclear family as inherently nurturing and supportive, one commentator wrote,

> In reality, many families 'nurture' unequal social relations between men and women, rich and poor, black and white, queer and straight… Women's subordination is reproduced in families where boys are raised to assume masculine dominance and girls are told (most recently by the president) that marriage and child rearing is their primary social role… The [document's] hallowed 'family' is often a pretty unsafe place. (Lynch & Morison, 2016, pp. 200–201).

Other commentators pointed out that children of gay and lesbian parents may be more tolerant of differences and thus well-adjusted to a multicultural society. Such arguments do not rely on proving that queer parents are "as good as" heterosexual parents or that their family lives will be the same.

Similarly, Brainer's (2019) fieldwork and interviews with LGBTQ people and their families in Taiwan ($n = 47$ LGBTQ people and 33 heterosexual parents and siblings) includes several queer parents who resist the normative gender and family roles that are imposed on their children by others. One $T$ (transmasculine) mother made a series of life-altering decisions after learning that her son is gay, among them ending her 20-year marriage to a man and breaking ties with family members who treated her poorly because of her masculinity. She explained that she did this to shield her son from family pressure and abuse and to encourage her son's relationship with his boyfriend as an alternative to heterosexual marriage. It was her intersecting roles as a T parent that empowered this mother to reject the social norms surrounding marital and family relationships. Another interviewee supported her adult daughter's polyamorous relationships with men, explaining that her own journey through heterosexual marriage and her developing identity as a *la ma* (lesbian mother) had altered her expectations for her child. For example, she now prioritized her daughter's sexual autonomy over conformity to cultural scripts. Both mothers described the differences embodied by their children and their support for such differences as evidence of their unique parenting *strengths* rather than deficits.

Glover, McKree, and Dyall (2009) used focus group interviews to study fertility issues and access to reproductive technologies in Maori (New Zealand indigenous) communities. Among *takatapui* (nonheterosexual) women interviewed, the issue of sperm donation was discussed at length. Some takatapui women reported that they preferred gay male sperm donors because they wanted to limit the influence of heterosexuality on their children and because they wanted to pass on the "gay gene" if such a thing should exist. The significance of these comments becomes more apparent when we consider the social and political climate in New Zealand, where the largest sperm bank banned gay donors until 2006. After the ban was lifted, a Professor of Genetics at New Zealand's Canterbury University said people who received sperm from gay men should be informed that a "gay gene" might be passed to their children (Glover et al., 2009, p. 305). In a context where discourse around the possible existence of a "gay gene" has been used to directly attack queer communities, takatapui mothers and prospective mothers offer a counter-discourse by constructing the "gay gene" as a positive and desirable trait.

Taken together, critiques of the same-sex/heterosexual typology and efforts to prove that these two types of families are virtually the same produce alternative ways to conceptualize the needs, desires, and social roles of LGBTQ parents. Some parents have not constructed a personal or collective identity based on the gender of their sexual partner(s). They have complicated relationships with the institution of marriage and may have heterosexual marriages and same-sex relationships concurrently. Comparative research often assumes structural difference while looking for similarity in child outcomes. Parents in the case studies we have presented seek precisely the opposite. Even as their households may look structurally similar to those of heterosexuals, many have made efforts to instill values and offer opportunities to their children that differ from widely held values in their countries and cultures of origin.

## Future Directions for Research and Practice

Banerjee and Connell (2018) call on social scientists to engage with conceptual work originating in the Global South and under conditions of colonialism and postcolonialism. This shift is not about collecting data in these areas, although that may be a part of the work. Rather, it is about incorporating theoretical insights that disrupt a still very deeply Western-centric canon (see Connell, 2007). Analytic approaches to LGBTQ parenting will be strongest when they shift in the ways that Banerjee and Connell describe. For instance, deploying a "solidarity-based approach" (p. 66) would allow us to analyze how coloniality has shaped LGBTQ parenting in the Global South and the Global North. This shift cautions scholars of the Global North against using the Global South merely as repository of data about LGBTQ parenting. Instead, Banerjee and Connell push us to change our perspectives to consider what we know about LGBTQ parenting in the Global South as a conscious body of knowledge that undoes our hegemonic and colonial understandings of parenting, queer sexuality, and family formations. There is still much that we do not know about queer sexuality and family formation in a majority of the world. The examples in this chapter complicate our understandings of, among other things, who "counts" as a queer or trans parent and what issues matter most to these parents and their children. These do more than diversify our empirical data. New theories and models are required to account for the ways that LGBTQ families are positioned within their societies as well as in global hierarchies.

We urge scholars and practitioners alike to broaden the definition of LGBTQ parenting to account for a greater variety of ways that people create families and bring children into those families. Current definitions exclude some practices that are especially prevalent among LGBTQ people of color, such as parenting children from a prior or ongoing heterosexual union and parenting children within extended family and community networks. We agree with scholars who argue that LGBTQ parenting and related laws and policies are matters of racial and economic justice (see Cahill, Battle, & Meyer, 2003; Cahill & Jones, 2001; Cianciotto, 2005; Dang & Frazer, 2004; DeFilippis, 2018; Schneebaum & Badgett, 2018). The work we have reviewed provides empirical support for intersectionality theories that challenge scholars to move beyond additive models of structural location. Experiences of LGBTQ families of color are not reducible to theories of race and racism, nor to theories of sexuality and heterosexism. It is imperative that we consider the racial implications of laws and policies around same-sex parenting and the implications for LGBTQ parents and children of structural racism and xenophobia.

Expanding research beyond predominately White, Western populations brings a fresh lens to ongoing conversations within LGBTQ family studies. Many of these parents challenge heteronormativity in deeper ways than a politics of sameness can accomplish. The construct of a "good mother" (and, in a smaller number of cases, a good father who "does the right thing") is one that came up in several of the studies we reviewed among parents of different racial and ethnic backgrounds (e.g., Herrera, 2009; Lewin, 2009; Moore, 2011a). But the ways that people think about and try to manifest "good" parenting—or are excluded from this category on the basis of their sexuality—vary by race, class, and other aspects of the parent's social location. As we have noted, even patterns that cut across racial groups often reveal meaningful variation that calls for different kinds of support.

Scholarship on race and ethnicity in the lives of LGBTQ parents and their children has grown substantially and LGBTQ scholars have made strides in centering parents and families of color. At the same time, there are many areas for growth. Transgender and especially bisexual parents of color are often lumped into studies of "LGBT" parents that focus on lesbians and gays see chapters "What Do We Now Know About Bisexual Parenting? A Continuing Call for Research", and "Transgender-Parent Families"). Multiracial families continue to be underrepresented in the literature despite their significant presence in our LGBTQ communities. When LGBTQ families are represented in popular culture and news media, it is still a White, wealthy lesbian or gay couple that is most common (Cavalcante, 2015; Ventura, Rodríguez-Polo, & Roca-Cuberes, 2019). It is important to get research about the diversity of LGBTQ families

out of the academy and into the broader society. Finally, we hope that future work will continue to move beyond a deficit model, attending to the challenges, strengths, and joys of LGBTQ families of color in all their complexity.

# References

Aarmo, M. (1999). How homosexuality became 'un-African': The case of Zimbabwe. In E. Blackwood & S. Wieringa (Eds.), *Female desires: Same-sex relations and transgender practices across cultures* (pp. 255–280). New York, NY: Columbia University Press.

Acosta, K. (2013). *Amiga y amantes: Sexually nonconforming Latinas negotiate family*. New Brunswick, NJ: Rutgers University Press.

Acosta, K. (2018). Queering family scholarship: Theorizing from the borderlands. *Journal of Family Theory & Review, 10*, 406–418. https://doi.org/10.1111/jftr.12263

Akerlund, M., & Cheung, M. (2000). Teaching beyond the deficit model: Gay and lesbian issues among African Americans, Latinos, and Asian Americans. *Journal of Social Work Education, 36*, 279–292. https://doi.org/10.1080/10437797.2000.10779008

Alimahomed, S. (2010). Thinking outside the rainbow: Women of color redefining queer politics and identity. *Social Identities, 16*, 151–168. https://doi.org/10.1080/13504631003688849

Allen, S., & Mendez, S. (2018). Hegemonic heteronormativity: Toward a new era of queer family theory. *Journal of Family Theory & Review, 10*, 70–86. https://doi.org/10.1111/jftr.12241

Androff, D., Ayon, C., Becerra, D., Gurrola, M., Salas, L., Krysik, J. Gerdes, K., & Segal, E. (2011). U.S. immigration policy and immigrant children's well-being: The impact of policy shifts. *Journal of Sociology & Social Welfare, 38*, 77–98. https://scholarworks.wmich.edu/jssw/vol38/iss1/5

Andreassen, R. (2019). *Mediated kinship: Gender, race, and sexuality in donor families*. New York, NY: Routledge.

Badgett, M. V. L., Durso, L., & Schneebaum, A. (2017). *New patterns of poverty in the lesbian, gay, and bisexual community*. Los Angeles, CA: The Williams Institute, UCLA School of Law.

Balsam, K. F., Molina, Y., Beadnell, B., Simoni, J., & Walters, K. (2011). Measuring multiple minority stress: The LGBT people of color microaggressions scale. *Cultural Diversity and Ethnic Minority Psychology, 17*, 163–174. https://doi.org/10.1037/a0023244

Banerjee, P., & Connell, R. (2018). Gender theory as southern theory. In B. Risman & W. Scarborough (Eds.), *Handbook of the sociology of gender* (pp. 57–68). New York, NY: Springer.

Battle, J., Pastrana, A., & Harris, A. (2017a). *An examination of Asian and Pacific Islander LGBT populations across the United States: Intersections of race and sexuality*. New York, NY: Palgrave Macmillan.

Battle, J., Pastrana, A., & Harris, A. (2017b). *An examination of Black LGBT populations across the United States: Intersections of race and sexuality*. New York, NY: Palgrave Macmillan.

Beckett, S., Mohummadally, A., & Pallotta-Chiarolli, M. (2014). Living the rainbow: 'Queerying' Muslim identities. In A. W. Ata (Ed.), *Education integration challenges: The case of Australian Muslims* (pp. 96–106). Melbourne, Australia: David Lovell Publishing.

Berkowitz, D. (2009). Theorizing lesbian and gay parenting: Past, present, and future scholarship. *Journal of Family Theory & Review, 1*, 117–132. https://doi.org/1 0.1111/j.1756-2589.2009.00017

Berkowitz D. (2013). Gay men and surrogacy. In A. Goldberg & K. Allen (Eds.), *LGBT-parent families* (pp. 71–85). New York, NY: Springer. https://doi. org/10.1007/978-1-4614-4556-2_5

Bible, J., Bermea, A., van Eeden-Moorefield, B., Benson, K., & Few-Demo, A. (2018). A content analysis of the first decade of the Journal of GLBT Family Studies. *Journal of GLBT Family Studies, 14*, 337–355. https:// doi.org/10.1080/1550428X.2017.1349626

Boston, J., & Duyvendak, J. W. (2015). People of color mobilization in LGBT movements in the Netherlands and the United States. In D. Paternotte & M. Tremblay (Eds.), *The Ashgate research companion to lesbian and gay activism* (pp. 135–148). New York, NY: Routledge.

Brainer, A. (2019). *Queer kinship and family change in Taiwan*. New Brunswick, NJ: Rutgers University Press.

Brandzel, A. (2016). *Against citizenship: The violence of the normative*. Urbana, IL: University of Illinois Press.

Brooks, D., Whitsett, D., & Goldbach, J. (2016). Interculturally competent practice with gay and lesbian families. In R. Fong & R. McRoy (Eds.), *Transracial and intercountry adoption: Cultural guidance for professionals* (pp. 90–125). New York, NY: Columbia University Press.

Cahill, S. (2010). Black and Latino same-sex couple households and the racial dynamics of antigay activism. In J. Battle & S. Barnes (Eds.), *Black sexualities: Probing powers, passions, practices and policies* (pp. 243–268). New Brunswick, NJ: Rutgers University Press.

Cahill, S., & Jones, K. (2001). *Leaving our children behind: Welfare reform and the gay, lesbian, bisexual and transgender community*. New York, NY: Policy Institute of the National Gay and Lesbian Task Force.

Cahill, S., Battle, J., & Meyer, D. (2003). Partnering, parenting, and policy: Family issues affecting Black lesbian, gay, bisexual, and transgender (LGBT) people. *Race and Society, 6*, 85–98. https://doi.org/10.1016/j. racsoc.2004.11.002

Carrillo, H. (2018). *Pathways of desire: The sexual migration of Mexican gay men*. Chicago, IL: University of Chicago Press.

Carroll, M. (2018a). Gay fathers on the margins: Race, class, marital status, and pathways to parenthood. *Family Relations, 67*, 104–117. https://doi. org/10.1111/fare.12300

Carroll, M. (2018b). Managing without moms: Gay fathers, incidental activism, and the politics of parental gender. *Journal of Family Issues, 39*, 3410–3435. https://doi.org/10.1177/0192513X18783229

Cavalcante, A. (2015). Anxious displacements: The representation of gay parenting on *Modern Family* and *The New Normal*. *Television & New Media, 16*, 454–471. https://doi.org/10.1177/1527476414538525

Chambers-Letson, J. (2018). *After the party: A manifesto for queer of color life*. New York, NY: NYU Press.

Chávez, K. (2013). *Queer migration politics: Activist rhetoric and coalitional possibilities*. Urbana, IL: University of Illinois Press.

Cho, J. (2009). The wedding banquet revisited: "Contract marriages" between Korean gays and lesbians. *Anthropological Quarterly, 82*, 401–422. https://doi. org/10.1353/anq.0.0069

Cianciotto, J. (2005). *Hispanic and Latino same-sex couple households in the United States: A report from the 2000 Census*. New York, NY: The National Gay and Lesbian Task Force Policy Institute.

Collins, P. H. (2000). *Black feminist thought: Knowledge, consciousness, and the politics of empowerment*. New York, NY: Routledge.

Collins, P. H. (2004). *Black sexual politics: African Americans, gender, and the new racism*. New York, NY: Routledge.

Compton, D., & Baumle, A. (2018). Demographics of gay and lesbian partnerships and families. In N. Riley & J. Brunson (Eds.), *International handbook on gender and demographic processes* (pp. 267–285). New York, NY: Springer.

Connell, R. (2007). *Southern theory: Social science and the global dynamics of knowledge in social science*. Boston, MA: Polity.

Conran, K., & Brown, T. (2017). *LGBT DREAMers and Deferred Action for Childhood Arrivals (DACA)*. Los Angeles, CA: The Williams Institute, UCLA School of Law.

Cross, C. (2018). Extended family households among children in the United States: Differences by race/ethnicity and socioeconomic status. *Population Studies, 72*, 235–251. https://doi.org/10.1080/00324728.2018. 1468476

Dang, A., & Frazer, S. (2004). *Black same-sex households in the United States: A report from the 2000 census*. New York, NY: Policy Institute of the National Gay and Lesbian Task Force and the National Black Justice Coalition.

Dang, A., & Vianney, C. (2007). *Living in the margins: A national survey of lesbian, gay, bisexual and transgender Asian and Pacific Islander Americans*. New York,

NY: The National Gay and Lesbian Task Force Policy Institute.

DasGupta, S., & DasGupta, S. D. (2010). Motherhood jeopardized: Reproductive technologies in Indian communities. In W. Chavkin & J.-M. Maher (Eds.), *The globalization of motherhood: Deconstructions and reconstructions of biology and care* (pp. 131–153). New York, NY: Routledge.

DeFilippis, J. (2016). What about the rest of us? An overview of LGBT poverty issues and a call to action. *Journal of Progressive Human Services, 27*, 143–174. https://doi.org/10.1080/10428232.2016.1198673

DeFilippis, J. (2018). A new queer liberation movement and its targets of influence, mobilization, and benefits. In J. DeFilippis, M. Yarbrough, & A. Jones (Eds.), *Queer activism after marriage equality* (pp. 81–107). New York, NY: Routledge.

Dozier, R. (2015). The power of queer: How "guy moms" challenge heteronormative assumptions about mothering and family. In B. Risman & V. Rutter (Eds.), *Families as they really are* (pp. 458–474). New York, NY: W. W. Norton.

Dreby, J. (2015). U.S. immigration policy and family separation: The consequences for children's well-being. *Social Science & Medicine, 132*, 245–251. https://doi.org/10.1016/j.socscimed.2014.08.041

Dunne, G. A. (2000). Opting into motherhood: Lesbians blurring the boundaries and transforming the meaning of parenthood and kinship. *Gender & Society, 14*, 11–35. https://doi.org/10.1177/089124300014001003

Engebretsen, E. L. (2009). Intimate practices, conjugal ideals: Affective ties and relationship strategies among lala (lesbian) women in contemporary Beijing. *Sexuality Research & Social Policy, 6*, 3–14. https://doi.org/10.1525/srsp.2009.6.3.3

Evans-Campbell, T., Fredriksen-Goldsen, K., Walters, K., & Stately, A. (2007). Caregiving experiences among American Indian Two-Spirit men and women: Contemporary and historical roles. *Journal of Lesbian and Gay Social Services, 18*, 75–92. https://doi.org/10.1300/J041v18n03_05

Farr, R., & Patterson, C. (2009). Transracial adoption by lesbian, gay, and heterosexual couples: Who completes transracial adoptions and with what results? *Adoption Quarterly, 12*, 187–204. https://doi.org/10.1080/10926750903313328

Few-Demo, A., Humble, Á., Curran, M., & Lloyd, S. (2016). Queer theory, intersectionality, and LGBT-parent families: Transformative critical pedagogy in family theory. *Journal of Family Theory & Review, 8*, 74–94. https://doi.org/10.1111/jftr.12127

Fong, R., & McRoy, R. (Eds.). (2016). *Transracial and intercountry adoption: Cultural guidance for professionals*. New York, NY: Columbia University Press.

Gates, G. (2013a). *LGBT adult immigrants in the United States*. Los Angeles, CA: The Williams Institute, UCLA School of Law.

Gates, G. (2013b). *LGBT parenting in the United States*. Los Angeles, CA: The Williams Institute, UCLA School of Law.

Gilley, B. J. (2006). *Becoming Two-Spirit: Gay identity and social acceptance in Indian country*. Lincoln, NE: University of Nebraska Press.

Glass, V. (2014). "We are with family": Black lesbian couples negotiate rituals with extended families. *Journal of GLBT Family Studies, 10*, 79–100. https://doi.org/10.1080/1550428X.2014.857242

Glover, M., McKree, A., & Dyall, L. (2009). Assisted human reproduction: Issues for takatapui (New Zealand indigenous non-heterosexuals). *Journal of GLBT Family Studies, 5*, 295–311. https://doi.org/10.1080/15504280903263702

Goldberg, A. (2019). *Open adoption and diverse families: Complex relationships in the digital age*. Oxford, UK: Oxford University Press.

Goldberg, A., Sweeney, K., Black, K., & Moyer, A. (2016). Lesbian, gay, and heterosexual adoptive parents' socialization approaches to children's minority statuses. *The Counseling Psychologist, 44*, 267–299. https://doi.org/10.1177/0011000015628055

Goldberg, A., & Smith, J. (2016). Predictors of race, adoption, and sexual orientation related socialization of adoptive parents of young children. *Journal of Family Psychology, 30*, 397–408. https://doi.org/10.1037/fam0000149

Goldberg, S., & Conron, K. (2018). *Adult LGBT American Indians and Alaskan Natives per region of the United States*. Los Angeles, CA: The Williams Institute, UCLA School of Law.

Gondouin, J. (2012). Adoption, surrogacy, and Swedish exceptionalism. *Critical Race and Whiteness Studies Journal, 8*, 1–20.

Grant, J., Mottet, L., Tanis, J., Harrison, J., Herman, J., & Keisling, M. (2011). *Injustice at every turn: A report of the national transgender discrimination survey*. Washington, DC: National Center for Transgender Equality and National Gay and Lesbian Task Force.

Hakim, N. H., Molina, L. E., & Branscombe, N. R. (2017). How discrimination shapes social identification processes and wellbeing among Arab Americans. *Social Psychological and Personality Science, 9*, 328–337. https://doi.org/10.1177/1948550617742192

Hamdi, N., Lachheb, M., & Anderson, E. (2018). Muslim gay men: Identity conflict and politics in a Muslim majority nation. *The British Journal of Sociology, 69*, 1293–1312. https://doi.org/10.1111/1468-4446.12334

Hammonds, E. M. (1997). Toward a genealogy of Black female sexuality: The problematic of silence. In M. J. Alexander & C. T. Mohanty (Eds.), *Feminist genealogies, colonial legacies, democratic futures* (pp. 170–182). New York, NY: Routledge.

Han, C. (2015). *Geisha of a different kind: Race and sexuality in Gaysian America*. New York, NY: New York University Press.

Han, C. (2017). Examining identity development among gay men of color. *Sociology Compass, 11*, 1–12. https://doi.org/10.1111/soc4.12503

Herrera, F. (2009). Tradition and transgression: Lesbian motherhood in Chile. *Sexuality Research & Social Policy, 6*, 35–51. https://doi.org/10.1525/srsp.2009.6.2.35

Hicks, S. (2011). *Lesbian, gay and queer parenting: Families, intimacies, genealogies*. Basingstoke, UK: Palgrave Macmillan.

Huang, S., & Brouwer, D. (2018). Negotiating performances of "real" marriage in Chinese queer xinghun. *Women's Studies in Communication, 41*, 140–158. https://doi.org/10.1080/07491409.2018.1463581

Huang, Y. P., Brewster, M., Moradi, B., Goodman, M., Wiseman, M., & Martin, A. (2010). Content analysis of literature about LGB people of color: 1998–2007. *The Counseling Psychologist, 38*, 363–396. https://doi.org/10.1177/0011000009335255

Jacobson, H. (2016). *Labor of love: Gestational surrogacy and the work of making babies*. New Brunswick, NJ: Rutgers University Press.

James, S. E., Brown, C., & Wilson, I. (2017). *2015 U.S. transgender survey: Report on the experiences of Black respondents*. Washington, DC and Dallas, TX: National Center for Transgender Equality, Black Trans Advocacy, & National Black Justice Coalition.

James, S. E., Jackson, T., & Jim, M. (2017). *2015 U.S. transgender survey: Report on the experiences of American Indian and Alaska Native respondents*. Washington, DC: National Center for Transgender Equality.

James, S. E., & Magpantay, G. (2017). *2015 U.S. transgender survey: Report on the experiences of Asian, Native Hawaiian, and Pacific Islander respondents*. Washington, DC and New York, NY: National Center for Transgender Equality & National Queer Asian Pacific Islander Alliance.

James, S. E., & Salcedo, B. (2017). *2015 U.S. transgender survey: Report on the experiences of Latino/a respondents*. Washington, DC and Los Angeles, CA: National Center for Transgender Equality and TransLatin@ Coalition.

Johnson, E. P. (2018). *Black. Queer. Southern. Women: An oral history*. Chapel Hill, NC: The University of North Carolina Press.

Karpman, H., Ruppel, E., & Torres, M. (2018). "It wasn't feasible for us": Queer women of color navigating family formation. *Family Relations, 67*, 118–131. https://doi.org/10.1111/fare.12303

Kastanis, A., & Gates, G. (2013a). *LGBT African Americans and African-American same-sex couples*. Los Angeles, CA: The Williams Institute, UCLA School of Law.

Kastanis, A., & Gates, G. (2013b). *LGBT Asian and Pacific Islander individuals and same-sex couples*. Los Angeles, CA: The Williams Institute, UCLA School of Law.

Kastanis, A., & Gates, G. (2013c). *LGBT Latino/a individuals and Latino/a same-sex couples*. Los Angeles, CA: The Williams Institute, UCLA School of Law.

Kastanis, A., & Wilson, B. (2014). *Race/ethnicity, gender, and socioeconomic wellbeing of individuals in same-sex couples*. Los Angeles, CA: The Williams Institute, UCLA School of Law.

Leibetseder, D. (2018). Queer reproduction revisited and why race, class, and citizenship still matter. *Bioethics, 32*, 138–144. https://doi.org/10.1111/bioe.12416

Lens, V. (2019). Judging the other: The intersection of race, gender, and class in family court. *Family Court Review, 57*, 72–87. https://doi.org/10.1111/fcre.12397

Lewin, E. (2009). *Gay fatherhood: Narratives of family and citizenship in America*. Chicago, IL: The University of Chicago Press.

Lynch, I., & Morison, T. (2016). Gay men as parents: Analysing resistant talk in South African mainstream media accounts of queer families. *Feminism & Psychology, 26*, 188–206. https://doi.org/10.1177/0959353516638862

Mays, V., Chatters, L., Cochran, S., & Mackness, J. (1998). African American families in diversity: Gay men and lesbians as participants in family networks. *Journal of Comparative Family Studies, 29*, 73–87. https://doi.org/10.3138/jcfs.29.1.73

Menjívar, C., Abrego, L., & Schmalzbauer, L. (2016). *Immigrant families*. Malden, MA: Policy Press.

Mohanty, C. (1984). Under Western eyes: Feminist scholarship and colonial discourses. *boundary 2, 12/13*, 333–350. https://doi.org/10.1057/fr.1988.42

Mohummadally, A. (2012). Pride and prejudice. *Daily Life*. Retrieved from http://www.dailylife.com.au/life-and-love/real-life/pride-and-prejudice-20120228-1u0ki.html

Moore, M. R. (2011a). *Invisible families: Gay identities, relationships, and motherhood among Black women*. Berkeley, CA: University of California Press.

Moore, M. R. (2011b). Two sides of the same coin: Revising analyses of lesbian sexuality and family formation through the study of Black women. *Journal of Lesbian Studies, 15*, 58–68. https://doi.org/10.1080/10894160.2010.508412

Moore, M., & Stambolis-Ruhstorfer, M. (2013). LGBT sexuality and families at the start of the twenty-first century. *Annual Review of Sociology, 39*, 491–507. https://doi.org/10.1146/annurev-soc-071312-145643

Moras, A., Shehan, C., & Berardo, F. (2007). African American families: Historical and contemporary forces shaping family life and studies. In H. Vera & J. Feagin (Eds.), *Handbook of the sociology of racial and ethnic relations* (pp. 145–160). New York, NY: Springer.

National Black Justice Coalition. (2012). *LGBT families of color: Facts at a glance*. Retrieved from http://

www.nbjc.org/sites/default/files/lgbt-families-of-color-facts-at-a-glance.pdf

Nebeling Petersen, M. (2018). Becoming gay fathers through transnational commercial surrogacy. *Journal of Family Issues, 39*, 693–719. https://doi.org/10.1177/0192513X16676859

Nixon, L. (2013). The right to (trans) parent: A reproductive justice approach to reproductive rights, fertility, and family-building issues facing transgender people. *William & Mary Journal of Women and the Law, 20*, 73–103.

Pande, A. (2015). Blood, sweat, and dummy tummies: Kin labour and transnational surrogacy in India. *Anthropologica, 57*, 53–62.

Pastrana, A., Battle, J., & Harris, A. (2017). *An examination of Latinx LGBT populations across the United States: Intersections of race and sexuality.* New York, NY: Palgrave Macmillan.

Patterson, C., & Tornello, S. (2010). Gay fathers' pathways to parenthood: International perspectives. *Journal of Family Research, 22*, 103–116. https://doi.org/10.2307/j.ctvdf0csb.11

Potgieter, C. (2003). Black South African lesbians: Discourses on motherhood and women's roles. *Journal of Lesbian Studies, 7*, 135–151. https://doi.org/10.1300/J155v07n03_10

Prendergast, S., & MacPhee, D. (2018). Family resilience amid stigma and discrimination: A conceptual model for families headed by same-sex parents. *Family Relations, 67*, 26–40. https://doi.org/10.1111/fare.12296

Purkayastha, B. (2012). Intersectionality in a transnational world. *Gender & Society, 26*, 55–66. https://doi.org/10.1177/0891243211426725

Pyke, K. (2000). "The normal American family" as an interpretive structure of family life among grown children of Korean and Vietnamese immigrants. *Journal of Marriage and Family, 62*, 240–255. https://doi.org/10.1111/j.1741-3737.2000.00240.x

Quiroz, P. (2007). *Adoption in a color-blind society.* Lanham, MD: Rowman & Littlefield.

Roberts, D. (2009). *Shattered bonds: The color of child welfare.* New York, NY: Basic Books.

Rodriguez, J. (2014). *Sexual futures, queer gestures, and other Latina longings.* New York, NY: NYU Press.

Romero, V. (2005). Asians, gay marriage, and immigration: Family unification at a crossroads. *Indiana International & Comparative Law Review, 15*, 337–347.

Ross, L., Epstein, R., Goldfinger, C., Steele, L., Anderson, S., & Strike, C. (2014). Lesbian and queer mothers navigating the adoption system: The impacts on mental health. *Health Sociology Review, 17*, 254–266. https://doi.org/10.5172/hesr.451.17.3.254

Rudrappa, S., & Collins, C. (2015). Altruistic agencies and compassionate consumers: Moral framing of transnational surrogacy. *Gender & Society, 29*, 937–959. https://doi.org/10.1177/0891243215602922

Ryan, M., & Berkowitz, D. (2009). Constructing gay and lesbian parent families beyond the closet. *Qualitative*

*Sociology, 32*, 153–172. https://doi.org/10.1007/s11133-009-9124-6

Ryan, M., & Moras, A. (2017). Race matters in lesbian donor insemination: Whiteness and heteronormativity in co-constituted narratives. *Ethnic and Racial Studies, 40*, 579–596. https://doi.org/10.1080/01419870.2016.1201581

Schneebaum, A., & Badgett, M. V. L. (2018). Poverty in US lesbian and gay couple households. *Feminist Economics.* https://doi.org/10.1080/13545701.2018.1441533

Singh, A., & Shelton, K. (2011). A content analysis of LGBT qualitative research in counseling: A ten-year review. *Journal of Counseling and Development, 89*, 217–226. https://doi.org/10.1002/j.1556-6678.2011.tb00080.x

Smith, D. (1993). The standard North American family: SNAF as an ideological code. *Journal of Family Issues, 14*, 50–65. https://doi.org/10.1177/0192513X93014001005

Spade, D., & Rohlfs, R. (2016). Legal equality, gay numbers and the (after?)math of eugenics. *The Scholar and Feminist Online, 13*, 1–25.

Stormhøj, C. (2018). Still much to be achieved: Intersecting regimes of oppression, social critique, and 'thick' justice for lesbian and gay people. *Sexualities.* Advance online publication. https://doi.org/10.1177/1363460718790873

Stotzer, R. (2013). *LGBTQI Hawai'i: A needs assessment of the lesbian, gay, bisexual, transgender, queer, and intersex communities in the state of Hawai'i. Supplement 2, findings by gender.* Honolulu, HI: Myron B. Thompson School of Social Work, University of Hawai'i at Mānoa.

Stotzer, R., Herman, J., & Hasenbush, A. (2014). *Transgender parenting: A review of existing research.* Los Angeles, CA: The Williams Institute, UCLA School of Law.

Strmic-Pawl, H., Jackson, B., & Garner, S. (2018). Race counts: Racial and ethnic data on the U.S. Census and the implications for tracking inequality. *Sociology of Race and Ethnicity, 4*, 1–13. https://doi.org/10.1177/2332649217742869

Sullivan, M. (2004). *The family of woman: Lesbian mothers, their children, and the undoing of gender.* Berkeley, CA: University of California Press.

Swarr, A., & Nagar, R. (2003). Dismantling assumptions: Interrogating 'lesbian' struggles for identity and survival in India and South Africa. *Signs: Journal of Women in Culture and Society, 29*, 491–516. https://doi.org/10.1086/378573

Tasker, F., & Rensten, K. (2019). Social science research on heterosexual relationship dissolution and divorce where one parent comes out as LGB. In A. Goldberg & A. Romero (Eds.), *LGBTQ divorce and relationship dissolution: Psychological and legal perspectives and implications for practice* (pp. 173–194). New York, NY: Oxford University Press.

Taylor, R., Forsythe-Brown, I., Lincoln, K., & Chatters, L. (2015). Extended family support networks of Caribbean Black adults in the United States. *Journal of Family Issues, 38*, 522–546. https://doi.org/10.1177/0192513X15573868

van Eeden-Moorefield, B., Few-Demo, A., Benson, K., Bible, J., & Lummer, S. (2018). A content analysis of LGBT research in top family journals 2000-2015. *Journal of Family Issues, 39*, 1374–1395. https://doi.org/10.1177/0192513X17710284

Ventura, R., Rodríguez-Polo, X., & Roca-Cuberes, C. (2019). "Wealthy gay couples buying babies produced in India by poor womb-women": Audience interpretations of transnational surrogacy in TV news. *Journal of Homosexuality, 66*, 609–634. https://doi.org/10.1080/00918369.2017.1422947

Vidal Ortiz, S., & Martínez, J. (2018). Latinx thoughts: Latinidad with an X. *Latino Studies, 16*, 384–395. https://doi.org/10.1057/s41276-018-0137-8

Vora, K. (2012). Limits of "labor": Accounting for affect and the biological in transnational surrogacy and service work. *South Atlantic Quarterly, 111*, 681–700. https://doi.org/10.1215/00382876-1724138

Wekker, G. (2006). *The politics of passion: Women's sexual culture in the Afro-Surinamese diaspora.* New York, NY: Columbia University Press.

Wyman-Battalen, A., Dow-Fleisner, S., Brodzinsky, D., & McRoy, R. (2019). Lesbian, gay, and heterosexual adoptive parents' attitudes towards racial socialization practices. *Journal of Evidence-Informed Social Work.* Advance online publication. https://doi.org/10.1080/23761407.2019.1576565

# LGBTQ-Parent Families in the United States and Economic Well-Being

Naomi G. Goldberg, Alyssa Schneebaum, Laura E. Durso, and M. V. Lee Badgett

Best estimates suggest that approximately 4.5% of adults in the United States identify as lesbian, gay, bisexual, and/or transgender (LGBT) (Newport, 2018), equating to approximately 11 million adults.[1] Several studies find that LGBT people are less likely to want to be parents and to actually be parents than their cisgender[2] heterosexual peers (Gates, Badgett, Macomber, & Chambers, 2007; Riskind & Patterson, 2010). Analyses of the 2008 and 2010 General Social Survey find that 37% of LGBT-identified people have had a child (Gates, 2013). Data from the 2016 American Community Survey (ACS) show that 23.9% of female same-sex couples and 8.1% of male same-sex couples were raising a child under the age of 18 (Goldberg & Conron, 2018). The 2015 US Transgender Survey shows that 18% of transgender people reported having a child of any age (James et al., 2016). A 2013 Pew survey similarly found that 35% of LGBT adults are parents compared to 14% of adults in the general public (Pew Research Center, 2013). Using these estimates, researchers suggest there are approximately 3 million LGBT adults who are parents in the United States (Gates, 2013). What is known about LGBTQ people who parent remains thin compared to the vast research about parents in general.

This chapter explores what is currently known about the economic well-being—or lack thereof—of LGBTQ parents and, more broadly, families headed by LGBTQ adults. This chapter also highlights the gaps in this knowledge that should drive crucial further research. More needs to be known about the economic well-being and financial security of LGBTQ-parent families, so that communities and policies can better support them.

Much of this chapter focuses on the economic status of (a) individuals who identify as LGBTQ and have children and (b) those who are in same-

---

[1] Applying Gallup's rate of 4.5% to the current estimates of the number of adults in the United States from the US Census Bureau.

[2] This term is used to refer to individuals who identify with a gender that is typically associated with the sex they were assigned at birth, as opposed to individuals who identify as transgender.

N. G. Goldberg (✉)
Movement Advancement Project, Boulder, CO, USA
e-mail: naomi@lgbtmap.org

A. Schneebaum
Department of Economics, Vienna University of Economics and Business, Vienna, Austria
e-mail: alyssa.schneebaum@wu.ac.at

L. E. Durso
Center for American Progress, Washington, DC, USA

M. V. L. Badgett
Department of Economics, University of Massachusetts Amherst, Crotty Hall, Amherst, MA, USA

Williams Institute, UCLA, Los Angeles, CA, USA
e-mail: lbadgett@econs.umass.edu

© Springer Nature Switzerland AG 2020
A. E. Goldberg, K. R. Allen (eds.), *LGBTQ-Parent Families*,
https://doi.org/10.1007/978-3-030-35610-1_6

sex couples and have a child under the age of 18 living in their homes. This is because these are the most frequent ways in which LGBTQ families are currently identifiable in large quantitative datasets (see chapter "The Use of Representative Datasets to Study LGBTQ-Parent Families: Challenges, Advantages, and Opportunities"). While these data sources are undoubtedly limited in their ability to explore the nuances and contours of all LGBTQ parents' economic lives, they provide a helpful starting place for discussions about the contours of the economic health of LGBTQ-parent families. Where possible and appropriate, we supplement the analysis with context and lessons from smaller-scale qualitative studies of the economic lives of LGBTQ people with children. These qualitative studies, while not representative of the populations they address, can give compelling information about some of the particulars of being LGBTQ and having a family. As an example, two qualitative studies address the particular concerns of LGBTQ parents in selecting their children's school and helping their children deal with the challenges of being "different" at school (Goldberg, Allen, Black, Frost, & Manley, 2018; Nixon, 2011). In particular, they show how sexual orientation interacts with class as well as race, location, and ability to present LGBTQ parents with unique challenges in raising their children, especially in terms of the children's educational opportunities. LGBTQ parents face a different set of concerns in choosing a school for their child, and they are sometimes less able to help their children deal with problems at school because of their own lack of acceptance by school employees. These types of stories cannot come out of the large datasets on which we base the core of our analysis below, but we refer back to them to give a voice to the story our large-scale data tell.

## Who Are "LGBTQ-Parent Families"?

When thinking about what LGBTQ-parent families' economic lives look like, it is important to define what is meant by "LGBTQ-parent families." In this chapter, we focus on one particular family configuration—families comprised of at least one child and at least one parent who identifies as LGBTQ. However, for reasons articulated further below, identifying such families or parents, particularly in surveys, is challenging and presents limitations in the current literature that need to be further examined in future research. LGBTQ-parent families with children may form in many ways, as discussed elsewhere in this book. There are LGBTQ-identified individuals who choose to intentionally parent either individually or with one or more other people. Paths to parenthood for so-called "intentional" LGBTQ parents could include using assisted reproductive technology, surrogacy, or adopting. A growing body of research explores how some LGBTQ-parent families involve more than two parents, such as including a third person who may be biologically related to a child like a sperm or egg donor or including significant individuals who are nonlegally or biologically related in "families of choice" (Robbins, Durso, Bewkes, & Schultz, 2017). There are also LGBTQ individuals who had children from a previous relationship *before* identifying to others as, or even recognizing their own identities as, LGBTQ (see chapter "LGBTQ Parenting Post-Heterosexual Relationship Dissolution").

## Measurement Challenges in Identifying LGBTQ-Parent Families

As a result of these various pathways to parenthood, it can be difficult to identify all families that contain at least one parent who is LGBTQ, particularly when any number of parents may or may not identify as LGBTQ. Take the example of a woman who has a biological child with a male partner, but they separate, and she then partners with a woman, with whom she parents the child independent of the involvement of the child's biological father. The woman in this example may have identified as bisexual throughout her life, but that identity may not be captured by survey instruments which collect data solely on relationship status and the gender of the individuals within those relationships. In this case, the woman may be incorrectly classified as straight while in her first relationship and incorrectly coded again as a lesbian in her second. While the measurement of relationships and household composition has improved over time, including recent changes to the decennial census which will allow same-sex couples to better indicate the legal status of their relationships (U.S. Census Bureau, 2018a), limitations in the measurement of sexual orientation challenge researchers' ability to identify the total universe of LGBTQ-parent families.

While federal surveys are often the gold standard tools used to define and understand the characteristics and needs of families in the United States, all too often these surveys do not include demographic questions about sexual orientation and gender identity. For example, the decennial census and the annual ACS are household surveys that are used as the foundation for much research about family composition and economic well-being. However, both surveys include household rosters that ask about relationship status to a single reference person but do not currently include questions about sexual orientation or gender identity. Given the structure of the surveys and the questions asked, researchers must focus on "same-sex couple" households, in which the householder and another adult are identified as the same sex on the form and the other adult is identified as a spouse or unmarried partner. Undoubtedly included in these "same-sex couple" households are couples in which one or both people identify as lesbian or gay, as bisexual, and/or as transgender. Similarly, in "different-sex couple" households (those in which one member of the couple identifies as male and one as female), there are undoubtedly some couples in which one or both members identify as bisexual and/or transgender.

We can see only hints of this kind of complexity in existing large datasets. Analysis of the 2014–2016 ACS data shows that in 68% of same-sex couples, the children were identified as the biological child(ren) of the householder, while in 16.3% of same-sex couples, the children were identified as stepchildren (Goldberg & Conron, 2018). These could be planned families, but a substantial number are likely children from a previous relationship (Gates, 2015a). Several analyses have found that LGB parents reported having their first child at earlier ages than heterosexual adults, suggesting that these children may have been the result of a previous different-sex relationship. These patterns are also consistent with LGB youth being more likely to experience unintended pregnancy or fatherhood than their heterosexual peers (Gates, 2011a). Finally, it is interesting to note an emerging trend toward fewer LGB people reporting parenthood, possibly because LGB people are coming out earlier and having earlier relationships with same-sex partners, making them less likely to have had children in previous different-sex relationships (Gates, 2011a). However, one recent study of LGBTQ people using a non-federal dataset indicates significant desire among LGBTQ millennials to become parents. Specifically, a study commissioned by the Family Equality Council found that 77% of LGBTQ people ages 18–35 are already parents or are considering having a child (Harris & Hopping-Winn, 2019).

## Rates of Cohabitation, Marital Status, and Related Demographics of LGBTQ People

Recent data from two surveys underscore the complexity of identifying LGBTQ people (and therefore LGBTQ parents) based on their cohabitation or what their family structures may look like. First, LGBTQ people are sometimes in same-sex couples, sometimes in different-sex couples, and sometimes living alone or in other family configurations. According to the Gallup Daily Tracking Poll from June 2016 to June 2017, of LGBT-identified adults in the United States, 10.2% are in a married same-sex couple; 6.6% are unmarried and living with a same-sex partner; 4.2% are unmarried and living with a different-sex partner; 13.1% are in a married different-sex couple; and the remaining 65.4% are not currently partnered or married (Jones, 2017). Analysis of the National Health Interview Survey (NHIS) from 2013 to 2016 finds higher rates of marriage cohabitation for LGB-identified people; 56.6% of lesbian women reported being married or cohabiting compared to 40.7% of bisexual women and 58.6% of heterosexual women (Badgett, 2018). A similar trend is seen in the NHIS among men, with 65.3% of heterosexual men reporting being married or cohabiting compared to 42.6% of gay men and 28.1% of bisexual men. Second, many—but not all—people in same-sex couples are LGB. In the same survey, 87% of women in married female same-sex couples identify as lesbian and 5% as bisexual; 96% of men in married same-sex couples identify as gay and none as bisexual (Badgett, 2018). A higher proportion of people in unmarried same-sex couples in the NHIS identify as bisexual: 9% of women in those couples identify as bisexual and 1% of men in those couples say that they are bisexual. (Some people in same-sex couples identify as heterosexual.) Certainly, given past research findings that bisexual adults comprise as much as half of LGB adults (Gates, 2011b), these data speak to the varying ways in which both gay lesbian people and bisexual people partner and form families (see chapter "What Do We Now Know About Bisexual Parenting? A Continuing Call for Research"). In fact, the 2013 NHIS revealed that 51% of bisexual-identified adults raising children were married with a different-sex partner; 11% had a different-sex unmarried partner; and 4% had a same-sex spouse or partner (Gates, 2014).

While many of the above studies include transgender people, there are fewer nationally representative surveys that include questions about transgender status or allow for the identification of transgender respondents. For example, in 2016, the Federal Interagency Working Group on Improving Measurement of Sexual Orientation and Gender Identity in Federal Surveys identified only six federal surveys which included at least one question assessing gender identity (2016). The Census Bureau alone collects data from more than 100 surveys (U.S. Census Bureau, 2019), and there are more than 200,000 federal datasets available on data.gov as of this writing (Data.Gov, 2019). While not every survey instrument is appropriate for the collection of gender identity data, there is a clear shortage of information available to identify transgender parents.

In their 2014 review of the literature about transgender people who are parents (51 studies), Stotzer, Herman, and Hasenbush found that between one-quarter and one-half of transgender and gender nonconforming respondents in these studies said they were parents, with higher rates overall for transgender women than for transgender men. A 2015 survey of more than 27,700 transgender and gender nonconforming individuals found that 18% reported being a parent to a child of any age (James et al., 2016). Looking just at respondents who had a legally related child (either through birth or legal adoption) under the age of 18 living with them, this number drops to 14% for all respondents, though 19% of respondents ages 18–24 had a related minor child living in their homes. Of these transgender parents, a majority were out to their children (69%; James et al., 2016). In the 2015–2016 California Health Interview Survey, 6.1% of transgender or gender nonconforming respondents reported having a child living in their home compared to 32.7% of cisgender respondents (Author analysis, 2018). In a 2011 survey of 6,400 transgender and gender nonconforming people, 38% of respondents indicated they were parents, with higher rates for American Indian and Latino/a respondents (45% and 40%). For respondents who had transitioned or come out later in life, 82% of respondents who came out or transitioned at age 55 or older had children (Grant et al., 2011).

## Theoretical Frameworks and Assumptions in the Literature

There are multiple considerations for contextualizing the available data on the economic health of LGBTQ-parent families. First is the approach to the assessment of economic instability. While we present here four different markers of economic instability, there are numerous other benchmarks that provide information about the relative economic stability of individuals and families, such as wealth and assets, homeownership, and insurance coverage (see, e.g., a list of 21 indicators of economic stability in the 2014 report, *Building Local Momentum for National Change: Half in Ten Annual Poverty and Inequality Indicators Report*, by the Center for American Progress Action Fund, Leadership Conference on Civil and Human Rights, and the Coalition for Human Needs, 2014). Unfortunately, there are currently limited data available to completely fill in the picture of the stability of LGBTQ-parent families using these metrics. In addition, data available for the present review include a standard measure of the poverty rate, which only takes into account an individual's income and household composition. Researchers and other practitioners have noted the limitations of this approach to measuring poverty and recommended using a calculation of poverty that takes additional variables into account (e.g., summarized in Dalaker, 2017). The poverty rates reviewed in the current chapter are also calculated at the individual level, and the available data do not allow for us to understand the impact of how economic instability within families of origin contribute to the lack of economic mobility for low and middle-income communities (e.g., Wagmiller & Adelman, 2009).

Second, much of the literature uses non-LGBTQ people or different-sex couples as the typical comparison group, which presumes that these individuals provide the standard by which LGBTQ people and families should be judged. This type of approach presumes that deviations from the standard are indicative of areas of concern and that the absence of a difference between the groups indicates the absence of a problem. Both assumptions limit our ability to determine what are meaningful differences across sexual orientation and gender identity, what strengths and resiliencies might be particularly valuable for LGBTQ people, and, for an outcome such as poverty, what might bias our thinking toward advancing policies and programs that close gaps rather than reducing economic instability for all. Similarly, much of the research reviewed here looks at family structures that closely resemble the traditional nuclear family—that is, a two-parent-headed household with minor children—and does not yet provide comprehensive information about alternative family structures, including chosen family.

Finally, there is extensive literature across a range of fields of study showing links between experiencing discrimination and negative outcomes like poor health and economic instability (e.g., Frost, Levahot, & Meyer, 2015; Kim & Fredriksen-Goldsen, 2017). As such, it is easy to try and look for causal pathways that incorporate the impact of institutional and/or interpersonal discrimination to understand how LGBTQ people and LGBTQ-parent families become less economically stable. While discrimination is undoubtedly a factor that helps explain the relative stability of some LGBTQ people and families, it is likely not the only factor which explains the outcomes reviewed in this chapter. For example, one may hypothesize that experiences of discrimination, or even the fear of discrimination, would result in lower reported rates of receiving public benefits such as nutrition assistance. However, as reviewed later, LGBTQ people tend to report higher rates of receipt of these benefits, indicating that the causal pathways are more complex and additional research is necessary to understand who is able to access these benefits and who may be continuing to experience barriers to access that are not readily identifiable when looking at rates of receipt. Assuming the significant impact of discrimination on the basis of sexual orientation and gender identity alone also risks ignoring the influence of other types of discrimination and oppression on LGBTQ people and their families. For example, intergenerational transfers of wealth have been shown to contribute to the maintenance of the racial wealth gap (McKernan, Ratcliffe, Simms, & Zhang, 2014), and this may help to explain why, for example, rates of poverty among children who live with Black male same-sex couples are startlingly high (Badgett, Durso, & Schneebaum, 2013).

## Higher Economic Insecurity for LGBTQ-Parent Families

The challenges of accurately reflecting the lives of LGBTQ people underscore the need for increased systematic data collection at the federal, state, and local levels focused on sexual orientation and gender identity. As noted above, large, nationally representative surveys like the decennial census and ACS rarely ask questions about sexual orientation and/or gender identity. That said, there are large, representative surveys that provide important information about the economic well-being of LGBTQ people, same-sex couples, and those raising children.

Overall, nationally representative surveys suggest that LGBTQ people and same-sex couples raising children face greater economic challenges compared to their non-LGBTQ and different-sex couple peers. There is evidence that some LGBTQ-parent families are more economically vulnerable than others, in part because of the broader patterns of social inequalities for various demographic groups of people. For example, Gates (2015b) finds that LGBT parents and same-sex couples raising children are more likely to be women (77% of the same-sex couples raising children are female), relatively young, and more likely to be people of color (34% of same-sex couples raising children)—all of which would point to lower overall incomes compared to men, older parents, and White parents, respectively (Gates, 2013). This next section summarizes the key findings on the economic security of LGBTQ families based on four key indicators: (a) household income, (b) poverty rates, (c) food insecurity, and (d) receipt of public benefits such as the Supplemental Nutrition Assistance Program (SNAP).

## Household Income

A growing body of research finds a disparity in the incomes of individual LGBTQ people compared to heterosexual, cisgender people (Badgett, 2018; Carpenter, Eppink, & Gonzalez, forthcoming; Newport, 2018). For example, the Gallup

Daily Tracking poll has included a single LGBT identity question for several years. One consistent finding of the survey is that people with lower incomes are more likely to report being LGBT, although we cannot say which characteristic is causing the other. For example, in the 2017 Gallup Daily Tracking poll, 6.2% of adults in the United States with annual household incomes less than $36,000 identified as LGBT, compared to 3.9% of adults with annual household incomes of $90,000 or more (Newport, 2018).

Complicating some of these findings are data from the US Census and other household roster-based surveys, which find that male same-sex couples report having higher household incomes than different-sex couples and female same-sex couples, while at the same time women in same-sex couples frequently earn more than women in different-sex couples and men in same-sex couples earn less than men in different-sex couples (Black, Sanders, & Taylor, 2007; Gates, 2015b; Klawitter, 2011, 2015). Much of this difference in household income could be related to the presence (or absence) of a female wage earner since, on the whole, men continue to be paid more than women in the United States (see Blau & Kahn, 2017). Yet, when examining household incomes together, these inequalities for men in same-sex couples and the individual advantage for women in same-sex couples translate into household advantages for households with two male earners or even one male earner and disadvantages for households with two female earners.

When looking specifically at LGBTQ-identified parents and same-sex couples with children, research finds that these families report lower household incomes than their peers. In the 2010 decennial census, the median household income of same-sex couples with minor children was $10,100 lower than different-sex couples with minor children (Gates, 2013). When considering different-sex and same-sex couples with only biological children in their household, Census Bureau analysis of 2009 ACS data shows that there are gaps in important economic outcomes for these two groups (Krivickas & Lofquist, 2011). Namely, the average gap in annual household income between married different-sex and same-sex couples with biological children was nearly $13,000. Further, those in married different-sex couples reported higher educational attainment than same-sex couples with children; 26.3% of different-sex parent couples and 20.8% of same-sex parent couples were comprised of two individuals who both had at least a bachelor's degree. These different-sex couples also reported higher labor force participation, with 59.4% of different-sex couples reporting that both spouses were employed, compared to 55.1% of same-sex couples. Different-sex couples with biological children also were more likely to own their homes than were same-sex couples (Krivickas & Lofquist, 2011).

## Poverty Rates

When examining household incomes, it is helpful to consider how many adults and children those incomes are supporting to better measure the economic resources that families have at their disposal. The federal poverty measure does just this—it sets a threshold for families considered "poor" based on the size of a family unit and the household income. In 2017, for a household with four people, including two children, the poverty threshold was $24,858 annually (U.S. Census Bureau, 2018c). Hence, reports of the percent of families below this threshold give us a clearer picture of families with very low incomes.

We start first with studies of data that compare same-sex couples and different-sex couples (Albelda, Badgett, Schneebaum, & Gates, 2009; Badgett et al., 2013; Schneebaum & Badgett, 2019). These studies show that female same-sex couples have higher rates of poverty than married different-sex couples (and sometimes than unmarried different-sex couples), while male same-sex couples generally have lower poverty rates than married different-sex couples. As noted earlier, that pattern largely reflects the gender gap in earnings that gives two men an income advantage on average over two women in a couple or a man and a woman. However, another consistent finding is that same-sex couples have a greater

risk of poverty compared to married different-sex couples after controlling for the many factors that predict poverty, such as education, employment status, race, age, and disability (Albelda et al., 2009; Badgett et al., 2013; Schneebaum & Badgett, 2019). In fact, it is likely that the poverty rates for same-sex couples would be even greater than currently observed, were it not for the protective effects of having higher average levels of education, higher rates of labor force participation, and fewer children compared to different-sex couples (Schneebaum & Badgett, 2019).

Studies that look at self-identified LGBTQ people find different patterns for the individual groups that make up the LGBTQ community. Lesbians and gay men appear to be as likely to be poor as are heterosexual people, while bisexual and transgender people are *more* likely to be poor than heterosexual or cisgender people, respectively (Badgett, 2018; Carpenter et al., forthcoming). A 2017 nationally representative survey conducted by the Center for American Progress found, for example, that 24% of bisexual men and 21% of bisexual women had household incomes below the federal poverty threshold compared to 13% of lesbians, 12% of gay men, 14% of straight women, and 6% of straight men (Mirza, 2018).

Mirroring measures in the broader population of families with children, LGBT individuals and same-sex couples with children have higher rates of poverty than childless same-sex couples or LGBT people (Albelda et al., 2009; Badgett et al., 2013; Badgett, 2018; Schneebaum & Badgett, 2019). However, in many surveys, LGBTQ-parent families report higher rates of having low incomes than other families with children. For example, in the 2012 Gallup Daily Tracking poll, 35.3% of single LGBT adults raising children had household incomes of $12,000 or less—near the poverty level for a one-person household, let alone a single adult raising one or more children—compared to 12.1% of single heterosexual people raising children (Badgett et al., 2013).

Analysis of the 2010 ACS showed that children under the age of 18 in same-sex couple families were more likely to live in poverty and to live in low-income families (200% of the federal poverty line) than were children living in households headed by married different-sex couples (Badgett et al., 2013). Specifically, 47.6% of children raised by male same-sex couples were living in families that are low income as were 38.7% of children raised by female same-sex couples. This compares to 31.7% of children raised by married different-sex couples. What is particularly remarkable about these findings is that, as noted above, typically male same-sex couples tend to have higher household incomes than both married different-sex couples and female same-sex couples, primarily due to having two male wage earners. But children in the homes of male same-sex couples are more likely to live in poverty or to be low income than married different-sex couples. This is likely due in part to the influence of structural racism and other factors which drive up the poverty rate for children living with male same-sex couples of color, particularly Black male same-sex couples, which is discussed further below.

## Food Insecurity

One frequently cited indicator of a family's economic resources is food insecurity: that is, how frequently during a set time period, typically the past month or the past year, a family did not have enough money for food. While some families who report food insecurity may also live at or below the poverty rate, families living in high-cost urban centers, for example, may have household incomes above the poverty rate but still struggle to consistently afford food. For example, in 2017, 30.8% of households with incomes at or below 185% of the poverty line were food insecure compared to 36.8% of households with incomes at or below the poverty line (U.S. Department of Agriculture, 2017). Hence, this measure is a helpful proxy for measuring broader economic insecurity beyond the poverty rate because it provides a measure of households' abilities to afford a basic necessity (food), and it takes into consideration a number of economic pressure points for families ranging from high

housing costs to energy and food prices to income (RTI International, 2014).

Again, mirroring the poverty findings, research shows that LGBT adults and individuals in same-sex couples are at an increased risk of food insecurity (Brown, Romero, & Gates, 2016), with those adults and families raising children at even high risk. For example, one-third (33%) of LGBT parents with minor children reported not having enough money for food in the past year compared to 20% of non-LGBT respondents, according to analysis of the June–December 2014 Gallup Daily Tracking poll (Brown et al., 2016). A multivariate analysis of the Gallup data reveals that LGBT adults with children are 1.7 times more likely to report not having enough money for food in the past year than non-LGBT adults with children. Similarly, in the 2014 NHIS, 17% of LGB people with children reported food insecurity in the past 30 days, compared to 12% of heterosexual adults—with both groups reporting increased food insecurity compared to those respondents without children (Brown et al., 2016).

## Receipt of Public Benefits

Eligibility for various public benefit programs designed to support low-income families varies. For example, the Supplemental Nutrition Assistance Program (SNAP) is the primary program designed to provide food assistance to individuals and families with low incomes—in most states incomes at or below 130% of the federal poverty level, which for a family of four is $2,790 in gross monthly income (U. S. Department of Agriculture, 2019). Receipt of SNAP benefits provides an indication of the extent to which individuals and families may be struggling economically and the extent to which they are connected to services and benefits.

A 2017 survey by the Center for American Progress examined reported receipt of several public programs including SNAP, Medicaid, unemployment insurance, and housing assistance for people who identified as LGBTQ and non-

LGBTQ respondents (Rooney, Whittington, & Durso, 2018). While the analyses do not specifically identify those respondents with minor children, these data show that LGBTQ people and their families (defined to include the survey respondent, the respondent's partner or spouse, and/or the partner's child) were generally more likely than non-LGBTQ people to receive these types of assistance in the year prior to the survey. For example, LGBTQ respondents were 1.6 times more likely than their peers to report that they or a member of their family had Medicaid coverage in the previous year. Moreover, LGBTQ people were more than twice as likely to have received SNAP benefits and 2.5 times more likely to receive public housing assistance.

Taking into consideration demographic characteristics such as sex, age, race, and educational attainment, LGB adults with children were 1.43 times more likely to participate in SNAP in the past year compared to heterosexual adults with children in the 2014 NHIS data (Brown et al., 2016). Analysis of the 2011–2013 National Survey of Family Growth shows that adult ages 18–44 have even higher rates of SNAP participation among LGB respondents with children; 46% of LGB adults with children reported participating in SNAP in the past year compared to 26% of heterosexual parents (Brown et al., 2016).

Mirroring the findings presented earlier that bisexual people, in general, have higher rates of poverty (Fredriksen-Goldsen, Kim, Barkan, Balsam, & Mincer, 2011; Pew Research Center, 2013), several studies have found that bisexual people, including parents, are more likely to receive public benefits. The 2017 Center for American Progress nationally representative survey found that 27% of bisexual women and their families had received SNAP and 21% had received Medicaid benefits in the past year compared to 10% of lesbians and their families (Mirza, 2018). In the 2014 NHIS, two in five bisexual adults with children had participated in SNAP in the past year compared to 26% of lesbians or gay men with children and 22% of straight adults with children (Brown et al., 2016).

In a multivariate analysis of 2014 ACS, same-sex couples with children were twice as likely to participate in SNAP in the past year compared to different-sex couples with children (Brown et al., 2016). Nearly one in four (24%) same-sex couples with children reported participating in SNAP in the past year compared to 14% of different-sex couples with children. Female same-sex couples raising children drive much of the disparity; 27% of female same-sex couples with children receive SNAP payments compared to 14% of male same-sex couples raising children.

In sum, available quantitative studies paint a picture of overall increased economic instability for LGBTQ-parent families, as demonstrated by income disparities, elevated relative rates of poverty and food insecurity, and higher reported receipt of public benefits. These data also suggest that not all LGBTQ-parent families may experience economic instability in the same way, which is covered in the next section. In the context of families, it is critical to keep in mind that economic resources are one of many factors that influence family and child well-being, ranging from parental time, quality of parent-child relationships, and the relationships among adults in a household to family stability. That said, families who struggle economically face added stress—both purely economic and also stress associated with the mental, emotional, and physical toll that food insecurity, concerns about safety and adequate housing, and more can take, all of which can make parenting more difficult and may affect family and child well-being (e.g., Mistry, Vandewater, Huston, & McLoyd, 2002).

## Economic Diversity Among LGBTQ-Parent Families: Who Is at Risk?

While the research summarized in the previous section repeatedly finds high rates of economic insecurity across four measures for LGBTQ-parent families, there is economic diversity within LGBTQ-parent families that mirrors the broader demographic diversity of these families. Certainly not every LGBTQ-parent family experiences economic insecurity. In fact, some LGBTQ-parent families report that they are thriving economically, with higher incomes than their heterosexual peers (Gates, 2015b). On the other hand, research finds that certain families are at increased risk for economic insecurity—frequently mirroring work from broader poverty studies in finding that women, Black and Hispanic people, unmarried and/or single parent families, and individuals with lower education attainment or lower labor force attachment all report higher rates of poverty (Fontenot, Semega, & Kollar, 2018).

## Race and Ethnicity

Existing research suggests clear patterns of the influence of race on rates of poverty for same-sex couples and, in particular, indicates impacts of the intersections of race, gender, and sexual orientation. Analysis of the 2010 ACS found large disparities for African American children in male same-sex households: 52.3% of African American children in same-sex male household were living in poverty as were 37.7% of African American children in female same-sex headed households (Badgett et al., 2013). These rates compare to 15.2% of African American children living with married different-sex parents. Similar disparities are not seen when comparing family type for White, Asian, or Hispanic children in the 2010 ACS, though rates are elevated for poor children in coupled families indicating "other races." Incredibly high rates of poverty for families headed by African American same-sex couples emphasize the need to think about the intersections of race, class, and sexual orientation and gender identity when conducting further research and designing policy interventions to improve family economic stability.

## Age of Children and Caregiving Specialization

Similar to other families, same-sex couples raising young children, in particular, experienced added economic strain. Analysis of 2010 ACS data reveal that poverty in same-sex couples is highest among families with young children—22.6% of children ages 0–5 in female same-sex couples lived in poverty, as did 24.2% of children that age in male same-sex couples.

These findings may speak to the economic strain of raising young children, particularly decisions around childcare and whether one parent may step out of the labor market entirely or reduce hours to provide care for young children. Since few parents have access to paid family leave in the United States, spending more time on caring labor in the home means the loss of one parent's income. Many families with children make these decisions, and same-sex couples may be similar in the ways they specialize in terms of time spent at work and time caring for children. For example, analysis of 2000 decennial census data revealed just as married women in different-sex couples work fewer hours per week and are less likely to work at all compared to men in different-sex couples, the same holds for one of the women in same-sex couples (Antecol & Steinberger, 2011). That is, same-sex couples and different-sex couples make similar choices about labor force participation once they have children.

## Marital Status

Much has been written about the economic benefits of marriage, while far fewer studies have examined the economic benefits for LGBTQ people and same-sex couples specifically (Badgett, 2009; Ramos, Goldberg, & Badgett, 2009). Broader research suggests that there is selection into marriage for individuals with increased individual incomes and other indicators of future financial security such as higher educational attainment and an increasing age at first marriage (e.g., Cherlin, 2018; Edin & Reed, 2005; Smock & Manning, 1997). As not all couples—both same-sex and different-sex—choose to legally marry, comparisons between married and unmarried individuals can be used to tease out the impacts of both sexual orientation and marital status on economic stability.

With the increasing availability of marriage to same-sex couples reaching full nationwide access in 2015, early indications are that similar trends hold for same-sex couples. In an examination of federal income tax returns filed by approximately 52.1 million joint filers between 2013 and 2015, both male and female same-sex couples who filed joint returns (an estimated 250,450 couples) had higher average incomes than did different-sex couple filers and were more likely to earn more than $150,000 annually, though male same-sex couples filing joint returns had more than $50,000 more in average adjusted gross income compared to different-sex filers (Fisher, Gee, & Looney, 2018).

Additional data to support this contention comes from an analysis of 2013 ACS data, which compared same-sex couples raising children who were married to those who were not (Gates, 2015b). These data show that married same-sex couples raising children have higher household incomes than those who are unmarried and raising children. Specifically, combining male and female couples, married same-sex couples with children reported median household incomes of $97,000, compared to $67,900 for unmarried same-sex couple households with children. When looking only at those children raised in married couple households, children raised by married different-sex couples had slightly higher rates of poverty than those raised by married same-sex couples (11% vs. 9%).

Complicating this narrative, however, is an analysis of the wages of men and women in same-sex couples versus those in different-sex couples *of the same marital status,* that is, comparisons of the wages of people in married same-sex couples with those of people in married different-sex couples and the wages of people in unmarried same-sex couples with those of people in unmarried different-sex couples (Schneebaum & Schubert, 2017). Analysis of 2013–2015 ACS data shows that the sexual orientation wage gap for individuals in couples differs by marital status. The sexual orientation wage penalty consistently observed for men in same-sex couples exists only for men in *married* same-sex couples, but not for men in unmarried same-sex couples.

At the same time, the wage premium typically seen for women in same-sex couples is lower for those who are in married same-sex couples than for those in unmarried same-sex couples. Thus, marriage seems to be associated with some wage disadvantage for individuals in same-sex couples.

## Path to Parenthood

Becoming a parent for some LGBTQ people is a choice and may require time intensive and costly assistance and interventions beyond what creating a family may require of heterosexual couples. Consider the example of two gay men intentionally choosing to parent. They may pursue a domestic or international adoption or a private adoption through an agency or adopting from the child welfare system, or they may pursue any number of biological reproduction options such as surrogacy or serving as a biological parent to the child of a friend (see chapter "Gay Men and Surrogacy"). All of these paths to parenthood require a great deal of time and commitment, as well as financial resources (National LGBT Health Education Center, 2016). Similar paths may exist for lesbian or bisexual women and certainly transgender parents. Because of the intentionality, time, and costs associated with creating an "intentional" family for some LGBTQ adults, it may be that the economic resources of these families are greater than those of both non-LGBTQ-parent families and LGBTQ people who became parents in a different way, such as through a previous relationship (Goldberg et al., 2014).

While exploring the economic realities for LGBTQ parents through the lens of their path to parenthood is certainly an area for further research (as discussed in more depth below), there is some indication that how LGBTQ adults become parents may both explain economic differences and be driven by those differences. For example, when examining households with only adopted or only stepchildren, same-sex couples report having more economic resources (Krivickas & Lofquist, 2011). In the 2009 ACS, same-sex couple households with *adopted* children reported $23,000 more in household income than did married different-sex couples with adopted children, and they were more likely to have both partners employed and to both have at least a bachelor's degree. This could indicate that families that are created intentionally through the process of adoption have greater economic resources. This may also be related to the fact that some adoptions, particularly private adoptions, are expensive and therefore couples with higher incomes may be more likely to adopt.

## Opportunities and Recommendations for Future Research

While the body of research about the economic situation of families headed by LGBTQ parents is growing and becoming richer thanks to more nationally representative surveys including questions about sexual orientation and gender identity and to more in-depth qualitative studies of same-sex couples with children, there is still more research needed to better understand the economics of LGBTQ families and how they differ from other families. This section highlights a few key areas for new research, which includes (a) deeper investigation into the diversity of LGBTQ families, their family formation practices, and their economic health in both quantitative and qualitative work; (b) the impact of family instability on the economic lives of LGBTQ parents and their children; (c) the impact of marriage and related access to legal parental recognition; (d) unique or added barriers for LGBTQ families in accessing public benefits designed to support low-income families; (e) the impact of employment discrimination; and (f) the extent to which LGBTQ families are accessing pro-family supports such as paid leave, childcare subsidies, and more.

## Investigate More Deeply the Diversity of LGBTQ Families

LGBTQ people are more likely than the general population to identify as people of color, with 40% of LGBT adults in the 2017 Gallup Daily Tracking poll identifying as people of color (Gates, 2017), and as noted above, research finds that LGBT people of color and people of color in same-sex couples are more likely to parent (Grant et al., 2011; Kastanis & Wilson, 2014). Yet, very little work has been done to investigate the ways in which paths to parenthood, challenges in parenting, and the economic challenges that many people of color in the United States experience impact the financial well-being of LGBTQ parents of color and their children.

There are LGBTQ families who are relatively invisible in the economic literature about LGBTQ families—perhaps because of their relatively small numbers amidst families as a whole, because of a lack of intentionality to include them in research, or because researchers have not specifically identified them. These families include "families on the margins" (Moore & Stambolis-Ruhstorfer, 2013), such as families including more than two parents, blended families, non-urban LGBTQ families, families of color, and transgender parents.

Geographic analysis of same-sex couples raising children challenges popular notions of where LGBTQ people and their families live—the idea that they are concentrated in coastal, urban centers. Rather, analysis of 2013 ACS data reveals that the share of same-sex couples raising children does not vary by region of the country (Gates, 2015b). Additional work is needed to understand the regional or urban vs. rural economic dynamics for LGBTQ parents given that LGBTQ parents and their children live across the entire United States, including in states lacking vital nondiscrimination protections (see chapter "LGBTQ-Parent Families in Community Context").

## Examine the Impact of Family Instability on the Economic Security of LGBTQ Parents

There are very few longitudinal studies of LGBTQ people such as Fredriksen-Goldsen's "Aging with Pride: National Health, Aging, Sexuality and Gender Study" (see Fredriksen-Goldsen, Kim, Jung, & Goldsen, 2019) and Lunn and Obedin-Maliver's (2019) "The PRIDE Study." There are also few studies of LGBTQ parents and their families, such as Farr's "Longitudinal Study of Lesbian, Gay, and Heterosexual Parent Adoptive Families" (see Farr, 2017), Gartrell's "US National Longitudinal Lesbian Family Study" (see Gartrell, Bos, & Koh, 2019), and Goldberg's longitudinal study of same-sex and different-sex two-parent families ("The Transition to Adoptive Parenthood Project"; see Goldberg & Garcia, 2016). As a result, it remains difficult to assess the extent to which family instability may contribute to economic challenges. Broader research about the economic stability of families with children highlights the impact of family instability, including divorce, separation, birth, adoption, and death (Hill, Romich, Mattingly, Shamsuddin, & Wething, 2017). Yet the extent to which LGBTQ-parent families are identified in surveys does not allow for this type of analysis. Given the suggestion that some LGBTQ-parent families formed through previous relationships, this may be a contributing factor to the economic disparities seen across a number of metrics.

## Investigate the Impact of the Changing Legal Landscape for Families

Undoubtedly, the 2015 US Supreme Court ruling in *Obergefell v. Hodges* drastically shifted the legal landscape for many LGBTQ families. Rather than being seen as legal strangers under the law and potentially disconnected from vital supports that flow through marriage and the related parental recognition, same-sex couples now have access to legal recognition through marriage, and parents nationwide can secure legal ties to the children they are raising. Research suggests that these legal changes have had some positive impacts on the lives of LGBTQ people (Lennox Kail, Acosta, & Wright, 2015; Riggle, Wickham, Rostosky, Rothblum, & Balsam, 2017; Rostosky, Riggle, Rothblum, & Balsam, 2016). Little of that research has looked specifically at the economics of LGBTQ parents and their children. Further work is needed to explore the short- and long-term impacts of marriage and related secured legal ties between parents and children.

## Identify and Eliminate Barriers or Challenges in Accessing Public Benefits

While some research shows that LGBTQ families are more likely to receive certain public benefits designed to support low-income families, there is little research examining the experiences of families in seeking and or receiving this type of assistance that would allow for improvements from the systems designed to help people maintain basic living standards. Given the higher rates of poverty found for same-sex couples with children and LGBTQ people with children, it is possible that some families do not seek assistance out of fear of discrimination or other barriers (see Shlay, Weinraub, Harmon, & Tran, 2004, for examples of barriers cited by low-income families generally). Some may have already experienced discrimination when trying to access benefits. Without stringent nondiscrimination policies at the federal, state, and local level, and because the recognition of same-sex couples' relationships by federal and state governments is relatively recent, some LGBTQ families may not think that they are eligible to apply. A 2017 national representative survey of LGBTQ people found that 6.1% of all LGBTQ people had avoided getting services they or their family needed out of fear of discrimination, with 17.0% of those having had experienced discrimination in the past year reporting the same avoidance behavior (Singh & Durso, 2017).

## Quantify the Impacts of Employment Discrimination on the Economic Lives of LGBTQ Parents

Evidence of employment discrimination against LGBTQ people is extensive, ranging from lower wages to reports of adverse employment action to rates of complaints being filed with government agencies (e.g., Sears & Mallory, 2011). These experiences of discrimination undoubtedly impact the economic well-being of LGBTQ people, whether resulting in bouts of unemployment or underemployment or reduced wages. The extent to which LGBTQ parents may experience employment discrimination in a unique way, by virtue of being parents, or whether employment discrimination is a driving factor for the economic disparities experienced by many LGBTQ parents and families is an area ripe for research. Existing literature suggests that parenthood has varying impacts on employment and earnings based on sex, with women frequently being penalized in the workplace for being a parent while men experience an advantage (Budig, 2014; Hodges & Budig, 2010). Future research should explore the changing employment experiences of LGBTQ people as they become parents.

## Explore Whether and to What Extent LGBTQ Families Access Pro-family Supports

Raising a family is hard work, and the USA lacks many pro-family supports that can ease the burden for families, such as extensive family leave, paid leave, a reasonable minimum wage, and childcare assistance. Given the ways in which LGBTQ families form—and the lack of legal recognition for many years—more research is needed about the ways in which LGBTQ families with children may or may not be able to fully access these supports in a country already limited in their availability. For example, currently just eight states and the District of Columbia have family leave laws that allow workers to take leave to care for a partner

to whom the worker is not *legally* related, and of these states, five states and the District of Columbia offer paid leave to care for a partner (Movement Advancement Project, 2019). Inclusive paid sick and paid family leave laws are incredibly important for LGBTQ people, more than 40% of whom report taking time off from work to care for friends or chosen family members with a health need (Robbins et al., 2017). While federal law permits a parent to take job-protected leave to care for a child for whom they are caring even if they are not legally recognized as a parent, only nine states and the District of Columbia provide leave beyond the federal minimum for such families, and just six states and the District of Columbia have provisions for paid leave in such circumstances (Movement Advancement Project, 2019).

## Examine Similarities and Differences with LGBTQ-Parent Families in Other Countries

This chapter focuses specifically on the economic well-being of LGBTQ-parent families in the USA. That said, there are likely similarities and differences with similarly constructed and structured families in other countries. Research that compares the experiences and economics of LGBTQ-parent families from various countries could allow for exploration of the extent to which various family laws and policies, and LGBTQ-affirming laws and policies, impact LGBTQ-parent families. For example, there is great variation in paid parental leave and non-discrimination protections around the world. That said, it is important to keep in mind the extent to which the USA has a particular economic and public benefits framework that may not be easily comparable. For example, data collected by the Organisation for Economic Co-operation and Development (OECD) indicated that in 2015, the USA spent 0.64% of annual GDP on public spending for family benefits compared to 1.46% in the Netherlands, which was the first country to allow same-sex couples to marry (OECD, 2019).

## The Impact of Economic Well-Being on LGBTQ-Parent Families

The research described in this chapter, much of it quantitative reports of economic resources or the lack thereof, presents the picture of some LGBTQ-parent families facing substantial economic insecurity and instability while others are thriving. While there is vast literature about family economic resources and the role they play in parent, child, and overall family well-being (e.g., Akee, Copeland, Costello, & Simeonova, 2018; Chaudry & Wimer, 2016), fewer studies have directly explored the relationship in LGBTQ-parent families.

For example, fewer economic resources can mean fewer choices for families. Goldberg and Smith (2014) explored preschool selection among lesbian, gay, and heterosexual adoptive parents. Not surprisingly, they found that parents with less income were more likely to consider cost in their selection and those with lower educations were more likely to consider location, speaking to the real constraints that the cost of early childhood education means for families. What this may mean for LGBTQ-parent families is that those who are more affluent can consider greater educational opportunities for their children, including schools that may have a higher share of LGBTQ-parent families. In a follow-up study with a subset of those participants, income was the cornerstone for decisions about schooling for lesbian and gay couples with adopted children (Goldberg et al., 2018).

In a case study of a poor single lesbian mother in a rural area in the United States, Mendez, Holman, Oswald, and Izenstark (2016) show that there are particular challenges to poverty based on sexual orientation, parenthood and marital status, and geographic location. The intersection of these various dimensions of minority status combines with living in poverty to have particularly strong negative effects on health and well-being. Facing discrimination or hate based on sexual orientation is more difficult when living in poverty, because the lack of economic resources constrains one's options to move to a more accepting place. The same case study shows how fragile the

receipt of public benefits is. Parents need to work in order to have income, but as soon as the income passes a particular threshold, the benefits are cut off—though the income may not be high enough to enable the family meet all its needs. Thus, while the quantitative data reflect the higher need of LGBTQ families to receive public assistance, case studies from the field suggest that the public assistance system could be made more helpful if the income threshold to receive the assistance were higher.

While studies of same-sex couples often find that they are more equitable in their distribution of household labor, particularly female same-sex couples (Chan, Brooks, Raboy, & Patterson, 1998; Kurdek, 1993; Kurdek, 2007; Patterson, Sutfin, & Fulcher, 2004), there is some evidence that this may be more true among higher-income couples and less true for lower-income and racially and ethnically diverse couples (Carrington, 1999; Goldberg, 2013; Moore, 2008). As the findings presented earlier from Antecol and Steinberger (2011) suggest, families with children, regardless of parental composition, may make different decisions about distribution of household labor, including child-rearing (e.g., Smart, Brown, & Taylor, 2017). For example, Goldberg and Perry-Jenkins (2007) found that biological mothers in lesbian couples with infants contributed more to childcare, while household work was divided equitably.

## Implications for Practice

In addition to better understanding the demographics, economic realities, and family dynamics of LGBTQ-parent families, additional research is needed to uncover strategies used by LGBTQ families to navigate economic challenges and to thrive financially. Some of those strategies may be useful teachings for other families. For example, the research reviewed in this chapter shows that LGBTQ-parent families are more likely to receive some forms of safety net assistance than other families but continue to have higher rates of economic insecurity. Perhaps these families are more comfortable seeking assistance, have less stigma about receiving assistance, or have something else that allows them to obtain assistance when they need it.

While answering the "why" of economic instability is crucial to designing and implementing meaningful policy change, there are a number of ways in which public policy could also alleviate some of the particular social and economic difficulties facing LGBTQ families that center on the implementation and evaluation of policies and programs. Areas of relevant public policy include advancing and evaluating the impact of inclusive paid family leave laws, childcare subsidies, a higher minimum wage, increased cash assistance and food assistance for low-income families, greater access to health insurance coverage and quality care, and stronger enforcement of nondiscrimination laws. Those policies would serve to strengthen all families and would also help to fill some of the gaps that are acutely felt by LGBTQ families.

## Conclusion

LGBTQ people face particular economic hardships and challenges and LGBTQ people with families even more so. The research shows that poverty rates in LGBTQ families are remarkably high; LGBTQ people heading families often have low incomes; they face food insecurity at higher rates than other families; and fear of and actual discrimination make it more difficult for LGBTQ people and their families to access the help and services they need. While there is increasing acceptance of and legal rights and protections for LGBTQ people, this chapter has shown some of the many ways in which LGBTQ families face economic hardship. It is thus important to recognize the unique circumstances and challenges of parenting while being LGBTQ. This chapter also highlights key areas for future research to help understand the "why" in terms of the economic challenges that LGBTQ families with children experience.

**Acknowledgments** Logan S. Casey, PhD, Policy Researcher, Movement Advancement Project.

Libby Hemphill, PhD, Director, Research Center for Minority Data, Inter-university Consortium for Policy and Social Research.

## References

Akee, R., Copeland, W., Costello, J. E., & Simeonova, E. (2018). How does household income affect child personality traits and behaviors? *American Economic Review, 108*, 775–827.

Albelda, R., Badgett, M. V. L., Schneebaum, A., & Gates, G. J. (2009, March). *Poverty in the lesbian, gay, and bisexual community*. Retrieved from The Williams Institute website: https://williamsinstitute.law.ucla.edu/wp-content/uploads/Albelda-Badgett-Schneebaum-Gates-LGB-Poverty-Report-March-2009.pdf

Antecol, H., & Steinberger, M. D. (2011). Labor supply differences between married heterosexual women and partnered lesbians: A semi-parametric decomposition approach. *Economic Inquiry, 51*, 783–805. https://doi.org/10.1111/j.1465-7295.2010.00363.x

Badgett, M. V. L. (2009). *When gay people get married: What happens when societies legalize same-sex marriage*. New York, NY: NYU Press.

Badgett, M. V. L. (2018). Left out? Lesbian, gay, and bisexual poverty in the U.S. *Population Research and Policy Review, 37*, 667–702. https://doi.org/10.1007/s11113-018-9457-5

Badgett, M. V. L., Durso, L. E., & Schneebaum, A. (2013, June). *New patterns of poverty in the lesbian, gay, and bisexual community*. Retrieved from The Williams Institute website: https://williamsinstitute.law.ucla.edu/wp-content/uploads/LGB-Poverty-Update-Jun-2013.pdf

Black, D. A., Sanders, S. G., & Taylor, L. J. (2007). The economics of lesbian and gay families. *Journal of Economic Perspectives, 21*, 53–70. https://doi.org/10.1257/jep.21.2.53

Blau, F. D., & Kahn, L. M. (2017). The gender wage gap: Extent, trends, and explanations. *Journal of Economic Literature, 55*, 789–865. https://doi.org/10.1257/jel.20160995

Brown, T. N. T., Romero, A. P., & Gates, G. J. (2016, July). *Food insecurity and SNAP participation in the LGBT community*. Retrieved from The Williams Institute website: https://williamsinstitute.law.ucla.edu/wp-content/uploads/Food-Insecurity-and-SNAP-Participation-in-the-LGBT-Community.pdf

Budig, M. J. (2014). *The fatherhood bonus & the motherhood penalty: Parenthood and the gender gap in pay*. Retrieved from Third Way website: https://thirdway.imgix.net/downloads/the-fatherhood-bonus-and-the-motherhood-penalty-parenthood-and-the-gender-gap-in-pay/NEXT_-_Fatherhood_Motherhood.pdf

Carrington, C. (1999). *No place like home: Relationships and family life among lesbians and gay men*. Chicago, IL: The University of Chicago Press.

Center for American Progress Action Fund, Leadership Conference on Civil and Human Rights, & Coalition for Human Needs. (2014, November). *Building local momentum for national change: Half in ten annual poverty and inequality indicators report*. Retrieved from Center for American Progress website: https://cdn.americanprogress.org/wp-content/uploads/2014/11/HiT2014-final.pdf

Chan, R. W., Brooks, R. C., Raboy, B., & Patterson, C. J. (1998). Division of labor among lesbian and heterosexual parents: Associations with children's adjustment. *Journal of Family Psychology, 12*, 402–419. https://doi.org/10.1037/0893-3200.12.3.402

Chaudry, A., & Wimer, C. (2016). Poverty is not just an indicator: The relationship between income, poverty, and child well-being. *Academic Pediatrics, 16*, S23–S29. https://doi.org/10.1016/j.acap.2015.12.010

Cherlin, A. J. (2018). How inequality drives family formation: The prima facie case. In N. R. Cahn, J. Carbone, L. F. DeRose, & B. Wilcox (Eds.), *Unequal family lives: Causes and consequences in Europe and the Americas* (pp. 69–82). Cambridge, UK: Cambridge University Press.

Dalaker, J. (2017, November 28). *The supplemental poverty measure: Its core concepts, development, and use.* Retrieved from Congressional Research Service website: https://crsreports.congress.gov/product/pdf/R/R45031/3

Data.Gov. (2019). *Federal government datasets.* Retrieved from https://www.data.gov/metrics

Edin, K., & Reed, J. M. (2005). Why don't they just get married? Barriers to marriage among the disadvantaged. *The Future of Children, 15*, 117–137. https://doi.org/10.1353/foc.2005.0017

Farr, R. H. (2017). Does parental sexual orientation matter? A longitudinal follow-up of adoptive families with school-age children. *Developmental Psychology, 53*, 252–264. https://doi.org/10.1037/dev0000228

Federal Interagency Working Group on Improving Measurement of Sexual Orientation and Gender Identity in Federal Surveys. (2016, August). *Current measures of sexual orientation and gender identity in federal surveys.* Retrieved from National Education Statistics website: https://nces.ed.gov/FCSM/pdf/current_measures_20160812.pdf

Fisher, R., Gee, G., & Looney, A. (2018, February 28). *Same-sex married tax filers after Windsor and Obergefell.* Retrieved from Tax Policy Center website: https://www.taxpolicycenter.org/sites/default/files/publication/153351/same-sex_married_tax_filers_after_windsor_and_obergefell_1.pdf

Fontenot, K., Semega, J., & Kollar, K. (2018). *Current population reports, P60–263, income and poverty in the United States: 2017.* Retrieved from U.S. Census Bureau website: https://www.census.gov/content/dam/Census/library/publications/2018/demo/p60-263.pdf

Fredriksen-Goldsen, K. I., Kim, H. J., Barkan, S. E., Balsam, K. F., & Mincer, S. L. (2011). Disparities in health-related quality of life: A comparison of lesbians and bisexual women. *American Journal of Public Health, 100*, 2255–2261. https://doi.org/10.2105/AJPH.2009.177329

Fredriksen-Goldsen, K. I., Kim, H. J., Jung, H., & Goldsen, J. (2019). The evolution of Aging with Pride – National Health, Aging, Sexuality/Gender Study: Illuminating the iridescent life course of LGBTQ adults aged 80 years and older in the United States. *The International Journal of Aging and Human Development, 88*, 380–404. https://doi.org/10.1177/0091415019837591

Frost, D. M., Levahot, K., & Meyer, I. H. (2015). Minority stress and physical health among sexual minority individuals. *Journal of Behavioral Medicine, 38*, 1–8. https://doi.org/10.1007/s10865-013-9523-8

Gartrell, N., Bos, H., & Koh, A. (2019). Sexual attraction, sexual identity, and same-sex sexual experiences of adult offspring in the US National Longitudinal Lesbian Family Study. *Archives of Sexual Behavior, 48*, 1495–1503. https://doi.org/10.1007/s10508-019-1434-5

Gates, G. J. (2011a). Family formation and raising children among same-sex couples. In *Family focus on… LGBT families, FF51*. Saint Paul, MN: National Council on Family Relations.

Gates, G. J. (2011b). *How many people are lesbian, gay, bisexual, and transgender?* Retrieved from The Williams Institute website: https://williamsinstitute.law.ucla.edu/wp-content/uploads/Gates-How-Many-People-LGBT-Apr-2011.pdf

Gates, G. J. (2013). *LGBT parenting in the United States.* Retrieved from The Williams Institute website: https://williamsinstitute.law.ucla.edu/wp-content/uploads/LGBT-Parenting.pdf

Gates, G. J. (2014). *LGB families and relationships: Analyses of the 2013 National Health Interview Survey.* Retrieved from The Williams Institute website: https://williamsinstitute.law.ucla.edu/wp-content/uploads/lgb-families-nhis-sep-2014.pdf

Gates, G. J. (2015a). Marriage and family: LGBT individuals and same-sex couples. *The Future of Children, 25*, 67–87. https://doi.org/10.1353/foc.2015.0013

Gates, G. J. (2015b). *Demographics of married and unmarried same-sex couples: Analyses of the 2013 American Community Survey.* Retrieved from The Williams Institute website: https://williamsinstitute.law.ucla.edu/wp-content/uploads/Demographics-Same-Sex-Couples-ACS2013-March-2015.pdf

Gates, G. J. (2017, January 11). *In U.S., more adults identifying as LGBT.* Retrieved from Gallup website: https://news.gallup.com/poll/201731/lgbt-identification-rises.aspx

Gates, G. J., Badgett, M. V. L., Macomber, J. E., & Chambers, K. (2007). *Adoption and foster care by gay and lesbian parents in the United States.* Retrieved Urban Institute website: https://www.urban.org/sites/default/files/publication/46401/411437-Adoption-and-Foster-Care-by-Lesbian-and-Gay-Parents-in-the-United-States.PDF

Goldberg, A. E. (2013). "Doing" and "undoing" gender: The meaning and division of housework in same-sex couples. *Journal of Family Theory & Review, 5*, 85–104. https://doi.org/10.1111/jftr.12009

Goldberg, A. E., Allen, K. R., Black, K. A., Frost, R. L., & Manley, M. H. (2018). "There is no perfect school": The complexity of school decision-making among lesbian and gay adoptive parents. *Journal of Marriage and Family, 80*, 684–703. https://doi.org/10.1111/jomf.12478

Goldberg, A. E., & Garcia, R. L. (2016). Gender-typed behavior over time in children with lesbian, gay, and heterosexual parents. *Journal of Family Psychology, 30*, 854–865. https://doi.org/10.1037/fam0000226

Goldberg, A. E., Gartrell, N. K., & Gates, G. (2014). *Research report on LGB-Parent families.* Retrieved from The Williams Institute website: https://williamsinstitute.law.ucla.edu/wp-content/uploads/lgb-parent-families-july-2014.pdf

Goldberg, A. E., & Perry-Jenkins, M. (2007). The division of labor and perceptions of parental roles: Lesbian couples across the transition to parenthood. *Journal of Social and Personal Relationships, 24*, 297–318. https://doi.org/10.1177/0265407507075415

Goldberg, A. E. & Smith, J. Z. (2014). Preschool selection considerations and experiences of school mistreatment among lesbian, gay, and heterosexual adoptive parents. *Early Childhood Research Quarterly, 20*, 64–75. https://doi.org/10.1016/j.ecresq.2013.09.006

Goldberg, S. K., & Conron, K. J. (2018, July). *How many same-sex couples in the U.S. are raising children?* Retrieved from The Williams Institute website: https://williamsinstitute.law.ucla.edu/wp-content/uploads/Parenting-Among-Same-Sex-Couples.pdf

Grant, J. M., Mottet, L. A., Tanis, J., Harrison, J., Herman, J. L., & Keisling, M. (2011). *Injustice at every turn: A report of the National Transgender Discrimination Survey.* National Center for Transgender Equality and National Gay and Lesbian Task Force. Retrieved from National Center for Transgender Equality website: https://www.transequality.org/sites/default/files/docs/resources/NTDS_Report.pdf

Harris, E., & Hopping-Winn, A. (2019). *LGBTQ family building survey.* Retrieved from Family Equality Council website: https://www.familyequality.org/wp-content/uploads/2019/02/LGBTQ-Family-Building-Study_Jan2019-1.pdf

Hill, H. D., Romich, J., Mattingly, M. J., Shamsuddin, S., & Wething, H. (2017). An introduction to household economic instability and social policy. *Social Service Review, 91*, 371–389. https://doi.org/10.1086/694110

Hodges, M., & Budig, M. J. (2010). Who gets the daddy bonus? Markers of hegemonic masculinity and the impact of first-time fatherhood on men's earnings. *Gender & Society, 24*, 717–745. https://doi.org/10.1177/0891243210386729

James, S. E., Herman, J. L., Rankin, S., Keisling, M., Mottet, L., & Anafi, M. (2016). *The report of the 2015 U.S. Transgender Survey.* Retrieved from National Center for Transgender Equality website: https://www.transequality.org/sites/default/files/docs/USTS-Full-Report-FINAL.PDF

Jones, J. M. (2017, June 22). *In U.S., 10.2% of LGBT adults now married to same-sex spouse.* Retrieved from Gallup website: https://news.gallup.com/poll/212702/lgbt-adults-married-sex-spouse.aspx

Kastanis, A., & Wilson, B. D. M. (2014). *Race/ethnicity, gender and socioeconomic wellbeing of individuals in same-sex couples.* Retrieved from The Williams Institute website: https://williamsinstitute.law.ucla.edu/wp-content/uploads/Census-Compare-Feb-2014.pdf

Kim, H. J., & Fredriksen-Goldsen, K. I. (2017). Disparities in mental health quality of life between Hispanic and non-Hispanic White LGB midlife and older adults and the influence of lifetime discrimination, social connectedness, socioeconomic status, and perceived stress. *Research on Aging, 39*, 991–1012. https://doi.org/10.1177/0164027516650003

Klawitter, M. (2011). Multilevel analysis of the effect of antidiscrimination policies on earnings by sexual orientation. *Journal of Policy Analysis and Management, 30*, 334–358. https://doi.org/10.1002/pam.20563

Klawitter, M. (2015). Meta-analysis of the effects of sexual orientation on earnings. *Industrial Relations, 54*, 4–32. https://doi.org/10.1111/irel.12075

Krivickas, K. M., & Lofquist, D. (2011). *Demographics of same-sex couple households with children* (SEHSD Working Paper 2011–11). Retrieved from U.S. Census Bureau website: https://www.census.gov/content/dam/Census/library/working-papers/2011/demo/SEHSD-WP2011-11.pdf

Kurdek, L. A. (1993). The allocation of household labor in gay, lesbian, and heterosexual married couples. *Journal of Social Issues, 49*, 127–139. https://doi.org/10.1111/j.1540-4560.1993.tb01172.x

Kurdek, L. A. (2007). The allocation of household labor by partners in gay and lesbian couples. *Journal of Family Issues, 28*, 132–148. https://doi.org/10.1177/0192513X06292019

Lennox Kail, B., Acosta, K. L., & Wright, E. R. (2015). State-level marriage equality and the health of same-sex couples. *American Journal of Public Health, 105*, 1101–1105. https://doi.org/10.2105/AJPH.2015.302589

Lunn, M. R., & Obedin-Maliver, J. (2019). *The PRIDE study.* Retrieved from https://pridestudy.org/team

McKernan, S. M., Ratcliffe, C., Simms, M., & Zhang, S. (2014). Do racial disparities in private transfers help explain the racial wealth gap? New evidence from longitudinal data. *Demography, 51*, 949–974. https://doi.org/10.1007/s13524-014-0296-7

Mendez, S. N., Holman, E. G., Oswald, R. F., & Izenstark, D. (2016). Minority stress in the context of rural economic hardship: One lesbian mother's story. *Journal of GLBT Family Studies, 12*, 491–511. https://doi.org/10.1080/1550428X.2015.1099493

Mirza, S. (2018, September 24). *Disaggregating the data for bisexual people.* Retrieved from Center for American Progress website: https://cdn.americanprogress.org/content/uploads/2018/09/21133117/BiCommunityStats-factsheet1.pdf

Mistry, R. S., Vandewater, E. A., Huston, A. C., & McLoyd, V. C. (2002). Economic well-being and children's social adjustment: The role of family process in an ethnically diverse low-income sample. *Child Development, 73*, 935–951. https://doi.org/10.1111/1467-8624.00448

Moore, M. R. (2008). Gendered power relations among women: A study of household decision making in black, lesbian stepfamilies. *American Sociological Review, 73*, 335–356. https://doi.org/10.1177/000312240807300208

Moore, M. R., & Stambolis-Ruhstorfer, M. (2013). LGBT sexuality and families at the start of the twenty-first century. *Annual Review of Sociology, 39*, 491–507. https://doi.org/10.1146/annurev-soc-071312-145643

Movement Advancement Project. (2019). *Family leave laws*. Retrieved from http://www.lgbtmap.org/equality-maps/fmla_laws

National LGBT Health Education Center, Fenway Institute. (2016). *Pathways to parenthood for LGBT people*. Retrieved from https://www.lgbthealtheducation.org/wp-content/uploads/Pathways-to-Parenthood-for-LGBT-People.pdf

Newport, F. (2018, May 22). *In U.S., estimate of LGBT population rises to 4.5%*. Retrieved from Gallup website: https://news.gallup.com/poll/234863/estimate-lgbt-population-rises.aspx

Nixon, C. A. (2011). Working-class lesbian parents' emotional engagement with their children's education: Intersections of class and sexuality. *Sexualities, 14*, 79–99. https://doi.org/10.1177/1363460710390564

OECD. (2019). *Family benefits public spending (indicator)*. Retrieved from the Organisation for Economic Co-operation and Development website: https://data.oecd.org/socialexp/family-benefits-public-spending.htm

Patterson, C. J., Sutfin, E. L., & Fulcher, M. (2004). Division of labor among lesbian and heterosexual parenting couples: Correlates of specialized versus shared patterns. *Journal of Adult Development, 11*, 179–189. https://doi.org/10.1023/B:JADE.0000035626.90331.47

Pew Research Center. (2013, June 13). *A survey of LGBT Americans: Attitudes, experiences and values in changing times*. Retrieved from https://www.pewsocialtrends.org/2013/06/13/a-survey-of-lgbt-americans/

Ramos, C., Goldberg, N. G., & Badgett, M. V. L. (2009, May). *The effects of marriage equality in Massachusetts: A survey of the experiences and impact of marriage on same-sex couples*. Retrieved from The Williams Institute website: https://williamsinstitute.law.ucla.edu/wp-content/uploads/Ramos-Goldberg-Badgett-MA-Effects-Marriage-Equality-May-2009.pdf

Riggle, E. D. B., Wickham, R. E., Rostosky, S. S., Rothblum, E. D., & Balsam, K. F. (2017). Impact of civil marriage recognition for long-term same-sex couples. *Sexuality Research and Social Policy, 14*, 223–232. https://doi.org/10.1007/s13178-016-0243-z

Riskind, R. G., & Patterson, C. J. (2010). Parenting intentions and desires among childless lesbian, gay, and heterosexual individuals. *Journal of Family Psychology, 24*, 78–81. https://doi.org/10.1037/a0017941

Robbins, K. G., Durso, L. E., Bewkes, F. J., & Schultz, E. (2017, October 30). *People need paid leave policies that cover chosen family*. Retrieved from Center for American Progress website: https://cdn.americanprogress.org/content/uploads/2017/10/26135206/UnmetCaregivingNeed-brief.pdf

Rooney, C., Whittington, C., & Durso, L. E. (2018, August 13). *Protecting basic living standards for LGBTQ people*. Retrieved from Center for American Progress website: https://cdn.americanprogress.org/content/uploads/2018/08/10095627/LGBT-BenefitCuts-report.pdf

Rostosky, S. S., Riggle, E. D. B., Rothblum, E. D., & Balsam, K. F. (2016). Same-sex couples' decisions and experiences of marriage in the context of minority stress: Interviews from a population-based longitudinal study. *Journal of Homosexuality, 63*, 1019–1040. https://doi.org/10.1080/00918369.2016.1191232

RTI International. (2014, July 14). *Current and prospective scope of hunger and food security in America: A review of current research*. Retrieved from https://www.rti.org/sites/default/files/resources/full_hunger_report_final_07-24-14.pdf

Schneebaum, A., & Badgett, M. V. L. (2019). Poverty in US lesbian and gay couple households. *Feminist Economics, 25*, 1–30. https://doi.org/10.1080/13545701.2018.1441533

Schneebaum, A., & Schubert, N. (2017, December). *Marriage (in)equality: Does the sexual orientation wage gap persist across marital status* (Working Paper No. 254). Vienna University of Economics and Business, Department of Economics. Retrieved from Vienna University website: https://epub.wu.ac.at/5964/1/wp254.pdf

Sears, B., & Mallory, C. (2011, July). *Documented evidence of employment discrimination & its effects on LGBT people*. Retrieved from The Williams Institute website: https://williamsinstitute.law.ucla.edu/wp-content/uploads/Sears-Mallory-Discrimination-July-20111.pdf

Shlay, A. B., Weinraub, M., Harmon, M., & Tran, H. (2004). Barriers to subsidies: Why low-income families do not use child care subsidies. *Social Science Research, 33*, 134–157. https://doi.org/10.1016/S0049-089X(03)00042-5

Singh, S., & Durso, L. E. (2017, May 2). *Widespread discrimination continues to shape LGBT people's lives in both subtle and substantial ways*. Retrieved from Center for American Progress website: https://www.americanprogress.org/issues/lgbt/news/2017/05/02/429529/widespread-discrimination-continues-shape-lgbt-peoples-lives-subtle-significant-ways/

Smart, M. J., Brown, A., & Taylor, B. D. (2017). Sex or sexuality? Analyzing the division of labor and travel in gay, lesbian, and straight households. *Travel Behaviour and Society, 6*, 75–82. https://doi.org/10.1016/j.tbs.2016.07.001

Smock, P. J., & Manning, W. D. (1997). Cohabiting partners' economic circumstances and marriage. *Demography, 34*, 331–341. https://doi.org/10.2307/3038287

Stotzer, R. L., Herman, J. L., & Hasenbush, A. (2014, October). *Transgender parenting: A review of exist-*

*ing research*. Retrieved from The Williams Institute website: https://williamsinstitute.law.ucla.edu/wp-content/uploads/transgender-parenting-oct-2014.pdf

U.S. Census Bureau. (2018a, March). *Questions planned for the 2010 Census and American Community Survey*. Retrieved from https://www2.census.gov/library/publications/decennial/2020/operations/planned-questions-2020-acs.pdf

U.S. Census Bureau. (2018b, August 28). *Table 17. Distribution of poor, by region*. Retrieved from https://www.census.gov/data/tables/time-series/demo/income-poverty/historical-poverty-people.html

U.S. Census Bureau. (2018c, September 6). *Poverty thresholds by size of family and number of children*. Retrieved from https://www.census.gov/data/tables/time-series/demo/income-poverty/historical-poverty-thresholds.html

U.S. Census Bureau. (2019). *Are you in a survey? List of all surveys*. Retrieved from https://www.census.gov/programs-surveys/are-you-in-a-survey/survey-list.html

U.S. Department of Agriculture. (2019). *What are the SNAP income limits?* Retrieved from https://www.fns.usda.gov/snap/eligibility#What%20are%20the%20SNAP%20income%20limits

U.S. Department of Agriculture, Economic Research Service. (2017). *Prevalence of food insecurity by selected household characteristics, 2017*. Retrieved from https://www.ers.usda.gov/media/9964/insecurity.xlsx

Wagmiller, R. L. & Adelman, R. M. (2009). *Childhood and intergenerational poverty: The long-term consequences of growing up poor*. Retrieved from National Center for Children in Poverty website: http://www.nccp.org/publications/pdf/text_909.pdf

# LGBTQ-Parent Families and Health

Amanda M. Pollitt, Corinne Reczek,
and Debra Umberson

Health disparities are defined as "gaps in health between segments of the population" (Centers for Disease Control and Prevention, 2013, p. 3). Health disparities encompass both physical (e.g., physical activity, diet and exercise, substance use, health-care-seeking, and sleep behaviors) and mental health (e.g., "a state of well-being in which every individual realizes his or her own potential, can cope with the normal stresses of life, can work productively and fruitfully, and is able to make a contribution to his or her community" [World Health Organization, 2014]) components. Sexual and gender minority people (or those who identify as lesbian, gay, bisexual, transgender, queer [LGBTQ], or some other non-heterosexual/noncisgender identity) report worse health than their heterosexual and cisgender peers (Institute of Medicine [IOM], 2011). This health disadvantage is attributed most commonly to gender and sexual minority stigma and dis-crimination, which in turn contribute to poorer access to health care and higher levels of stress (Meyer, 2003). Because LGBTQ-parent families consist of one or more parents who identify as LGBTQ, these health disparities have implications for the health and well-being of both parents and children in LGBTQ-parent families.

In this chapter, we summarize the literature on physical and mental health outcomes of parents and children under the age of 18 in LGBTQ-parent families using a family resilience approach (Prendergast & MacPhee, 2018). We first describe the family resilience theoretical framework as well as other frameworks that can be and have been commonly used to study the health of LGBTQ people and their families. Then, we review the broad findings of past research on physical and mental health in LGBTQ-parent families, acknowledging that there has been much less research on LGBTQ parents compared to research on their children. We address physical and mental health outcomes in separate sections; however, because most studies in this area have examined mental health, we highlight the broad literature on LGBTQ physical health disparities and how these findings could be applied to LGBTQ-parent families. We then describe the literature on parenting stress/stigma and peer victimization mechanisms and the physical and mental health outcomes related to these mechanisms. Finally, we explore specific social and family contexts of LGBTQ-parent families as

A. M. Pollitt (✉)
Population Research Center, University of Texas at
Austin, Austin, TX, USA
e-mail: apollitt@utexas.edu

C. Reczek
Department of Sociology, The Ohio State University,
Columbus, OH, USA
e-mail: reczek.2@osu.edu

D. Umberson
Department of Sociology, University of Texas at
Austin, Austin, TX, USA
e-mail: umberson@utexas.edu

© Springer Nature Switzerland AG 2020
A. E. Goldberg, K. R. Allen (eds.), *LGBTQ-Parent Families*,
https://doi.org/10.1007/978-3-030-35610-1_7

intersections that may be related to physical and mental health. We summarize literature conducted since 2000 considering major societal changes in LGBTQ rights in the USA and globally. In each section, we also identify gaps in the literature and describe how there is much more to learn about health disparities, resilience, and outcomes for all members of LGBTQ-parent families.

## Theoretical Frameworks for Understanding the Health of LGBTQ-Parent Families

Most studies on sexual minority health disparities have utilized the minority stress model (Meyer, 2003) as a theoretical framework for understanding high rates of negative physical and mental health outcomes among sexual minority people. The minority stress model posits that sexual minority people experience stigma-related stressors, above and beyond everyday stressors that all people experience, and these additional stressors result in poorer health. Though this model is a deficit-based approach to understanding LGBTQ health, research in this area has been used to combat views that sexual minority people are fundamentally mentally ill and to instead put the focus on stigma as a source of stress that contributes to physical and mental health disparities among LGBTQ people (Meyer, 2013). Similarly, most past research on health outcomes in LGBTQ-parent families has taken a deficit-based approach by examining similarities and differences between children of same-sex and different-sex parents. In this approach, different-sex parents are the "gold standard" by which researchers surmise that children of same-sex parents are healthy if they report outcomes similar to children of different-sex parents (Stacey & Biblarz, 2001). This approach is likely why many studies in this area have relied on nontheoretical perspectives such as public policy and controversy concerns (Farr, Tasker, & Goldberg, 2017) and focused on the mental health outcomes of children in LGBTQ-parent families, with less research on physical health or the health of LGBTQ parents.

Fortunately, recent theoretical and empirical research has moved well beyond a deficit approach to examine pathways of health in LGBTQ-parent families (Goldberg & Gartrell, 2014; Manning, Fettro, & Lamidi, 2014; Reczek, Spiker, Liu, & Crosnoe, 2016), though most research has continued to focus on mental health outcomes for children. A particularly promising theoretical framework for advancing our understanding of health as experienced by LGBTQ-parent families is a model of family resilience offered by Prendergast and MacPhee (2018). This model, which situates families within the minority stress model (Meyer, 2003), asks, "When examining the family system, which processes reduce the effects of discrimination on (a) psychological well-being; (b) family cohesion, coherence, flexibility, and adaptability; (c) parenting practices and relations; and (d) child behavioral and academic outcomes in LG families?" (Prendergast & MacPhee, 2018, p. 27). Thus, the model serves as a guiding framework for examining vulnerability (i.e., minority stressors) and resilience (i.e., protective factors) for negative physical and mental health outcomes in LGBTQ-parent families.

## Physical and Mental Health Outcomes in LGBTQ-Parent Families

### Physical Health Outcomes

LGBTQ people are at higher risk than cisgender heterosexual people for numerous negative health behaviors and physical health outcomes, including alcohol use, tobacco use, obesity, and cancer (IOM, 2011). LGBTQ people and their families also have less access to health insurance and health care, which increases the likelihood of physical health problems over time (Buchmueller & Carpenter, 2010). Despite clear evidence of physical health disparities in LGBTQ populations, we found it difficult to identify literature that examined physical health outcomes among LGBTQ parents and children. In one of the only papers that examined physical health, Goldberg, Smith, McCormick, and Overstreet (2019) examined predictors of health and health behaviors in a sample of same-sex parents and found that parenting stress and internalized homophobia were associated with poorer physical health. In a study on children's physical and mental health outcomes, Reczek et al. (2016); Reczek, Spiker, Liu, and Crosnoe (2017) found that children of same-sex parents did not differ from children of different-sex parents on parent-rated health, lost school days due to illness or injury, or behavior problems. However, they found that children of married same-sex parents were more likely to report activity limitations than children of same-sex cohabiting, different-sex married, and different-sex cohabiting parents, which the authors suggested might be a function of adoption of special needs children by same-sex married parents. These studies offer preliminary insight into the physical health of LGBTQ-parent families, but there is much more work to do in this area.

Instead, the vast majority of studies have examined mental health outcomes of children of same-sex parents. Thus, our review focuses on mental health because of this limitation in the literature; however, we would like to stress that physical health plays an important role in families, and physical and mental health are often closely intertwined. Examining the mental health of members of LGBTQ-parent families is critical for understanding physical health because poorer mental health and higher stress predict worse physical health across the lifespan (Ohrnberger, Fichera, & Sutton, 2017). At the same time, poor physical health strains mental health and exacerbates stressors related to mental health (Cohen, Janicki-Deverts, & Miller, 2007). We encourage researchers in this area to not only focus on physical health outcomes but to also explore the ways in which physical and mental health interact in LGBTQ-parent families.

## Mental Health Outcomes

Research finds significant and consistent mental health disparities between heterosexual and LGBTQ people on outcomes such as depressive

symptoms, anxiety, and suicide (IOM, 2011). Negative mental health outcomes may also be elevated among LGBTQ parents; however, the few studies that have directly examined mental health among same-sex parents have found no sexual orientation differences (Goldberg & Smith, 2008; Goldberg & Smith, 2011; Shapiro, Peterson, & Stewart, 2009). In comparison, there is a large literature on the mental health of children of LGBTQ parents—specifically lesbian and gay or same-sex parents—and multiple meta-analyses synthesizing this literature have found no differences in mental health or psychosocial adjustment compared to children of different-sex parents (Crowl, Ahn, & Baker, 2008; Fedewa, Black, & Ahn, 2015; Miller, Kors, & Macfie, 2017). Studies that utilize community or convenience samples (e.g., Baiocco et al., 2015; Golombok et al., 2003), representative samples (e.g., Reczek et al., 2016, 2017; Wainwright & Patterson, 2006, 2008), and systematic and narrative reviews (e.g., Anderssen, Amlie, & Ytterøy, 2002; Goldberg & Gartrell, 2014; Moore & Stambolis-Ruhstorfer, 2013; Telingator & Patterson, 2008) also point to the same general conclusion that children in same-sex parent families fare as well as children in different-sex parent families. However, research on broad sexual minority populations and recent work on same-sex parent families point to unique stressors experienced by LGBTQ-parent families that may contribute to physical and mental health outcomes. Next, we consider these stressors in relation to health outcomes of parents and children in LGBTQ-parent families.

## Pathways of Physical and Mental Health in LGBTQ-Parent Families

LGBTQ parents and their children are at risk of experiencing stigma related to their family structure, which has implications for the physical and mental health of LGBTQ-parent families (Meyer, 2003; see chapters "Clinical Work with LGBTQ Parents and Prospective Parents" and "Clinical Work with Children and Adolescents Growing Up with LGBTQ Parents"). We present literature on two relatively highly researched minority stress pathways that likely impact the physical and mental health of parents and children in LGBTQ-parent families, respectively: parenting stigma/stress and peer victimization. Because we take a family resilience approach (Prendergast & MacPhee, 2018) to reviewing the literature on stigma, we also focus on potential protective and resilience factors that may mitigate negative health outcomes related to these stressors.

## Parental Stigma, Parenting Distress, and Social Support

The key premise of the minority stress model is that sexual minority stigma-related stress, such as discrimination and internalized homophobia, results in poorer overall health among LGBTQ people (Meyer, 2003). Indeed, LGBTQ people report unique stigma-based stressors during and after the transition to parenthood, including lack of family support (Goldberg, 2010; Goldberg & Smith, 2014; Reczek, 2014; Tornello, Farr, & Patterson, 2011), unsupportive social and legal policies (Goldberg & Smith, 2011; Lick, Tornello, Riskind, Schmidt, & Patterson, 2012; Shapiro et al., 2009), and discrimination during adoption and custody processes (Goldberg, Moyer, Kinkler, & Richardson, 2012), which are related to poorer physical (Goldberg et al., 2019) and mental health outcomes (Goldberg & Smith, 2011; Shapiro et al., 2009). However, there is little research suggesting that stigma and its resultant health outcomes among same-sex parents undermine the mental health of children. For example, Baiocco et al. (2015) compared children of different-sex and same-sex parents in Italy; despite strong anti-gay attitudes and a highly unfavorable legal environment (same-sex couples cannot marry or adopt in Italy), they found no differences in children's well-being. Even direct experiences of stigma appear unrelated to children's mental health outcomes: Crouch, Waters, McNair, Power, and Davis (2014) found that though Australian children whose same-sex attracted parents experienced stigma reported poorer mental health and emo-

tional problems than children whose parents did not, these children did not report poorer mental health compared to children of different-sex parents.

Further, few studies find differences between same-sex and different-sex parents in parenting stress (often measured using the Parenting Stress Index; Abidin, 1990), suggesting that stigma might not strongly impact parenting stress in same-sex parent families (Farr, 2017; Goldberg & Gartrell, 2014; Golombok et al., 2003; Golombok et al., 2014), thus explaining healthy outcomes among children. For example, Golombok et al. (2003) found no differences in parenting stress or socioemotional development between lesbian mothers and different-sex parents in a national sample of parents from the Avon Longitudinal Study of Parents and Children in the UK. Although some studies show that parenting stress is associated with child mental health such as emotional difficulties and externalizing behaviors, these pathways did not differ for same-sex and different-sex parents (Farr, 2017; Golombok et al., 2003; Golombok et al., 2014). Interestingly, studies that do find higher reports of parenting stress among same-sex parents compared to different-sex parents find no differences in child mental health (Bos, Knox, van Rijn-van Gelderen, & Gartrell, 2016; Golombok et al., 2014).

Research with children of same-sex parents suggests a number of positive factors that explain why stigma does not have a strong influence on parenting stress among same-sex parent families. High-quality parent-child relationships marked by warmth, closeness, and cohesion reduce the stress of parenting and predict better mental health and adjustment of children (Baiocco et al., 2015; Baiocco, Carone, Ioverno, & Lingiardi, 2018; Bos et al., 2016; Bos, van Balen, & van den Boom, 2007; Crouch et al., 2014; Farr, 2017; Fedewa et al., 2015; Tornello & Patterson, 2018). Other studies have suggested that more egalitarian attitudes and shared divisions of labor among same-sex parents reduce parenting stress (Miller et al., 2017). Lesbian mothers often report greater satisfaction with co-parenting with their female partners than do heterosexual mothers with their male partners; and, in turn, mothers' greater satisfaction has been linked to lower internalizing and externalizing behavior among children (Bos et al., 2007; Farr & Patterson, 2013).

## Peer Victimization and Coping

One of the major arguments against allowing same-sex couples to have or adopt children has been that children in these families will experience bullying or victimization from peers, resulting in poor outcomes (Clarke, Kitzinger, & Potter, 2004; van Gelderen, Gartrell, Bos, & Hermanns, 2009). Whether children of same-sex parents are at greater risk for victimization compared to children of different-sex parents is unclear. The proportion of children in LGBTQ-parent families who experience peer victimization varies in the literature, with estimates ranging as low as 8% in some studies (Farr, Oakley, & Ollen, 2016) and as high as 43% in others (Bos, Gartrell, Peyser, & van Balen, 2008; Gartrell, Rodas, Deck, Peyser, & Banks, 2005). Nationally representative samples of children of lesbian mothers and children of different-sex parents from the US National Longitudinal Study of Adolescent to Adult Health (Add Health), matched on numerous demographic and family characteristics, reported similar levels of victimization (i.e., how often they had been shot at, cut, or jumped; had a gun or knife pulled on them; or had seen someone shot or stabbed; Wainright & Patterson, 2006) and relationships with peers (Wainright & Patterson, 2008). Rivers, Poteat, and Noret (2008) also found similarities between families with a school-based sample of children of lesbian compared to heterosexual mothers.

The literature on peer victimization as a minority stress mechanism for poor mental health has shown that bias-based bullying and victimization strongly predict mental health among LGBTQ children and youth (Poteat, Mereish, DiGiovanni, & Koenig, 2011; Russell, Sinclair, Poteat, & Koenig, 2012); this research has implications for the health of children in LGBTQ-parent families who face stigma about their

families. Peer victimization of children in LGBTQ-parent families often occurs at school, particularly in elementary school, where children report experiencing disapproving comments, annoying questions, exclusion, and, most commonly, abusive language and being teased (van Gelderen, Gartrell, Bos, van Rooij, & Hermanns, 2012). Studies show that experiences of peer victimization among children of same-sex parents, whether in the form of stigmatization, homophobia, or bullying, are associated with lower self-esteem (Bos & van Balen, 2008) and internalizing and externalizing behaviors in childhood (Bos, Gartrell, van Balen, Peyser, & Sandfort, 2008; Farr et al., 2016; Gartrell et al., 2005) and adolescence (Bos & Gartrell, 2010; Gartrell & Bos, 2010; van Rijn-van Gelderen, Bos, & Gartrell, 2015).

However, even when children of same-sex parents report that peer victimization "hurts their feelings" (Gartrell et al., 2005, p. 522), their mental health (measured using the Child Behavior Checklist; Achenbach, 1991) is still relatively on par with children of different-sex parents (Gartrell et al., 2005). This finding may be related to individual and social characteristics (i.e., resiliency factors) that play important roles in reducing the association between peer victimization and mental health. Children who had contact with friends or other children with lesbian or gay parents (Bos & van Balen, 2008) were exposed to LGBTQ curricula and history (Bos, Gartrell, Peyser, et al., 2008; Short, 2007), had mothers involved in lesbian communities (Bos, Gartrell, Peyser, et al., 2008; Short, 2007), and reported family compatibility in adolescence (Bos & Gartrell, 2010) fared better in the face of victimization than those who did not. However, recent qualitative work also shows that children of same-sex parents may cope with peer victimization in maladaptive ways, particularly through avoidance (e.g., concealment of their family situation, ignoring victimization, avoiding social contact; Kuvalanka, Leslie, & Radina, 2014; van Gelderen, Gartrell, et al. 2012). Though these coping strategies may be beneficial in the short term, research shows that concealment and denial of stigma can lead to negative mental health outcomes over time

(Pachankis, 2007). Thus, although children of same-sex parents appear to function well in the face of peer victimization and bullying, maladaptive or harmful ways of coping could be detrimental to children's mental health.

## Intersections of Family Contexts for Physical and Mental Health Outcomes

Although decades of research have established physical and mental health disparities between LGBTQ and heterosexual people (IOM, 2011), recently there has been increased attention on and numerous calls for the consideration of within-group understandings of sexual minority health (e.g., Fish & Russell, 2018; Pollitt, Brimhall, Brewster, & Ross, 2018) and a focus on intersectionality (e.g., Cole, 2009; IOM, 2011; Prendergast & MacPhee, 2018). Intersectionality theory posits that people have multiple, intersecting identities that are embedded within broader social contexts (Crenshaw, 1989) with implications for their health and well-being. Similarly, identities or contexts that LGBTQ parent families embody, such as gender, race, or class, intersect with family status to further influence physical and mental health through dynamics within and outside the family, access to resources, and reduced or exacerbated stressors. These intersecting contexts may also foster resilience to physical and mental health outcomes in the face of stigmatization and stress. In this next section, we describe particular contexts that can influence how stigma and stress impact physical and mental health outcomes in LGBTQ-parent families and understudied areas that require additional research.

### Parent Gender and Sexual Identity

Initial debates about the legality and morality of same-sex marriage and parenting relied on similar arguments that children of same-sex parents, specifically lesbian mothers, would face poorer health and well-being than children of different-sex parents (Goldberg & Gartrell, 2014; Patterson, 2017). The political focus on the capabilities of lesbian mothers to raise healthy children, in tandem with a lesbian baby boom, led to a rise in research on the mental health of children of lesbian mothers (Goldberg & Gartrell, 2014; Patterson, 2017; Tasker, 2010). Specifically, anti-marriage equality arguments were based on underlying, societal assumptions that raising healthy children requires both mothers and fathers and that the absence of fathers has a large impact on children's adjustment (Biblarz & Stacey, 2010; Goldberg & Allen, 2007). Multiple scholars have argued that there is little logic to the assumption that motherhood and fatherhood are distinct constructs and that children will have worse functioning without both mothers and fathers (Biblarz & Stacey, 2010; Reczek, 2016). Indeed, Golombok et al. (2014) explicitly tested for differences between gay fathers and lesbian mothers and found no differences in anxiety, depression, parenting stress, family dynamics, conflict, or child adjustment. Thus, this research suggests that the genders of parents do not play a central role in children's mental health outcomes.

Though the literature on transgender parents has been growing, there has been much less research on the physical and mental health of transgender parents and their children compared to the literature on same-sex parents (see chapter "Transgender-Parent Families"). Research suggests that transgender parents experience many of the same stressors reported by lesbian and gay parents that might influence parenting stress and thus physical and mental health: the fear that their children will be bullied, the dissolution of their relationships because of their gender transition, and the restructuring of family and gender roles (Haines, Ajayi, & Boyd, 2014; Pyne, Bauer, & Bradley, 2015). Greater risk for negative mental health among children of transgender parents before and after their parent's transition (White & Ettner, 2007) appears related to stressors in their parents' relationship: elevated conflict in and potential dissolution of their parents' relationship, including transphobic comments from the nontransgender parent, have significant effects on the well-being of children (Freedman, Tasker, & Di Ceglie, 2002; Haines et al., 2014; Hines, 2006; White & Ettner, 2007). In addition, transgender parents face significant discrimination in custody determinations in which they may be unable to see their children (Pyne et al., 2015); this loss of the parent-child relationship can be devastating for both parents and children, particularly if it results in instability and grief for the child. However, much of the research on mental health among children of transgender parents is with clinical samples (Freedman et al., 2002; White & Ettner, 2004, 2007). Additional research with transgender parents from the general population is needed to better understand children's well-being and how best to support transgender parent families with the stress and instability that occur during transitions.

Bisexual people report worse mental and physical health than both their lesbian/gay and heterosexual peers (Dyar et al., 2019; Pompili et al., 2014; Ross et al., 2018; Salway et al., 2019; see chapter "What Do We Now Know About Bisexual Parenting? A Continuing Call for Research") as the result of stigma-based stressors including erasure/invalidation of their sexual identity and perceptions that bisexual people are promiscuous and cannot be monogamous (Israel & Mohr, 2004). However, because bisexual people are more likely to be in different-sex relationships and thus not categorized as sexual minority parents (Herek, Norton, Allen, & Sims, 2010), there have been fewer studies on the health of bisexual parents and their children despite the fact that they are more likely to be parents than lesbian/gay people (Gates, 2014; Herek et al., 2010). Though bisexual parents in different-sex relationships and their children might not face the same stigma that children of lesbian, gay, or bisexual parents in same-sex relationships experience, research shows that experiences of biphobia prevent these parents from disclosing their bisexual identities to others, including their children (Bartelt, Bowling, Dodge, & Bostwick, 2017; Tasker & Delvoye, 2015). It is conceivable that bisexual parents could have worse physical and mental health due to experiences with these unique stigma and

stressors with implications for their children's health as well. For example, Calzo et al. (2017) found that children of bisexual parents had higher externalizing behaviors than children of heterosexual, lesbian, or gay parents; this result disappeared once the authors accounted for parents' psychological distress. As the population of people identifying as bisexual continues to grow (Copen, Chandra, & Febo-Vazquez, 2016)—and may begin to outnumber people who identify as lesbian or gay (Gates, 2014)—it will be critical to understand the unique experiences of bisexual parents and their children and their impact on physical and mental health.

## Race/Ethnicity

Research generally on LGBTQ-parents of color is quite limited (see chapter "Race and Ethnicity in the Lives of LGBTQ Parents and Their Children: Perspectives from and Beyond North America"). Few quantitative studies reviewed for this chapter included substantive numbers of parents of color despite the fact that LGBTQ people of color are more likely to be parents than LGBTQ White people (Gates, 2015). Thus, less is known about the health and well-being of parents of color in LGBTQ-parent families. Available research suggests important stressors and stigma at the intersection of sexual orientation, family status, and race/ethnicity that could have implications for physical and mental health outcomes of LGBTQ-parents of color and their children. Gay fathers of color describe feeling isolated and ignored in gay communities as well as conflict within their racial/ethnic communities (Carroll, 2018). Family welfare policies and systems are often discriminatory against both LGBTQ parents and parents of color, such as increased vigilance of families of color from child protective services and laws that ban same-sex parents from adopting from foster care (Cahill, Battle, & Meyer, 2003). There are also ways in which racial/ethnic families are resilient; for example, gay fathers of color often feel like pioneers who are well prepared to face any stigma they or their children might experience (Carroll,

2018) and often have extended, supportive kinship networks for raising children (Cahill et al., 2003). More research on the health of LGBTQ-parents of color and their children, in light of these potential stressors, is needed.

It is also important to note that adoptive LGBTQ-parent families are often multiracial considering that same-sex couples are more likely to be interracial (Farr & Patterson, 2009) and are more likely to adopt children of color than different-sex parents (Farr & Patterson, 2009; Raleigh, 2012). Though these families might face multiple forms of discrimination, research shows that White lesbian parents who adopt children of color are aware of the struggles that their children may face and feel better equipped to prepare their children for coping with stigma because of their own experiences with discrimination (Richardson & Goldberg, 2010). This is a ripe area of research for understanding how the intersection of identities in families, such as sexual identity and race, might allow parents to better help their children cope with both heterosexism and racism (Farr & Patterson, 2009; Wyman Battalen, Farr, Brodzinsky, & McRoy, 2019) as a protective factor for health.

## Social Class

One intersectional context that threads through, and underlies, many of these other contexts is socioeconomic status (SES). Though variation in SES among LGBTQ-parent families is largely unexamined, and nationally representative research shows inconsistencies in whether same-sex parents report higher SES than different-sex parents (Crouch et al., 2014; Gates, 2015; Reczek et al., 2016, 2017), social class is one of the most important predictors of health and well-being in families, including LGBTQ-parent families. Parents in the general population who are unemployed, live in poverty, and have lower education levels report lower well-being and are more likely to report that their children have emotional difficulties and behavioral problems (Reczek et al., 2016, 2017). Some studies show that higher SES

mitigates mental health disparities between children of same-sex and different-sex parents (Gartrell & Bos, 2010; Wainright & Patterson, 2006). Higher financial status might provide stability and other resources, such as access to health care and health insurance, which are associated with better physical and mental health for LGBTQ parents and their children (Buchmueller & Carpenter, 2010). Higher social class might also play a role in protecting children of LGBTQ-parents from peer victimization because higher SES families have greater resources to choose the geographical or political areas in which they live, to place their children in higher-quality schools (Goldberg, Allen, Black, Frost, & Manley, 2018), and to feel that they can advocate for their children when they experience bullying (Kosciw & Diaz, 2008; Nixon, 2011). However, LGBTQ-parent families with lower SES likely have unique strengths that result in better health and adjustment; for example, LGBTQ parents with less financial capital may invest more emotional and social capital in their families with benefits to health (Nixon, 2011). Additional research on identifying important resilience factors among families with lower SES is needed (see chapter "LGBTQ-Parent Families in the United States and Economic Well-Being").

## Routes to Parenthood

LGBTQ people become parents through numerous pathways, and the ways in which LGBTQ people become parents intersect with gender, sexuality, and social class. Prior to increased positive attitudes toward LGBTQ people and an expansion of rights such as marriage equality, stigmatization, and desire for children led some LGBTQ people to conceal their identities in different-sex marriages (Gates, 2015; See chapter "LGBTQ Parenting Post-Heterosexual Relationship Dissolution"). Thus, many LGBTQ-parent families formed in the context of a different-sex relationship ended in divorce (Gates, 2014; Goldberg & Gartrell, 2014; Patterson, 2006; Tasker, 2005). The finding in earlier studies that children of divorced lesbian and gay parents had worse mental health outcomes than children of different-sex parents did not consider the impact of divorce (Gates, 2015). Reevaluation of these studies, and more recent studies that took divorce into account, whether by controlling for divorce or comparing children with divorced same-sex parents to children with divorced different-sex parents, found no differences in child mental health (Patterson, 2006; Stacey & Biblarz, 2001; Tasker, 2005; Telingator & Patterson, 2008). Thus, if family formation is related to mental health among children in LGBTQ-parent families, it is likely due to family instability and stability, which are critical for the mental health of all children (Waldfogel, Craigie, & Brooks-Gunn, 2010).

Further, instability related to singlehood might play a role in children's mental health: Studies have found more differences in psychological adjustment between single- and two-parent families, regardless of sexual orientation or family status, than differences between same-sex and different-sex parents (Calzo et al., 2017; Golombok et al., 2003; Shechner, Slone, Lobel, & Shechter, 2013). However, it is important to note that instability is not inherent in divorced or single-parent families, and these families often show remarkable resilience. For example, some studies have found no differences in problem behavior between planned biological children whose lesbian mothers remained together and those whose mothers had separated (though it is unclear whether these mothers remarried; Gartrell & Bos, 2010; van Gelderen, Bos, Gartrell, Hermanns, & Perrin, 2012).

Pathways of stress and mental health among same-sex parents formed through adoption appear similar to those of different-sex adoptive parents. For example, gay fathers who adopted with previous partners reported higher parenting stress than those who adopted with their current partner or as a single parent; similarly, fathers who adopted from foster care reported higher parenting stress than those who went through private, public, or religious adoption (Tornello et al., 2011). This research shows few differences in children's mental health based on adoption through international, private domestic, or public

domestic adoption (Goldberg & Smith, 2013). Instead, relationship conflict, preparation for adoption, and parent depressive symptoms predicted internalizing and externalizing behaviors among adopted children, regardless of whether their parents were lesbian, gay, or heterosexual (Goldberg & Smith, 2013).

Social class selection into intentional parenthood could also play a role in physical and mental health outcomes in LGBTQ-parent families. It is likely that LGBTQ people with higher SES, especially those in same-sex relationships, are better able to plan to become parents than LGBTQ people with lower SES because access to conception and adoption methods particularly surrogacy requires substantial financial and legal resources. Families formed through surrogacy are characterized by high incomes and levels of education (Carone, Lingiardi, Chirumbolo, & Baiocco, 2018; Miller et al., 2017), which has implications for family health. For example, in a recent study of Italian same-sex parent families, Carone et al. (2018) suggest that the significant amount of planning required for surrogacy, combined with fathers' higher SES, might explain their finding of better adjustment among children of gay fathers than lesbian mothers. The few studies on the health of these families show either similar or better psychological adjustment compared to families formed through other methods (Baiocco et al., 2015, 2018; Crouch et al., 2014; Golombok et al., 2018; van Rijn-van Gelderen et al., 2017). However, social class may become a stronger predictor of health in LGBTQ-parent families over time as fewer LGBTQ people have children in different-sex marriages and rely more heavily on adoption or alternative conception methods (Gates, 2015).

## Directions for Future Research

The research covered in this review suggests that how researchers define "LGBTQ parents" matters when examining the physical and mental health outcomes of LGBTQ-parent families and that these families come in a large variety of forms. Though the majority of research has studied the health of children of same-sex couples who are parents, there are many other understudied forms of LGBTQ-parent families. We know less, for example, about the health of self-identified LGBTQ people raising children in same- or different-sex relationships, residential versus nonresidential LGBTQ parents, and LGBTQ single parents and stepparents. Moreover, the definitions, categorization, and study populations of LGBTQ parents used in research can influence findings on children's mental health because there might be differences in stigma and social support among particular groups. For example, bisexual parents are often not included as sexual minorities in most research because parents are often categorized based on relationship status (i.e., same or different-sex parents), and bisexual people are more likely to be partnered to someone of a different-sex. Studies such as the one conducted by Calzo et al. (2017), which included multiple forms of LGBTQ-parent families and examined whether children of lesbian, gay, bisexual, and heterosexual parents in same-sex or different-sex, one-parent or two-parent families differed on psychological adjustment, are excellent examples of including multiple types of families. Thus, major areas for future research are in the areas of physical and mental health outcomes of bisexual and transgender parents and their children, particularly given elevated health disparities and unique relationship and stigma experiences of these groups.

The majority of studies in the area of LGBTQ-parent families and health have focused on the mental health and well-being of minor children of same-sex parents; as children and parents begin to age, there is a unique opportunity for researchers to study the intergenerational relationships of LGBTQ parents and their adult children. There is ample evidence that the relationship between parents and adult children impacts the health of both generations (Lowenstein, Katz, & Biggs, 2011; Reczek, 2016); this is a particularly important area for studying physical health factors given that physical health declines over the life course. Initial research in this area shows that gay men and lesbian women have relationships

with their parents and parents-in-law marked by both conflict and support, with implications for relationship quality (Reczek, 2016). Understanding how strain and support in relationships between LGBTQ parents, their parents (i.e., grandparents), and children over time could illuminate risk and protective factors for LGBTQ physical health disparities. Further, it is unknown how relationships between adult LGBTQ children and their parents shape the transition of LGBTQ adults to parenthood, nor how relationships between LGBTQ parents and their own children matter for parental health and well-being (Reczek, 2016).

Researchers have begun to examine the experiences of LGBTQ children of LGBTQ parents, also known as "second-generation" LGBTQ children (see chapter "The "Second Generation:" LGBTQ Youth with LGBTQ Parents"). These youth have unique experiences that can confer advantages and disadvantages to mental health, particularly compared to LGBTQ children of different-sex parents. For example, disclosure to parents might be less stressful for second-generation LGBTQ youth; however, these youth might be reluctant to reinforce stereotypes that LGBTQ parents raise LGBTQ children (Kuvalanka & Goldberg, 2009). Little research has been conducted on the health and well-being of second-generation LGBTQ children, and it is unclear whether LGBTQ health disparities are attenuated or exacerbated in this population. Thus, the experiences of second-generation LGBTQ youth are rich areas for future research, particularly to deepen understandings of how minority stress influences health.

The literature covered in this chapter also points to the importance of including sexual and gender identity questions in population-based surveys of families, particularly those that assess health (Wolff, Wells, Ventura-DiPersia, Renson, & Grov, 2017). Until recently, much of the research in this area has had to rely on community or convenience samples to accurately capture LGBTQ parents; these studies, such as the US National Longitudinal Lesbian Family Study, have been particularly important for studying the well-being of lesbian mothers and their children. However, it is difficult for researchers to account for selection bias in these studies, and participants are more likely to be White and have higher SES (Patterson, 2006). In comparison, the number of population-based surveys of health that researchers can use to identify same-sex parents is quite small (these include Add Health, the National Longitudinal Survey of Youth 1979 and 1997, the Avon Longitudinal Study of Parents and Children, and the National Health Interview Survey), and precisely identifying them can be difficult (DeMaio, Bates, & O'Connell, 2013). Now that marriage equality is legal in many countries, including the USA, the UK, and Australia, oversampling for LGBTQ people, particularly parents, in nationally representative datasets would improve researchers' abilities to capture the experiences and health of broader, more diverse samples of families.

Now that the field has reached general consensus on the mental health of children of LGBTQ parents and begun to move beyond a deficit-based approach (Goldberg & Gartrell, 2014; Manning et al., 2014), this is an exciting opportunity to examine the complexity of family dynamics on health in LGBTQ-parent families using advanced statistical methods, especially as data on sexual and gender identity and LGBTQ parents improve (Umberson, Thomeer, Kroeger, Lodge, & Xu, 2015). Statistical methods such as structural equation modeling can easily model complex longitudinal, mediational processes between large numbers of variables while accounting for measurement error. Multilevel modeling (also known as hierarchical linear modeling) can also answer longitudinal research questions while taking into account the interdependence between parents, partners, and children. For example, Farr (2017) conducted hierarchical linear modeling to examine how family functioning in same- and different-sex parent families predicted parent and teacher reports of children's health outcomes over time. These models were nested within couples and time such that they accounted for the interdependence between the two reports from both parents, reports from teachers, and repeated measure-ment. Such studies extend the literature by providing nuanced, precise estimates of complex family processes and health.

## Implications for Practice

The practical implications of this research are clear: though LGBTQ-parent families are vulnerable to negative physical and mental health as the result of societal stigma, research shows substantial resiliency such that the majority of these families are functioning well. Clinicians should not assume that children in LGBTQ-parent families face poorer outcomes simply because of their family structure. Maladaptive coping with stigma-related stress by children of LGBTQ parents appears to be related to negative mental health outcomes; thus, clinicians should capitalize on the strengths that these families have in order to cope with external and internal stressors. Though few studies have shown differences in children's mental health by family formation method, clinicians can be aware that LGBTQ-parent families are formed in a multitude of ways and can support children in how they understand their families (Telingator & Patterson, 2008). It is also particularly important for clinicians to help LGBTQ-parent families through transitions related to disclosure, relationship dissolution (if it occurs), and gender transition (in the case of transgender parents; Haines et al., 2014; White & Ettner, 2004).

Supportive school environments can mitigate the stress of peer victimization and mental health outcomes related to it among children in LGBTQ-parent families. Teachers, principals, and other staff members can be advocates for children of LGBTQ parents by ensuring that their classrooms and schools are free from bias-based bullying. Research on LGBTQ youth shows that perceived school support is associated with higher feelings of safety in the presence of school harassment (McGuire, Anderson, Toomey, & Russell, 2010; Russell, Horn, Kosciw, & Saewyc, 2010). Enumerated anti-bullying policies that include protections against discrimination based on family status or structure, in addition to sexual orientation and gender identity, would provide school personnel with the ability to intervene in peer victimization based on family status.

## Conclusion

In this chapter, we have reviewed the research on the physical and mental health of parents and children in LGBTQ-parent families with a focus on the health-shaping mechanisms of vulnerability and resilience in families. In doing so, we highlight the importance of mental health disparities that result from homophobic and transphobic stigma and stress, especially for parents, and the mental health resiliency of children of same-sex families. We show that it is not being in a same-sex family, per se, that shapes child well-being but rather potential instability in family relationships that contribute to poor child health. Future research should examine physical health outcomes to determine further health disparities and should attend to the experiences of LGBTQ-parent families of color and bisexual and transgender parent families in particular. Overall, policy makers, clinicians, and social institutions such as schools can play an important role in facilitating better health by understanding the root causes of health disparities for both children and adults in LGBTQ-parent families.

## References

Abidin, R. (1990). *Parenting Stress Index test manual.* Charlottesville, VA: Pediatric Psychology Press.

Achenbach, T. M. (1991). *Manual for the Child Behavior Checklist/4–18 and 1991 Profile.* Burlington, VT: University of Vermont, Department of Psychiatry.

Anderssen, N., Amlie, C., & Ytterøy, E. A. (2002). Outcomes for children with lesbian or gay parents. A review of studies from 1978 to 2000. *Scandinavian Journal of Psychology, 43,* 335–351. https://doi.org/10.1111/1467-9450.00302

Baiocco, R., Carone, N., Ioverno, S., & Lingiardi, V. (2018). Same-sex and different-sex parent families in Italy: Is parents' sexual orientation associated with child health outcomes and parental dimensions? *Journal of Developmental & Behavioral Pediatrics, 39,* 555–563. https://doi.org/10.1097/DBP.0000000000000583

Baiocco, R., Santamaria, F., Ioverno, S., Fontanesi, L., Baumgartner, E., Laghi, F., & Lingiardi, V. (2015). Lesbian mother families and gay father families in Italy: Family functioning, dyadic satisfaction, and child well-being. *Sexuality Research and Social Policy, 12,* 202–212. https://doi.org/10.1007/s13178-015-0185-x

Bartelt, E., Bowling, J., Dodge, B., & Bostwick, W. (2017). Bisexual identity in the context of parenthood: An exploratory qualitative study of self-identified bisexual parents in the United States. *Journal of Bisexuality, 17,* 378–399. https://doi.org/10.1080/15299716.2017.1384947

Biblarz, T. J., & Stacey, J. (2010). How does the gender of parents matter? *Journal of Marriage and Family, 72,* 3–22. https://doi.org/10.1111/j.1741-3737.2009.00678.x

Bos, H., & Gartrell, N. (2010). Adolescents of the USA National Longitudinal Lesbian Family Study: Can family characteristics counteract the negative effects of stigmatization? *Family Process, 49,* 559–572. https://doi.org/10.1111/j.1545-5300.2010.01340.x

Bos, H. M., Gartrell, N. K., Peyser, H., & van Balen, F. (2008). The USA national longitudinal lesbian family study (NLLFS): Homophobia, psychological adjustment, and protective factors. *Journal of Lesbian Studies, 12,* 455–471. https://doi.org/10.1080/10894160802278630

Bos, H. M., Gartrell, N. K., van Balen, F., Peyser, H., & Sandfort, T. G. (2008). Children in planned lesbian families: A cross-cultural comparison between the United States and the Netherlands. *American Journal of Orthopsychiatry, 78,* 211–219. https://doi.org/10.1037/a0012711

Bos, H. M., Knox, J. R., van Rijn-van Gelderen, L., & Gartrell, N. K. (2016). Same-sex and different-sex parent households and child health outcomes: Findings from the National Survey of Children's Health. *Journal of Developmental & Behavioral Pediatrics, 37,* 179–187. https://doi.org/10.1097/DBP.0000000000000288

Bos, H. M., & van Balen, F. (2008). Children in planned lesbian families: Stigmatisation, psychological adjustment and protective factors. *Culture, Health & Sexuality, 10,* 221–236. https://doi.org/10.1080/13691050701601702

Bos, H. M., van Balen, F., & van den Boom, D. C. (2007). Child adjustment and parenting in planned lesbian-parent families. *American Journal of Orthopsychiatry, 77,* 38–48. https://doi.org/10.1037/0002-9432.77.1.38

Buchmueller, T., & Carpenter, C. S. (2010). Disparities in health insurance coverage, access, and outcomes for individuals in same-sex versus different-sex relationships, 2000–2007. *American Journal of Public Health, 100,* 489–495. https://doi.org/10.2105/AJPH.2009.160804

Cahill, S., Battle, J., & Meyer, D. (2003). Partnering, parenting, and policy: Family issues affecting Black lesbian, gay, bisexual, and transgender (LGBT) people. *Race and Society, 6,* 85–98. https://doi.org/10.1016/j.racsoc.2004.11.002

Calzo, J. P., Mays, V. M., Björkenstam, C., Björkenstam, E., Kosidou, K., & Cochran, S. D. (2017). Parental sexual orientation and children's psychological well-being: 2013–2015 National Health Interview Survey. Child Development. Advance online publication. doi:https://doi.org/10.1111/cdev.12989

Carone, N., Lingiardi, V., Chirumbolo, A., & Baiocco, R. (2018). Italian gay father families formed by surrogacy: Parenting, stigmatization, and children's psychological adjustment. Developmental Psychology, 54, 1904–1916. https://doi.org/10.1037/dev0000571

Carroll, M. (2018). Gay fathers on the margins: Race, class, marital status, and pathway to parenthood. Family Relations, 67, 104–117. https://doi.org/10.1111/fare.12300

Centers for Disease Control and Prevention. (2013). CDC health disparities and inequalities report—United States, 2013. Morbidity and Mortality Weekly Report, 62, 1–187. Retrieved from https://www.cdc.gov/mmwr/pdf/other/su6203.pdf

Clarke, V., Kitzinger, C., & Potter, J. (2004). 'Kids are just cruel anyway': Lesbian and gay parents' talk about homophobic bullying. British Journal of Social Psychology, 43, 531–550. https://doi.org/10.1348/0144666042565362

Cohen, S., Janicki-Deverts, D., & Miller, G. E. (2007). Psychological stress and disease. Journal of the American Medical Association, 298, 1685–1687. https://doi.org/10.1001/jama.298.14.1685

Cole, E. R. (2009). Intersectionality and research in psychology. American Psychologist, 64, 170–180. https://doi.org/10.1037/a0014564

Copen, C. E., Chandra, A., & Febo-Vazquez, I. (2016). Sexual behavior, sexual attraction, and sexual orientation among adults aged 18–44 in the United States: Data from the 2011–2013 National Survey of Family Growth. National Health Statistics Reports, 88, 1–14. Retrieved from https://www.cdc.gov/nchs/data/nhsr/nhsr088.pdf

Crenshaw, K. (1989). Demarginalizing the intersection of race and sex: A Black feminist critique of antidiscrimination doctrine, feminist theory, and antiracist politics. The University of Chicago Legal Forum, 139–167.

Crouch, S. R., Waters, E., McNair, R., Power, J., & Davis, E. (2014). Parent-reported measures of child health and wellbeing in same-sex parent families: A cross-sectional survey. BMC Public Health, 14, 635. https://doi.org/10.1186/1471-2458-14-635

Crowl, A., Ahn, S., & Baker, J. (2008). A meta-analysis of developmental outcomes for children of same-sex and heterosexual parents. Journal of GLBT Family Studies, 4, 385–407. https://doi.org/10.1080/15504280802177615

DeMaio, T. J., Bates, N., & O'Connell, M. (2013). Exploring measurement error issues in reporting of same-sex couples. Public Opinion Quarterly, 77, 145–158. https://doi.org/10.1093/poq/nfs066

Dyar, C., Taggart, T. C., Rodriguez-Seijas, C., Thompson, R. G., Elliott, J. C., Hasin, D. S., & Eaton, N. R. (2019). Physical health disparities across dimensions of sexual orientation, race/ethnicity, and sex: Evidence for increased risk among bisexual adults. Archives of Sexual Behavior, 48, 225–242. https://doi.org/10.1007/s10508-018-1169-8

Farr, R. H. (2017). Does parental sexual orientation matter? A longitudinal follow-up of adoptive families with school-age children. Developmental Psychology, 53, 252–264. https://doi.org/10.1037/dev0000228

Farr, R. H., Oakley, M. K., & Ollen, E. W. (2016). School experiences of young children and their lesbian and gay adoptive parents. Psychology of Sexual Orientation and Gender Diversity, 3, 442–447. https://doi.org/10.1037/sgd0000187

Farr, R. H., & Patterson, C. J. (2009). Transracial adoption by lesbian, gay, and heterosexual couples: Who completes transracial adoptions and with what results? Adoption Quarterly, 12, 187–204. https://doi.org/10.1080/10926750903313328

Farr, R. H., & Patterson, C. J. (2013). Coparenting among lesbian, gay, and heterosexual couples: Associations with adopted children's outcomes. Child Development, 84, 1226–1240. https://doi.org/10.1111/cdev.12046

Farr, R. H., Tasker, F., & Goldberg, A. E. (2017). Theory in highly cited studies of sexual minority parent families: Variations and implications. Journal of Homosexuality, 64, 1143–1179. https://doi.org/10.1080/00918369.2016.1242336

Fedewa, A. L., Black, W. W., & Ahn, S. (2015). Children and adolescents with same-gender parents: A meta-analytic approach in assessing outcomes. Journal of GLBT Family Studies, 11, 1–34. https://doi.org/10.1080/1550428X.2013.869486

Fish, J. N., & Russell, S. T. (2018). Queering methodologies to understand queer families. Family Relations, 67, 12–25. https://doi.org/10.1111/fare.12297

Freedman, D., Tasker, F., & Di Ceglie, D. (2002). Children and adolescents with transsexual parents referred to a specialist gender identity development service: A brief report of key developmental features. Clinical Child Psychology and Psychiatry, 7, 423–432. https://doi.org/10.1177/1359104502007003009

Gartrell, N., & Bos, H. (2010). US National Longitudinal Lesbian Family Study: Psychological adjustment of 17-year-old adolescents. Pediatrics, 126, 1–9. https://doi.org/10.1542/peds.2009-3153

Gartrell, N., Rodas, C., Deck, A., Peyser, H., & Banks, A. (2005). The National Lesbian Family Study: 4. Interviews with the 10-year-old children. American Journal of Orthopsychiatry, 75, 518–524. https://doi.org/10.1037/0002-9432.75.4.518

Gates, G. J. (2014). LGBT demographics: Comparisons among population-based surveys. Retrieved from University of California Los Angeles School of Law, Williams Institute: http://williamsinstitute.law.ucla.edu/wp-content/uploads/lgbt-demogs-sep-2014

Gates, G. J. (2015). Marriage and family: LGBT individuals and same-sex couples. The Future of Children, 25(2), 67–87. https://doi.org/10.1353/foc.2015.0013

Goldberg, A. E. (2010). Lesbian and gay parents and their children: Research on the family life cycle. Washington,

DC: American Psychological Association. https://doi.org/10.1037/12055-000

Goldberg, A. E., & Allen, K. R. (2007). Imagining men: Lesbian mothers' perceptions of male involvement during the transition to parenthood. *Journal of Marriage and Family, 69*, 352–365. https://doi.org/10.1111/j.1741-3737.2007.00370.x

Goldberg, A. E., Allen, K. R., Black, K. A., Frost, R. L., & Manley, M. H. (2018). "There is no perfect school": The complexity of school decision-making among lesbian and gay adoptive parents. *Journal of Marriage and Family, 80*, 684–703. https://doi.org/10.1111/jomf.12478

Goldberg, A. E., & Gartrell, N. K. (2014). LGB-parent families: The current state of the research and directions for the future. *Advances in Child Development and Behavior, 46*, 57–88. https://doi.org/10.1016/B978-0-12-800285-8.00003-0

Goldberg, A. E., Moyer, A. M., Kinkler, L. A., & Richardson, H. B. (2012). "When you're sitting on the fence, hope's the hardest part": Experiences and challenges of lesbian, gay, and heterosexual couples adopting through the child welfare system. *Adoption Quarterly, 15*, 1–28. https://doi.org/10.1080/10926755.2012.731032

Goldberg, A. E., & Smith, J. Z. (2008). Social support and psychological well-being in lesbian and heterosexual preadoptive couples. *Family Relations, 57*, 281–294. https://doi.org/10.1111/j.1741-3729.2008.00500.x

Goldberg, A. E., & Smith, J. Z. (2011). Stigma, social context, and mental health: Lesbian and gay couples across the transition to adoptive parenthood. *Journal of Counseling Psychology, 58*, 139–150. https://doi.org/10.1037/a0021684

Goldberg, A. E., & Smith, J. Z. (2013). Predictors of psychological adjustment in early placed adopted children with lesbian, gay, and heterosexual parents. *Journal of Family Psychology, 27*, 431–442. https://doi.org/10.1037/a0032911

Goldberg, A. E., & Smith, J. Z. (2014). Predictors of parenting stress in lesbian, gay, and heterosexual adoptive parents during early parenthood. *Journal of Family Psychology, 28*, 125–137. https://doi.org/10.1037/a0036007

Goldberg, A. E., Smith, J. Z., McCormick, N., & Overstreet, N. (2019). Health behaviors and outcomes of parents in same-sex couples: An exploratory study. *Psychology of Sexual Orientation & Gender Diversity*. Advance online publication. doi:https://doi.org/10.1037/sgd0000330

Golombok, S., Blake, L., Slutsky, J., Raffanello, E., Roman, G. D., & Ehrhardt, A. (2018). Parenting and the adjustment of children born to gay fathers through surrogacy. *Child Development, 89*, 1223–1233. https://doi.org/10.1111/cdev.12728

Golombok, S., Mellish, L., Jennings, S., Casey, P., Tasker, F., & Lamb, M. E. (2014). Adoptive gay father families: Parent–child relationships and children's psychological adjustment. *Child Development, 85*, 456–468. https://doi.org/10.1111/cdev.12155

Golombok, S., Perry, B., Burston, A., Murray, C., Mooney-Somers, J., Stevens, M., & Golding, J. (2003). Children with lesbian parents: A community study. *Developmental Psychology, 39*, 20–33. https://doi.org/10.1037/0012-1649.39.1.20

Haines, B. A., Ajayi, A. A., & Boyd, H. (2014). Making trans parents visible: Intersectionality of trans and parenting identities. *Feminism & Psychology, 24*, 238–247. https://doi.org/10.1177/0959353514526219

Herek, G. M., Norton, A. T., Allen, T. J., & Sims, C. L. (2010). Demographic, psychological, and social characteristics of self-identified lesbian, gay, and bisexual adults in a U.S. probability sample. *Sexuality Research and Social Policy, 7*, 176–200. https://doi.org/10.1007/s13178-010-0017-y

Hines, S. (2006). Intimate transitions: Transgender practices of partnering and parenting. *Sociology, 40*, 353–371. https://doi.org/10.1177/0038038506062037

Institute of Medicine. (2011). *The health of lesbian, gay, bisexual and transgender people: Building a foundation for better understanding*. Washington, DC: National Academies Press.

Israel, T., & Mohr, J. J. (2004). Attitudes toward bisexual women and men: Current research, future directions. *Journal of Bisexuality, 4*, 117–134. https://doi.org/10.1300/J159v04n01_09

Kosciw, J. G., & Diaz, E. M. (2008). *Involved, invisible, ignored: The experiences of lesbian, gay, bisexual and transgender parents and their children in our nation's K–12 schools*. New York, NY: GLSEN.

Kuvalanka, K. A., & Goldberg, A. E. (2009). "Second generation" voices: Queer youth with lesbian/bisexual mothers. *Journal of Youth and Adolescence, 38*, 904–919. https://doi.org/10.1007/s10964-008-9327-2

Kuvalanka, K. A., Leslie, L. A., & Radina, R. (2014). Coping with sexual stigma: Emerging adults with lesbian parents reflect on the impact of heterosexism and homophobia during their adolescence. *Journal of Adolescent Research, 29*, 241–270. https://doi.org/10.1177/0743558413484354

Lick, D. J., Tornello, S. L., Riskind, R. G., Schmidt, K. M., & Patterson, C. J. (2012). Social climate for sexual minorities predicts well-being among heterosexual offspring of lesbian and gay parents. *Sexuality Research and Social Policy, 9*, 99–112. https://doi.org/10.1007/s13178-012-0081-6

Lowenstein, A., Katz, R., & Biggs, S. (2011). Rethinking theoretical and methodological issues in intergenerational family relations research. *Aging and Society, 31*, 1077–1083. https://doi.org/10.1017/S0144686X10000991

Manning, W. D., Fettro, M. N., & Lamidi, E. (2014). Child well-being in same-sex parent families: Review of research prepared for American Sociological Association Amicus Brief. *Population Research and Policy Review, 33*, 485–502. https://doi.org/10.1007/s11113-014-9329-6

McGuire, J. K., Anderson, C. R., Toomey, R. B., & Russell, S. T. (2010). School climate for transgender youth: A mixed method investigation of student experiences and school responses. *Journal of Youth and Adolescence, 39*, 1175–1188. https://doi.org/10.1007/s10964-010-9540-7

Meyer, I. H. (2003). Prejudice, social stress, and mental health in lesbian, gay, and bisexual populations: Conceptual issues and research evidence. *Psychological Bulletin, 129*, 674–697. https://doi.org/10.1037/0033-2909.129.5.674

Meyer, I. H. (2013). Prejudice, social stress, and mental health in lesbian, gay, and bisexual populations: Conceptual issues and research evidence. *Psychology of Sexual Orientation and Gender Diversity, 1*, 3–26. https://doi.org/10.1037/2329-0382.1.S.3

Miller, B. G., Kors, S., & Macfie, J. (2017). No differences? Meta-analytic comparisons of psychological adjustment in children of gay fathers and heterosexual parents. *Psychology of Sexual Orientation and Gender Diversity, 4*, 14–22. https://doi.org/10.1037/sgd0000203

Moore, M. R., & Stambolis-Ruhstorfer, M. (2013). LGBT sexuality and families at the start of the twenty-first century. *Annual Review of Sociology, 39*, 491–507. https://doi.org/10.1146/annurev-soc-071312-145643

Nixon, C. A. (2011). Working-class lesbian parents' emotional engagement with their children's education: Intersections of class and sexuality. *Sexualities, 14*, 79–99. https://doi.org/10.1177/1363460710390564

Ohrnberger, J., Fichera, E., & Sutton, M. (2017). The relationship between physical and mental health: A mediation analysis. *Social Science & Medicine, 195*, 42–49. https://doi.org/10.1016/j.socscimed.2017.11.008

Pachankis, J. E. (2007). The psychological implications of concealing a stigma: A cognitive-affective-behavioral model. *Psychological Bulletin, 133*, 328–345. https://doi.org/10.1037/0033-2909.133.2.328

Patterson, C. J. (2006). Children of lesbian and gay parents. *Current Directions in Psychological Science, 15*, 241–244. https://doi.org/10.1111/j.1467-8721.2006.00444.x

Patterson, C. J. (2017). Parents' sexual orientation and children's development. *Child Development Perspectives, 11*, 45–49. https://doi.org/10.1111/cdep.12207

Pollitt, A. M., Brimhall, A. L., Brewster, M. E., & Ross, L. E. (2018). Improving the field of LGBTQ psychology: Strategies for amplifying bisexuality research. *Psychology of Sexual Orientation and Gender Diversity, 5*, 129–131. https://doi.org/10.1037/sgd0000273

Pompili, M., Lester, D., Forte, A., Seretti, M. E., Erbuto, D., Lamis, D. A., … Girardi, P. (2014). Bisexuality and suicide: A systematic review of the current literature. *The Journal of Sexual Medicine, 11*, 1903–1913. https://doi.org/10.1111/jsm.12581

Poteat, V. P., Mereish, E. H., DiGiovanni, C. D., & Koenig, B. W. (2011). The effects of general and homophobic victimization on adolescents' psychosocial and educational concerns: The importance of intersecting identities and parent support. *Journal of Counseling Psychology, 58*, 597–609. https://doi.org/10.1037/a0025095

Prendergast, S., & MacPhee, D. (2018). Family resilience amid stigma and discrimination: A conceptual model for families headed by same-sex parents. *Family Relations, 67*, 26–40. https://doi.org/10.1111/fare.12296

Pyne, J., Bauer, G., & Bradley, K. (2015). Transphobia and other stressors impacting trans parents. *Journal of GLBT Family Studies, 11*, 107–126. https://doi.org/10.1080/1550428X.2014.941127

Raleigh, E. (2012). Are same-sex and single adoptive parents more likely to adopt transracially? A national analysis of race, family structure, and the adoption marketplace. *Sociological Perspectives, 55*, 449–471. https://doi.org/10.1525/sop.2012.55.3.449

Reczek, C. (2014). The intergenerational relationships of gay men and lesbian women. *Journals of Gerontology Series B: Psychological Sciences and Social Sciences, 69*, 909–919. https://doi.org/10.1093/geronb/gbu042

Reczek, C. (2016). Re-envisioning why fathers matter beyond the gender binary: A case for gay fathers. In S. M. McHale, V. King, J. Van Hook, & A. Booth (Eds.), *Gender and couple relationships* (pp. 181–186). Cham: Springer. https://doi.org/10.1007/978-3-319-21635-5_11

Reczek, C., Spiker, R., Liu, H., & Crosnoe, R. (2016). Family structure and child health: Does the sex composition of parents matter? *Demography, 53*, 1605–1630. https://doi.org/10.1007/s13524-016-0501-y

Reczek, C., Spiker, R., Liu, H., & Crosnoe, R. (2017). The promise and perils of population research on same-sex families. *Demography, 54*, 2385–2397. https://doi.org/10.1007/s13524-017-0630-y

Richardson, H. B., & Goldberg, A. E. (2010). The intersection of multiple minority identities: Perspectives of White lesbian couples adopting racial/ethnic minority children. *Australian and New Zealand Journal of Family Therapy, 31*, 340–353. https://doi.org/10.1375/anft.31.4.340

Rivers, I., Poteat, V. P., & Noret, N. (2008). Victimization, social support, and psychosocial functioning among children of same-sex and opposite-sex couples in the United Kingdom. *Developmental Psychology, 44*, 127–134. https://doi.org/10.1037/0012-1649.44.1.127

Ross, L. E., Salway, T., Tarasoff, L. A., MacKay, J. M., Hawkins, B. W., & Fehr, C. P. (2018). Prevalence of depression and anxiety among bisexual people compared to gay, lesbian, and heterosexual individuals: A systematic review and meta-analysis. *The Journal of Sex Research, 55*, 435–456. https://doi.org/10.1080/00224499.2017.1387755

Russell, S. T., Horn, S., Kosciw, J., & Saewyc, E. (2010). Safe schools policy for LGBTQ students. *Social Policy Report, 24*, 1–25. https://doi.org/10.1002/j.2379-3988.2010.tb00065.x

Russell, S. T., Sinclair, K. O., Poteat, V. P., & Koenig, B. W. (2012). Adolescent health and harassment based on discriminatory bias. *American Journal of Public Health, 102*, 493–495. https://doi.org/10.2105/AJPH.2011.300430

Salway, T., Ross, L. E., Fehr, C. P., Burley, J., Asadi, S., Hawkins, B., & Tarasoff, L. A. (2019). A systematic review and meta-analysis of disparities in the prevalence of suicide ideation and attempt among bisexual populations. *Archives of Sexual Behavior, 48*, 89–111. https://doi.org/10.1007/s10508-018-1150-6

Shapiro, D. N., Peterson, C., & Stewart, A. J. (2009). Legal and social contexts and mental health among lesbian and heterosexual mothers. *Journal of Family Psychology, 23*, 255–262. https://doi.org/10.1037/a0014973

Shechner, T., Slone, M., Lobel, T. E., & Shechter, R. (2013). Children's adjustment in non-traditional families in Israel: The effect of parental sexual orientation and the number of parents on children's development. *Child: Care, Health and Development, 39*, 178–184. https://doi.org/10.1111/j.1365-2214.2011.01337.x

Short, L. (2007). Lesbian mothers living well in the context of heterosexism and discrimination: Resources, strategies and legislative change. *Feminism and Psychology, 17*, 57–74. https://doi.org/10.1177/0959353507072912

Stacey, J., & Biblarz, T. (2001). (How) does the sexual orientation of parents matter? *American Sociological Review, 66*, 159–183. https://doi.org/10.2307/2657413

Tasker, F. (2005). Lesbian mothers, gay fathers, and their children: A review. *Developmental and Behavioral Pediatrics, 26*, 224–240. https://doi.org/10.1097/00004703-200506000-00012

Tasker, F. (2010). Same-sex parenting and child development: Reviewing the contribution of parental gender. *Journal of Marriage and Family, 72*, 35–40. https://doi.org/10.1111/j.1741-3737.2009.00681.x

Tasker, F., & Delvoye, M. (2015). Moving out of the shadows: Accomplishing bisexual motherhood. *Sex Roles, 73*, 125–140. https://doi.org/10.1007/s11199-015-0503-z

Telingator, C. J., & Patterson, C. (2008). Children and adolescents of lesbian and gay parents. *Journal of the American Academy of Child and Adolescent Psychiatry, 47*, 1364–1386. https://doi.org/10.1097/CHI.0b013e31818960bc

Tornello, S. L., Farr, R. H., & Patterson, C. J. (2011). Predictors of parenting stress among gay adoptive fathers in the United States. *Journal of Family Psychology, 25*, 591–600. https://doi.org/10.1037/a0024480

Tornello, S. L., & Patterson, C. J. (2018). Adult children of gay fathers: Parent–child relationship quality and mental health. *Journal of Homosexuality, 65*, 1152–1166. https://doi.org/10.1080/00918369.2017.1406218

Umberson, D., Thomeer, M. B., Kroeger, R. A., Lodge, A. C., & Xu, M. (2015). Challenges and opportunities for research on same-sex relationships. *Journal of Marriage and Family, 77*, 96–111. https://doi.org/10.1111/jomf.12155

van Gelderen, L., Bos, H. M., Gartrell, N., Hermanns, J., & Perrin, E. C. (2012). Quality of life of adolescents raised from birth by lesbian mothers: The US National Longitudinal Family Study. *Journal of Developmental & Behavioral Pediatrics, 33*, 17–23. https://doi.org/10.1097/DBP.0b013e31823b62af

van Gelderen, L., Gartrell, N., Bos, H., & Hermanns, J. (2009). Stigmatization and resilience in adolescent children of lesbian mothers. *Journal of GLBT Family Studies, 5*, 268–279. https://doi.org/10.1080/15504280903035761

van Gelderen, L., Gartrell, N., Bos, H. M., van Rooij, F. B., & Hermanns, J. M. (2012). Stigmatization associated with growing up in a lesbian-parented family: What do adolescents experience and how do they deal with it? *Children and Youth Services Review, 34*, 999–1006. https://doi.org/10.1016/j.childyouth.2012.01.048

van Rijn-van Gelderen, L., Bos, H. M., & Gartrell, N. K. (2015). Dutch adolescents from lesbian-parent families: How do they compare to peers with heterosexual parents and what is the impact of homophobic stigmatization? *Journal of Adolescence, 40*, 65–73. https://doi.org/10.1016/j.adolescence.2015.01.005

van Rijn-van Gelderen, L., Bos, H. W. M., Jorgensen, T. D., Ellis-Davies, K., Winstanley, A., Golombok, S., … Lamb, M. E. (2017). Wellbeing of gay fathers with children born through surrogacy: A comparison with lesbian-mother families and heterosexual IVF parent families. *Human Reproduction, 33*, 101–108. https://doi.org/10.1093/humrep/dex339

Wainright, J. L., & Patterson, C. J. (2006). Delinquency, victimization, and substance use among adolescents with female same-sex parents. *Journal of Family Psychology, 20*, 526. https://doi.org/10.1037/0893-3200.20.3.526

Wainright, J. L., & Patterson, C. J. (2008). Peer relations among adolescents with female same-sex parents. *Developmental Psychology, 44*, 117–126. https://doi.org/10.1037/0012-1649.44.1.117

Waldfogel, J., Craigie, T., & Brooks-Gunn, J. (2010). Fragile families and child wellbeing. *The Future of Children, 20*, 87–112. https://doi.org/10.1353/foc.2010.0002

White, T., & Ettner, R. (2004). Disclosure, risks and protective factors for children whose parents are undergoing a gender transition. *Journal of Gay & Lesbian Psychotherapy, 8*, 129–145. https://doi.org/10.1007/s00787-006-0591-y

White, T., & Ettner, R. (2007). Adaptation and adjustment in children of transsexual parents. *European Child & Adolescent Psychiatry, 16*, 215–221. https://doi.org/10.1007/s00787-006-0591-y

Wolff, M., Wells, B., Ventura-DiPersia, C., Renson, A., & Grov, C. (2017). Measuring sexual orientation: A review and critique of U.S. data collection efforts and implications for health policy. *The Journal of Sex Research, 54*, 507–531. https://doi.org/10.1080/00224499.2016.1255872

World Health Organization. (2014). *Mental health: A state of well-being*. Retrieved from https://www.who.int/features/factfiles/mental_health/en/

Wyman Battalen, A., Farr, R. H., Brodzinsky, D. M., & McRoy, R. G. (2019). Socializing children about family structure: Perspectives of lesbian and gay adoptive parents. *Journal of GLBT Family Studies, 15*, 235–255. https://doi.org/10.1080/1550428X.2018.1465875

# Part II

# Understudied Areas

# Gay Men and Surrogacy

Dana Berkowitz

The visibility of gay fathers[1] is on the rise, with growing numbers adopting children, sharing parenting with lesbian women, and having children through surrogacy arrangements. The increase in the number of gay fathers who choose to construct their families outside of heterosexual unions is a result of a combination of factors. These include, but are not necessarily limited to, recent developments in reproductive technology, changing legalities in the adoption system, greater acceptance of lesbians and gay men, and broader changes in the diversity of American families (Gamson, 2015; Goldberg, 2010a, 2012; Goldberg, Downing, & Moyer, 2012; Stacey, 2006). Changes in the social, historical, and political context for gay men have increased the visibility of gay fathering, and gay fathers are much less likely to be viewed as the anomaly they once were.

Alongside their increasing visibility is a burgeoning body of research on gay fathers, specifically on the cohort of gay men who became parents after coming out rather than in the context of a previous heterosexual relationship (see Berkowitz & Marsiglio, 2007; Carone, Baiocco, & Lingiardi, 2017; Goldberg, 2010a; Greenfeld & Seli, 2011; Lewin, 2009; Petersen, 2018; Stacey, 2006). However, scholars are just beginning to understand the diversity of structures, arrangements, and practices within gay father-headed family constellations, as there are several paths to parenthood for this emerging cohort—including domestic and international adoption, fostering, surrogacy arrangements, and creative kinship ties that often entail sharing parenting with a LGBQ woman or women. Developing a more nuanced understanding of gay fathers is necessary to better understand the unique family experiences embedded within each of these family forms.

This chapter provides an overview of the scholarship on one particularly understudied group of this new cohort of gay fathers—gay men who have become parents through the assistance of a surrogate mother. Questions that I address in this chapter are: For those gay men using surrogacy, how is the transition to parenthood unique when compared with adoption, fostering, and shared parenting with lesbian women? To what extent do gender, sexuality, social class, race, ethnicity, and nation intersect in surrogacy arrangements? How does the importance of biological relatedness to the

---

[1]Consistent with the majority of research in this area, I use the term gay fathers throughout this chapter to serve as an umbrella term for sexual minority fathers. That said, however, it is important to note that the overwhelming majority of research on sexual minority men, fatherhood, and surrogacy has been conducted with gay fathers, not bisexual or transgender fathers.

D. Berkowitz (✉)
Department of Sociology and Program in Women's and Gender Studies, Louisiana State University, Baton Rouge, LA, USA
e-mail: dberk@lsu.edu

© Springer Nature Switzerland AG 2020
A. E. Goldberg, K. R. Allen (eds.), *LGBTQ-Parent Families*,
https://doi.org/10.1007/978-3-030-35610-1_8

child shape the decision-making processes of those gay men pursuing surrogacy? How are the identities of the egg donor and/or surrogate mother implicated in the process of building a family and, later, for doing family? How do changing legalities shape gay men's decision-making processes and experiences with surrogacy? Answering these fundamental questions about gay fathers and surrogacy provides a starting point for understanding the diversity in routes to gay parenthood and the variety of family structures formed. I expect that this chapter will be of value to researchers and students interested in the intersections of sexuality, gender, and reproduction. Lawyers, policy makers, educators, clinicians, and practitioners who work with sexual minority parents and assisted reproductive technologies may also see this chapter as a valuable source of information. Finally, this chapter should be of interest to current gay fathers who have used surrogacy and gay prospective fathers who are interested in pursuing surrogacy arrangements.

I begin by outlining some of the guiding theoretical perspectives that have been used to frame the scholarship on sexual minority parenting and assisted reproductive technologies. Next, I detail the different types of surrogacy arrangements and the demographic profiles of those gay men who use surrogacy. I review the studies on gay fathers and surrogacy, exploring the rationales behind men's choice to construct their family using this pathway; the relationships that develop between expectant fathers, surrogate mothers, and their children; and, finally, the consequences for family formation. Then, I discuss the rise and fall of reproductive outsourcing, consider the current legal issues facing gay fathers who use surrogacy, and conclude by offering suggestions for research, theory, policy makers, and practitioners. Of note is that I use the term "gay fathers" because that is the subject of the overwhelming majority of the research on sexual minority men, fatherhood, and surrogacy. As I discuss at the end of this chapter, research on other sexual minority fathers is needed in order to better understand how other sexually marginalized men construct and experience surrogate family constellations.

# Theoretical Frameworks

Several complementary theoretical perspectives have guided the scholarship on sexual minority parenting and surrogacy. Oftentimes these perspectives integrate one or more of the following: symbolic interactionism (Berkowitz, 2007; Berkowitz & Marsiglio, 2007), social constructionism (Stacey, 2006), feminism (Ehrenshaft, 2005; Ryan & Berkowitz, 2009; Stacey, 2006), and intersectionality (Gamson, 2015; Mamo & Alston-Stepnitz, 2015; Petersen, 2018; Stacey, 2006). Symbolic interactionism assumes that human beings possess the ability to think and imbue their world with meaning. Such a perspective has been used to emphasize how gay men develop their self-as-father identities and how meanings of self, parent, child, and family emerge from gay men's interactions with surrogates, egg donors, agencies, extended families, and interlopers (Blumer, 1969; Mead, 1934). Similarly, a social constructionist perspective turns the spotlight on the extent to which families, gender, and sexualities are socially and materially constructed (Oswald, Blume, & Marks, 2005). When gay fathers conceive children with egg donors and surrogates, they expose the socially constructed reality behind taken-for-granted assumptions about parenting, fathering, and family. Moreover, gay fathers actively disentangle heterosexuality from parenthood, and in so doing, they disrupt fundamental notions about family. Gay men who choose to parent can challenge normative definitions of family, fatherhood, and even established gender and sexual norms of the mainstream gay subculture. Thus, viewing gay fathers' involvement with their children through these lenses illuminates the fluidity of family, gender, and sexuality.

Much of the work on sexual minority parenting has been spearheaded by feminist scholars who have long challenged "the ideology of the monolithic family and the notion that any one family arrangement is natural, biological, or functional in a timeless way" (Goldberg & Allen, 2007, p. 354). Feminist scholarship has been instrumental in highlighting how gay fathers who become parents via surrogacy do not represent the disintegration of family, but rather constitute new, creative, and valid family constellations. Some more recent work on gay men and surrogacy uses an intersectional feminist analysis (Collins, 1990) to unpack how gay fathers who are able to use surrogacy are embedded within wider systems of economic, historical, and political structures (Gamson, 2015; Petersen, 2018). Throughout this chapter I will demonstrate how privilege and subordination intersect in gay families constructed through surrogacy in complex ways (Baca-Zinn, 1994). Taking seriously the interlocking systems of privilege and oppression in the lived experiences of gay fathers who use surrogacy illuminates how these men's class, race, and Western privilege allows them to buy their way out of discriminatory adoptive policies and stake out a 9-month lease on a surrogate mother's womb in order to construct a genetically related, and sometimes a genetically engineered, child (Dillaway, 2008).

Some newer interdisciplinary research has grounded analyses in communication, family stress, and child development theories to conceptualize how gay men make decisions about surrogacy and to better understand the experience of surrogate families for gay fathers and their children. For example, one study used uncertainty reduction theory (URT), a framework that theorizes how communication patterns among partners can be used to reduce uncertainty as they form impressions with one another and to explore how gay-intended fathers communicated with potential surrogate mothers and egg donors on an online forum (May & Tenzek, 2016).

Some of this new literature has even moved beyond theorizing the surrogacy process to include thoughtful analyses about the experiences of raising children in gay surrogate families. One study of parental well-being among gayfather-headed families with infants born through surrogacy used family stress theory to gage how the introduction of an infant impacted family and relationship dynamics in gay surrogate families (Van Rijn van Gelderen et al., 2018). The authors found that in addition to the normal stress of an infant, gay fathers confronted additional stressors, specifically those that accompany being

a sexual minority and those related to the unknowns of surrogacy. Another study that explored the adjustment of children born to gay fathers through surrogacy grounded their research in a developmental contextual systems approach (Overton, 2015), whereby they examined children's development in terms of the bidirectional relations between the children, the family, and the wider social world (Golombok et al., 2018).

## Gay Fathers Using Surrogacy

Surrogacy is an assisted reproductive technology (ART) in which the prospective parent(s) forge a contract with a woman to carry their child (Bergman, Rubio, Green, & Padron, 2010). There are two different types of surrogacy arrangements: traditional genetic surrogacy and gestational surrogacy. Traditional genetic surrogacy is when the surrogate mother is implanted with the sperm of a man, carries the fetus to term, and births a child, of whom she is genetically related (Bergman et al., 2010). Gestational surrogacy, which is also called in vitro fertilization (IVF) surrogacy, occurs when another woman's ovum is fertilized by one of the man's sperm using IVF and the resulting embryo is transplanted into another woman's womb (Bergman et al., 2010; Growing Generations, 2019). In the latter case, the surrogate who carries the fetus to term and births the child is not genetically related to the child. Gestational surrogacy has become increasingly more common and accounts for approximately 95% of all surrogate pregnancies in the USA (Smerdon, 2008).

Surrogacy practitioners and agencies that cater to gay fathers generally recommend gestational surrogacy over traditional surrogacy, as it provides fathers certainty over legal parentage (American Society for Reproductive Medicine, 2012). Moreover, using gestational surrogacy allows gay men to bypass fears that surrogates who are genetically related to the baby will be more attached to their baby and thus more likely to change their minds about the arrangement— although of note is that there is no evidence to support this. In a study of interviews with gay fathers about their motivations to pursue surrogacy, the overwhelming majority (36 out of 40) opted for a gestational over genetic surrogacy arrangement, and half of these men chose to do so because they felt that there was a greater risk that the arrangement would fail if the surrogate had a genetic link to the baby (Blake et al., 2017). The other most popular reason gay men mentioned for this choice was that gestational surrogacy was recommended to them by their agency, a finding that exposes how the institutionalized attitudes of agencies can profoundly influence gay men's individual decision-making around surrogacy (Blake et al., 2017).

Gay men's experience with the surrogacy process is mediated by other institutions as well. For example, in 2006, the Ethics Committee of the American Society for Reproductive Medicine concluded that requests for assisted reproduction should be treated without regard for sexual orientation. However, simply because the Ethics Committee issued a statement of sexual inclusivity does not necessarily require individual surrogacy agencies to comply with such an endorsement. Indeed, despite the fact that multiple organizational bodies have endorsed adoption by sexual minorities (e.g., the American Psychological Association, the American Academy of Pediatrics, and others), the legal and interpersonal barriers that gay men and lesbians face in adopting have been well documented by scholars (Brodzinsky, Patterson, & Vaziri, 2002; see chapters "LGBTQ Adoptive Parents and Their Children" and "LGBTQ Foster Parents"). Thus, the extent to which the committee's statement is effective in pressuring surrogacy agencies to work with gay men is still unknown. Future research is needed that further explores the practices and policies of individual surrogacy agencies and personnel.

It is impossible to provide a definitive number of gay men who have become fathers through surrogacy. However, in 2018, when I contacted a representative from Growing Generations, the oldest and largest agency specializing in surrogacy arrangements for gay men, he told me that since its inception in 1996, it has worked with approximately 2000 clients. In 2013, the agency reported on its website that it had worked with 1000 clients. Thus, the number of clients had presumably doubled in only 5 years. In addition, the *Chicago Tribune* recently commissioned and reported on an informal survey of fertility clinics conducted by FertilityIQ (a website where patients assess their fertility physicians), which revealed that 10–20% of donor eggs are going to gay men having babies via gestational surrogacy (Schoenberg, 2016). Moreover, where we do not have exact numbers, it is reasonable to assume that the amount of gay men using surrogacy to have children is on the rise. The same survey from FertilityIQ reported that in some cities, the numbers have increased to 50% in the last 5 years (Schoenberg, 2016). Furthermore, in the recent study that explored how gay-intended fathers used classified ads on an online community created and maintained by surrogate mothers and intended parents, the authors noted that the number of gay men seeking the services of surrogates on websites is on the rise (May & Tenzek, 2016).

## Research on Gay Fathers and Surrogacy

When I wrote the first edition of this chapter in 2013, there were only two empirical studies on gay fathers and surrogacy (seeBergman et al., 2010 ; Greenfeld & Seli, 2011). By 2019, the number of empirical studies had increased at least fivefold (see Baiocco et al., 2015; Blake et al., 2017; Carone et al., 2018; Green, Rubio, Bergman, & Katuzny, 2015; Golombok et al., 2018; May & Tenzek, 2016; Petersen, 2018; Tornello, Kruczkowski, & Patterson, 2015; Van Rijn-van Gelderen et al., 2018). Despite this exponential growth, however, there is still only a handful of scholarly research studies on this topic, much of which is based on small convenience samples of White upper-class men. Nonetheless, the body of research on gay fathers and surrogacy has documented a wide range of dimensions, including gay men's motivations for having a child through surrogacy (Blake et al., 2017), the decision-making processes involved in their path to parenthood (Blake et al., 2017), the transition to parenthood (Bergman et al., 2010; Greenfeld & Seli, 2011), relationships with potential and actual surrogates and egg donors (Carone et al., 2018; Greenfeld & Seli, 2011; May & Tenzek, 2016), decisions about disclosing information about surrogates and donors to their children (Carone et al., 2018), the division of household labor among bio-genetic and non-biogenetic fathers (Tornello et al., 2015), parental adjustment (Van Rijn-van Gelderen et al., 2018), children's psychological adjustment (Baiocco et al., 2015; Golombok et al., 2018; Green et al., 2015), single gay men and surrogacy (Carone et al., 2017), and gay men's experiences with transnational commercial surrogacy (Petersen, 2018). It is worth noting that a significant strength of this research is that it is being produced by a diverse group of international scholars, including but not limited to the USA, the UK, the Netherlands, Spain, and Italy.

In addition to these studies is a handful of empirical qualitative studies on gay fathers that have included men who became fathers through surrogacy in their samples (Berkowitz, 2007; Berkowitz & Marsiglio, 2007; Mitchell & Green, 2007; Ryan & Berkowitz, 2009; Stacey, 2006). Finally, although not empirical studies per se, Joshua Gamson, a sociologist, wrote about his own experience with surrogacy in his book, *Modern Families* (2015), and Arlene Istar Lev (2006), a social worker, chronicled her experiences meeting and interacting with gay fathers who have used surrogacy. Diane Ehrenshaft (2000, 2005), a clinical and developmental psychologist who specializes in psychotherapy and consultation with families formed through assisted reproductive technologies, has written about surrogacy in the context of both heterosexual and gay and lesbian-parent families. The findings from these studies and clinical and experiential reports form the foundation of much of this chapter.

## The High Cost of Surrogacy

Surrogacy arrangements can be made independently between a gay male couple (or individual) and a female surrogate without the assistance of an agency. Legally, however, this is quite risky and can create a host of potential legal problems regarding custody of the child (Lev,

2006). Prior to the recent rise of agencies like Growing Generations (https://www.growinggenerations.com) and Creative Family Connections (https://www.creativefamilyconnections.com) which are willing to work with single gay men and gay couples, gay men were forced to find surrogate mothers through placing ads in newspapers or through other informal channels like inviting friends or family members to serve as surrogates (Lev, 2006). However, now many gay men choose to work through an agency, despite the fact that this increases the cost of surrogacy exponentially (Lev, 2006). Working with an agency can be beneficial in that agency personnel assist fathers with introductions to possible surrogate mothers, screen the surrogate mother medically and psychologically, provide counseling for all involved parties, and help to navigate convoluted bureaucratic red tape (Lev, 2006). However, commercial surrogacy, as mediated through an agency, is typically the most expensive route to parenthood for gay men and costs upward of $150,000 (http://www.growinggenerations.com, May & Tenzek, 2016). Commercial traditional surrogacy involves financing the participation of the surrogate, the services of an agency, physician services, legal fees, and health insurance to cover all procedures. Yet, as detailed above, practitioners and agencies that cater to gay fathers generally recommend gestational surrogacy over traditional surrogacy. This requires financing the participation of the egg donor, the services of both an egg donor agency and a surrogate agency, IVF physician services, and health insurance to cover all procedures.

The high costs of surrogacy mean that it is only an option for a small number of relatively affluent gay men, a fact that is illustrated by the demographic composition of the participants in any of the empirical studies that included information about income. In one study, the mean household income was $270,000 (Bergman et al., 2010),[2] in another, the average income was $230,000 (Tornello et al., 2015) and in a third, the mean annual family income was $370,000 (Blake et al., 2017). These incomes are vastly above the

---

[2]This number is only reflective of the 37 out of 40 men in the study who answered the question on income.

national average and far above the mean household income of gay men adopting children, which is approximately $100,000 (Gates, Badgett, Macomber, & Chambers, 2007). Moreover, in the Bergman et al. (2010) study, 14 out of the 40 fathers in the sample already had children currently enrolled in a private preschool at an average cost of $8764 annually, and 67% planned on sending their children to private schools in the near future. Furthermore, 68% of the men in the sample reported using some type of childcare assistance, ranging from au pairs to nannies to housekeepers.

In addition, the majority of gay men who pursue fatherhood through surrogacy are White. In the Bergman et al. (2010) sample, 80% were White, in the Greenfeld and Seli (2011) sample, 90% identified as White, in the Tornello et al. (2015) sample, over 90% (2015) were White, and in the Blake et al. (2017) sample, 84% were White. This pattern is also true for gay fathers in other countries. In Petersen's (2018) study of gay men in Denmark who had used transnational surrogacy, all were White, and in a multinational study conducted in the UK, Denmark, and France, 96% of the British and Dutch parents were White (no race information was collected on French parents) (Van Rijn-van Gelderen et al., 2018).

The gay fathers in these samples are also different from gay men who become parents through adoption in terms of their racial and ethnic diversity. Using US Census data, Gates et al. (2007) estimated that among gay male adoptive parents, 61% were White, 15% were African American, 15% were Latino, 4% were Asian/Pacific Islander, 1% were American Indian, and 4% reported some other race/ethnicity. Thus, these studies confirm the extent to which surrogacy is a procreative pathway only available to a racially and economically privileged minority.

## Thinking About Parenting: Surrogacy as an Option

Research has documented that gay men become parents for many of the same reasons as heterosexual men: Both cite the desire for nurturing children, the constancy of children in their lives, the achievement of some sense of immortality via children, and the sense of family that children help to provide (Berkowitz & Marsiglio, 2007; Goldberg et al., 2012; Mallon, 2004). However, the social and psychological dimensions of gay men's reproductive decision-making are additionally complicated by internalized homophobia, anxieties about raising properly gendered (and heterosexual) children, and structural obstacles such as lack of information and navigating legal barriers (Berkowitz & Marsiglio, 2007; Brinamen & Mitchell, 2008; Goldberg, 2010a). Moreover, unlike the majority of their heterosexual counterparts who couple, become pregnant, and give birth, gay men who wish to parent must carefully consider a variety of other variables when contemplating parenthood. Such considerations include deciding on how they should go about creating a family: that is, whether it should be through adoption, foster parenting, kinship ties, or through surrogacy arrangements. Embedded in these decisions are issues of cost, access, and the extent to which a genetic relationship is perceived as important by men in their conceptualizations of family.

Oftentimes, those gay men who choose surrogacy are motivated by the higher degree of control they have in the process when compared with adoption, feel that the presence of a genetic link to their child is an important factor for the creation of family ties, and worry about the psychological stress a child may experience as a result of being adopted (Blake et al., 2017; Carone et al., 2017; Goldberg, 2010a; Lev, 2006). For example, one man told Lev (2006) that he chose surrogacy because "it was the only way our child would be born without sadness as a part of his life story, i.e., there was someone who had to give you up, didn't want you, couldn't care for you" (p. 76). In viewing an adopted child as always already wounded, or psychologically damaged, this man sets up a hierarchical pattern of families wherein those not formed through such privileged means like surrogacy are deemed less valuable. It is important that scholars studying sexual minority parenting do not mirror these patterns and are careful not to privilege biogenetic ties over other kinds of family formations. Gay men's families constructed through surrogacy can be respected without treating them as any more privileged than families constructed through adoption, fostering, or kinship ties.

Nevertheless, it is important to keep in mind that the legal and interpersonal barriers that gay men face in adopting have been well documented (Goldberg, 2012) and are well known to gay men pursuing parenthood. In one study that interviewed 74 fathers about their decision-making processes and motivations for having a child through surrogacy, the authors found that almost two-thirds felt that adoption was a less preferable and/or feasible path to parenthood and slightly over half expressed a desire to have a genetic connection with their child (Blake et al., 2017). One man told the authors:

> We liked surrogacy really because what we had read about adoption it seemed like quite a random process, and you weren't in control. Even after the child was born, there were all sorts of stipulations and criteria by which you, for no reason of your own, lose your child. (p. 864)

In another study that interviewed single gay fathers in Italy, most men expressed that they chose surrogacy because they felt that it was more secure than adoption (Carone et al., 2017). One man explained:

> It just seemed like adoption was too much a random process. . .mental health issues could arise, the child could be born with genetic defects and stuff like that. There is a great deal of unknown with adoption and I didn't want that. With surrogacy it is much more of a guarantee, and it seemed like the most promising way to have my family. (p. 1876)

These narratives mirror Goldberg and Scheib's (2015) findings in their interviews with 50 lesbian women who became mothers using donor insemination. The authors found that women preferred DI because of perceived structural barriers and problems with adoption, a desire to be pregnant, and a desire for genetic parenthood. These findings are not surprising, given that reigning social norms in all Western nations establish biological relatedness as critical for defining family. Moreover, this tendency may be especially pronounced in certain countries/cultures, such as Italy, where gay men are still denied legal recognition of their families. And so many men in the study by Carone et al. (2017) said they wanted a genetic link to their child. One man told the authors, "I felt that a genetic child would really be my child...it is DNA, there is nothing we can say or do about it" (p. 186). Even in countries like the USA that have legal recognition of same-sex families, cultural and social recognition lag far behind. It is thus not surprising that the presence of a genetic relationship is an oft-cited reason that gay men choose surrogacy (Lev, 2006).

## The Family Tree: Gay Fathers, Surrogate Mothers, Egg Donors, and Their Children

Surrogacy is similar to donor insemination (DI) in that it allows for one parent to be genetically related to the child, and it involves a biological "other" to provide the other half of the genetic material. However, in the case of surrogacy, there is an added dimension not present in DI wherein another person—a female body—also carries the fetus to term and births the child. Thus, a critical difference between DI and surrogacy is that surrogacy always includes a physically present (female) body. However, despite this crucial departure, many of the complexities that accompany DI are also relevant in the context of surrogacy (see Goldberg & Scheib, 2015). For example, while surrogacy provides one parent a genetic link, it also introduces a genetic asymmetry such that only one partner has a biological bond to the child (Goldberg, 2010a). This of course may prompt couples to wonder how this biological connection will shape parent-child bonding and can even provoke jealous feelings in the partner who is not genetically related to the child (Ehrenshaft, 2005). Moreover, questions about the source of the sperm can privilege one partner in a gay male couple. Where some gay fathers choose to find out whose sperm actually impregnated the surrogate (or, in many cases, the egg donor), many others report creatively bypassing this issue by mixing their sperm before insemination and choose not to find out whose sperm was ultimately responsible for conception following the birth of their child (Blake et al., 2017; Ryan & Berkowitz, 2009).

For many, the decision of whose sperm should be used to impregnate the egg donor or surrogate is a significant one. In making these decisions, fathers typically consider factors such as their age, health, and the presence of any hereditary conditions or disorders (Blake et al., 2017; Greenfeld & Seli, 2011). There are a handful of studies that provide some initial evidence for how gay men using surrogacy make decisions about which partner should supply the sperm. In the Greenfeld and Seli (2011) sample, 12 couples (80%) deliberately chose who would inseminate the egg donor. Decisions were made with the following considerations in mind: Six couples agreed that the older partner should provide the sperm, two couples had a partner who had already fathered children in a previous heterosexual relationship and thus thought that the other partner should have this opportunity as well, two couples chose the partner who had a stronger desire to be a biological parent, and two couples reported that they decided to go with the partner who had "better genes" (p. 227). In the remaining three couples, both partners had equivalent desires for biological parenthood and thus inseminated equal numbers of eggs. Two of these three couples produced twins who were half-siblings. With regard to the one couple who had a single child, the authors did not report whether the couple ultimately discovered who was the genetic parent (Greenfeld & Seli, 2001).

Similarly, in Blake et al. (2017) study of 74 fathers that addressed gay men's decision-making processes and motivations for having a child through surrogacy, the authors found that in half of the respondents, both men donated sperm, leaving biogenetic fatherhood to chance. In the other families, only one father donated sperm. For 22% of these men, having a genetic tie to their child was more important to one partner than the other, 12% planned to take turns in who would have a genetic tie to their babies, 4% cited medical reasons in who provided sperm, and in a small number of cases (5%) one man provided the sperm because they had decided to use a sister as an egg donor (Blake et al., 2017).

Just like researchers have documented in studies on lesbian couples and DI (Chabot & Ames, 2004; Goldberg, 2006; Goldberg & Scheib, 2015), some researchers have indicated that choices about who should supply the sperm and have a genetic relationship to the child might be contingent upon one partner's belief that their family of origin is more likely to accept a child who is genetically related to them (Goldberg, 2012). In fact, there is some evidence that when only one parent has a genetic link to the child, some families of origin may be slow to accord full parental status to the other partner (Mitchell & Green, 2007). Sometimes families of the biological parent see the child as belonging only to their own family, and families of the non-genetically related parent neglect to see the child as a part of their family. However, recent research on gay families constructed through surrogacy suggests that these patterns might be changing. Where Blake et al. (2017) did not look at long-term relationships among families, they did find that family members' reactions to gay men's parenthood intentions were no different for genetic compared to nongenetic fathers. The majority of fathers in their sample described their family's reactions as supportive, regardless of the genetic relationship. However, future research is still needed to see how gay men's families of origin relate to and bond with children conceived and birthed through surrogacy, particularly in those cases where a father is unable to secure a biological or legal relationship to the child.

## Who Are the Surrogate Mother and/or Egg Donor?

Researchers have interrogated how those who use assisted reproductive technologies like surrogacy and DI make decisions about gestational carriers and egg and sperm donors. Regardless of gender or sexual identity, individuals and couples using these kinds of ARTs share a motivation distinguished by the high level of control they have in choosing what their child will look like. Additionally, studies have shown that these individuals carefully and often meticulously evaluate the characteristics of the surrogate mother and/or egg and sperm donors (Blake et al., 2017; Carone et al., 2017; Ehrenshaft, 2005; Goldberg & Scheib, 2015; Ryan & Berkowitz, 2009). For example, prospective parents often look for surrogates who resemble themselves or their partners in terms of race, ethnicity, religious affiliation, vocational interests, personal characteristics, and appearance (Mitchell & Green, 2007; Ryan & Berkowitz, 2009). The most common request from the men in Greenfeld and Seli's sample (2011) was for an egg donor who was tall, attractive, educated, and closely resembled the non-inseminating partner.

Increasingly, intended gay fathers interested in surrogacy are using virtual communities to facilitate the matching process with surrogates and/or egg donors. In an innovative study, May and Tenzek (2016) investigated how gay-intended fathers strategically disclosed information about themselves in a sample of 29 online classified ads on surromomsonline.com, the official website of Surrogate Mothers Online, LLC. They found that gay-intended parents used what the authors called "proactive disclosure," as they shared intimate details and personal feelings in an attempt to reduce uncertainty and initiate further interaction with surrogates and egg donors. The authors concluded:

> Generally speaking, the more specific IPs [intended parents] can be about their preferences, the more uncertainty can be reduced as the surrogate mother reads that ad and vice versa. By addressing these logistical considerations during the initial matching process, intended parents can bypass "nonqualified" surrogates and focus on the strongest matches. (pp. 444–445)

Findings from May and Tenzek's study revealed that gay-intended parents looking for a surrogate and/or egg donor emphasized their long-term desire to father a child, and some even disclosed their past failed attempts in their journey to fatherhood. Many also accentuated their relationship stability in order to diffuse any stereotypes

the potential surrogate might have about gay men's evasion of monogamy. In addition, several highlighted their financial stability in order to communicate their ability to compensate the surrogate and provide for their future child. In terms of what they were looking for in a surrogate, the most common request from the men in their study was for a surrogate who was "young, healthy, and experienced [as a surrogate]" (p. 444). Some men also emphasized an openness to carry multiples, and others sought surrogates who had their own private health insurance with no surrogacy exclusions.[3]

Only 1 of the 29 ads in this study explicitly mentioned race, and this couple expressed a preference for a traditional surrogate who was White or Latino. However, other research has revealed that as gay-prospective fathers evaluate their surrogates-to-be, they carefully cogitate on the importance of racial and ethnic matching, speculating how adding another dimension like racial differences to their already publicly perplexing family might confuse their child or encumber interactions with curious interlopers (deBoer, 2009; Ryan & Berkowitz, 2009). Prospective fathers often consider the extent to which they are willing to make what is already a conspicuous gay family even more conspicuous by becoming an interracial family (deBoer, 2009).

Making separate choices about an egg donor and a gestational surrogate allows intended parents to choose among a wider pool of egg donors. It also facilitates intended parents' ability to select a donor whose physical, cultural, and biographical characteristics are more similar to themselves or their partners. Since there is a significantly smaller pool of gestational surrogates than egg donors, once the genetic concerns associated with the selection of the egg donor have been addressed, the choice of the surrogate is less constrained (Mitchell & Green, 2007). Thus, commercial surrogacy and egg donation makes it such that those men who can afford to do so "can literally purchase the means to eugenically reproduce White

---

[3]Although most health insurance companies regularly cover pregnancy-related expenses, some have started to add "surrogacy-exclusion" provisions to their policies.

infants in their own idealized image, selecting desired traits in egg donors…with whom to mate their own DNA" (Stacey, 2006, p. 39). In fact, in her advice to parents seeking assisted reproductive technologies, Ehrenshaft (2005) writes that "you can feel that you have the whole world in your hands" as you "discover the power to craft the child that will be yours" (p. 42). This gives affluent gay men who wish to become parents the ability to regain control of their reproductive options.

In the process of deciding on a surrogate and/or egg donor, gay-prospective parents thoughtfully peruse websites with pictures and descriptions before actually meeting face-to-face. This initial screening happens within a context in which babies are increasingly viewed as precious commodities. Ehrenshaft (2005) argues that this commodification is further magnified for those using assisted reproductive technologies since these intended parents have spent months, even years, searching for a donor or surrogate and draining financial resources paying for expensive procedures.

For gay men, this process is further intensified since they are not only limited by the reproductive limits of their bodies, but have been told by religious, political, and cultural institutions that fatherhood was never an option for them. When viewed through a heteronormative lens, the idea of shopping for a child's features among potential egg donors or searching for a surrogate with the healthiest possible womb may be viewed as an unnecessary luxury akin to crafting a perfect child. However, for gay men using surrogacy, this process takes on a whole new meaning, as it is one of the few ways that they are able to manage the discord between dominant heterosexual reproductive scripts and their own reproductive experiences. Moreover, many gay-prospective parents pursuing surrogacy do not experience their journey to parenthood as one ensconced in privilege; rather, they focus on the challenges and lack of control associated with the process. In his interviews with White Danish gay men about their experiences with transnational surrogacy, Petersen (2018) observed that these men felt like they had little control over the various obstacles

in the surrogacy process, including the high numbers of failed IVF cycles, miscarriages, and rapidly changing global legalities.

## How Can We Trust Her? What Are Her Motives?

Surrogacy makes it such that the gay male couple, or the gay man, wait for a child to be birthed by a woman they may barely know. Moreover, because a surrogate mother cannot maintain the same anonymity that a sperm donor can, surrogacy involves an enormous amount of trust, even with accompanying legal protections. Some gay fathers may express anxiety about the child potentially developing a bond to the surrogate, while others may wonder about the woman's attachment to the child she is carrying (Ehrenshaft, 2000; Lev, 2006). Some gay fathers have reported that an important criterion for a desirable surrogate was her ability to not bond with the child she is carrying (Lev, 2006).

Alongside an evaluation of the surrogate mother's age, race, physical attractiveness, medical history, intelligence, athleticism, and artistic ability, gay men also inquire about her motives. Although surrogates are offered compensation packages of anywhere between $42,000 to $58,000, depending on the state (see https://www.growinggenerations.com/surrogacy-program/surrogates/surrogate-mother-pay/), the majority report that they are not motivated solely by money, but rather by altruism, selflessness, and a desire to help a family have a child (Lev, 2006). In their analysis of online classified ads, May and Tenzek (2016) found that many ads from surrogates stressed helping someone "fulfill their dream" of becoming parents and expressed a personal longing to help those who were not able to have children on their own.

Yet, it is reasonable to believe that money is a substantial factor in motivating surrogate mothers, even if an altruistic motive is also present. One study conducted at the Infertility Center of New York found that 89% of surrogate mothers acknowledged that they would not agree to serve as a surrogate mother unless they were paid a substantial fee (Dillaway, 2008). People desiring children through surrogacy often grapple with whether the surrogate mother is motivated purely by financial means or by an inclination to help people in need of children (Ehrenshaft, 2005). Gay men, having few other options for birthing children, may be especially worried about this motivation. However, in Stacey's (2006) ethnographic research on gay men and kinship, she found that some surrogates actually preferred to work with gay men because there was no mother in the picture who might potentially be dealing with feelings of jealousy, infertility, and exclusion. Moreover, unlike heterosexual couples, for which assisted reproductive technologies are usually a last resort, gay fathers turn to surrogacy joyfully as a pathway to parenthood (Carone et al., 2017; Stacey, 2006). Because such assisted technologies are universally necessary for gay men who wish to create their own biological offspring, they carry none of the stigma or sense of failure of many infertile heterosexual couples (Mitchell & Green, 2007). As such, some studies report that gay men can and do enjoy harmonious relationships with surrogates (Carone et al., 2017).

## Weaving in the Identities of the Surrogate Mother and Egg Donor

The experiences of gay fathers show the contradictory status of the surrogate mother and egg donor's relationship to the family as simultaneously present and absent figures (Ehrenshaft, 2005). For some families, they are *present* via the recognition of the important contribution of their genetic material, their physical bodies, and their contribution to their family. But they can also be *absent* in terms of a conventional social relationship to their kin (Ehrenshaft, 2005). Although the paradoxical notion of presence and absence can be expected in any family arrangement that relies on assisted reproduction or adoption, it is especially evident in gay father-headed families because of the constant societal reminder that this third party was a necessity in creating their families.

Gay men who use gestational surrogacy are more likely to care about their possible future contact with the surrogate more so than the egg donor and are more likely to maintain a relationship with her in the future (Blake et al., 2017; Carone et al., 2018; Greenfeld & Seli, 2011). Because it is the surrogate mother who is pregnant with and births the child, it is she who the fathers generally forge long-term relationships with, and the vast majority of men not only meet her but also have long-standing relationships with her. Interestingly, whereas the egg donor supplies the genetic link and is carefully scrutinized for her medical history and physical characteristics, she is primarily an absent figure in the family following conception. For example, in Blake and colleagues' (2017) study of 40 American gay father surrogacy families, a greater percentage of fathers had met with the surrogate (83%) than had met with the egg donor (25%) after the birth of the child. Fathers were also more likely to have met with the surrogate in the past year (53%) compared with the egg donor (6%). What is more, in the two cases where fathers had met with the egg donor in the past year, she was previously known to the couple — in one case she was a friend and another, a sister. Of the 11 parents in this sample who continued to have regular contact with egg donors following the birth of their child, nine of these were open-identity egg donors, and the other two were the friend and sister mentioned above. It is important to point out that while egg donors were often absent figures when children were young, some fathers reported intentionally choosing an egg donor with whom there would be the possibility of contact, as to ensure that their child could learn about their ancestry, if they were curious in the future.

That fathers were more likely to maintain a relationship with the surrogate than with the egg donor is likely because egg retrieval is a brief procedure when compared with the bonding time that surrogates and intended parents have with one another during the course of the pregnancy. Moreover, while the basis of commercial surrogacy is a financial arrangement, the realities are such that this is often a relationship characterized by appreciation, mutual respect, and gratitude, with many gay fathers often forging deep bonds with their surrogates (Mitchell & Green, 2007).

The limited empirical research on gay fathers who have used surrogacy suggests that they cultivate ways to share in the pregnancy experience of their surrogate. Some document their experience with scrapbooks or by giving their surrogate mother a video camera, while others use social media platforms, e-mail, FaceTime, and Skype to keep up-to-date with belly growth, fetal development, ultrasound pictures, and doctor's appointments (Berkowitz & Marsiglio, 2007; Carone et al., 2017). Even well after the pregnancy and birth, many gay fathers choose to have ongoing relationships with their surrogates and, in some cases, with their egg donors (Carone et al., 2017; Mitchell & Green, 2007). These relationships, once maintained through letters, are now primarily maintained through social media (Carone et al., 2017). A few of the fathers that Lev (2006) interviewed were so close with their surrogate that they named her godmother to their child. Although this pattern of designating the surrogate as a godmother was relatively rare, the majority of gay fathers told Lev (2006) that they shared a distant, albeit caring relationship with their surrogates.

## Constructing Family Stories with and for Children

The notion of the birth mother who helps make the possibility of a baby come true weaves in and out of the entire lifespan of any family using surrogacy (Berkowitz, 2006; Mitchell & Green, 2007). Like those families constructed through DI, surrogacy raises questions about a "symbolic other" necessary for the creation of a family that parents, children, extended family members, and other social actors must constantly negotiate. One commonality shared by families constructed through surrogacy and DI is that parents may struggle with when and how to tell their children the story of their inception. Perhaps because surrogacy involves a pregnancy that is trickier to

hide, downplay, or ignore, research has found that compared with other families constructed through assisted reproductive technologies, such as DI, families formed through surrogacy are more open about the origin of their family, regardless of parents' sexual orientation (Carone et al., 2017).

For example, in one American study, 83% of the gay fathers in the sample had started the disclosure process to their children by the time they were 5.5 years old (Blake et al., 2017). In a study of gay father families conducted in Italy, all of the children older than 6 years of age had learned that their births were a result of planned surrogacies (Carone et al., 2017). Slightly over half of the children interviewed for this study demonstrated a clear understanding of their conception and were cognizant that one woman had donated an egg and another woman had carried them in her body. The rest of the children exhibited some knowledge of their origin, and even though they did not explicitly mention a surrogate or egg donor, they were able to explain that their fathers needed help in creating them (Carone et al., 2017).

One way that parents communicate the uniqueness of their family to their children is by celebrating a child's conception day in addition to the child's actual birthday, as this becomes an important date that gay fathers who created their families though surrogacy are unique in knowing (Mitchell & Green, 2007). How gay fathers answer personal queries about their child's conception ultimately serves as a model for how their children will deal with similar situations and construct their own family stories. As these children grow older, they cannot rely on a legacy of cultural givens, but rather must establish on their own the meanings and significance of their extended family (Mitchell & Green, 2007). Like their parents, children raised with an understanding of assisted reproductive technologies like that of surrogacy may be less inclined to conflate sex and reproduction and thus may have a unique ability to challenge these taken-for-granted connections among their peers. Future research is needed on how children born to gay fathers and surrogate mothers negotiate dominant two-parent heteronormative family ideology as they understand their family stories and communicate these stories to others.

## The Family Experience for Children and Their Fathers

Like all sexual minority parents, gay fathers who have constructed their families through surrogacy and their children must contend with the "hegemonic shadow of the heterosexual paradigm" (deBoer, 2009, p. 333). However, recent research indicates that both children and parents can flourish in this family setting despite having to continuously navigate societal heteronorms. For example, a recent American study based on 40 gay father families created through surrogacy and 55 lesbian mother families created through donor insemination assessed children's adjustment using a combination of methods, including interviews, video-recorded observations, and standardized questionnaires, which were administered to parents, children, and teachers (Golombok et al., 2018). Children in both family types were described as having high levels of adjustment, and children in gay father families showed considerably lower levels of internalizing problems than children in lesbian mother families (Golombok et al., 2018). Other studies have revealed low levels of parent-reported adjustment problems among children born to gay fathers through surrogacy (Baiocco et al., 2015), especially internalizing problems (e.g., depression, anxiety; Green et al., 2015). An Italian study found that gay father families formed through surrogacy had similar parent-reported family functioning, emotional regulation, and adjustment of children when compared with groups of lesbian mother families formed through donor insemination and heterosexual parent families with naturally conceived children (Baiocco et al., 2015). Similarly, a survey of 68 gay father families with 3- to 10-year-old children born through gestational surrogacy found that the children of gay fathers had point-

edly lower levels of adjustment problems compared with data obtained from the wider population. Furthermore, the daughters of the gay fathers showed particularly low levels of internalizing problems (Green et al., 2015).

Like their children, gay men who create their families through surrogacy also report faring well. One study found that gay men who became fathers via surrogacy communicated high levels of satisfaction with their relationships (Tornello et al., 2015). In a multinational study that interrogated the differences in levels of parental well-being between gay father families with infants born through surrogacy, lesbian mother families with infants born through DI, and heterosexual parent families with infants born through IVF, the authors found that the gay fathers reported relatively levels of parental stress, anxiety, and depression (Van Rijn-van Gelderen et al., 2018).

Where much of the research has revealed that gay men who become parents using surrogacy experience similar life changes as heterosexual fathers, there are some notable differences that likely arise from their sexual minority status. Many fathers in the Bergman et al. (2010) study described shifting their schedules and their priorities to accommodate their childcare responsibilities and their new role as parents. Fathers reported lessening work hours and switching jobs, and some even became stay-at-home dads. Sometimes these changes resulted in a decrease in household income. Other studies have documented how gay men who become fathers via surrogacy share more equally in the division of household labor than their heterosexual counterparts. For example, Tornello et al. (2015) found that the men in their sample reported egalitarian ways of dividing and choosing to divide unpaid family labor and showed no variance in the division of labor patterns as a function of parents' biological relatedness to the child. By decreasing their ties to paid labor, increasing their presence in the home, and dividing unpaid family labor more evenly, these men challenge socially constructed cultural narratives that assume men are incompetent nurturers and that gay men are anti-family and irresponsible.

Such findings are not unique to those gay men who become fathers through surrogacy. Research conducted with gay fathers who became parents through adoption and fostering has documented similar findings (Lassiter, Dew, Newton, Hays, & Yarbrough, 2006; Mallon, 2004; Schacher, Auerbach, & Silverstein, 2005). However, other scholars have argued that the assumption that gay men's marginalized location from traditional family life means that gay fathers always resist and transform traditional notions of gayness, fathering, and family is overly reductionistic (Goldberg, 2010b). Such reasoning fails to account for the diversity within these families and the role of contextual variables like institutional support and the broader sociopolitical and legal milieu (Goldberg, 2010b). Take, for example, the fact that 68% of the men in Bergman et al.'s (2010) sample relied on hired help to assist with childcare and domestic duties. Clearly, although many gay fathers challenge stereotypes of men as primary caregivers, many are also able to buy their way out of domesticity, a finding intimately tied to both their class position in society and their ability as male-bodied parents to continue to rely on the privilege granted to the traditional father-as-breadwinner status. Moreover, because surrogacy is only available to an economically privileged minority of gay men, it seems reasonable to believe that a larger proportion of gay men who have become fathers through surrogacy are more likely to outsource domestic help than those who became fathers through adoption, fostering, or through kinship ties. Future research is needed to see if this is indeed the case.

Bergman et al. (2010) reported that one of the most striking findings from their study on gay men who became fathers through surrogacy was men's description of heightened self-esteem from having and raising children. In addition, these men reported an increase in support and acceptance from both their families of origin and their partners' families of origin since they had become parents, even in cases where families of origin were not biologically related to new children—a finding similarly documented among new lesbian mothers (Goldberg, 2006). With the initiation of the parenting role comes a shift in adult gay children's relationships with their aging parents who often take pride in their new identities as grandparents (deBoer, 2009). Where this is certainly an experience shared by most parents, there is an added dimension for gay fathers since there is a lack of ceremonial and legal validation of their relationships.

## Gay Fathers, Surrogacy, and Reproductive Outsourcing

Although reproductive outsourcing, or the trend of paying for overseas surrogates from countries in the Global South, is no longer an option for gay men (except in the case where men from Western nations come to the USA to pursue surrogacy), the rise and fall of this controversial phenomenon exposes how global privilege and marginalization collide in profoundly complicated ways (Mamo & Alston-Stepnitz, 2015; Petersen, 2018). Even before its demise, the legalities of reproductive outsourcing seemed to change overnight. India was once the top destination spot for gay-intended fathers, but that ended in 2013 when new regulations for medical visas were introduced that required intended parents be in a heterosexual marriage (Petersen, 2018). By early 2014, gay men were at the vanguard of a highly unregulated transnational commercial surrogacy boom in Thailand (Petersen, 2018). However, in August of the same year, an Australian couple left a child born with Down syndrome with the surrogate mother, and the country faced international condemnation for their unregulated status of surrogacy; in turn, Thailand outlawed commercial surrogacy completely. In the wake of these new directives in India and Thailand, many of the Indian agencies forced to close a year earlier began to open branches in Nepal, which quickly became the destination for gay couples (Petersen, 2018). However, that ended when the government issued a ban on surrogacy in 2015 (Petersen, 2018). At that point, the only remaining place where gay men could pursue transnational surrogacy was the state of Tabasco in Mexico, where commercial surrogacy was unregulated. But, when the legislature of Tabasco elected to curtail surrogacy for foreigners in December 2015, all of gay men's options to pursue commercial surrogacy abroad were terminated (Petersen, 2018). Currently, the USA is the only destination legally accessible to gay men interested in using surrogacy to birth children (Petersen, 2018).

Where surrogacy has always been a practice marred with class distinctions, the phenomenon of fertility tourism, or paying for surrogates in less privileged nations (Smerdon, 2008), magnified the inequality between commissioning parent and surrogate (and/or egg donor). It is not surprising then that many were skeptical of fertility tourism from the start, seeing it as a system that allowed "wealthy infertile couples" to treat third parties from disenfranchised groups as "passports" to reproduction (Smerdon, 2008, p. 24). However, as Petersen (2018) observed in his study of White Danish gay men about their experiences with transnational surrogacy, rather than seeing these men as unequivocally privileged, the "ambiguities and contradictions that form the men's positions within a racialized, sexualized, and procreative hierarchy" reveal how intersections of privilege and inequality uniquely shaped the experiences of transnational surrogacy for gay men (p. 713). The rapidly shifting legalities in each of these countries impacted gay men "harder and more frequently than their heterosexual counterparts" and left them "immobile with reproductive matter trapped in different geographies" (Petersen, 2018, p. 713).

## Legal Issues Facing Gay Surrogate Families in America

Despite a number of advances in recent years, the legal landscape is still a challenging terrain for many LGBTQ parents. Although commercial surrogacy is highly regulated in the USA by private industry with "rigorous procedures such as psychological testing and interviews, genetic histories, and careful matching of donors and surrogates" (Bergman et al., 2010, p. 117), the federal government does not regulate surrogacy

at all, and control and oversight of surrogacy arrangements is relinquished to individual state jurisdiction. Thus, those pursuing this procreative pathway are often left to navigate inconsistencies among state laws, legislative action, and court decisions (Smerdon, 2008). Additionally, in traditional surrogacy, the surrogate is considered the biological mother of the child; in turn, gay-intended parents must obtain a pre-birth parentage order that allows both parents to be listed on the child's birth certificate at birth, regardless of the biological relationship to the child (Gays with Kids, February 28, 2018). In some states that do not allow pre-birth parentage orders, intended fathers may establish legal parentage following the birth. However, in states with ambiguous laws, the nonbiological father may be required to undergo adoption proceedings (Gays with Kids, February 28, 2018).

According to Creative Family Connections, a gay-friendly surrogacy agency and law firm that has an interactive map of legalities by state on its website (2016), in 10 states (CA, CT, DC, DE, ME, NH, NJ, NV, RI, TX), married same-sex couples are permitted to enter into surrogacy contracts (https://www.creativefamilyconnections.com/us-surrogacy-law-map). These states also grant pre-birth orders and allow both parents to be named on the birth certificate. The vast majority of states (35), however, have vague, unclear, or inconsistent laws, and while surrogacy is not technically illegal, potential legal hurdles can ensue. In these states, it may be more difficult, if not impossible, to obtain a pre-birth parentage order. In Arizona and Indiana, surrogacy is practiced and courts will issue parentage orders. However, surrogacy contracts can be made invalid by statute. Louisiana, Michigan, New York, and Washington all prohibit surrogacy. In August of 2016, Louisiana passed a bill restricting all surrogacy contracts to married heterosexual couples. In addition to legal inconsistencies and hurdles in the USA, at the time of writing, the current administration is denying citizenship to children of gay parents if they are born abroad, a policy shift that could potentially implicate families conceived via overseas surrogacy arrangements (Bollinger, 2019).

Overall, the legal aspects surrounding surrogacy and sexual minority parents are for the most part rather unsettled. Gay men who are considering surrogacy should be aware of different state-by-state and global regulations. Moreover, they should find an agency that is not only open to working with sexual minorities but also one that understands how to traverse the state-by-state surrogacy laws.

## Implications for Future Research

Commercial surrogacy is certainly one of the most high-tech and expensive paths to gay parenthood. The relatively high cost of surrogacy means that those men who create their families through this route typically have significantly higher incomes than men who may opt to become parents through adoption, fostering, or kinship ties. Gay men who become fathers using surrogacy are unique in that they are primarily White affluent men who have a biological tie to their child. These interlocking privileged positions can shield them from some of the vulnerabilities that gay men of color, gay men with lesser incomes, and gay men who adopt all too often encounter. Nonetheless these men are similar to gay fathers in other contexts like adoption or fostering in that their path to parenting entails a great deal of thought, planning, and decision-making.

Scholars are beginning to understand more about the transition to parenthood and the parenting experiences of gay men who choose surrogacy. However, future research is still needed. Comparative studies with samples of gay fathers in other contexts and with heterosexual fathers and mothers who became parents through surrogacy are necessary. Moreover, additional research on gay families constructed through surrogacy is needed to better understand the extent to which the genetic connection between one of the fathers and the child affects the family dynamics, the division of domestic and paid labor, and relationships with family of origin. Scholars should further examine the degree and types of contact that exist between the surrogate and/or egg donor and the gay parents and their children after the birth of the child. Finally, additional work is needed to explore how gay fathers using surrogacy deal with their growing visibility in their diverse communities.

Additionally, research on other sexual minority fathers who do not identify as gay is needed in order to better understand how other sexually marginalized men construct and experience surrogate family constellations. Finally, further theorizing is required to better understand how constructions of race, nation, family, and sociopolitical power are embedded in the relationships among gay fathers, surrogates, egg donors, and their children. As Rothman (1989) observed over two decades ago, surrogate motherhood was not brought to us by scientific progress; rather it was brought to us by brokers who saw the potential of a new market.

## Implications for Policy and Practice

Policy makers need to be aware that gay men are having children through assisted reproductive technologies like that of surrogacy. At a basic level, surrogacy agencies, lawyers, fertility specialists, and other healthcare professionals must continue to communicate a philosophy of inclusion and acceptance for gay-prospective fathers. Also, clinicians need to acknowledge that surrogate parenthood is increasingly common for gay men, both in the USA and abroad. Clinicians should assist gay men using surrogacy in their family planning, with special attention to the areas that uniquely define their transition to parenthood. Furthermore, for those couples that choose to have half of the eggs fertilized by one partner and half by the other, counseling should include considerations about the possible consequences that might result from this option. For example, the couple should be made aware of the genetic asymmetry that will result if they birth a single child and of the possibility of having twins that share the same maternal genetics but different paternal genetics (Greenfeld & Seli, 2011).

## Conclusion

The parenting and family landscape is changing rapidly before our eyes, and we now have extraordinary technological advances that combine eggs and sperm in what were until very recently unimaginable ways. Gay fathers choosing surrogacy are at the cutting edge of pushing society to reassess its assumptions and constructions about sex, reproduction, and parenthood. We can be certain that as more and more people are thinking about creative ways to have babies, the lessons learned from this emerging cohort of gay men who have become fathers through surrogacy will impact how we engage the new family forms of the twenty-first century.

## References

American Society for Reproductive Medicine (2012). https://www.connect.asrm.org/home.

Baca-Zinn, M. (1994). Feminist thinking from racial-ethnic families. In S. Fergusen (Ed.), *Shifting the center: Understanding contemporary families* (pp. 18–27). Boston, MA: McGraw Hill.

Baiocco, R., Santamaria, F., Ioverno, S., Fontanesi, L., Baumgartner, E., Laghi, F., & Lingiardi, V. (2015). Lesbian mother families and gay father families in Italy: Family functioning, dyadic satisfaction, and child well-being. *Sexuality Research and Social Policy, 12,* 202–212. https://doi.org/10.1007/s13178-015-0185-x

Bergman, K., Rubio, R. J., Green, R. J., & Padron, E. (2010). Gay men who become fathers via surrogacy: The transition to parenthood. *Journal of GLBT Family Studies, 6,* 111–141. https://doi.org/10.1080/15504281003704942

Berkowitz, D. (2006). *Gay men: Negotiating procreative, father, and family identities.* (Unpublished doctoral dissertation). Gainesville, FL: University of Florida.

Berkowitz, D. (2007). A sociohistorical analysis of gay men's procreative consciousness. *Journal of GLBT Family Studies, 3,* 157–190. https://doi.org/10.1300/J461v03n02_07

Berkowitz, D., & Marsiglio, W. (2007). Gay men: Negotiating procreative, father, and family identities. *Journal of Marriage and Family, 69,* 366–381. https://doi.org/10.1111/j.1741-3737.2007.00371.x

Blake, L., Carone, N., Raffanello, E., Slutsky, J., Ehrhardt, A. A., & Golombok, S. (2017). Gay fathers' motivations for and feelings about surrogacy as a path to parenthood. *Human Reproduction, 32,* 1–8. https://doi.org/10.1093/humrep/dex026

Blumer, H. (1969). *Symbolic interactionism: Perspective and method.* Englewood Cliffs, NJ: Prentice-Hall.

Bollinger, A. (May, 2019). The Trump administration is denying citizenship to the kids of gay parents if they're born abroad. LGBT Nation. Retrieved from https://www.lgbtqnation.com/2019/05/trump-administration-denying-citizenship-kids-gay-parents-theyre-born-abroad/?fbclid=IwAR3xTsNIonCYUa7pA4GJv6-KSu1WjfHL26zq8EqkOAYrhRu4f3P73edzFwk

Brinamen, C. F., & Mitchell, V. (2008). Gay men becoming fathers: A model of identity expansion. *Journal of GLBT Family Studies, 4,* 521–541. https://doi.org/10.1080/15504280802191772

Brodzinsky, D., Patterson, C., & Vaziri, M. (2002). Adoption agency perspectives on lesbian and gay prospective parents: A national study. *Adoption Quarterly, 5,* 5–23. https://doi.org/10.1300/J145v05n03_02.

Carone, N., Baiocco, R., & Lingiardi, V. (2017). Single fathers by choice using surrogacy: Why men decide to have a child as a single parent. *Human Reproduction, 32*(9), 1871–1879. https://doi.org/10.1093/humrep/dex245

Carone, N., Baiocco, R., Manzi, D., Antoniucci, C., Caricato, V., Pagliarulo, E., & Lingiardi, V. (2018). Surrogacy families headed by gay men: Relationships with surrogates and egg donors, fathers' decisions over disclosure and children's views on their surrogacy origins. *Human Reproduction, 33,* 248–257. https://doi.org/10.1093/humrep/dex362

Chabot, J. M., & Ames, B. D. (2004). "It wasn't 'let's get pregnant and do it'": Decision-making in lesbian couples planning motherhood via donor insemination. *Family Relations, 53,* 348–356. https://doi.org/10.1111/j.0197-6664.2004.00041.x

Collins, P. H. (1990). *Black feminist thought: Knowledge, consciousness, and the politics of empowerment.* New York, NY: Routledge.

Creative Family Connections: Surrogacy Agency and Law Firm. Retrieved from https://www.creativefamilyconnections.com/

deBoer, D. (2009). Focus on the family: The psychosocial context of gay men choosing fatherhood. In P. L. Hammack & B. J. Cohler (Eds.), *The story of sexual identity: Narrative perspectives on the gay and lesbian life course* (pp. 327–346). New York, NY: Oxford University Press.

Dillaway, H. E. (2008). Mothers for others: A race, class, and gender analysis of surrogacy. *International Journal of Sociology of the Family, 34,* 301–326.

Ehrenshaft, D. (2000). Alternatives to the stork: Fatherhood fantasies in donor insemination Families. *Studies in Gender and Sexuality, 1,* 371–397. https://doi.org/10.1080/15240650109349165

Ehrenshaft, D. (2005). *Mommies, daddies, donors, surrogates: Answering tough questions and building strong families.* New York, NY: Guilford Press.

Gamson, J. (2015). *Modern families: Stories of extraordinary journeys to kinship.* New York, NY: NYU Press.

Gates, G., Badgett, M. V. L., Macomber, J. E., & Chambers, K. (2007). *Adoption and foster care by gay and lesbian parents in the United States.* Washington, DC: The Urban Institute.

Goldberg, A. E. (2006). The transition to parenthood for lesbian couples. *Journal of GLBT Family Studies, 2*, 13–42. https://doi.org/10.1300/J461v02n01_02

Goldberg, A. E. (2010a). *Lesbian and gay parents and their children: Research on the family life cycle.* Washington, DC: American Psychological Association. https://doi.org/10.1037/12055-000

Goldberg, A. E. (2010b). Studying complex families in context. *Journal of Marriage and Family, 72*, 29–34. https://doi.org/10.1111/j.1741-3737.2009.00680.x

Goldberg, A. E. (2012). *Gay dads: Transitions to adoptive fatherhood.* New York, NY: NYU Press.

Goldberg, A. E., & Allen, K. R. (2007). Imagining men: Lesbian mothers' perceptions of male involvement during the transition to parenthood. *Journal of Marriage and Family, 69*, 352–365. https://doi.org/10.1111/j.1741-3737.2007.00370.x

Goldberg, A. E., Downing, J. B., & Moyer, A. M. (2012). Why parenthood and why now? gay men's motivations for pursuing parenthood. *Family Relations, 61*, 157–174. https://doi.org/10.1111/j.1741-3729.2011.00687.x

Goldberg, A. E., & Scheib, J. E. (2015). Why donor insemination and not adoption? Narratives of female-partnered and single mothers. *Family Relations, 64*, 726–742. https://doi.org/10.1111/fare.12162

Golombok, S., Blake, L., Slutsky, J., Raffanello, E., Roman, G. D., & Ehrhardt, A. (2018). Parenting and the adjustment of children born to gay fathers through surrogacy. *Child Development, 89*, 1223–1233. https://doi.org/10.1111/cdev.12728

Green, R.-J., Rubio, R. J., Bergman, K., & Katuzny, K. (2015, August). Gay fathers by surrogacy. Prejudice, parenting, and well-being of female and male children. Paper presented at the American Psychological Association Annual Convention, Toronto, Ontario, Canada.

Greenfeld, D. A., & Seli, E. (2011). Gay men choosing parenthood through assisted reproduction: Medical and psychosocial considerations. *Fertility & Sterility, 95*, 225–229. https://doi.org/10.1016/j.fertnstert.2010.05.053

Growing Generations (2019). https://www.growinggenerations.com/

Lassiter, P. S., Dew, B. J., Newton, K., Hays, D. G., & Yarbrough, B. (2006). Self-defined empowerment for gay and lesbian parents: A qualitative explanation. *The Family Journal, 14*, 24–252. https://doi.org/10.1177/1066480706287274

Lev, A. I. (2006). Gay dads: Choosing surrogacy. *Lesbian & Gay Psychology Review, 7*, 73–77.

Lewin, E. (2009). *Gay fatherhood: Narratives of family and citizenship in America.* Chicago, IL: University of Chicago Press.

Mallon, G. P. (2004). *Gay men choosing parenthood.* New York, NY: Columbia University Press.

Mamo, L., & Alston-Stepnitz, E. (2015). Queer intimacies and structural inequalities: New directions in stratified reproduction. *Journal of Family Issues, 36*, 519–540. https://doi.org/10.1177/0192513X14563796

May, A., & Tenzek, K. (2016). "A gift we are unable to create ourselves": Uncertainty reduction in online classified ads posted by gay men pursuing surrogacy. *Journal of GLBT Family Studies, 12*, 430–450. https://doi.org/10.1080/1550428X.2015.1128860

Mead, G. H. (1934). *Mind, self, and society.* Chicago, IL: University of Chicago Press.

Mitchell, V., & Green, R. J. (2007). Different storks for different folks: Gay and lesbian parents' experiences with alternative insemination and surrogacy. *Journal of GLBT Family Studies, 3*, 81–104. https://doi.org/10.1300/J461v03n02_04

Oswald, R. F., Blume, L. B., & Marks, S. R. (2005). Decentering heteronormativity: A proposal for family studies. In V. Bengtson, A. Acock, K. Allen, P. Dilworth-Anderson, & D. Klein (Eds.), *Sourcebook of family theories and methods: An interactive approach* (pp. 143–165). Newbury Park, CA: Sage.

Overton, W. F. (2015). Processes, Relations, and Relational-Developmental-Systems. In Handbook of Child Psychology and Developmental Science, R.M. Lerner (Ed.). https://doi.org/10.1002/9781118963418.childpsy102.

Petersen, M. N. (2018). Becoming gay fathers through transnational commercial surrogacy. *Journal of Family Issues, 39*, 693–719. https://doi.org/10.1177/0192513X16676859

Rothman, B. K. (1989). *Recreating motherhood: Ideology and technology in a patriarchal society.* New York, NY: W. W. Norton.

Ryan, M., & Berkowitz, D. (2009). Constructing gay and lesbian families 'beyond the closet. *Qualitative Sociology, 32*, 153–172. https://doi.org/10.1007/s11133-009-9124-6

Schacher, S., Auerbach, C. F., & Silverstein, L. B. (2005). Gay fathers. Expanding the possibilities for all of us. *Journal of GLBT Family Studies, 1*, 31–52. https://doi.org/10.1300/J461v01n03_02

Schoenberg, N. (2016, November 23). Gay men increasingly turn to surrogates to have babies. Chicago Tribune. Retrieved from www.chicagotribune.com/lifestyles/health/sc-gay-men-having-babies-health-1130-20161123-story.html

Smerdon, U. R. (2008). Crossing bodies, crossing borders: International surrogacy between the U.S. and India. *Cumberland Law Review, 39*, 15–85.

Stacey, J. (2006). Gay parenthood and the decline of paternity as we knew it. *Sexualities, 9*, 27–55. https://doi.org/10.1177/1363460706060687

Tornello, S. L., Kruczkowski, S. M., & Patterson, C. J. (2015). Division of labor and relationship quality among male same-sex couples who became fathers via surrogacy. *Journal of GLBT Family Studies, 11*, 375–394. https://doi.org/10.1080/1550428x.2015.1018471

Van Rijn-van Gelderen, L. V., Bos, H. W., Jorgensen, T. D., Ellis-Davies, K., Winstanley, A., Golombok, S., . . . Lamb, M. E. (2018). Wellbeing of gay fathers with children born through surrogacy: A comparison with lesbian-mother families and heterosexual IVF parent families. Human Reproduction, 33, 101–108. doi:https://doi.org/10.1093/humrep/dex339

# LGBTQ Foster Parents

Damien W. Riggs

This chapter focuses on LGBTQ foster parents. It begins by providing a brief history of formal foster care in the context of Australia, the UK, and the USA, given these are the three countries where the research reviewed in this chapter has been undertaken. This background information is important as it provides a context to the differing ways in which formal foster care is utilized within the statutory child protection systems of each country. The chapter then considers the extant literature on LGBTQ foster parents, grouped under five key themes: (a) the silencing of sexuality, (b) the pathologizing of sexuality, (c) the expectation that LGBTQ foster parents demonstrate "appropriate" gender role models, (d) the resistance to placement matching of LGBTQ children in foster care, and (e) the expectation that LGBTQ foster parents educate child protection staff. The chapter finishes by exploring gaps in the literature, opportunities for future research, and the implications of the existing research for both policy and practice.

## Brief History of Formal Foster Care

Across the world, the history of formal foster care is far reaching. Formal foster care here refers to the statutory removal of children from their birth parents due to concerns about abuse and/or neglect and their placement with foster families, either with the aim of reunifying children with their birth parents or their subsequent placement in either long-term foster care or adoption. In countries such as Australia, the UK, and the USA, informal care for other people's children has been commonplace for centuries, though the advent of formal foster care began in the nineteenth century (Scott & Swain, 2002). Beyond these three countries, practices of foster care are central to kinship in many geographic regions, dating back tens of thousands of years (Carsten, 2004).

Formalized foster care in Australia, the UK, and the USA shares something of a similar trajectory, before diverging in the late twentieth century. As noted above, caring for other people's children in informal arrangements was historically common. With population growth, however, came an increased demand for homes for children who were orphaned or whose parents could not care for them (Scott & Swain, 2002).

In response to this increased demand, benevolent organizations in the early twentieth century turned their attention to child welfare, with the aim of placing children with families

D. W. Riggs (✉)
College of Education, Psychology and Social Work, Flinders University, Adelaide, SA, Australia
e-mail: damien.riggs@flinders.edu.au

© Springer Nature Switzerland AG 2020
A. E. Goldberg, K. R. Allen (eds.), *LGBTQ-Parent Families*,
https://doi.org/10.1007/978-3-030-35610-1_9

161

(Gowan, 2014). In each country, however, a series of scandals in relation to "baby farming" brought into question the efficacy of informal fostering arrangements, in addition to problems associated with the costs of state involvement in the care of children (Zelizer, 1994). The rise of orphanages was one attempt at reducing the trafficking of children and the treatment of children as indentured labor; however, this too was a cost to the public purse. Additionally, it was slowly acknowledged that outcomes for children raised in orphanages were often poor and that many children experienced considerable abuse or neglect in orphanages due to underfunding and the (often negative) views of staff charged with the care of children (Gowan, 2014).

One answer to the "problem" of rising costs of state care and the abuse of children in orphanages was adoption. The legal transfer of parentage was one way to shift the cost of children from the state to adoptive parents, and it was also thought to hold the possibility of shifting the prevailing logic away from seeing children as indentured labor, instead framing them as loved family members (Zelizer, 1994). At the same time, however, extinguishing the rights of birth parents was increasingly recognized as problematic. This has meant, particularly in the USA, that foster care still has a major role to play in the child protection system. As a result, in the USA children removed from their birth parents may live for a considerable period of time in foster care or with other birth family members before then being placed for adoption (Riggs & Due, 2018).

In Australia and the UK, foster care continues to play a significant role in child protection systems. In the UK, foster care was the most common form of care for children who could not live with their birth parents throughout the second half of the twentieth century. Since the turn of the millennium, however, adoption has been the preferred mode of placement for children who cannot live with their birth parents, yet significant numbers of children still live in foster placements either due to short-term orders or while awaiting an adoptive placement (Riggs & Due, 2018). In

Australia, by contrast, foster care remains the primary form of placement (Riggs, Bartholomaeus, & Due, 2016). It has been argued that this is due to histories of adoption in Australia that have involved the forced removal of Indigenous (i.e., First Nations) children (Cuthbert & Quartly, 2012), recognition of which has cast adoption as inherently problematic. In recent years, however, certain legislatures in Australia have turned their focus to adoption and have amended laws to increase the likelihood that children in long-term foster placements will be adopted (Murphy, Quartly, & Cuthbert, 2009).

This background information is important when turning to consider the experiences of LGBTQ people as foster parents. Specifically, and depending on the country, foster care may be a transitional family context situated between reunification with birth parents and placement for adoption, or it may be a permanent arrangement until a child turns 18. When we consider the literature on LGBTQ foster parents, however, and despite differences across countries in terms of foster care practice, we see many similarities, specifically with regard to ongoing discrimination. While, as will be shown in this chapter, this appears to be slowly changing, a culture of suspicion continues to predominate when it comes to LGBTQ foster parents.

## Research on LGBTQ Foster Parents

In terms of the number of LGBTQ people who are foster parents, data on population sizes are scarce. No such information is available in the Australian context or for the UK. In the USA, Gates, Badgett, Macomber, and Chambers (2007) provided an estimate of the number of children living with lesbian or gay foster parents, suggesting that at the time over 14,100 children lived with such parents, constituting 6% of children living with foster parents who are not birth family members.

With regard to how gender and sexuality have been theorized in research on LGBTQ foster parents, early research tended to focus on homophobia as experienced by lesbian and gay foster parents (e.g., Ricketts, 1991). Homophobia, in this research, focused on affect, and specifically the emotional reactions that heterosexual people have when interacting with or considering interactions with people who are not heterosexual (Hudson & Ricketts, 1980). As such, this early research theorized something of a direct (causal) relationship between the existence of lesbian and gay foster parents and other people's responses to them. Beginning with the work of Hicks (1996), however, research on lesbian and gay foster parents has increasingly sought to theorize how reactions to lesbian and gay foster parents are the result of normative accounts of gender and sexuality that circulate within a broader framework of heteronormativity. Drawing on Butler's (1990) conceptualization of the "heterosexual matrix," Hicks and others have explored how lesbian and gay foster parents are often positioned outside of normative accounts of gender by default of not being heterosexual. This focus on heteronormativity has allowed for a broader focus on the positioning of lesbian and gay foster parents in society, rather than the specific interpersonal context of homophobia.

The sections below present a thematic review of research that has almost solely focused on lesbian and gay foster parents. The thematic areas reported are those that predominate in the literature and are relatively consistent across the literature. Comment is made where the findings within a given thematic area appear to have shifted across time.

## Silencing of Sexuality

This first theme refers to research that has focused on how discussions of lesbian or gay sexualities are silenced by child protection workers. In the UK, Hicks (2000) conducted interviews with 30 social workers who reported that a "good" lesbian foster care applicant accepted the idea that lesbian sexuality should be silenced or minimally spoken of. In the USA, Patrick and Palladino (2009) interviewed nine lesbian or gay foster par-

ents and similarly found that agency staff rarely spoke about lesbian or gay sexuality, which included refraining from or refusing to speak with both foster children and birth parents about foster parent sexuality prior to a placement occurring. In the Australian context, Riggs (2007), drawing on the assessment reports of five lesbian or gay foster parents, reported a contradiction between silence and deception. On the one hand, applicants were expected to mute discussions about their sexuality, yet on the other hand applicants were treated as deceptive if they did not speak openly about their sexuality as part of the assessment process.

In addition to child protection staff often refraining from talking about lesbian or gay sexualities, previous research also suggests that such sexualities are silenced via what Wilton (1995) refers to as "heterosexualization." Heterosexualization occurs when nonheterosexual relationships are depicted as "just like" heterosexual relationships or when nonheterosexual people are encouraged to present themselves publically as heterosexual. In his research on gay foster parents, for example, Hicks (2006) suggests that gay men may be rendered palatable as foster parents through their depiction as "maternal men." While in some ways this depicts gay men as failed men (i.e., men are not normatively expected to be maternal), in other ways the maternal men narrative constructs gay men as non-threatening through being positioned as just like heterosexual mothers. The research summarized in this theme spans two decades, suggesting that discomfort with, or opposition to, the voicing of lesbian and gay sexualities has been relatively consistent within the context of child protection.

## Pathologization of Sexuality

In addition to lesbian or gay sexualities being silenced, research also suggests that such sexualities may be brought to the fore by child protection staff in order to question or pathologize them. In the study by Patrick and Palladino (2009) summarized above, some participants reported that birth parents used knowledge about lesbian or gay sexualities to make false allegations of child abuse by foster parents in order to pathologize their sexuality. In their survey of 60 lesbian, gay, or bisexual foster parents living in the USA, Downs and James (2006) found that a significant proportion hid their sexuality from birth parents for fear that it would be pathologized. In his work on gay foster parents, Hicks (2000) suggests that while in some contexts gay men are depicted as maternal men, in other contexts they are depicted as "perverts," with suspicious motives to provide care. Riggs (2011a) also found this in his examination of five films featuring gay foster parents, in which gay sexualities were depicted as perverse and a risk to children.

In terms of explicit pathologization, early research by Skeates and Jabri (1988) in the UK found that of the 11 lesbian or gay foster parents they studied, those who were out about their sexuality to agency staff experienced prejudice. Almost a decade later, in Hicks' (1996) interviews with 11 lesbians or gay men assessed to become foster or adoptive parents, participants reported that assessment workers displayed a prurient interest in their sexualities. A decade later again, and in the Australian context, Riggs and Augoustinos (2009) found in their interviews with ten lesbian or gay foster parents that many reported experiencing homophobia from child protection staff. By contrast, recent research conducted in the UK by Wood (2015) with 24 lesbian or gay foster or adoptive parents found that none had been refused assessment, none experienced a prurient focus on (or silencing of) their sexuality, and none reported experiencing discrimination. This may reflect changes in the ways that lesbian and gay foster carers are positioned by foster care agencies or may potentially be a product of regional differences in recruitment strategies.

Research spanning three decades has consistently found that lesbian and gay foster parents experience pathogizing responses from birth parents and child protection staff. However, the most recent research suggests that such pathologization may be less common, indicating perhaps something of a shift in the acceptability of the explicit voicing of homophobia.

## Expectation to Demonstrate "Appropriate" Gender Role Models

Consistent across the literature is an emphasis upon lesbian and gay foster parents reporting that they are expected to demonstrate that they will provide "appropriate" gender role models to foster children. Hicks (2000), for example, found that social workers reported that they expected lesbian applicants to demonstrate that they were not anti-men, that they were not militant in their feminism, and that they would adopt traditional female gender roles within the home. While as noted above, Wood (2015) found that her participants had not experienced overt discrimination, they nonetheless were still asked by assessment workers how they would provide appropriate gender role models. Notably, her participants were attuned to this expectation, yet felt that they had no capacity to question or resist the expectation given reasonable fears about not being approved or having children placed with them.

This theme of a focus on lesbian and gay foster parents being expected to provide "appropriate" gender role models links very much to the broader literature on LGBTQ parenting. The literature has consistently documented the expectation that lesbian mothers in particular account for how they will provide male role models to their children (e.g., Clarke, 2006; Clarke & Kitzinger, 2005). This may reflect the predominance of research on lesbian mothers, though it may also reflect a particular concern that children, and in particular boys, need "male role models." It is thus perhaps unsurprising that the literature on lesbian and gay foster parents echoes this expectation.

## Resistance to Placement Matching for LGBTQ Children in Care

Different to the expectation that LGBTQ foster parents should provide "appropriate" gender role models to children in their care, this theme focuses on how LGBTQ foster parents have at times been depicted as inherently *inappropriate* role models for LGBTQ children in care. For example, Australian interview research by Riggs (2011b) with 30 lesbian and gay foster parents reported that participants felt they were perceived by child protection staff as inappropriate role models for LGBTQ children specifically, and participants were denied requests to have LGBTQ children placed with them. This is concerning given research findings on the experiences of LGBTQ children in the context of child protection and the views of heterosexual foster parents with regard to caring for LGBTQ children. For example, in the USA, Mallon (2001) interviewed 54 young people about their experiences of foster care and found that some reported that heterosexual foster parents terminated a placement upon learning that a child was lesbian or gay. Drawing from interviews with ten LGBQ youth, Gallegos et al. (2011) reported that just under half felt that being placed with an LGBTQ foster parent was important to them. Those who felt it would be important to be placed with an LGBTQ foster parent noted that this would make it more likely that they would be supported rather than discriminated against in care.

In regard to the views of heterosexual and/or cisgender foster parents, Clements and Rosenwald (2007), drawing on focus groups conducted with 25 foster parents living in the USA, found that many held misconceptions about LGBTQ children, including a fear that LGBTQ children placed with them would abuse their children, religious beliefs that positioned homosexuality as a sin, and a view of lesbian or bisexual children as safe, while gay male children were seen as a risk. Of the seven participants who previously had an LGBTQ child placed with them, six had terminated the placement on the basis of views about the child's gender or sexuality. Finally, survey research by Bucchio (2012) conducted in the USA with 304 foster mothers found that 40.8% of the sample reported that they were unwilling to accept a placement for a sexual minority youth.

Given these findings with regard to the relative unwillingness of heterosexual and/or cisgender foster parents to care for LGBTQ children, and given estimates made by Wilson and Kastanis (2015) that in Los Angeles alone approximately 19% of children in care are LGBTQ, it is concerning that there appears to be an unwillingness to place such children with LGBTQ foster parents. This may reflect ongoing systemic discrimination toward LGBTQ foster parents, or it may reflect a lack of awareness by child protection staff of the benefits of placement matching to LGBTQ children in care.

## Expectation to Educate Child Protection Staff

The final theme evident across the literature is the expectation that LGBTQ foster parents should educate child protection staff in order to facilitate their inclusion and acceptance in foster care assessment and practice. In interview research conducted by Wood introduced above (2015), for example, her lesbian and gay participants reported no discrimination. Yet this may be because they felt compelled to disclose their sexuality early in the assessment process and to do so in ways that demonstrated that it would not negatively impact upon children potentially placed with them. In so doing, the participants were educating child protection staff about a very particular version of lesbian or gay families that was most likely to be seen as palatable (i.e., that they were in stable monogamous relationships).

Research by Riggs (2010a) in the Australian context introduced above has also suggested that many of the participants felt compelled to accept "pragmatic imbalances." Riggs used the term "pragmatic imbalances" to refer to the ways in which many of his participants felt compelled to put aside their own political views so as to educate child protection staff about a specifically palatable and hence acceptable version of lesbian or gay sexualities. Willingness to do so was explained by participants as a focus on the needs of children—needs that had to be weighed against any personal desire to speak more openly with child protection staff about lesbian and gay politics. Riggs (2007) also notes how lesbian or gay foster care applicants are expected to educate child protection staff about lesbian or gay sexualities in order to warrant their own inclusion. A failure to do so was experienced by some participants as risking a poor assessment and thus the potential of not being approved to provide care.

This theme suggests that the expectation for LGBTQ foster parents to educate child protection staff is subtle but ongoing. In having to educate staff, LGBTQ foster parents not only must have an informed opinion on the lives of LGBTQ people to share with child protection staff, but may also feel compelled to present a particular normative image of LGBTQ people. This may come at the expense of a more inclusive, nuanced, and diverse account of LGBTQ people's lives.

## Directions for Future Research

Despite the relatively consistent findings reported in the research summarized above, there are also some consistent gaps in this work, primarily pertaining to gender, sexuality, race, location (i.e., urban or regional), nationality, and religion. Of the studies reviewed, only one included bisexual participants, yet the authors note that given the sample included 30 gay men, 25 lesbians women, and 5 bisexual people, analysis of the latter was not undertaken separately and that "casual inspection of the data suggested no obvious differences" (Downs & James, 2006, p. 286). A closer and more focused analysis of the data might, however, have identified unique experiences pertaining to bisexual foster parents.

Previous literature is almost entirely silent on queer or transgender foster parents. One policy document produced for the Human Rights Campaign Foundation in the USA was identified that focused on transgender or nonbinary foster and adoptive parents and did include the views of a small number of such parents (Perry, 2017), but these were not analyzed systematically nor was a research method reported in the document. The second edition of Hicks and McDermott's (2018) edited collection on lesbian and gay foster carers also includes one story by a transgender foster parent, Dylan, who noted that he was treated well by his assessing foster care agency, but was treated poorly by a medical professional who was

required to provide an assessment. Queer foster parents are not mentioned at all in the previous literature, though as noted above queer foster children have been the focus of recent research on LGBTQ children in care (Gallegos et al., 2011).

Also largely overlooked in previous literature are the topics of race and class. This is of particular concern given the high rates of Black and Indigenous children in care in the three countries focused on in this chapter (Roberts, 2009; Tilbury, 2009). While the research samples reviewed in this chapter almost exclusively included White lesbian or gay foster parent, this does not explain why the whiteness of such participants is not a topic of investigation, nor why the race of their foster children was not explored. As Riggs (2006) has noted, as much as White LGBTQ foster parents may experience discrimination on the basis of their gender or sexuality, they likely also experience considerable privileges on the basis of their race. Hicks and McDermott (1999, 2018) note this specifically in both editions of their collection that documents the experiences of lesbian or gay foster and adoptive parents living in the UK. Black foster parents, Barbara and Shazia, who contributed their stories to Hicks and McDermott's (2018) collection, noted that racism and homophobia intersected in the child protection system, shaping the placements they were offered, and the supports they had access to. In the Australian context, Riggs (2012) reports on a single case study of a non-Indigenous gay man caring for an Indigenous child. Riggs notes the ways in which the man actively attended to his race privilege, which included making concessions to birth families, based on awareness of cultural differences, with regard to their views on his sexuality (i.e., he accepted some degree of negative affect directed toward him as a gay man, given his awareness of specific Indigenous cultural values in regard to the community from which the child was removed).

Given histories of forced removal of children, and particularly First Nations and Black children, further attention is required to examine complicity with, or resistance to, colonization and racism on the part of White LGBTQ foster parents.

Complicity may occur when White LGBTQ foster parents accept placements for Black or First Nations children without questioning placement principles that, in countries such as Australia, emphasize the importance of children being placed within their own communities (Kee & Tilbury, 1999). Such foster parents are no more inherently outside of racialized systems of power and control than are White heterosexual foster parents. As such, research examining how LGBTQ foster parents, and particularly White LGBTQ foster parents, understand racialized power imbalances and their impact upon child protection systems is important. This is important so as to identify best practice for White LGBTQ foster parents in supporting non-white children placed with them where this is the only placement option available.

Other topics that might provide useful avenues for future research are indicated in some of the previous literature. Both Hicks and McDermott (1999; 2018) and Riggs (2011a, 2011b) suggest that there might be unique benefits to children being raised by LGBTQ foster parents. These include providing same-gender only households for children who have previously experienced abuse from someone of a different gender or conversely providing opportunities for positive interactions with someone of a different gender. Research on the potential advantages of placement matching for all children, and here specifically LGBTQ children, would benefit from adopting an intersectional approach (Crenshaw, 1990), so as to explore how matching based on, for example, gender, sexuality, race, and class might serve to promote positive outcomes for both children and parents. Research may also usefully explore in closer detail the views of child protection staff, including perceived advantages and barriers to placement matching for LGBTQ foster parents and children.

In terms of children, it is notable that to date no research has been undertaken with children of LGBTQ foster parents, including LGBTQ children—although some work on LGBTQ youth with LGBTQ adoptive parents has been conducted (see chapter "LGBTQ Adoptive Parents and Their Children"). This is in some ways surprising, given the now extensive body of research on children of LGBTQ parents more broadly. It is, however, perhaps less surprising if we consider how narratives of "vulnerability" serve to inform research with children in foster care (Riggs, King, Delfabbro, & Augoustinos, 2009) and perhaps particularly children placed with LGBTQ parents. Nonetheless, listening to the views of children placed with LGBTQ foster parents is important, as it offers the possibility to either affirm or extend on the views previously expressed in research with LGBTQ foster parents.

Also in terms of avenues for future research, the findings of Wood (2018) in her research with 25 lesbian or gay foster or adoptive parents suggest that lesbian and gay foster parents might be uniquely attuned to the needs of birth parents and more willing than other foster parents to work on developing positive relationships with birth parents. This possibility is also suggested by research on lesbian and gay adoptive parents (e.g., Goldberg, Kinkler, Richardson, & Downing, 2011). Given the importance of best connections with birth parents for children in care, this is an area deserving of closer attention in the future.

Given the ongoing demand for foster parents, and the increased recognition that LGBTQ people can meet this demand, future research might usefully focus on how LGBTQ people perceive becoming foster parents—that is, the challenges, barriers, and benefits. Given the known barriers and challenges identified in the research summarized above, it will be important that child protection systems understand what LGBTQ people make of such barriers and challenges and how they may be addressed in terms of welcoming LGBTQ people as prospective foster parents.

Finally, this chapter has focused on research undertaken in Australia, the UK, and the USA. A likely explanation for the predominance of these locales is the use of formal foster care in each and the relative visibility of LGBTQ people as potential research participants. It is not the case, however, that formal foster care is absent in other locales, nor that other forms of care (such as informal foster care or kinship care) do not occur (see chapter "Race and Ethnicity in the Lives of

LGBTQ Parents and Their Children: Perspectives from and Beyond North America"). While in certain locales accessing LGBTQ research participants may be somewhat more difficult, it will be important that into the future researchers attempt to address the gap in the literature constituted by the sole focus on Australia, the UK, and the USA. It will also be important that future research seeks to engage other research methodologies in addition to the primarily interview and focus group-based research reviewed in this chapter. This might include using dynamic methodologies such as photo elicitation or walk and talk approaches and may also involve the use of large-scale quantitative surveys (see chapters "Qualitative Research on LGBTQ-Parent Families" and "The Use of Representative Datasets to Study LGBTQ-Parent Families: Challenges, Advantages, and Opportunities").

## Implications for Practice

Beyond empirical research, there are a growing number of publications that focus on specific practice and policy issues pertaining to LGBTQ foster parents. Researchers such as Mallon (2011, 2015) have advocated for the need for a holistic approach to engagement with LGBTQ foster parents, one that begins with how agencies promote their services and advertise for foster applicants, through to the assessment process, the placement process, and the subsequent support of placements. Other policy and practice recommendations include the need to assess whether agency materials are heteronormative (and cisgenderist), the importance of LGBTQ support groups, and the need to avoid heteronormative (and cisgenderist) assumptions in placement matching (Cosis Brown, Sebba, & Luke, 2015). Finally, it has long been acknowledged that for many LGBTQ people kinship extends beyond birth families, with friends often included as kin (Weston, 1997). Child protection agencies might usefully engage with the ways in which friendships may be unique sources of strength and support for LGBTQ foster parents (Riggs, 2010b).

Beyond these general recommendations for policy and practice, there are specific recommendations that focus on transgender and nonbinary foster parents. A recent US policy document (Perry, 2017) outlines the importance of proactive inclusivity by agencies for transgender and nonbinary foster parents (such as flags or reading materials), the provision of a space in registration forms to speak about gender history, gender identity or gender expression being discussed in policy documents, the use of affirming language by staff; gender neutral bathrooms available at agencies, agencies advertising in community magazines, agencies having transgender and nonbinary staff members, the inclusion of transgender and nonbinary people in training materials, and not asking questions beyond the interview schedules used in assessments that would suggest personal curiosity about transgender and nonbinary people's lives.

In terms of lesbian and gay foster parents specifically, and drawing from Wood (2015), it is important to acknowledge that while her participants did not experience overt discrimination, many felt that they were expected to present a very specific image of lesbian and gay families. This would suggest the importance of child protection staff being aware of and welcoming of a diversity of family forms. Wood's participants also highlighted that the training materials they were exposed to almost exclusively included heterosexual foster parents. The inclusion of a diversity of foster parents in training materials, including racially diverse foster parents, and bisexual, transgender, and queer foster parents, is thus an important way of ensuring the inclusion of LGBTQ foster parents.

In conclusion, LGBTQ people bring with them unique experiences and strengths that may be seen as assets in their role as foster parents. Importantly, however, the inclusion of LGBTQ people in the child protection system should not be solely based on what they uniquely have to offer. Rather, the inclusion of LGBTQ people should be premised upon recognition of the heteronormative and cisgenderist views that have historically precluded the inclusion of LGBTQ people as foster parents, undoubtedly to the detriment of both LGBTQ people and children needing foster placements. In this sense, then, LGBTQ people are not merely an untapped resource for child protection systems. Rather, LGBTQ people as foster parents are part of a wider child protection system that should have as its central focus the well-being of children, which necessitates a diversity of placement options so as to best meet their needs.

# References

Bucchio, J. D. (2012). *Characteristics of foster parents willing to care for sexual minority youth*. Unpublished doctoral thesis, University of Tennessee.

Butler, J. (1990). *Gender trouble: Feminism and the subversion of identity*. New York, NY: Routledge.

Carsten, J. (2004). *After kinship*. Cambridge, UK: Cambridge University Press.

Clarke, V. (2006). 'Gay men, gay men and more gay men': Traditional, liberal and critical perspectives on male role models in lesbian families. *Lesbian & Gay Psychology Review, 7*, 19–35.

Clarke, V., & Kitzinger, C. (2005). 'We're not living on planet lesbian': Constructions of male role models in debates about lesbian families. *Sexualities, 8*, 137–152. https://doi.org/10.1177/1363460705050851

Clements, J. A., & Rosenwald, M. (2007). Foster parents' perspectives on LGB youth in the child welfare system. *Journal of Gay and Lesbian Social Services, 19*, 57–69. https://doi.org/10.1300/J041v19n01_04

Cosis Brown, H., Sebba, J., & Luke, N. (2015). *The recruitment, assessment, support and supervision of lesbian, gay, bisexual and transgender foster carers*. Oxford, UK: Rees Centre.

Crenshaw, K. (1990). Mapping the margins: Intersectionality, identity politics, and violence against women of color. *Stanford Law Review, 43*, 1241–1298.

Cuthbert, D., & Quartly, M. (2012). 'Forced adoption' in the Australian story of national story of national regret and apology. *Australian Journal of Politics and History, 58*, 82–96. https://doi.org/10.1111/j.1467-8497.2012.01625.x

Downs, A. C., & James, S. E. (2006). Gay, lesbian, and bisexual foster parents: Strengths and challenges for the child welfare system. *Child Welfare, 85*, 281–298.

Gallegos, A., Roller White, C., Ryan, C., O'Brien, K., Pecora, P. J., & Thomas, P. (2011). Exploring the experiences of lesbian, gay, bisexual, and questioning adolescents in foster care. *Journal of Family Social Work, 14*, 226–236. https://doi.org/10.1080/10522158.2011.571547

Gates, G., Badgett, M. V. L., Macomber, J., & Chambers, K. (2007). *Adoption and foster care by gay and lesbian parents in the United States*. Los Angeles, CA: The Williams Institute.

Goldberg, A. E., Kinkler, L. A., Richardson, H. B., & Downing, J. B. (2011). Lesbian, gay, and heterosexual couples in open adoption arrangements: A qualitative study. *Journal of Marriage and Family, 73*, 502–518. https://doi.org/10.1111/j.1741-3737.2010.00821.x

Gowan, B. G. M. (2014). Historical evolution of child welfare services. In G. P. Mallon & P. McCartt Hess (Eds.), *Child welfare for the twenty-first century: A handbook of practices, policies and programs* (pp. 11–44). New York, NY: Columbia University Press.

Hicks, S. (1996). The 'last resort'?: Lesbian and gay experiences of the social work assessment process in fostering and adoption. *Practice, 8*(2), 15–24. https://doi.org/10.1080/09503159608415357

Hicks, S. (2000). 'Good lesbian, bad lesbian...': Regulating heterosexuality in fostering and adoption assessments. *Child & Family Social Work, 5*(2), 157–168. https://doi.org/10.1046/j.1365-2206.2000.00153.x

Hicks, S. (2006). Maternal men – perverts and deviants? Making sense of gay men as foster carers and adopters. *Journal of GLBT Family Studies, 2*, 93–114. https://doi.org/10.1300/J461v02n01_05

Hicks, S., & McDermott, J. (1999). Editorial essay. In S. Hicks & J. McDermott (Eds.), *Lesbian and gay fostering and adoption: Extraordinary yet ordinary* (pp. 147–198). London, UK: Jessica Kingsley.

Hicks, S., & McDermott, J. (2018). *Lesbian and gay foster care and adoption* (2nd ed.). London, UK: Jessica Kingsley.

Hudson, W. W., & Ricketts, W. A. (1980). A strategy for the measurement of homophobia. *Journal of Homosexuality, 5*, 357–372. https://doi.org/10.1300/J082v05n01_02

Kee, M. A., & Tilbury, C. (1999). The aboriginal and Torres Strait islander child placement principle is about self determination. *Children Australia, 24*(3), 4–8. https://doi.org/10.1017/S1035077200009196

Mallon, G. P. (2001). Sticks and stones can break your bones: Verbal harassment and physical violence in the lives of gay and lesbian youths in child welfare settings. *Journal of Gay and Lesbian Social Services, 13*, 63–81. https://doi.org/10.1300/J041v13n01_06

Mallon, G. P. (2011). Lesbian and gay prospective foster and adoptive families: The home study assessment process. In D. Brodzinsky & A. Pertman (Eds.), *Adoption by lesbians and gay men: A new dimension in family diversity* (pp. 130–149). New York, NY: Oxford University Press.

Mallon, G. P. (2015). *Lesbian, gay, bisexual and trans foster and adoptive parents: Recruiting, assessing, and supporting untapped family resources for children and youth*. Washington, DC: Child Welfare League of America.

Murphy, K., Quartly, M., & Cuthbert, D. (2009). "In the best interests of the child": Mapping the (re) emergence of pro-adoption politics in contemporary Australia. *Australian Journal of Politics & History, 55*, 201–218. https://doi.org/10.1111/j.1467-8497.2009.01516a.x

Patrick, D., & Palladino, J. (2009). The community interactions of gay and lesbian foster parents. In T. J. Socha & G. Stamp (Eds.), *Parents and children communicating with society: Managing relationships outside of the home* (pp. 323–342). New York, NY: Routledge.

Perry, J. R. (2017). *Promising practices for serving transgender and non-binary foster and adoptive parents.* Washington, DC: The Human Rights Campaign Foundation.

Ricketts, W. (1991). *Lesbians and gay men as foster parents.* Portland, ME: University of Southern Maine.

Riggs, D. W. (2006). *Priscilla, (white) queen of the desert: Queer rights/race privilege.* New York, NY: Peter Lang.

Riggs, D. W. (2007). Reassessing the foster care system: Examining the impact of heterosexism on lesbian and gay applicants. *Hypatia, 22,* 132–148. https://doi.org/10.1111/j.1527-2001.2007.tb01153.x

Riggs, D. W. (2010a). Pragmatic imbalances: Australian lesbian and gay foster carers negotiating the current legal context. *Law in Context: A Socio-Legal Journal, 28,* 65–73.

Riggs, D. W. (2010b). Perceptions of support among Australian lesbian and gay foster carers. In T. Morrison, A. Morrison, M. A. Carrigan, & D. T. McDermott (Eds.), *Sexual minority research in the new millennium* (pp. 93–106). New York, NY: Nova Science.

Riggs, D. W. (2011a). 'Let's go to the movies': Filmic representations of gay foster and adoptive parents. *Journal of GLBT Family Studies, 7,* 297–312. https://doi.org/10.1080/1550428X.2011.564948

Riggs, D. W. (2011b). Australian lesbian and gay foster carers negotiating the child protection system: Strengths and challenges. *Sexuality Research and Social Policy, 8,* 215–216. https://doi.org/10.1007/s13178-011-0059-9

Riggs, D. W. (2012). Non-indigenous lesbians and gay men caring for Indigenous children: An Australian case study. In C. Phellas (Ed.), *Researching non-heterosexual sexualities* (pp. 201–214). Surrey, UK: Ashgate.

Riggs, D. W., & Augoustinos, M. (2009). Institutional stressors and individual strengths: Policy and practice directions for working with Australian lesbian and gay foster carers. *Practice: Social Work in Action, 21*(2), 77–90. https://doi.org/10.1080/09503150902875919

Riggs, D. W., Bartholomaeus, C., & Due, C. (2016). Public and private families: A comparative thematic analysis of the intersections of social norms and scrutiny. *Health Sociology Review, 25,* 1–17. https://doi.org/10.1080/14461242.2015.1135071

Riggs, D. W., & Due, C. (2018). Support for family diversity: A three-country study. *Journal of Infant and Reproductive Psychology, 36,* 192–206. https://doi.org/10.1080/02646838.2018.1434491

Riggs, D. W., King, D., Delfabbro, P. H., & Augoustinos, M. (2009). "Children out of place": Representations of foster care in the Australian news media. *Journal of Children and Media, 3,* 234–248. https://doi.org/10.1080/17482790902999918

Roberts, D. (2009). *Shattered bonds: The color of child welfare.* New York, NY: Civitas Books.

Scott, D., & Swain, S. (2002). *Confronting cruelty: Historical perspectives on child protection in Australia.* Melbourne, Australia: Melbourne University Press.

Skeates, J., & Jabri, D. (1988). *Fostering and adoption by lesbians and gay men.* London, UK: London Strategic Policy Unit.

Tilbury, C. (2009). The over-representation of indigenous children in the Australian child welfare system. *International Journal of Social Welfare, 18*(1), 57–64. https://doi.org/10.1111/j.1468-2397.2008.00577.x

Weston, K. (1997). *Families we choose: Lesbians, gays, kinship.* New York, NY: Columbia University Press.

Wilson, B. D., & Kastanis, A. A. (2015). Sexual and gender minority disproportionality and disparities in child welfare: A population-based study. *Children and Youth Services Review, 58,* 11–17. https://doi.org/10.1016/j.childyouth.2015.08.016

Wilton, T. (1995). *Immortal, invisible: Lesbians and the moving image.* London, UK: Routledge.

Wood, K. (2015). 'It's all a bit pantomime': An exploratory study of gay and lesbian adopters and foster carers in England and Wales. *The British Journal of Social Work, 46,* 1708–1723. https://doi.org/10.1093/bjsw/bcv115

Wood, K. (2018). Families beyond boundaries: Conceptualising kinship in gay and lesbian adoption and fostering. *Child & Family Social Work, 23,* 155–162. https://doi.org/10.1111/cfs.12394

Zelizer, V. A. (1994). *Pricing the priceless child: The changing social value of children.* Princeton, NJ: Princeton University Press.

# Polyamorous Parenting in Contemporary Research: Developments and Future Directions

Maria Pallotta-Chiarolli, Elisabeth Sheff,
and Ruby Mountford

Anne: What do you think requires further research
      [about polyfamilies?]
Pete: Apart from everything? (PolyVic polypar-
      enting group)

Children raised in polyamorous families (or *polyfamilies*) have parents who may identify with any sexual or gender orientation, are of diverse cultures and social classes, are in openly negotiated intimate sexual relationships with more than one partner, and may or may not cohabitate, share finances, or expect sexual exclusivity among a group larger than two (Pallotta-Chiarolli, 2010a; Pallotta-Chiarolli, Haydon, & Hunter, 2013; Sheff, 2013, 2016a). Parents who agree to only be in sexual relationships with each other and closed to relationships outside the group are in *polyfidelitous* families. Many *polycules*—chosen family networks of people associated through polyamorous relationships (Creation, 2019)—have members that

maintain *polyaffective* relationships that are emotionally intimate and nonsexual (Sheff, 2016b). Because polyamory and other forms of consensual non-monogamies (CNM) are becoming increasingly common in both LGBTIQ+ (especially among gay male and bisexual folks, see Levine, Herbenick, Martinez, Fu, & Dodge, 2018) and heterosexual populations in the twenty-first century (Moors, 2017), researchers and family service providers require more information to adequately understand and serve these multiple and sometimes shifting configurations of multiparent families (Anapol, 2010; Barker & Langdridge, 2010; Sheff, 2013). Most polycules contain LGBTQ+ members, and research has documented an especially strong link between bisexuality and polyamory (Anderlini-D'Onofrio, 2009; Pallotta-Chiarolli, 2014, 2016a). While polyamorous parenting is gaining momentum in research, it remains under-researched and under-resourced in health services and education sectors (Goldfeder & Sheff, 2013; Raab, 2018).

This chapter begins with an overview of academic research and theoretical development on polyparenting since the 2013 edition of this book and then focuses on the authors' ongoing research. Given the continued dearth of existing research on polyfamilies, we take care to identify what remains unknown or understudied and con-

M. Pallotta-Chiarolli (✉)
Deakin University, Melbourne, VIC, Australia
e-mail: mariapc@deakin.edu.au

E. Sheff
Sheff Consulting, Chattanooga, Tennessee,
USA

R. Mountford
Melbourne Bisexual Network,
Melbourne, VIC, Australia

© Springer Nature Switzerland AG 2020
A. E. Goldberg, K. R. Allen (eds.), *LGBTQ-Parent Families*,
https://doi.org/10.1007/978-3-030-35610-1_10

clude with a brief discussion of some directions for further research and implications for practice in education, healthcare, and the law.

## Erasure, Exclusion by Inclusion, and the Absence of Intersectionality: Ongoing Polyparenting Research Issues

There are four larger issues that form the backdrop for the academic and social conversations about polyfamilies. These are very similar and often interwoven with the concerns summarized by Pallotta-Chiarolli (2016b) in relation to bisexualities in health and education policies and practice. First, the *erasure* of polyfamilies in academic discourse continues to reflect and influence the similar ignorance of polyfamilies in social, legal, health, and educational realms. Some scholars adapt to the absence of theorizing and data about polyfamilies and their children by utilizing research on children from same-sex parent families to help articulate and explain what children from polyfamilies experience (Sheff, 2011). While understandable, this second issue of *exclusion by inclusion* is also problematic because the experiences of polyfamilies are distinct and children in polyfamilies may face even more heightened levels of invisibility and stigmatization, compared to children of same-sex parents.

Third, extant research continues to be severely limited by its reliance on White middle-class samples. Both Pallotta-Chiarolli (2006, 2010b) and Sheff and Hammers (2011) recognized this *absence of intersectionality* as a major limitation in their own earlier research, reflecting the ongoing concern that most research methods fail to access larger representations of people of diverse and intersectional socioeconomic, cultural, and religious locations, as well as transgender, intersex, and gender diverse identities (Cardoso, 2019; Noel, 2006; see Haritaworn, Chin-ju, & Klesse, 2006). Most participants in polyfamilies research continue to be White, middle-class, college-educated individuals who identify as cisgendered male or female and who have high levels of

cyberliteracy which allows them to participate in social and support groups and thereby find themselves participating in our research. While Pallotta-Chiarolli's (2010a, 2016a) research provides specific sections on cultural and religious diversity (see also the personal stories by Raven and Anthony Lekkas in Pallotta-Chiarolli, 2018), we recognize and acknowledge the impact that a predominantly homogeneous privileged group of people has on research findings and the implications for practice.

Fourth, another issue of erasure and exclusion is the absence of the perspectives, experiences, and insights of children and adults who have grown up in polyfamilies, as well as the ways in which growing up in a polyamorous household affects children's well-being, later relationships, and education. Scholars such as Strassberg (2003) have long considered this lack a major hindrance to the development of legal, health, and educational policies and practices that support these children and their families. As this chapter will outline with preliminary findings, Sheff's (forthcoming) current wave of data addresses this to some extent, though her longitudinal sample continues to consist mostly of White participants.

## Comparison to Monogamous Families, Bisexualities, and Clinical Research: Recent Developments in Polyparenting Research

Despite the above identified concerns in research with polyfamilies, there have been significant strides toward establishing the study of polyamorous and other consensually non-monogamous (CNM) families. This section first provides an overview on recent polyfamily research and then summarizes the authors' contributions to that field.

It is evident that since 2013 (the first edition of this book), researchers have expanded their examination of polyamorous families in comparison to the experiences of monogamous families. Klesse (2018) provides a comprehensive review of the available research on polyfamilies and identifies three themes that structured many of the findings in the available research: the wider range of parenting practices, the experience and impact of social and legal discrimination, and parental response to stigmatization. Other recent research includes the ways in which polyamory could "oxygenate" marriage (Conley & Moors, 2014), the lessons the same-sex marriage debate holds for polyamory (Aviram & Leachman, 2015), and the issues that arise in the dissolution of polyamorous families (Argentino & Fiore, 2019). An example that covers the identified themes and issues is Boyd's (2017a, 2017b) Canadian study of the demographic characteristics of polyamorous families. Boyd found that polyamorists are younger, better educated, and have a higher income than the national norm; they tend to make decisions together as a family; and they have challenges with family laws and institutional regulations. For instance, in many nations laws prohibit more than two people from becoming legal spouses or adopting children together.

Two other themes are increasingly appearing in polyfamily research. First, there is a greater awareness of bisexual polyparenting within polyfamilies and CNM research (Bartelt, Bowling, Dodge, & Bostwick, 2017; Delvoye & Tasker, 2015; see chapter "What Do We Now Know About Bisexual Parenting? A Continuing Call for Research"). Second, and particularly pertinent for practice implications, is the research undertaken by clinicians and other health service providers. Therapists have documented the pernicious effects of therapeutic bias and sex negativity with polyamorous clients (Henrich & Trawinski, 2016), the critical incidents that assist or hinder people from developing polyamorous identities (Duplassie & Fairbrother, 2018), and family therapists' attitudes toward polyamorous relationships (Sullivan, 2017). Bevacqua's (2018) instructional case study equipped nurses who want to provide competent and informed care for children from polyamorous families with the data they require to do so.

The four research issues we identify and the literature we review also draw attention to how polyfamilies face significant discriminations and hardships and mostly rely on the assistance of their communities and resilient relationship practices. Pallotta-Chiarolli and Sheff are among the primary long-term researchers in this field, contributing foundational studies. In a quantitative analysis of the *Loving More Polyamory Survey* of over 1000 participants from the USA), Pallotta-Chiarolli (2002, 2006) examined the educational experiences of children, teachers, and parents from polyfamilies. This was followed by the US and Australian qualitative research with 29 bisexual and/or polyamorous adolescents and young adults, 40 polyparents, and 14 adolescents and young adults who had polyparents, in relation to their educational, health, sociocultural, familial concerns, contexts, and strengths (Pallotta-Chiarolli, 2010a, 2010b).

Beginning in 1996, Sheff's *Longitudinal Polyamorous Family Study* (LPFS) has undertaken four waves of qualitative data collection and thematic analysis on children growing up in polyamorous families. Via interviews, participant observation at polycommunity events, and interacting with the Internet polyamorous community online, the LPFS has completed the children's interviews and half of the adults' interviews for the fourth wave. Overall, Sheff interviewed 206 people in polyamorous families, 37 of them children. Building on the findings from waves one through three (Sheff, 2010, 2011, 2015a), emerging findings from the fourth wave of data collection indicate these parents tend to employ a free-range parenting style, sustain permeable family boundaries, and use flexibility to create resilience over time. Other research themes include people's experiences in polyfamilies (Sheff, 2015b), coming out to family of origin as polyamorous (Sheff, 2016a), polyparenting strategies (Sheff, 2010, 2013), a comparison with same-sex families (Sheff, 2011), legal issues facing polyfamilies with children (Goldfeder & Sheff, 2013), endings and transitions in relationships (Sheff, 2014), and polyamorous family resilience (Sheff, 2016b). Sheff's emerging findings continue to indicate that polyamorous families, while not perfect, can be positive environments that support adults across the life span and raise confident, healthy children.

Pallotta-Chiarolli et al. (2013) conducted the *PolyVic study*, collecting data with members of the PolyVic parenting group (a support and social group in Victoria, Australia). Upon invitation to participate in an audio-taped group discussion, 13 polyparents (9 cisgender women and 4 cisgender men aged 35–50 years, of unspecified sexualities) attended. More recently, as part of the *Women with Bisexual Male Partners* (WWBMP) study with 68 sexually diverse women between 2002 and 2012 (Pallotta-Chiarolli, 2014, 2016a; Pallotta-Chiarolli & Lubowitz, 2003), Pallotta-Chiarolli (2016a) conducted semi-structured interviews with four heterosexual and six bisexual mothers who stated they were in polyfamilies raising children with bisexual men. Three primary themes emerged from the findings of Pallotta-Chiarolli's PolyVic and WWBMP studies: (a) managing disclosure and exposure to children and external systems such as schools, (b) parents' concerns regarding their polyfamilies, and (c) the strength and resilience of polyfamilies against external stigmatization.

In the next section we present a more detailed overview of the similar and differing themes from the fourth wave of Sheff's (forthcoming) LPFS, Pallotta-Chiarolli et al.'s (2013) PolyVic study, and Pallotta-Chiarolli's (2016a) WWBMP study. While Sheff's research predominantly explores the workings of polyfamilies themselves, Pallotta-Chiarolli's research predominantly explores the strategies required of polyfamilies in the management of their external worlds.

## Emerging Findings: Inside the Polyfamily

### Free-Range Parenting Style

Most polyparents report using a parenting style that some would label as *free-range* (Skenazy, 2009). Free-range parenting involves allowing children to make choices and have age-appropriate freedoms while gaining the tools or skills to navigate the world. Thus, via free-range parenting,

polyparenting is closely akin to the ways in which previous generations were parented, in contrast to the highly safety-conscious and restrictive parenting style popular today, termed "helicopter parenting," in White affluent families (Darlow, Norvilitis, & Schuetze, 2017). The LPFS data shows that one of the ways in which polyparents encourage free-range children is to allow them to make age-appropriate choices. This can involve anything from allowing a 4-year-old to select their clothing for the day to letting a teenager spend the night at someone else's house. Sometimes this extends to homeschooling, which can also emphasize the learner's choice in directing their own search for knowledge. Significant for the poly-family version of free-range parenting, polyparents also tend to emphasize the consequences of children's actions. For instance, allowing a tween to select their clothing for the day also means that they must bear the discomfort if they select something that is too warm or too cold for the weather. Contrary to the helicopter parenting style in which a parent would make the child dress in a specific way or deliver more appropriate clothing to the school (Darlow et al., 2017), the free-range parent would require that the child endure the discomfort in order to learn to make more appropriate choices in the future. The degree and severity of the consequences change as the child ages—older children can make more complex and higher stake choices, but the consequences for young children's choices should not be too severe.

### Collaborative Parenting

One of the primary ways in which polyparents practice free-range parenting is to share responsibilities among a group of adults, what Pallotta-Chiarolli et al.'s (2013) PolyVic research participants identified as *collaborative parenting*.

> Bronwyn: It takes a village to raise a child. They have input from a variety of adults with a variety of beliefs, a variety of religious backgrounds, of political views, just all sorts of things that they bring as an adult to children's life.
> Eve: The [mainstream] attitude's kind of, "Oh why aren't YOU looking after YOUR child?" whereas in this kind of poly community I think you often

find that it's "these are our children". . . collaborative parenting.

The sharing and distribution of parenting duties among a group of adults has thus far revealed two functions: (a) access to free time and privacy, something that is crucial for managing the complex schedules which may arise among people with multiple partners, metamours (partners' partners who are not sexually or romantically involved), and other chosen family members and to pursue individual careers and interests and (b) to encourage free-range children to be responsible for themselves and still have access to adult assistance when required. Collaborative parenting requires not only scheduling the adults' time to ensure there is always someone available to the children but also for the adults to discuss their individual boundaries of interactions with the children. For example, discipline was especially important for polyparents and their wider communities of care to agree upon, and many supporting adults preferred to let the primary parents (usually the biological parents) handle consequences as much as possible (Sheff, 2015a, b).

Thus far the LPFS, VicPoly, and WWBMP data indicate that this collaborative parenting is mostly positive for both children and adults. Research participants generally report that self-directed play, peer and sibling interactions, and self-directed activities produce independent young people capable of making choices and dealing with social interactions. Undoubtedly, some disadvantages emerge which require ongoing navigation and negotiation, such as multiple contestations over child-rearing practices and the blending of step-siblings, but they have not yet clarified as trends or patterns in the data at this point beyond what serial monogamous blended families experience.

## Permeable Family Boundaries and Extended Kinship

Parents' permeability is most evident in two ways: admitting additional adults and adopting children. Much like LGBTIQ+ parent families, some of which are polyamorous, polyfamilies tend to construct their emotional intimates following a chosen kinship style in which biological and legal relationships are not necessarily the hallmark of "real" relationships, but rather family is built around those who prove to be reliable, loving, trustworthy, and helpful (Weston, 1997). These families of choice can include biological and legal family members, current and former lovers, metamours, and close friends. Polyfamilies can offer adults who have not had children the opportunity to become important in a child's life and, as previously presented, can offer children a range of adults for advice, role models, and support. Sheff (2013) has described these chosen adults as otherfathers (akin to othermothers, Burton & Hardaway, 2012), and Pallotta-Chiarolli's PolyVic research participants label them oddparents (Pallotta-Chiarolli et al., 2013). The construction of new kinship terms or the reintroduction of pre-Industrial or non-Western kinship terms is possibly sparked by the growing Western awareness and appreciation of traditional precolonial First Peoples' diversity of families, communities, and lifestyles (Anderlini-D'Onofrio, 2009; Pallotta-Chiarolli, 2019).

> Lisa: [Being a] tribal aunt's been a really cool thing and very empowering.
> Eve: [My child] has an oddfather, not a godfather. . . and he's a fairy oddfather.

The above discussion on the expansion of family members and the invention or reintroduction of kinship terms or "queer bonds" indicate a significant facet of polyparenting which requires much more research (Anapol, 2010; Iantaffi, 2006).

Polyfamilies' permeable boundaries extend to adopting children, both socially/unofficially and legally. The LPFS found that, in some cases, children befriend a peer who has a negative family environment or is homeless and bring that peer home to the polyfamily. Initially the peer is usually "just staying for a while," and eventually it becomes clear that the family is taking the child in as nonlegal kin. In other cases, the adults notice a child in need or a child approaches the family to ask for admittance. While some polyfamilies proceed to officially adopt the child, others simply integrate the child into the family and do not necessarily use the term adoption. Not all adoptions and integrations are absolute or long term, with some lasting for a period of time and/or living separately and others lasting for years and including putting the child through college.

## Flexible Resilience

Resilience theory is a strengths-based perspective that emphasizes the role of communication, flexibility, and emotional intimacy as key elements that distinguish those families able to face significant hardship and come through stronger together, from those families which are distant and/or dissolved during or after facing similar heartache (Patterson, 2002). In addition to the importance of communication skills for family function and positive parenting, communication skills allow parents to retain evolving relationships with children as they age into young adulthood, or shifting life circumstances bring new familial configurations. Using the skills refined in their romantic relationships in developing resilience against external risks, polyparents attempt to communicate with children in honest and age-appropriate ways that change over time as the child matures. When this communication works well, resilient polyfamilies are able to provide each other with the kind of support, flexibility, and wide safety net that helps children and adults survive difficulty and thrive through adversity. Of particular importance to family resilience is what Sheff (2016b) terms polyaffectivity wherein adults retain emotional and kinship connections when no longer sexually connected. This enduring connection outside of sexual interaction allows for positive co-parenting and continued reliance and resilience for both the adults and children.

When considered together, the above three themes emphasize the optimistic side of poly-family life, which is often erased from external mainstream critiques of polyparenting (Kurtz, 2003; Marquardt, 2007). From inside the poly-family, while some participants in the LPFS experienced significant life hardship, family con-

flict, and nasty divorces, it is important to note that none assigned polyamory any culpability in their various catastrophes. Rather, most emphasized the role of lovers, metamours, children, and other chosen kin in helping them navigate and survive the above and other vagaries of life. There are (at least) three possible reasons for this optimism. First, these respondents could be engaging in image maintenance in front of a researcher, using the most positive interpretation in order to make polyamory seem more socially acceptable against overwhelming external negativity and stereotyping. Second, the volunteer nature of the samples, and in particular the ones who stayed connected to Sheff's study and remained willing to discuss polyamory for 23 years, may have resulted in a bias toward optimism. Those long-term respondents, who Sheff (2015a, b) labels "the persistent polyamorists," are more likely to have positive experiences than those who no longer identify as polyamorous or are less willing to respond to requests for another interview. Third, respondents might emphasize the positive elements of polyamory because it really does work for them, contributing support, intimacy, love, sex, and a wide social safety net to help when things go wrong. Terry, age 16, from the WWBMP research (Pallotta-Chiarolli, 2016a) felt disillusioned and angry that his parents' livelihood could be severely jeopardized if he spoke about his bisexual father and polyfamily at his school within their small rural community. Thus, he passed his family as hetero-monogamous while he stated that his "real education" was occurring outside the school gates:

> I feel lucky to tell you the truth, that I've got such an open family and I look around and see all these people who are living with this very small mind, and I can look around with this wide-open view and see the real world.

## Emerging Findings: Outside the Polyfamily

In the PolyVic (Pallotta-Chiarolli et al., 2013) and WWBMP (Pallotta-Chiarolli, 2016a) studies, the following themes arose in relation to disclosing to children, and these were inextricably linked to the reactions of disclosure and exposure from the polyfamilies' external communities, services, and schools. First, telling the children was essential and wanted in order to foster family health and closeness, foster the child's understanding of sexual and family diversity, and develop confidence and resilience in the wider world. Second, telling the children required negotiating the child's level of outness with others such as peers, schools, health service providers, family members, and the wider society. Third, when to tell the children was determined by a range of factors such as the child's age/maturity, gender, health status, resilience to external discrimination, and closeness of the relationship with the parents and parents' partners. Fourth, for some polyparents, disclosure to children was not an option due to the inherent risks this would evoke for the children and parents from external sectors such as the law, custody arrangements, and child protection agencies. The following conversation from the PolyVic group exemplifies these various positions:

> Juliet: It's nothing that the school has to know about.
> Bronwyn: If I had a comment I would address it. The children haven't been asked any questions [when they say something about their family at school].
> Nigel: One of my children was told [at secondary school by the year level co-ordinator] not to discuss poly or my bisexuality with any school friends or on the school grounds. . .they would be ostracised or they'd be picked on, that it was not relevant for school. . . .The advice was ignored [by my daughter] (laughter) which I'm quite proud of. . . . We actually contacted the teacher and said "No, that's wrong. We will be encouraging our daughter to be herself and to do what she wants."

Confirming the findings of earlier researchers (see Constantine & Constantine, 1976; Davidson, 2002; Strassberg, 2003), Pallotta-Chiarolli (2010a) found that preschool youngsters can handle disclosure in a more matter-of-fact way, while school-age children, who have had exposure to monogamist constructions of families within schools and among a wider range of peers and mainstream media discourses, tend to experience

varying degrees of embarrassment and discomfort and may feel conflicted when hearing outsiders' discriminatory remarks about their parents. Adolescents are likely to experience the strongest anxieties and confusions as they are facing puberty issues in regard to their own sexualities, relationships, and identities and may feel heightened sensitivity to peer attitudes against nonnormative sexualities and families. They are also the most likely age group to keep their polyfamilies secret, given that they are also more aware of wider dominant moral, political, or social discourses that construct cultural understandings of what constitutes a healthy family (see Weitzman, 2006, 2007).

## Passing, Bordering, and Polluting

Overall, a major anxiety that most polyparents talked about in Pallotta-Chiarolli's (2010a, 2010b) research is the fear that being out about their families would lead to harassment and stress for their children. Many tried to prepare their children for the consequences of their public disclosure and provided them with verbal, mental, and emotional strategies to counteract or deflect negativity so that they would be active agents rather than passive victims in educational and health institutions. Pallotta-Chiarolli (2010a, 2010b, 2016a) has theorized and explored how polyfamilies will border, pass, or pollute in external settings like schools. In other words, how and to what extent do polyfamilies undertake self-surveillance and self-regulation for protection from external surveillance and regulation?

**Passing** Some families will endeavor to pass as heterosexual or same-sex couple parent families, using commonplace normative labels such as "auntie," "godparent," or "friend" for polyfamily members to avoid external scrutiny of and discrimination against their polyhome. These strategies of editing, scripting, and concealment may provide protection and the ability to live out family realities with little external surveillance or interference. Likewise, many polyfamilies will pass as monogamous to their own children in order to protect children from the cognitive and emotional dissonance inherent in keeping secrets.

**Bordering** Many polyfamilies and their children feel like border dwellers, on the margins of multiple spaces and contexts, constantly navigating and negotiating their positions and degrees of outness between home and various sites in the external world in order to minimize harm and discrimination. Thorson (2009) uses Petronio's (2002) work on communication privacy management (CPM) to offer some insight into the negotiation of these border zones. Parents and children negotiate "information ownership" and privacy rules and enact "protection and access rules" (Thorson, 2009, p. 34) for any processes of disclosure. Jeremy, a PolyVic father of two school-aged children, discussed the outcomes of CPM strategies: "They'll [our children] get to the point of going, 'With this person I can share this, and with this person I don't' . . .we trust in their commonsense."

Thus, polyfamilies need to negotiate which forms of CPM may work best in harm minimization: withdrawing from potentially harmful external settings and engaging in affirming settings; compartmentalizing, segregating, or bordering the worlds of home and external settings; cloaking certain realities so that they are invisible or pass as normative; or fictionalizing certain aspects of one's life and family (Richardson, 1985).

**Polluting** Some polyparents and their children see themselves as polluting outside worlds (Douglas, 1966) by coming out and presenting their relationships as legitimate and worthy of official affirmation. Thus, they not only claim public space but compel institutions to adapt to new and expanding definitions of family. This resonates with how Cardoso (2019) demonstrates "the political is personal" (p. 1), whereby poly-activism is shaped by the personal experiences and strategies of polyfamilies as well as what is collectively possible within their environments.

Proactive polyparents undertake subversive strategies such as gaining positions of parent power and decision-making in schools and other communities or establishing solid working relationships and friendships within neighborhood, church, and school communities. These strategies consolidate their security, provide access to policy making, community thinking, and action, as well as making it possible to forge strong trusting bonds with other "deviant" minority persons in the community. Nevertheless, polyparents need to weigh up the dangers and the positives of having children polluting their schools with knowledge and "sassiness" about their polyfamilies. In summary, most polyfamilies need to weigh up passing, bordering, and polluting strategies according to context, setting, and time, as is evident in the following section of conversation from the PolyVic parenting group:

> Anne: [Passing] Not having to deal with the judgement of people outside about the impact that your poly-amory is having on your family.
> Robyn: [Polluting] It's good to teach your child that she should do what she wants and. . .not be worried about what other people think of her.
> Daryl:[Bordering] I know at least three of the [schoolfriends'] families are okay but at least another one of them I'm thinking, they might be a bit weirded out about it.

Sometimes, the best a polyparent could do was minimize the potential for harm by selecting the better of bad options. Rosemary, a heterosexual mother in the WWBMP study (Pallotta-Chiarolli, 2016a), voiced her decision not to send her children to a religious school to protect her children from "screwed up" religious beliefs, on top of mainstream social values:

> We feel that would probably be one of the worst environments for them to go to in terms of the church's stand on a lot of these things....I just don't want my children paying the price for somebody else's screwedupness.

## Polyfamilies and Schools

What negotiations and silences surround polyfamilies within school communities? How do children from polyfamilies experience school? Apart from Pallotta-Chiarolli's (2006) research, these questions remain unasked in most recent research with polyfamilies. The little research there shows that sensationalized stereotypes about polyrelationships conspire with silence about diverse family realities to perpetuate ignorance, misrepresentation, and stigmatization in school settings.

## Surveillance in Health, Welfare, and Legal Services

The pathologization and problematization of polyfamilies by legal, welfare, and health service providers and government agencies, and the lack of substantial research into what polyfamilies require from these services and systems has been a continuing research and practice concern (Firestein, 2007; Weber, 2002; Weitzman, 2006, 2007). For polyfamilies, their assumed pathology is often closely linked to actual or feared surveillance via city, county, and state mechanisms such as Child Protective Services.

A related theme that has consistently arisen in research since the 1970s is the question of whether disclosure may risk having children taken away from their families by Child Protection Services (see Anapol, 2010; Sheff, 2010; Walston, 2001; Watson & Watson, 1982). Many parents in our research stressed the need for polyfamilies to collect documentation and legal papers in order to protect themselves and their children should any situation arise with child and social welfare services. Child welfare service providers could also benefit from additional education regarding children of sex and gender minorities, among them children from polyfamilies.

The above consistent findings across studies raise a major question which requires further research and awareness of its implications for practice: To what extent is the low rate of visibility of polyfamilies due to their concealment from outside structures such as health, education, and family services for fear of the ramifications of disclosure?

## Polyfamilies in the Media

Another parental concern that has been consistent throughout the available research is the need to incorporate positive representations of polyfamilies in texts, arts, media, and popular culture for both polyparents and their children (Pallotta-Chiarolli, 2010a, 2016a). These representations will then provide public points of reference and examples that would facilitate both wider societal visibility and polyfamilies' confidence to disclose to their own children and the external society (Smith, 2015; Taormino, 2008; Trask, 2007). Many polyparents and their offspring also called for novels and picture books for children. Pallotta-Chiarolli's (2008) novel for adolescents, young adults, and adults, *Love You Two*, with its multicultural, multisexual, and multipartnered characters, is based on her research over 15 years. These findings again raise the question requiring further research: To what extent is the ongoing low degree of disclosure to one's children and outside social institutions due to the erasure or absence of positive images in popular culture which provide a discourse that affirms polyfamilies and thereby the emotional and social health and well-being of their children?

## Toward Visibility, Inclusion, and Intersectionality: Directions for Future Research and Implications for Practice

Throughout this chapter, we have provided an overview of the available research on polyfamilies since 2013 and summarized our recent findings from three studies—Sheff's LPFS, Pallotta-Chiarolli et al's PolyVic study, and Pallotta-Chiarolli's WWBMP—which concur with previous findings. Our studies demonstrate striking similarities and consistency in our findings regarding erasure, exclusion by inclusion, and the absence of intersectionality even though the data were collected by separate researchers, continents apart, in widely different social contexts. For example, the connection between lack of polyfamily visibility and polyfamilies' fear of both surveillance and disclosure was significant. We also discussed how this theme was manifested in interactions with education, health, and legal services and the erasures and absences in the media. We conclude that the above themes require further research from the perspectives of both the polyfamilies and the above sectors in order to develop comprehensive and useful resources for practice in service provision.

Another major similarity between our studies is the emphasis of our research participants on the optimistic side and strengths of polyfamily life. While some research participants in all of the studies experienced significant life hardship, family conflict, and dissolution, none assigned polyamory any culpability. Rather, most emphasized the role of extended kinship and children in helping them navigate and survive the above and other vagaries of life. In this chapter, we posited three reasons for this optimism and recommend addressing two questions in future polyresearch methodologies: (a) Are respondents engaging in image maintenance in front of a researcher and why? and (b) How do we broaden our samples and develop methods so that volunteers who have experienced difficulties with polyamory feel able to divulge their experiences and trust that the researchers will provide empathy and empowerment?

Further research with children will also be useful in deepening the understanding of polyparenting and its outcomes and may address the above methodological concerns. However, given the difficulty of gaining Human Research Ethics (HRE) or Institutional Research Board (IRB) approval for research on children in general, much less children in sex and gender minority families, it is not a surprise that few academics have focused on children. Sheff's experience with the IRB was emblematic of this challenge: After 3 years of almost weekly meetings with IRB compliance specialists in which Sheff painstakingly addressed all of the IRB concerns regarding including the children of polyfamilies in her research, Sheff and the chair of her department were summoned before the entire board to account for the need to include children in the sample. During this meeting IRB members commented to Sheff that "The parents will tell you what the children think, so you only really need to talk to them," and that "We already know about kids in gay families, why do we need to know about kids in polyamorous families, too?" Sheff maintains that parents do not always know what their children truly think and that polyfamilies and gay families are so distinct as to merit individual examination. Nevertheless, strategies such as undertaking family history and ethnographic research with young adults who were raised in polyfamilies are increasingly possible, given that this is a numerically increasing and visible cohort (Creation, 2019; Smith, 2015).

This chapter also highlighted the major concerns that reliance on participants who are almost always White and middle class results in exclusion by inclusion: A potentially wider variance of insights are collapsed or subsumed into White-centric and middle-class universalisms. We strongly recommend adopting and creating research designs with an intersectional lens which addresses the interweavings of genders, sexualities, ethnicities, indigeneities, socioeconomic status, age, and (dis)abilities. We also recommend challenging Anglocentrism in research publication and a stronger engagement with innovative and groundbreaking research being undertaken beyond the Australian, Canadian, UK, and US assemblage. For instance, Vasallo (2018) from Spain intersects a critique of monogamy with a critique of Islamophobia; and researchers from Brazil explore the positioning of polyfamilies within domestic partnership laws (Sá & Viecili, 2014; Santiago, 2015; Silva, 2014). Related to an intersectional approach is the need to adopt a decolonizing approach whereby we engage with non-Western countries which may have had their precolonial diversity of genders, sexualities, and familial relationships erased or stigmatized in historical colonialism and contemporary neocolonialism (Pallotta-Chiarolli, 2019; Smith, 2012).

**Acknowledgments** To the wonderful group of parents from PolyVic and the women in the Women with Bisexual Male Partners research. Many thanks to Peter Haydon and

Anne Hunter with whom some of this work was published in the first edition (2013) of this book. And many thanks to Sara Lubowitz with whom the Women with Bisexual Male Partners research was conducted.

Maria Pallotta-Chiarolli and Ruby Mountford

Thank you to all of the participants in the Longitudinal Polyamorous Families Study, your candor and willingness to take time for participation have made the research possible.

Elisabeth Sheff

# References

Anapol, D. (2010). *Polyamory in the 21st century: Love and intimacy with multiple partners*. New York, NY: Rowman and Littlefield.

Anderlini-D'Onofrio, S. (2009). *Gaia and the new politics of love: Notes from a polyplanet*. Berkeley, CA: North Atlantic Books.

Argentino, J. A., & Fiore, C. (2019). Dissolution of polyamorous relationships, multiple parent families, and other complex arrangements. In A. E. Goldberg & A. P. Romero (Eds.), *LGBTQ divorce and relationship dissolution: Psychological and legal perspectives and implications for practice* (pp. 422–440). Oxford, UK: Oxford University Press.

Aviram, H., & Leachman, G. M. (2015). The future of polyamorous marriage: Lessons from the marriage equality struggle. *Harvard Women's Law Journal, 38*, 269–336.

Barker, M., & Langdridge, D. (2010). *Understanding non-monogamies*. London, UK: Routledge.

Bartelt, E., Bowling, J., Dodge, B., & Bostwick, W. (2017). Bisexual identity in the context of parenthood: An exploratory qualitative study of self-identified bisexual parents in the United States. *Journal of Bisexuality, 17*, 378–399. https://doi.org/10.1080/152 99716.2017.1384947

Bevacqua, J. (2018). Adding to the rainbow of diversity: Caring for children of polyamorous families. *Journal of Pediatric Health Care, 32*, 490–493. https://doi.org/10.1016/j.pedhc.2018.04.015

Boyd, J. P. (2017a). *Polyamorous relationships and family law in Canada*. Alberta, Canada: Canadian Research Institute for Law and the Family. Retrieved from http://www.crilf.ca/Documents/Polyamorous%20 Relationships%20and%20Family%20Law%20-%20 Apr%202017.pdf

Boyd, J. P. (2017b). *Polyamory in Canada: Research on an emerging family structure*. Alberta, Canada: Canadian Research Institute for Law and the Family. Retrieved from https://vanierinstitute.ca/polyamory-in-canada-research-on-an-emerging-family-structure/

Burton, L. M., & Hardaway, C. R. (2012). Low-income mothers as "othermothers" to their romantic partners' children: Women's coparenting in multiple partner fertility relationships. *Family Process, 51*, 343–359. https://doi.org/10.1111/j.1545-5300.2012.01401.x

Cardoso, D. (2019). The political is personal: The importance of affective narratives in the rise of poly-activism. *Sociological Research Online, 24*, 1–18. https://doi.org/10.1177/1360780419835559

Conley, T. D., & Moors, A. C. (2014). More oxygen please!: How polyamorous relationship strategies might oxygenate marriage. *Psychological Inquiry, 25*, 56–63. https://doi.org/10.1080/1047840X.2014.876908

Constantine, L., & Constantine, J. (1976). *Treasures of the island: Children in alternative families*. Beverly Hills, CA: Sage.

Creation, K. (2019). *This heart holds many: My life as the nonbinary millennial child of a polyamorous family*. Portland, OR: Thorntree Press.

Darlow, V., Norvilitis, J. M., & Schuetze, P. (2017). The relationship between helicopter parenting and adjustment to college. *Journal of Child and Family Studies, 26*, 2291–2298. https://doi.org/10.1007/s10826-017-0751-3

Davidson, J. (2002). Working with polyamorous clients in the clinical setting. *Electronic Journal of Human Sexuality, 5*, 8.

Delvoye, M., & Tasker, F. (2015). Narrating self-identity in bisexual motherhood. *Journal of GLBT Family Studies, 12*, 5–23. https://doi.org/10.1080/15504 28X.2015.1038675

Douglas, M. (1966). *Purity and danger: An analysis of concepts of pollution and taboo*. London, UK: Routledge

Duplassie, D., & Fairbrother, N. (2018). Critical incidents that help and hinder the development and maintenance of polyamorous relationships. *Sexual and Relationship Therapy, 33*, 421–439. https://doi.org/10.1080/146819 94.2016.1213804

Firestein, B. A. (Ed.). (2007). *Becoming visible: Counseling bisexuals across the lifespan*. New York, NY: Columbia University Press.

Goldfeder, M., & Sheff, E. (2013). Children of polyamorous families: A first empirical look. *Journal of Law & Social Deviance, 5*, 150–243.

Haritaworn, J., Chin-ju, L., & Klesse, C. (2006). Poly/logue: A critical introduction to polyamory. *Sexualities, 9*, 515–529. https://doi.org/10.1177/1363460706069963

Henrich, R., & Trawinski, C. (2016). Social and therapeutic challenges facing polyamorous clients. *Sexual and Relationship Therapy, 31*, 376–390. https://doi.org/10.1080/14681994.2016.1174331

Iantaffi, A. (2006). Polyamory and parenting: Some personal reflections. *Lesbian and Gay Psychology Review, 7*(1), 70–72.

Klesse, C. (2018). Polyamorous parenting: Stigma, social regulation, and queer bonds of resistance, *Sociological Research Online*, 1–19.

Kurtz, S. (2003, March 12). Heather has 3 parents. *National Review Online*. http://www.nationalreview.com/kurtz/kurtz031203.asp

Levine, E. C., Herbenick, D., Martinez, O., Fu, T. C., & Dodge, B. (2018). Open relationships, nonconsensual nonmonogamy, and monogamy among U.S. adults: Findings from the 2012 National Survey of Sexual Health and Behavior. *Archive of Sexual Behavior, 47*, 1439–1450. https://doi.org/10.1007/s10508-018-1178-7

Marquardt, E. (2007, July). *16*. When three really is a crowd. *New York Times*.

Moors, A. C. (2017). Has the American public's interest in information related to relationships beyond "the couple" increased over time? *The Journal of Sex Research, 54*, 677–684. https://doi.org/10.1080/00224499.2016.1178208

Noel, M. J. (2006). Progressive polyamory: Considering issues of diversity. *Sexualities, 9*, 602–620. https://doi.org/10.1177/1363460706070003

Pallotta-Chiarolli, M. (2002). Polyparents having children, raising children, schooling children. *Loving More Magazine, 31*, 8–12.

Pallotta-Chiarolli, M. (2006). Polyparents having children, raising children, schooling children. *Lesbian and Gay Psychology Review, 7*(1), 48–53.

Pallotta-Chiarolli, M. (2008). *Love you two*. Sydney, NSW: Random House.

Pallotta-Chiarolli, M. (2010a). *Border families, border sexualities in schools*. New York, NY: Rowman & Littlefield.

Pallotta-Chiarolli, M. (2010b). To pass, border or pollute: Polyfamilies go to school. In M. Barker & D. Langdridge (Eds.), *Understanding non-monogamies* (pp. 182–187). London, UK: Routledge.

Pallotta-Chiarolli, M. (2014). New rules, no rules, old rules or our rules': Women designing mixed-orientation marriages with bisexual men. In M. Pallotta-Chiarolli & B. Pease (Eds.), *The politics of recognition and social justice: Transforming subjectivities and new forms of resistance*. London, UK: Routledge.

Pallotta-Chiarolli, M. (2016a). *Women in relationship with bisexual men: Bi men by women*. New York, NY: Rowman & Littlefield.

Pallotta-Chiarolli, M. (Ed.). (2016b). *Bisexuality in education: Erasure, exclusion by inclusion, and the absence of intersectionality*. London, UK: Routledge.

Pallotta-Chiarolli, M. (Ed.). (2018). *Living and loving in diversity: An anthology of Australian multicultural queer adventures*. Adelaide, SA: Wakefield Press.

Pallotta-Chiarolli, M. (2019). Pre-colonial actualities, post-colonial amnesia and neo-colonial assemblage. In Z. Davy, A. C. Santos, C. Bertone, R. Thoreson, & S. Wieringa (Eds.), *Handbook of global sexualities*. London, UK: Sage.

Pallotta-Chiarolli, M., Haydon, P., & Hunter, A. (2013). These are our children': Polyamorous parenting. In A. E. Goldberg & K. R. Allen (Eds.), *LGBT-parent families: Innovations in research and implications for practice* (pp. 117–131). New York, NY: Springer.

Pallotta-Chiarolli, M., & Lubowitz, S. (2003). Outside belonging: Multi-sexual relationships as border exis-tence. *Journal of Bisexuality, 3*, 53–86. https://doi.org/10.1300/J159v03n01_05

Patterson, J. M. (2002). Understanding family resilience. *Journal of Clinical Psychology, 58*, 233–246. https://doi.org/10.1002/jclp.10019

Petronio, S. (2002). *Boundaries of privacy: Dialectics of disclosure*. New York, NY: SUNY Press.

Raab, M. (2018). Care in consensually non-monogamous relationship networks: Aspirations and practices in a contradictory field. *Graduate Journal of Social Science, 14*, 10–27.

Richardson, L. (1985). *The new other woman*. New York, NY: The Free Press.

Sá, C. F. S., & Viecili, M. (2014). As novas famílias: Relações poliafetivas. *Revista Eletrônica de Iniciação Científica, 5*(1), 137–156.

Santiago, R. S. (2015). *Poliamor e direito das famílias: Reconhecimento e consequências jurídicas*. Curitiba, Spain: Juruá.

Sheff, E. (2006). Poly-hegemonic masculinities. *Sexualities, 9*, 621–642. https://doi.org/10.1177/1363460706070004

Sheff, E. (2010). Strategies in polyamorous parenting. In M. Barker & D. Langdridge (Eds.), *Understanding non-monogamies* (pp. 169–181). London, UK: Routledge.

Sheff, E. (2011). Polyamorous families, same-sex marriage, and the slippery slope. *Journal of Contemporary Ethnography, 40*, 487–520. https://doi.org/10.1177/0891241611413578

Sheff, E. (2013). *The polyamorists next door: Inside multiple-partner relationships and families*. New York, NY: Rowman & Littlefield.

Sheff, E. (2014). Not necessarily broken: Redefining success when polyamorous relationships end. In T. S. Weinberg & S. Newmahr (Eds.), *Selves, symbols, and sexualities: An interactionist anthology* (pp. 201–214). Thousand Oaks, CA: Sage.

Sheff, E. (2016a). *When someone you love is polyamorous*. Portland, OR: Thorntree Press.

Sheff, E. (2016b). Resilient polyamorous families. In P. Karian (Ed.), *Critical & experiential: Dimensions in gender and sexual diversity* (pp. 257–280). Eastliegh, UK: Resonance Publications.

Sheff, E., & Hammers, C. (2011). The privilege of perversities: Race, class and education among polyamorists and kinksters. *Psychology & Sexuality, 2*, 198–223. https://doi.org/10.1080/19419899.2010.537674

Silva, B. J. (2014). Expressões contemporâneas das relações afetivo amorosas: A emergência do Poliamor. *Getpol – Anais Colóquio do Grupo de Estudos de Teoria Política, 2*(1). Retrieved from http://periodicos.ufes.br/getpol/article/view/8158

Sheff, E. (2015a). Polyamorous parenting. In G. Abbie (Ed.), *The Sage Encyclopedia of LGBTQ Studies*. Thousand Oaks, CA: Sage.

Sheff, E. (2015b). *Stories from the polycule: Real life in polyamorous families*. Portland, OR: Thorntree Press.

Skenazy, L. (2009). *Free-range kids: Giving our children the freedom we had without going nuts with worry.* Hoboken, NJ: John Wiley & Sons.

Smith, B. (2015). I grew up in a polyamorous household. Vice, 2 June. Retrieved from www.vice.com/en_us/article/9bgy5z/i-grew-up-in-a-polyamorous-household-528

Smith, L. T. (2012). *Decolonizing methodologies: Research and indigenous peoples.* London, UK: Zed Books.

Strassberg, M. I. (2003). The challenge of post-modern polygamy: Considering polyamory. *Capital University Law Review, 31*(439), 1–122.

Sullivan, S. M. (2017). Marriage and family therapists' attitudes and perceptions of polyamorous relationships. (Doctoral dissertation, Purdue University).

Taormino, T. (2008). *Opening up: A guide to creating and sustaining open relationships.* San Francisco, CA: Cleis Press.

Thorson, A. R. (2009). Adult children's experiences with their parent's infidelity: Communicative protection and access rules in the absence of divorce. *Communication Studies, 60,* 32–48. https://doi.org/10.1080/10510970802623591

Trask, R. (2007). PolyParents, PolyKids. *Loving More Magazine, 37,* 16–17.

Vasallo, B. (2018). *Pensamiento monógamo, terror poliamoroso.* Brasilia, Brazil: La Oveja Roja.

Walston, J. (2001). Polyamory: An exploratory study of responsible multi-partnering. Paper presented at the Institute of 21st-Century Relationships Conference, Washington, DC.

Watson, J., & Watson, M. A. (1982). Children of open marriages: Parental disclosure and perspectives. *Alternative Lifestyles, 5,* 54–62.

Weber, A. (2002). Survey results: Who are we? And other interesting impressions. *Loving More Magazine, 30,* 4–6.

Weitzman, G. D. (2006). Therapy with clients who are bisexual and polyamorous. *Journal of Bisexuality, 6*(1/2), 138–164. https://doi.org/10.1300/J159v06n01_08

Weitzman, G. D. (2007). Counseling bisexuals in polyamorous relationships. In B. A. Firestein (Ed.), *Counseling bisexuals across the lifespan* (pp. 312–335). New York, NY: Columbia University Press.

Weston, K. (1997). *Families we choose: Lesbians, gays, kinship.* New York, NY: Columbia University Press.

# Asexuality and Its Implications for LGBTQ-Parent Families

## Megan Carroll

As a marginalized sexual orientation category, asexuality has much to offer discussions of LGBTQ parenting. Asexuality signifies an absence of sexual attraction to people of any gender, challenging dominant paradigms of love, sex, and relationships. Asexual individuals find intimacy and emotional fulfillment through a variety of partnership models, challenging the idea that sexual activity legitimates a relationship or that romantic love should be privileged above platonic love (Scherrer, 2010a). Yet asexualities have long been ignored, to the extent that many continue to associate the "A" in LGBTQIA+ with "ally" rather than "asexual" (Mollet & Lackman, 2018). Often referred to as "the invisible orientation" (Decker, 2014), asexuality is especially understudied in comparison to other sexual orientations. Yet an understanding of asexuality in the context of LGBTQIA+ family research can help scholars and practitioners adapt to an increasingly diverse, complex, and fluid landscape of gender and sexuality.

This chapter is structured around two key questions: (1) What is asexuality? How is the definition and measurement of asexuality evolving? (2) What are asexual people's experiences, especially regarding sex, romance, and parent-

ing? How are their experiences characterized by overlapping systems of inequality, especially gender, race, class, and disability? These questions are designed to offer guidance on the intersections of asexuality and LGBTQ parenting and highlight new avenues of research into this understudied topic.

This chapter is informed by theories of intersectionality and postmodernism. Intersectionality theory posits that individual experiences are influenced by multiple axes of one's social location (Collins, 1990). It examines how identity categories and their associated hierarchies interact and create interlocking systems of oppression (Collins, 1990; Crenshaw, 1991; Yuval-Davis, 2006). Many family scholars have been reluctant to incorporate intersectionality as a dominant paradigm, but intersectionality offers a theoretical framework to understand how systems of sexuality, gender, race, and other axes of inequality interact and shape family life (Baca Zinn, 2012).

Postmodernism broadly refers to the erosion of shared meanings in society. In the context of families, postmodernism provides a framework for understanding how taken-for-granted associations between marriage, sexuality, and kinship have been challenged by new technologies, demographic changes, and shifting cultural norms (Aveldanes, Pfeffer, & Augustine, 2018; Stacey, 1996). Whereas sexuality was once more closely associated with one's family life, post-

M. Carroll (✉)
Department of Sociology, California State University – San Bernardino, San Bernardino, CA, USA

modern sexualities are defined neither by love nor sexual reproduction, allowing eroticism to exist for its own sake (Bauman, 1998). Postmodern concepts of sexuality and family have therefore created the necessary conditions for asexuality to emerge as a self-concept defined by one's distance from eroticism and sexual relationships.

## What Is Asexuality?

There is a widespread misconception in society that all humans experience sexual attraction and sexual desire (Carrigan, 2012; Przybylo, 2011). Asexuality is an umbrella term for the identity category that challenges those assumptions. Given the relatively recent emergence of asexuality as a sexual orientation category, the precise definition of asexuality itself remains in flux (Chasin, 2011). The most common definition of asexual—"someone who does not experience sexual attraction"—comes from the Asexual Visibility and Education Network (AVEN), an organization and online resource founded by David Jay in 2001. AVEN has played an important role de-stigmatizing asexuality, and their message boards served as the birthplace of the asexual community by creating a hub for online communication between asexual individuals (Jones, Hayter, & Jomeen, 2017). AVEN's definition of asexuality appears in much of the literature and is used by many self-identified asexual individuals (Brotto, Knudson, Inskip, Rhodes, & Erskine, 2010; Jones et al., 2017; Van Houdenhove, Gijs, T'Sjoen, & Enzlin, 2015a). Alternatively, some prefer to describe their asexuality as a lack of interest in sex, not necessarily connected to attraction (Scherrer, 2008). The definition of asexuality is often discussed and contested within online spaces, as not all asexual individuals agree on what "lack of sexual attraction" means (Mitchell & Hunnicutt, 2019; Scherrer, 2008).

Most research on asexuality uses AVEN's definition, defining asexuality by its relationship to sexual attraction. Van Houdenhove et al. (2015a), who studied the interaction between identity,

attraction, and behavior among 566 asexual survey respondents aged 18–72, conclude that "lack of sexual attraction" is the most appropriate and most commonly shared definition. A few other studies support the idea that asexuality should be defined by a lack of sexual desire or excitement, rather than attraction (Aicken, Mercer, & Cassell, 2013; Prause & Graham, 2007). Behavioral definitions of asexuality are especially rare (see Brotto et al., 2010 for one exception), as asexual discourses actively differentiate asexuality (a sexual orientation) from celibacy (a choice) (Cerankowski & Milks, 2010). Individuals who experience attraction but choose not to engage in sexual activity, e.g., for religious reasons, would be considered celibate but not asexual (Decker, 2014).

## Measuring Asexuality

Data from a national probability sample in Great Britain suggests that about 1% of the population is asexual, defined as having no sexual attraction to either men or women (Bogaert, 2004). This number is often used as a benchmark in research on asexualities, though it has been difficult for researchers to replicate. Aicken et al. (2013), also using data from British probability surveys, found that 0.4% of respondents had never experienced sexual attraction. Nurius (1983), using a sample of 689 undergraduate and graduate students, found that 5% of men and 10% of women were asexual, defined as those who report not feeling sexual attraction to either men or women.

Methodological limitations in the measurement and identification of sexuality create significant obstacles to gathering data on asexual people as a population. Sexuality is typically measured using criterion of behavior, attraction, and identity that do not translate well for asexualities (Poston & Baumle, 2010). For example, asexual respondents' sexual behavior tends to vary, making behavior a less reliable metric to identify asexual respondents (Van Houdenhove et al., 2015a). Some researchers may expect asexual respondents to be those who have never had sex (Poston & Baumle, 2010), but in one study of

79 asexual respondents, 40% of asexual men and 34% of asexual women had sex, with 25% of men and 19% of women reporting that they "always enjoyed having sex" (Aicken et al., 2013, p. 121). Behavioral metrics also potentially conflate asexuality and celibacy (Poston & Baumle, 2010).

Popular instruments of sexual attraction are also unreliable as they tend to measure responses to gendered object of desire, assuming that attraction exists for all respondents equally. For example, the National Survey of Family Growth (NSFG), widely considered to be the most robust and inclusive national survey for measurements of sexuality, asks respondents to decide whether they are (a) only attracted to the opposite sex, (b) mostly attracted to the opposite sex, (c) equally attracted to the opposite sex and the same sex, (d) mostly attracted to the same sex, (e) only attracted to the same sex, or (f) not sure (Poston & Baumle, 2010). Ostensibly, asexual survey respondents may select "not sure," but the wording of the question is ambiguous and laden with the assumption that all individuals experience sexual attraction (Poston & Baumle, 2010).

It is also very rare for asexuality to be included in the identity categories provided on large-scale national surveys. Few people are familiar with the term "asexual" (MacInnis & Hodson, 2012). Data that has included asexuality as an option has led to significant errors with survey respondents who are ignorant of asexual terminology, creating issues with reliability (M. Hoban, American College Health Association, June 19, 2018, personal communication). More research is needed to identify solutions that would improve reliability of surveys with "asexual" as an identity category option.

## Developing an Asexual Vocabulary

As an umbrella term, "asexual" represents a range of sexual and romantic dispositions that fall outside the norm. Just as binary constructs of gender, sex, and sexuality have been replaced by the understanding that each falls along a spectrum, asexuality is also conceptualized as a spectrum (Decker, 2014). Gendered objects of desire ("male" and "female") at the extremes of more familiar spectrums of sexuality are replaced on the asexual spectrum with the presence of desire itself. In this way, there is a diversity of attitudes toward sex within the asexual community, with some falling closer to one extreme in which they have never experienced sexual attraction and reject the notion of engaging in any sexual activity and others experiencing attraction in very limited circumstances and perhaps even favoring sexual activity in their lives (Carrigan, 2011). Identity categories that have emerged to describe asexual people on the latter end of the spectrum include gray-asexual, in which sexual attraction is experienced rarely or under specific circumstances, and demisexual, in which sexual attraction only occurs after an emotional bond has been formed (Carrigan, 2011; Decker, 2014).

Attitudes toward romance vary significantly among asexual individuals, and the emerging discourse within asexual communities regularly disaggregates sexual and romantic attraction (Carrigan, 2011; Jones et al., 2017). This discourse serves to explain that one can be romantically interested in another person and not desire to have sex with them. Just as sexual attraction falls across a spectrum, leading to a proliferation of terms that asexual people use to describe their sexual identities, romantic attraction also occurs along a spectrum. Some asexual individuals are aromantic, meaning they do not experience romantic attraction or have romantic feelings for others, whereas others may strongly desire romantic relationships in their lives (Brotto et al., 2010; Decker, 2014; Van Houdenhove, Gijs, T'Sjoen, & Enzlin, 2015b).

Within the asexual community, the specific terms for asexual individuals' sexual orientations are regularly combined with terms that describe the individual's romantic orientation (Carrigan, 2011). These romantic orientation identity labels tend to center around gendered object choices, even though sexual activity is ostensibly removed from the equation (Scherrer, 2008). For example, asexual individuals sometimes describe themselves as heteroromantic (romantically attracted to those of a different gender), homoromantic (romantically attracted to those of the same gender), biromantic (romantically attracted to more than one gender), panromantic (romantically attracted to people regardless of gender), and so on (Decker, 2014). When combined with their sexual identity labels, these romantic orientation categories create multi-term identities that asexual individuals may use to describe themselves, such as aromantic gray-asexual, grayromantic demisexual, or panromantic asexual. This phenomenon is not necessarily limited to asexual individuals. Troia (2018), in her analysis of millennials' sexual identities, found that multi-term identities, nonbinary identities, and "asterisk identities" (i.e., qualifying the subjective meanings of identity labels to communicate a more specific understanding of their sexuality; p. 1) were common patterns among young respondents situated within a postmodern era of sexual fluidity.

## Connections to the LGBTQ Community

Asexuality is one of many sexual identities that has emerged or gained prominence in the postmodern era. Meanings of sexuality have been shifting to accommodate a wider range of perspectives, and people with similar experiences are able to form meaningful connections online, contributing to a growth in (a)sexual identities and communities (Callis, 2014; Carrigan, 2011; Troia, 2018). Carrigan (2011) notes that the asexual community, which primarily manifests in online spaces, has a remarkable ability to create community cohesion while articulating diverse, individual differences surrounding romantic orientations and attitudes toward sex. But integrating asexuality with the broader LGBTQ community has been challenging (Mollet & Lackman, 2018).

Mollet and Lackman (2018) found that not all self-identified asexual individuals consider themselves to be part of the LGBTQ umbrella, and many have encountered rejection and isolation from within the LGBTQ community (Dawson, Scott, & McDonnell, 2018; Mollet & Lackman,

2018). While asexual individuals and LGBTQ individuals share the experience of marginalization within a heterosexist society, some asexual individuals have reported that their ability to "pass" as heterosexual and having an identity defined by a "lack" of something depressed their motivation to participate in collective action (Dawson et al., 2018, p. 387). Some asexual people have found common ground in the LGBTQ community based on their romantic orientations, whereas others feel that being immersed in a sexual community, even an LGBTQ one, is alienating and oppressive (Mollet & Lackman, 2018). Whether institutional support systems included "asexual" within their LGBTQIA+ lexicon (as opposed to "ally") has also been influential in asexual individuals' sense of belonging (Mollet & Lackman, 2018; Scherrer, 2008). Further research is needed to investigate how specific shared experiences—such as pathologizing, medicalized narratives, or mechanisms of discrimination—have created opportunities for community cohesion between asexual individuals and others within the LGBTQIA+ community.

## From Pathology to Identity

Asexuality is not a new phenomenon. The Kinsey Report of 1948 famously created a 7-point scale of sexual orientation that described respondents as exclusively heterosexual (0), exclusively homosexual (6), or somewhere in between (Bogaert, 2012). Less widely known is Kinsey's category "X," reserved for those who could not be placed on the Kinsey Scale because they did not experience sexual attraction (Bogaert, 2012; Decker, 2014). The road from Kinsey to the modern asexual identity movement stretches about 50 years, during which time asexuality has been pathologized, dismissed, and invalidated by conventional approaches to human sexuality.

Characteristics of asexuality overlap with ideas about abnormal sexual functioning. Since the 1980s, the third edition of the *Diagnostic and Statistical Manual of Mental Disorders (DSM)*

has included psychosexual disorders that focus on sexual desire. "Hypoactive sexual desire disorder" (HSDD) is characterized by the *DSM* as a deficiency or absence of sexual fantasies and desire for sexual activity that causes distress or interpersonal difficulty (Brotto, 2010; Prause & Graham, 2007). This entry in the *DSM* has become controversial as it imposes a pathology onto asexual individuals and assumes that "normal" or healthy sexual functioning necessitates sexual desire and sexual fantasies (Flore, 2013; Hinderliter, 2013). Asexual individuals have challenged the idea that they qualify for an HSDD diagnosis, arguing that people with HSDD continue to experience sexual attraction, whereas asexual people do not (Brotto et al., 2010). Researchers have argued that asexual individuals do not meet the *DSM*'s criteria for HSDD because their lack of sexual desire does not cause "distress," which asexual discourses also reflect (Bishop, 2013; Hinderliter, 2013). Furthermore, data measuring women's vaginal pulse amplitude (VPA) and self-reported arousal to erotic stimuli has suggested that asexual women have the same capacity for sexual arousal as other women, challenging the idea that asexuality is equivalent to sexual dysfunction (Brotto & Yule, 2011).

Another pathologizing narrative about asexuality is the misconception that it represents an aversion to sex stemming from exposure to sexual trauma. Research has disputed this assumption, finding that asexual people do not avoid sex due to a fear of sexual activity or forced sexual activity (Brotto et al., 2010; Prause & Graham, 2007). Rather, asexual people simply have no interest in sexual activity (Brotto et al., 2010). Medicalized, pathologizing narratives that explain non-heterosexualities as either disorders of sexual desire or responses to sexual trauma are not unique to asexuality (Cvetkovich, 2003; Hinderliter, 2013). The history of homosexuality is also strongly characterized by violence under the guise of medicalization, which continues today in the form of conversion therapy (Waidzunas, 2015).

In addition to a history of clinical approaches that have marginalized asexualities, popular assumptions about "human nature" have also pathologized asexuality. Sexual desire is often framed in the public imagination as an innate and universal experience among human beings (Gupta, 2017). As a result, research has shown that asexual individuals—or those who do not experience sexual desire—are viewed as "less human" (MacInnis & Hodson, 2012, p. 725). As asexual communities have formed and gained visibility, pathologizing narratives about human nature and normal sexual functioning have been publicly challenged (Gressgård, 2013). Asexual people have been careful to distinguish asexuality as a sexual orientation, much like gay, lesbian, and bisexual, each of which describe the orientation of one's sexual attractions (Brotto et al., 2010; Brotto & Yule, 2017). In doing so, asexual people are creating a novel identity category and incorporating asexuality as part of a normal spectrum of healthy human sexuality (Foster & Scherrer, 2014; Gressgård, 2013).

A common theme within the asexuality literature is the validation of asexual identities through community engagement (Jones et al., 2017). AVEN and other online communities have made it possible for anyone with an Internet connection to find information about asexuality and communicate with asexual-identified people, creating affirming spaces around asexual identities and raising awareness of asexuality (Jones et al., 2017; MacNeela & Murphy, 2015). AVEN has been especially instrumental in helping asexual people express themselves and find a sense of belonging given the dearth of representations of asexuality in media (Brotto et al., 2010; Jones et al., 2017). AVEN has also helped social scientists discover and recruit asexual people for research, and some study participants have reported that they only began to identify as asexual once they discovered the language and community surrounding asexuality via the Internet and AVEN specifically (Scherrer, 2008). Even the word "asexual" has been inaccessible for many people, leading to moments of personal satisfaction and meaning when respondents discovered it (MacNeela & Murphy, 2015; Scott, McDonnell, & Dawson, 2016). Similar experiences of validation have been found in studies of transgender, bisexual, and other populations whose identity labels are rendered invisible within the public sphere (Cashore & Tuason, 2009; Levitt & Ippolito, 2014).

Carrigan (2011) describes a pattern among asexual experiences: individuals begin with a feeling of individual difference, which is followed by self-questioning and assumed pathology before arriving at self-clarification and communal identity. In other words, asexual individuals receive the same messages that the rest of society receives about normative sexualities. As they discover that they do not fit the normative prescription of wanting sex or experiencing sexual attraction, they begin questioning themselves, seeking explanations for those differences, often arriving at pathologizing conclusions—that is, "something must be wrong with me" (Carrigan, 2011; Van Houdenhove et al., 2015b). Both asexual identity labels and community support, most of which are online and accessible to a wide range of people, serve a function of counteracting those pathologizing narratives and expanding the possibilities of human sexuality, allowing asexual people to understand their feelings and sexual dispositions within a framework that embraces and validates their experience.

## What Are Asexual People's Experiences?

### Intersections with Gender, Race, Class, and Disability

One characteristic of the asexual community that has emerged through small, qualitative samples is its unique gender composition. There have been consistent findings that the asexual spectrum includes more cisgender women than men (Bogaert, 2004; MacNeela & Murphy, 2015), as well as disproportionate numbers of individuals under the transgender umbrella (Bauer et al., 2018; Van Houdenhove et al., 2015a). Some research suggests that cisgender men may be inhibited from identifying as asexual, noting that there is especially intense social pressure on asexual men (MacNeela & Murphy, 2015; Przybylo, 2014; Vares, 2018). One respondent,

for example, described feelings of being "less of a man because I'm asexual, like it's a weakness or a failure" (MacNeela & Murphy, 2015, p. 807). While men may face greater pressure to conform to norms of sexual dominance, theoretical approaches to the intersections of gender and asexuality have also pointed to inequalities in men and women's sexual autonomy, which has granted men more permission to refuse sex and control their own sexual destinies (Fahs, 2010; Gupta, 2018).

As noted above, disproportionate numbers of asexual individuals exist under the transgender umbrella (Bauer et al., 2018; Van Houdenhove et al., 2015a). The reasons for the overlap between asexualities and transgender embodiments are undertheorized, but the interaction between gender identity and asexuality is a popular topic of discussion within online asexual communities (MacNeela & Murphy, 2015). While some within the asexual community view their gender and sexual identities as distinct and separate, others described their asexual identities as freeing them from traditional gender expectations (MacNeela & Murphy, 2015). The gender composition of asexual communities raises many questions within the sociology of sexualities that can help extend theoretical insights into the interaction between gender and sexuality and how cisnormativity and heteronormativity operate to marginalize transgender asexual people (Sumerau, Barbee, Mathers, & Eaton, 2018).

The race and class dynamics of the asexual community are also undertheorized. Bogaert's (2004) probability sample suggested that asexual people had lower levels of education and socioeconomic status and were less likely to be Caucasian than non-asexual respondents, yet the community that manifests through online forums like AVEN is disproportionately White and college-educated (Bauer et al., 2018). Income and education have been used as control variables in some quantitative studies of asexuality (e.g., Brotto et al., 2010); in turn, much more research is needed that explicitly explores the intersection of socioeconomic status and asexuality. Owen (2014, 2018) has analyzed asexuality in the context of racialized sexual scripts that have historically maintained whiteness and white supremacy. For example, Owen (2018, p. 70) writes about the asexual construction of the "mammy" figure, an ideological and political device mapped onto Black bodies that is "undesiring and undesirable," thus representing an overlap between asexuality and Blackness. Additional theoretical approaches that can illuminate the relationship between asexuality, race, and class, as well as empirical studies of race and class within the asexual community, are needed.

The literature has also begun to explore intersections of asexuality and disability. Kim (2011) observes that disabled persons are structurally desexualized and stereotyped as asexual, leading to counternarratives from disability social movements that demand sexual rights and perpetuate the idea that sexual desire is universal and innate. At the same time, asexual communities are careful to deny that there is any causal link between asexuality and disability (Cuthbert, 2017). Asexual disabled individuals are then caught between two communities— disabled individuals and asexual individuals—who are actively distancing themselves from each other (Cuthbert, 2017; Kim, 2011). Kim (2011) explains that progressive narratives of disability and asexuality overlap in that both refer to embodiments that do not need to be eliminated or cured.

## Parenting

There has been extremely limited research on asexual parents. One study found that 34% of asexual men and 21% of asexual women had children, and similar proportions were married or cohabiting with a partner (Aicken et al., 2013). Yet few researchers have explored more details of asexual parenting. We do not yet know how most asexual individuals come to be parents or whether the desire to have children varies between romantic and aromantic asexual individuals. It is possible that, like most children raised by LGBTQ parents, most children of asexual parents are born into heterosexual unions (Gates, 2015). But given the variation in sexual behavior among the asexual population, it is also possible that children

and families are more easily embraced as consistent with asexual identities.

Asexuality poses a challenge for our understandings of romantic and sexual relationships, so parenting relationships are a necessary next step for researchers. The lack of research on asexual parenting may be indicative of an infantilization of asexuality, much like the social construction of disability (Kim, 2011). It may also be indicative of a general invisibility and misunderstand of asexuality, especially given how often it is conflated with celibacy (Cerankowski & Milks, 2010). As researchers continue to investigate details of asexual individuals' intimate relationships, it is important to consider how asexual parenting can also further our understanding of diverse expressions of love and family formation.

## Intimate Relationships

The emerging literature on asexuality has strived to understand the romantic and sexual histories and interests of asexual individuals. For example, some asexual individuals express interest in physical intimacy, like hugging, kissing, or cuddling, as part of their ideal relationship and sufficient for their satisfaction (Scherrer, 2008, 2010b; Van Houdenhove et al., 2015b). Others, especially those identifying as aromantic, describe their ideal relationship as similar to a "close friendship," where emotional intimacy is achieved without any physical intimacy (Scherrer, 2008, p. 629; Van Houdenhove et al., 2015b). Overall, friendship has been identified as a key source of both emotional and physical intimacy for asexual individuals (Dawson, McDonnell, & Scott, 2016; Scherrer, 2010b). These findings are reminiscent of the "romantic friendships" that characterized Boston marriages in the late nineteenth century, which have since been interpreted as lesbian partnerships (Faderman, 1991, p. 18; Rothblum & Brehony, 1993). Given the large proportions of cisgender women within the asexual community, the sociohistorical connections between Boston marriages and contemporary constructs of asexuality are worthy of further exploration.

Some quantitative researchers have identified patterns of romantic and intimate relationships within the asexual population. Brotto et al.'s (2010) sample revealed that 70% of respondents had been in a romantic relationship at some point in their lives, with 9% of men and 29% of women reporting relationships that lasted longer than 5 years. Many asexual people in Brotto et al.'s (2010) qualitative sample craved the intimacy, companionship, and connection that romantic relationships could provide. Although some expressed concern that their asexuality would prevent them from finding meaningful relationships with accepting partners, asexual individuals with romantic interests often find themselves in romantic relationships with non-asexual partners (Van Houdenhove et al., 2015b). In such situations, the type and frequency of sexual activities are often negotiated between partners and vary based on asexual individuals' attitudes toward sexual activity (Brotto et al., 2010; Chasin, 2015; Van Houdenhove et al., 2015b).

The phrase "unwanted but consensual" appears in the literature to describe the sexual encounters that asexual respondents have with their non-asexual partners (Brotto et al., 2010; Prause & Graham, 2007, p. 346). Sexually active asexual individuals have described their reasons for having sex as a "sacrifice" for the relationship, a way of showing love for their partner, or something that seemed like a normal course for the relationship (Dawson et al., 2016; Van Houdenhove et al., 2015b). Asexual respondents in Brotto et al.'s (2010) study explained that what set them apart from non-asexual people was the lack of excitement or anticipation leading up to sexual experiences. Sex did not help asexual respondents feel closer to their partners, even if it helped their non-asexual partners feel closer to them. Some described needing to focus on something else during sex, which prevented them from creating emotional intimacy (Brotto et al., 2010).

While some asexual individuals pursue romantic relationships with non-asexual partners, others prefer to stay single—or find similarly asexual partners—rather than make sexual compromises in their relationships (Scherrer, 2010a; Van Houdenhove et al., 2015b; Vares, 2018).

Some asexual individuals also report negotiating non-monogamous sexual relationships with their non-asexual partners, often with the condition that their emotional relationship remains closed (Brotto et al., 2010; Copulsky, 2016; Scherrer, 2010b). Asexual people in relationships with another asexual person have described the benefits of not needing to deal with the "messiness" of sexual relationships, expressing appreciation for being able to be naked and physically close to each other without being pressured to have sex (Brotto et al., 2010).

## Sexual Activity

The concept of asexuality has generated much curiosity about asexual individuals' sexual activity and functioning, outside of the context of intimate relationships. Asexual individuals' need for sexual release, specifically their sex drives and experiences of masturbation, are frequent topics of inquiry in the literature. People who identify as asexual can appear in many places along the continuum of experiencing sexual desire (Bogaert, 2004; Brotto et al., 2010). For example, a minority of respondents in Van Houdenhove et al.'s (2015b) study report "normal" libido levels, with one individual expressing annoyance that "that's just my body" (p. 272). Some asexual individuals in Brotto et al.'s (2010, p. 609) study argued that their sexual desire and arousal were not "directed" at anyone because they did not experience sexual attraction.

Attitudes toward sexual activity vary considerably within the asexual community. Some asexual individuals are disgusted by the idea of sex, whereas others are merely disinterested (Van Houdenhove et al., 2015b). Regardless of their level of interest in having sex with other people, the literature suggests that masturbation is common among self-identified asexual individuals, including those with lower libido levels (Jones et al., 2017). Brotto et al. (2010) found that a majority of asexual respondents in their quantitative sample masturbated at least once a month. Yet Brotto et al. (2010) also found that when discussing sexual intercourse, masturbation, or their bodies, asexual respondents used language that was less colored by emotion and more focused on the technical language or mechanics of sex. Many described their genitals as "just there," expressing neither disgust nor excitement over genitalia (Brotto et al., 2010). Emotionally charged language was still used when discussing other aspects of their lives and behaviors, suggesting that their choice of language uniquely reflects respondents' relationship to sex. More research is needed to understand the variation of sexual activity within the asexual community and asexual individuals' engagement with specific practices (such as BDSM) that are coded as sexual (Sloan, 2015; Vares, 2018).

## Marginalization

The emerging literature on asexualities has begun tracing the contours of asexual marginalization. Marginalization emerges in different ways across the life course for asexual individuals, which may have implications for asexual parenting. For example, many report marginalization in the form of feeling different from their peers during adolescence. The emergence of asexual identities has occurred in tandem with the rise in hookup culture and pervasive sexual content in media and advertising (Przybylo, 2011; Vares, 2018). Many asexual people report that they did not understand "what the fuss was about" and could not relate to their friends' interest in sex (Brotto et al., 2010, p. 610). As asexual individuals age, their alienation from dating networks can turn into alienation from social networks based on parenting and children as their peers create families (MacNeela & Murphy, 2015). Aromantic asexual individuals may be especially alienated from a culture that overwhelmingly portrays individuals without romantic attachments as misanthropic and deeply flawed (MacNeela & Murphy, 2015).

A common theme within this literature is the denial and dismissal of asexual identities that occurs through interactions with peers, family members, and providers. Asexual respondents report expectations of bias from medical and mental health practitioners, many of whom (perhaps inadvertently) make dismissive or pathologizing comments that fail to affirm their sexual orientation (Chasin, 2015; Foster & Scherrer, 2014). Pathologizing reactions from family members and others in asexual individuals' personal lives are also common (Mitchell & Hunnicutt, 2019). In addition to the framing of asexuality as a disorder, whether it be biomedical or a psychological repression of sexual desire, asexual people are often presumed to be immature or just needing to meet the "right person" (MacNeela & Murphy, 2015). Asexual women are dismissed through gender stereotypes suggesting that women in general are disinterested in sex (MacNeela & Murphy, 2015). Each of these narratives denies asexuality as a legitimate, meaningful identity category and sexual orientation.

Measuring other forms of harassment and marginalization has been challenging, but in one survey, verbal insults, anti-asexual remarks, and derogatory names were among the most common forms of discrimination reported by asexual individuals, each of which were found to increase stress on respondents (Gazzola & Morrison, 2012). Sexual violence in the form of corrective rape has also been identified as an experience shared between asexual women, lesbian women, and transgender men, among other gender and sexual minorities (Doan-Minh, 2019). Through these acts of violence, attackers frame their assaults as attempts to "fix" their victims, thus violating both their bodily autonomy and their sexual identity (Doan-Minh, 2019).

Further research is needed to identify how these forms of marginalization affect asexual parents and their children. It is possible that, like other LGBTQ parents, asexual parents socialize their children to recognize the rich diversity of sexual identities and orientations and actively build resilience for their children through their parenting practices (Bos & Gartrell, 2010; see chapter "Lesbian-Mother Families Formed Through Donor Insemination"; Oswald, 2002). But it is also possible that the characteristics of asexuality and asexual discrimination affect children in ways that are unique from other LGBTQ parents.

## Implications for LGBTQ-Parent Families

New paradigms of love and sex emerging from the asexual community have implications for researchers and practitioners working with LGBTQ-parent families. First, asexuality encourages broader recognition of different forms of intimacy (Gressgård, 2013). Asexual individuals find intimacy and emotional fulfillment through friendship, non-sexual romantic partnerships, open and polyamorous relationships, and dyadic, monogamous romantic relationships (Scherrer, 2010a, 2010b). To be more inclusive of asexual parents and families, practitioners must be willing to challenge the idea that sexual activity legitimates a relationship or that romantic love should be privileged above platonic love (Scherrer, 2010a). Researchers should also consider how the heterogeneity of asexual relationships may shape parenting practices within the asexual community. Much more research is necessary to understand how and why asexual people have children, as well as how those children may be impacted by asexual parents' marginalization.

Practitioners should also be critical of widespread assumptions that sexual or romantic attraction is essential to the human experience (Carrigan, 2012). The same-sex marriage movement has played a role in perpetuating myths of a universal and innate need for sex and romantic love, emphasizing these desires as common to both heterosexual and LGBTQ lives (Hinderliter, 2013; Scherrer, 2010a). Research on asexuality suggests that a life well lived need not include sex and romance, and people lacking interest in these dimensions are not deficient or broken in any way (Bishop, 2013; Bogaert, 2012; Gressgård, 2013).

Finally, the process through which asexual individuals negotiate their sexual relationships has implications for people of all sexual orientations (Chasin, 2015). Asexual individuals in relationships with non-asexual partners have found ways to set boundaries, create mutual agreements, and establish consent through open communication with each other (Brotto et al., 2010; Vares, 2018). In doing so, they may be creating new models of mindful, healthy interactions between intimate partners (Chasin, 2015; Scherrer, 2010b).

## Directions for Future Research

The body of knowledge on asexuality is still in its infancy, creating many opportunities for researchers to explore and contribute to a growing field. One major challenge impeding additional research on asexualities is the ability to identify asexual respondents through surveys and qualitative recruitment strategies. Online communities like AVEN are governed by specific norms that may not reflect the experiences of all asexual individuals, yet finding asexual respondents outside of these asexual-specific online spaces is very difficult (Brotto & Yule, 2009; Chasin, 2011; Hinderliter, 2009). Methods of recruitment that can triangulate a diverse population of asexual subjects are needed. More research is also needed on how survey instruments can capture asexual respondents when the option "asexual" is sometimes selected erroneously by celibate, non-asexual individuals (M. Hoban, American College Health Association, June 19, 2018, personal communication). It is possible that defining sexual orientation labels on surveys could be helpful, though creating rigid definitions may also have unintended consequences on how different age groups interpret the survey (Williams Institute, 2009).

More research is also needed to explore intersections of gender, race, and class with asexuality. The data on race within asexual communities has been inconsistent, and few researchers have begun to explore connections between asexuality and racialized sexual stereotypes that might marginalize asexual people of color (Owen, 2014). Higher proportions of cisgender women and transgender individuals within asexual communities also raise more questions than have been answered (Gupta, 2018; MacNeela & Murphy, 2015; Sumerau et al., 2018). Given the contentious and contradictory relationship that has historically existed between women's sexuality and the feminist movement, asexuality can open new doors to thinking about the relationship between sex and power from a feminist perspective (Cerankowski & Milks, 2010; Fahs, 2010). The relationship between the rise in online communication and emerging asexual identities also carries important implications for socioeconomic class within the asexual community (Jones et al., 2017; MacNeela & Murphy, 2015). At a time when advances in LGBTQ family policy changes disproportionately benefit White, middle-class couples, more research is needed to understand how class variation within the asexual community impacts asexual parents (Scherrer, 2010a).

The relationship between asexuality and the larger LGBTQ community is also an area in need of further research. Although Mollet and Lackman (2018) found that asexual-identified people report rejection and isolation from the LGBTQ community, more research is needed to understand points of connection and disruption for asexual and LGBTQ communities and to identify social contexts in which commonalities between asexual and LGBTQ people are most salient. For example, asexual people report experiences of marginalization in the form of discrimination, verbal insults, and pathologizing, medicalizing narratives, all of which are familiar patterns within the LGBTQ community (Gazzola & Morrison, 2012). Similarly, the development of asexual vocabularies and the validation some report after finding the term "asexual" may also be a relevant point of connection (Cashore & Tuason, 2009; Levitt & Ippolito, 2014; Scott et al., 2016). More research is also needed to understand the specific sexual practices of asexual individuals and the prominent overlap between asexual and transgender embodiments (Bauer et al., 2018; Sloan, 2015; Van Houdenhove et al., 2015a; Vares, 2018).

Connections between asexuality and the larger LGBTQ community can also shed light on the diverse forms of partnership within the asexual community. Asexual individuals who are in same-sex couples have received extremely limited attention, yet they raise interesting questions about gender and sexuality. For example, findings on asexual men have found that expectations of sexual dominance inhibit men from identifying as asexual (MacNeela & Murphy, 2015; Przybylo, 2014). How do these identity conflicts extend for asexual men in same-sex relationships, who are stereotyped as especially promiscuous? For asexual women in same-sex relationships, does the history of Boston marriages provide a framework through which they can interpret their relationship (Faderman, 1991; Rothblum & Brehony, 1993)? Or do other stereotypes unique to lesbian relationships (e.g., "lesbian bed death") create additional challenges (Nichols, 2004, p. 363)? The vast heterogeneity of romantic and sexual interests within the asexual community creates many opportunities for researchers to explore the diversity of LGBTQ families.

## References

Aicken, C. R. H., Mercer, C. H., & Cassell, J. A. (2013). Who reports absence of sexual attraction in Britain? Evidence from national probability surveys. *Psychology & Sexuality, 4*, 121–135. https://doi.org/10.1080/19419899.2013.774161

Aveldanes, J. M., Pfeffer, C. A., & Augustine, J. (2018). Postmodern families. *Oxford Bibliographies Online.* https://doi.org/10.1093/obo/9780199756384-0159

Baca Zinn, M. (2012). Patricia Hill Collins: Past and future innovations. *Gender & Society, 26*, 28–32. https://doi.org/10.1177/0891243211426873

Bauer, C., Miller, T., Ginoza, M., Guo, Y., Youngblom, K., Baba, A., … Adroit, M. (2018). *The 2016 Asexual Community Survey summary report.* Retrieved from https://asexualcensus.files.wordpress.com/2018/11/2016_ace_community_survey_report.pdf. The Asexual Community Survey Team.

Bauman, Z. (1998). On postmodern uses of sex. *Theory, Culture & Society, 15*, 19–33. https://doi.org/10.1177/02632764980015003002

Bishop, C. (2013). A mystery wrapped in an enigma – Asexuality: A virtual discussion. *Psychology & Sexuality, 4*, 195–206. https://doi.org/10.1080/19419899.2013.774168

Bogaert, A. F. (2004). Asexuality: Prevalence and associated factors in a national probability sample. *The Journal of Sex Research, 41*, 279–287. https://doi.org/10.1080/00224490409552235

Bogaert, A. F. (2012). *Understanding asexuality.* Plymouth, England: Rowman & Littlefield.

Bos, H., & Gartrell, N. (2010). Adolescents of the USA National Longitudinal Lesbian Family Study: Can family characteristics counteract the negative effects of stigmatization? *Family Process, 49*, 559–572. https://doi.org/10.1111/j.1545-5300.2010.01340.x

Brotto, L. A. (2010). The DSM diagnostic criteria for hypoactive sexual desire disorder in women. *Archives of Sexual Behavior, 39*, 221–239. https://doi.org/10.1007/s10508-009-9543-1

Brotto, L. A., Knudson, G., Inskip, J., Rhodes, K., & Erskine, Y. (2010). Asexuality: A mixed-methods approach. *Archives of Sexual Behavior, 39*, 599–618. https://doi.org/10.1007/s10508-008-9434-x

Brotto, L. A., & Yule, M. A. (2009). Reply to Hinderliter (2009). *Archives of Sexual Behavior, 38*, 622–623. https://doi.org/10.1007/s10508-009-9514-6

Brotto, L. A., & Yule, M. A. (2011). Physiological and subjective sexual arousal in self-identified asexual women. *Archives of Sexual Behavior, 40*, 699–712. https://doi.org/10.1007/s10508-010-9671-7

Brotto, L. A., & Yule, M. (2017). Asexuality: Sexual orientation, paraphilia, sexual dysfunction, or none of the above? *Archives of Sexual Behavior, 46*, 619–627. https://doi.org/10.1007/s10508-016-0802-7

Callis, A. (2014). Bisexual, pansexual, queer: Non-binary identities and the sexual borderlands. *Sexualities, 17*, 63–80. https://doi.org/10.1177/1363460713511094

Carrigan, M. (2011). There's more to life than sex? Difference and commonality within the asexual community. *Sexualities, 14*, 462–478. https://doi.org/10.1177/1363460711406462

Carrigan, M. A. (2012). "How do you know you don't like it if you haven't tried it?" Asexual agency and the sexual assumption. In T. G. Morrison, M. A. Morrison, M. A. Carrigan, & D. T. McDermott (Eds.), *Sexual minority research in the new millennium* (pp. 3–20). New York, NY: Nova Science Publishers.

Cashore, C., & Tuason, M. T. G. (2009). Negotiating the binary: Identity and social justice for bisexual and transgender individuals. *Journal of Gay & Lesbian Social Services, 21*, 374–401. https://doi.org/10.1080/10538720802498405

Cerankowski, K. J., & Milks, M. (2010). New orientations: Asexuality and its implications for theory and practice. *Feminist Studies, 36*, 650–664. Retrieved from http://www.jstor.org/stable/27919126

Chasin, C. D. (2011). Theoretical issues in the study of asexuality. *Archives of Sexual Behavior, 40*, 713–723. https://doi.org/10.1007/s10508-011-9757-x

Chasin, C. D. (2015). Making sense in and of the asexual community: Navigating relationships and identities in a context of resistance. *Journal of Community & Applied Social Psychology, 25*, 167–180. https://doi.org/10.1002/casp.2203

Collins, P. H. (1990). *Black feminist thought: Knowledge, consciousness, and the politics of empowerment.* New York, NY: Routledge.

Copulsky, D. (2016). Asexual polyamory: Potential challenges and benefits. *Journal of Positive Sexuality, 2*, 11–15.

Crenshaw, K. (1991). Mapping the margins: Identity, politics and violence against women of color. *Stanford Law Review, 43*, 1241–1299. https://doi.org/10.2307/1229039

Cuthbert, K. (2017). You have to be normal to be abnormal: An empirically grounded exploration of the intersection of asexuality and disability. *Sociology, 51*, 241–257. https://doi.org/10.1177/0038038515587639

Cvetkovich, A. (2003). *An archive of feelings: Trauma, sexuality, and lesbian public cultures.* Durham, NC: Duke University Press.

Dawson, M., McDonnell, L., & Scott, S. (2016). Negotiating the boundaries of intimacy: The personal lives of asexual people. *The Sociological Review, 64*, 349–365. https://doi.org/10.1111/1467-954X.12362

Dawson, M., Scott, S., & McDonnell, L. (2018). "'Asexual' isn't who I am": The politics of asexuality. *Sociological Research Online, 23*, 374–391. https://doi.org/10.1177/1360780418757540

Decker, J. S. (2014). *The invisible orientation: An introduction to asexuality.* New York, NY: Skyhorse Publishing.

Doan-Minh, S. (2019). Corrective rape: An extreme manifestation of discrimination and the state's complicity in sexual violence. *Hastings Women's Law Journal, 30*, 167–196. Retrieved from https://repository.uchastings.edu/hwlj/vol30/iss1/8

Faderman, L. (1991). *Odd girls and twilight lovers: A history of lesbian life in twentieth-century America.* New York, NY: Penguin Books.

Fahs, B. (2010). Radical refusals: On the anarchist politics of women choosing asexuality. *Sexualities, 13*, 445–461. https://doi.org/10.1177/1363460710370650

Flore, J. (2013). HSDD and asexuality: A question of instruments. *Psychology & Sexuality, 4*, 152–166. https://doi.org/10.1080/19419899.2013.774163

Foster, A. B., & Scherrer, K. S. (2014). Asexual-identified clients in clinical settings: Implications for culturally competent practice. *Psychology of Sexual Orientation and Gender Diversity, 1*, 422–430. https://doi.org/10.1037/sgd0000058

Gates, G. J. (2015). Marriage and family: LGBT individuals and same-sex couples. *The Future of Children, 25*, 67–87.

Gazzola, S. B., & Morrison, M. A. (2012). Asexuality: An emergent sexual orientation. In T. G. Morrison, M. A. Morrison, M. A. Carrigan, & D. T. McDermott (Eds.), *Sexual minority research in the new millennium* (pp. 21–44). New York, NY: Nova Science Publishers.

Gressgård, R. (2013). Asexuality: From pathology to identity and beyond. *Psychology & Sexuality, 4*, 179–192. https://doi.org/10.1080/19419899.2013.774166

Gupta, K. (2017). "And now I'm just different, but there's nothing actually wrong with me": Asexual marginalization and resistance. *Journal of Homosexuality, 64*, 991–1013. https://doi.org/10.1080/00918369.2016.1236590

Gupta, K. (2018). Gendering asexuality and asexualizing gender: A qualitative study exploring the intersections between gender and asexuality. *Sexualities.* Advance online publication., 22, 1197. https://doi.org/10.1177/1363460718790890

Hinderliter, A. C. (2009). Methodological Issues for Studying Asexuality. *Archives of Sexual*

*Behavior, 38*, 619–621. https://doi.org/10.1007/s10508-009-9502-x

Hinderliter, A. (2013). How is asexuality different from hypoactive sexual desire disorder? *Psychology & Sexuality, 4*, 167–178. https://doi.org/10.1080/19419899.2013.774165

Jones, C., Hayter, M., & Jomeen, J. (2017). Understanding asexual identity as a means to facilitate culturally competent care: A systematic literature review. *Journal of Clinical Nursing, 26*, 3811–3831. https://doi.org/10.1111/jocn.13862

Kim, E. (2011). Asexuality in disability narratives. *Sexualities, 14*, 479–493. https://doi.org/10.1177/1363460711406463

Levitt, H. M., & Ippolito, M. R. (2014). Being transgender: The experience of transgender identity development. *Journal of Homosexuality, 61*, 1727–1758. https://doi.org/10.1080/00918369.2014.951262

MacInnis, C. C., & Hodson, G. (2012). Intergroup bias toward "Group X": Evidence of prejudice, dehumanization, avoidance, and discrimination against asexuals. *Group Processes & Intergroup Relations, 15*, 725–743. https://doi.org/10.1177/1368430212442419

MacNeela, P., & Murphy, A. (2015). Freedom, invisibility, and community: A qualitative study of self-identification with asexuality. *Archives of Sexual Behavior, 44*, 799–812. https://doi.org/10.1007/s10508-014-0458-0

Mitchell, H., & Hunnicutt, G. (2019). Challenging accepted scripts of sexual "normality": Asexual narratives of non-normative identity and experience. *Sexuality & Culture, 23*, 507–524. https://doi.org/10.1007/s12119-018-9567-6

Mollet, A. L., & Lackman, B. R. (2018). Asexual borderlands: Asexual collegians' reflections on inclusion under the LGBTQ umbrella. *Journal of College Student Development, 59*, 623–628. https://doi.org/10.1353/csd.2018.0058

Nichols, M. (2004). Lesbian sexuality/female sexuality: Rethinking 'lesbian bed death'. *Sexual and Relationship Therapy, 19*, 363–371. https://doi.org/10.1080/14681990412331298036

Nurius, P. S. (1983). Mental health implications of sexual orientation. *The Journal of Sex Research, 19*, 119–136. https://doi.org/10.1080/00224498309551174

Oswald, R. F. (2002). Resilience within the family networks of lesbians and gay men: Intentionality and redefinition. *Journal of Marriage and Family, 64*, 374–383. https://doi.org/10.1111/j.1741-3737.2002.00374.x

Owen, I. H. (2014). On the racialization of asexuality. In K. J. Cerankowski & M. Milks (Eds.), *Asexualities: Feminist and queer perspectives* (pp. 119–135). New York, NY: Routledge.

Owen, I. H. (2018). Still, nothing: Mammy and black asexual possibility. *Feminist Review, 120*, 70–84. https://doi.org/10.1057/s41305-018-0140-9

Poston, D. L., & Baumle, A. K. (2010). Patterns of asexuality in the United States. *Demographic Research, 23*, 509–530. https://doi.org/10.4054/DemRes.2010.23.18

Prause, N., & Graham, C. A. (2007). Asexuality: Classification and characterization. *Archives of Sexual Behavior, 36*, 341–356. https://doi.org/10.1007/s10508-006-9142-3

Przybylo, E. (2011). Crisis and safety: The asexual in sexusociety. *Sexualities, 14*, 444–461. https://doi.org/10.1177/1363460711406461

Przybylo, E. (2014). Masculine doubt and sexual wonder: Asexually-identified men talk about their (a)sexualities. In K. J. Cerankowski & M. Milks (Eds.), *Asexualities: Feminist and queer perspectives* (pp. 225–247). New York, NY: Routledge.

Rothblum, E. D., & Brehony, K. A. (Eds.). (1993). *Boston marriages: Romantic but asexual relationships among contemporary lesbians*. Boston, MA: University of Massachusetts Press.

Scherrer, K. S. (2008). Coming to an asexual identity: Negotiating identity, negotiating desire. *Sexualities, 11*, 621–641. https://doi.org/10.1177/1363460708094269

Scherrer, K. S. (2010a). What asexuality contributes to the same-sex marriage discussion. *Journal of Gay and Lesbian Social Services, 22*, 56–73. https://doi.org/10.1080/10538720903332255

Scherrer, K. S. (2010b). Asexual relationships: What does asexuality have to do with polyamory? In M. Barker & D. Langdridge (Eds.), *Understanding non-monogamies* (pp. 154–159). London, UK: Routledge.

Scott, S., McDonnell, L., & Dawson, M. (2016). Stories of non-becoming: Non-issues, non-events and non-identities in asexual lives. *Symbolic Interaction, 39*, 268–286. https://doi.org/10.1002/SYMB.215

Sloan, L. J. (2015). Ace of (BDSM) clubs: Building asexual relationships through BDSM practice. *Sexualities, 18*, 548–563. https://doi.org/10.1177/1363460714550907

Stacey, J. (1996). *In the name of the family: Rethinking family values in the postmodern age*. Boston, MA: Beacon Press.

Sumerau, J. E., Barbee, H., Mathers, L. A. B., & Eaton, V. (2018). Exploring the experiences of heterosexual and asexual transgender people. *Social Sciences, 7*, 162–178. https://doi.org/10.3390/socsci7090162

Troia, B. (2018). "You're the one that put me in a box": Integration, cultural constraints, and fluid LGBTQ+ millennial identities. Paper presented at the 113th Annual Meeting of the American Sociological Association, Philadelphia, PA.

Van Houdenhove, E., Gijs, L., T'Sjoen, G., & Enzlin, P. (2015a). Asexuality: A multidimensional approach. *The Journal of Sex Research, 52*, 669–678. https://doi.org/10.1080/00224499.2014.898015

Van Houdenhove, E., Gijs, L., T'Sjoen, G., & Enzlin, P. (2015b). Stories about asexuality: A qualitative study on asexual women. *Journal of Sex & Marital Therapy, 41*, 262–281. https://doi.org/10.1080/0092623X.2014.889053

Vares, T. (2018). "My [asexuality] is playing hell with my dating life": Romantic identified asexuals negotiate the dating game. *Sexualities, 21*, 520–536. https://doi.org/10.1177/1363460717716400

Waidzunas, T. (2015). *The straight line: How the fringe science of ex-gay therapy reoriented sexuality.* Minneapolis, MN: University of Minnesota Press.

Williams Institute. (2009). *Best practices for asking questions about sexual orientation on surveys* [Research Report]. Retrieved from http://williamsinstitute. law.ucla.edu/wp-content/uploads/SMART-FINAL-Nov-2009.pdf

Yuval-Davis, N. (2006). Intersectionality and feminist politics. *European Journal of Women's Studies, 13,* 193–209. https://doi. org/10.1177/1350506806065752

# Transgender-Parent Families

## Carla A. Pfeffer and Kierra B. Jones

Researchers of sex, gender, and sexuality have gone to great lengths to disentangle each of these concepts from one another, yet in everyday life experience, they often remain highly interrelated. Given shifts in societal acceptance of gay and lesbian identities and relationships, along with conflation of sex, gender, and sexual orientation, some children of a transgender parent may even implore, "Why can't you just be gay?!" (Israel, 2005). It is important to consider that sex, gender, and sexuality are also highly dependent upon one another for meaning. For example, sexual orientation requires a specification of one's own gender identity in relation to the gender identity (or identities) of individuals to whom one is attracted (e.g., "I'm a trans woman who is attracted to other women"). Specifying one's sexual identity may become particularly challenging when individual partners' sex or gender identities fall outside the binary—such as for those who are intersex, genderqueer, gender nonbinary ("enby"), or gender nonconforming. In this chapter, we explore the relatively under-researched area of transgender-parent families. In doing so,

we consider the diverse array of transgender and nonbinary parents as well as how particular intersections of sex, gender, and sexuality may produce both challenges and opportunities for transgender-parent families.

## Becoming a Parent

### Pathways to Parenthood

Transgender (trans) families, like cisgender (cis) families, are not a monolith; they are diverse in their structure and contours. They include single parents, two parents, or multiple parents and parents who live co-residentially with their children or not. Trans parents raising children may be gay, lesbian, bisexual, asexual, or queer. Trans parents span across the age spectrum. Some trans parents may have a disability. Trans-parent families may include extended family members or extended family may be estranged from them. Their families may include members of choice rather than (or in addition to) members who are biologically related. Trans parents raising children with a partner may be doing so in the context of monogamous or polyamorous partnerships, and those partnerships may be sexual or nonsexual. Some trans-parent families may be legally recognized or documented while others are not; and in some cases, documented status of family members may differ (see chapter "LGBTQ-Parent Immigrant

Carla A. Pfeffer and Kierra B. Jones contributed equally to this chapter.

C. A. Pfeffer (✉) · K. B. Jones
Department of Sociology, University of South Carolina, Columbia, SC, USA
e-mail: pfefferc@mailbox.sc.edu; kbjones@email.sc.edu

© Springer Nature Switzerland AG 2020
A. E. Goldberg, K. R. Allen (eds.), *LGBTQ-Parent Families*,
https://doi.org/10.1007/978-3-030-35610-1_12

Families: We're Here, We're Queer, We're Invisible"). Some trans parents may be religious while others are not, and the religious affiliations of family members may differ; political beliefs and affiliations may also vary within and across families. Trans parents may be divorced or widowed and span across the socioeconomic spectrum. Their children may be biologically related to them or not (and may be adopted or not). Trans-parent families include partners and/or children whose race and ethnicity match one another and/or whose do not.

Trans people, like cis people, have a number of possible pathways to becoming a parent and building families: adoption; giving birth to biologically related offspring with or without the use of assisted reproductive technologies; gestational surrogacy using one's own or donor gametes; fostering or guardianship of children who are or who are not biologically related; and step-parenthood in the context of blended families. Across each of these pathways, trans people and their partners may face additional struggles and challenges due largely to social stigma and discrimination against trans people. There are important differences among trans people connected to parental intentions, with transgender women reporting stronger intention to become parents through adoption and transgender men reporting stronger intention to become parents in ways that would result in biological relatedness to their children—including pregnancy (Tornello & Bos, 2017).

It must be understood, of course, that parenthood intentions do not arise in a social vacuum and that systemic barriers to particular pathways to parenthood for some groups may overdetermine reported intentions. In the context of children born prior to a parent's transition, a divorce following one's coming out as transgender too often involves legal cases that challenge trans people's fitness to retain custody and visitation rights or that figure them as unfit parents when attempting to adopt (Dierckx, Mortelmans, Motmans, & T'Sjoen, 2017; Stotzer, Herman, & Hasenbush, 2014). Other reports of transgender people's intentions and experiences related to parenthood reveal challenges around being

legally named and listed as parents in the context of a child's birth or adoption (Cahill & Tobias, 2006; Pyne, Bauer, & Bradley, 2015; Sabatello, 2011; Stotzer et al., 2014).

## Medically Assisted Reproduction

Transgender people also report negative experiences and heightened scrutiny by some medical professionals when seeking reproductive services and assisted reproductive technologies (Beatie, 2008; James-Abra et al., 2015; Pyne et al., 2015). In one interesting finding, trans men who gave birth to their children were more likely than the general population to rely upon nonphysicians and nonhospital locations when giving birth (Light, Obedin-Maliver, Sevelius, & Kerns, 2014). Additional research would do well to assess if this is a trend as well as to ascertain whether this reduced likelihood of physician and hospital utilization among trans men during childbirth is driven by fears of discrimination and stigma or other factors—such as greater interest in de-medicalized birthing sites (e.g., home) and support professionals (e.g., midwives and doulas).

Some of the challenges that aspiring trans parents face when seeking assisted reproductive technologies include language on forms that excludes their identity and experiences; providers' assumptions that their clients are nontransgender and heterosexual; care refusal by providers upon learning a potential patient is trans; and provider beliefs that some pathways to pregnancy should not be available to some trans people (e.g., that trans men should not gestate because it is inconsonant with normative male social roles) (James-Abra et al., 2015; More, 1998; Murphy, 2012, 2015). Some health professionals—including those specializing in reproductive health—may fail to consider or discuss the possibility that their transgender patients may wish to become parents in the future (Pyne et al., 2015). This is particularly troubling considering that many trans people and their partners do indeed express the desire to become parents (Pfeffer, 2017; Wierckx et al., 2012).

Until quite recently, research literatures on transgender reproduction tended to focus on ethical debates connected to reproduction that place transgender people in the center as spectacle and slippery-slope cautionary tales rather than as individuals and families (Murphy, 2010; Pyne et al., 2015). These literatures somehow render obscure the socially mediated desire that some transgender people have to pursue family building and becoming parents as most people do—through means that will establish some degree of biological relatedness (Mamo & Alston-Stepnitz, 2015; Pyne et al., 2015).

Transgender patients seeking assisted reproductive technologies report both needing to engage in self-advocacy in order to have needs met safely and effectively yet also feared that such self-advocacy might endanger the ability to receive care—causing some individuals not to advocate for themselves, even in the context of receiving trans-incompetent reproductive healthcare services (James-Abra et al., 2015). Too often, assisted reproductive technologies are explored without provider consideration of how the recommended protocols (such as temporary discontinuation of testosterone therapy for trans men) and hormonal shifts of pregnancy and postpartum may significantly impact their patient's well-being or potentially trigger gender dysphoria and/or postpartum depression (dickey, Ducheny, & Ehrbar, 2016; Ellis, Wojnar, & Pettinato, 2014; Light et al., 2014; Obedin-Maliver & Makadon, 2016).

Further, accessing assisted reproductive technologies may also be difficult or impossible for trans people who do not have insurance or whose insurance does not provide such services or will not provide them unless a patient has documented infertility (which is challenging to document if a trans man is partnered with someone who does not produce sperm) (dickey et al., 2016). The process of becoming a trans parent often brings with it intrusive questioning from strangers, colleagues, and family members alike about how children were conceived; genetic contributions of each parent; gestational details; childbirth plans; infant feeding plans; and legal connections between parents and their children (Ellis et al., 2014).

## Demographics of Trans-parent Families

Determining the size, composition, and structure of families with at least one transgender parent is a challenging task due to the dearth of research on trans-parent families and large-scale data collection on gender identity (Biblarz & Savci, 2010; Meier & Labuski, 2013). Only in recent decades, with increased visibility of trans individuals through media coverage and ongoing public discussions of trans rights, have researchers started to make significant progress in the collection of these data. A crucial part of the issue in gathering such information has been the sheer lack of questions regarding gender identity on surveys that would make these calculations possible (Crissman, Berger, Graham, & Dalton, 2017; Pyne et al., 2015).

One of the most widely cited estimates of US transgender population comes from the *National Transgender Discrimination Survey* (NTDS). Estimates of the transgender population vary, but with updated measures, most estimates range between 0.5% and 0.6% of the US adult population (Crissman et al., 2017; Flores, Herman, Gates, & Brown, 2016; Grant et al., 2011). Within this population, it is estimated that trans women outnumber trans men and gender-nonconforming people (Crissman et al., 2017). Younger adults (18–24 years of age) also appear more likely to identify as transgender and as nonbinary than older adults (25 years of age and older) (Flores et al., 2016). This finding may be an indication of shifting social norms and increased acceptance of diverse gender identities in younger cohorts.

In a review of 51 studies of transgender parenting, all of which used nonprobability sampling techniques, between 25% and 50% respondents reported being parents (Stotzer et al., 2014). Of the estimated US transgender population, Grant et al. (2011) found that 38% were parents and 18% claimed at least one dependent. Individuals who transitioned later in life were more likely to have children than younger individuals. Specifically, 82% of those 55 years or older were parents compared to 38% of those 25–44 years. This parallels findings in some other research on trans families. For example, in a large probability sample of trans individuals in Ontario, Canada, researchers found that many (73.3%) transgender parents were 35 years or older (Pyne et al., 2015). Gender differences in parenting may also exist, as trans women report higher rates of parenting than the rates of both trans men and gender-nonconforming individuals; however, trans women in the sample were also significantly older than other respondents (Pyne et al., 2015). Given the correlation of age with parenthood, it is likely that age differences in the sample at least partially explain these reported differences in parenthood status.

Less information is known about trans-parent families and parenting rates across racial and ethnic lines (see chapter "Race and Ethnicity in the Lives of LGBTQ Parents and Their Children: Perspectives from and Beyond North America"). Most small-scale qualitative studies have disproportionately represented White, college-educated, middle-class individuals, offering an incomplete picture of what trans families look like today. Of the larger transgender population, Indigenous Americans have both higher rates of parenting (45%) and higher rates of dependent children in comparison to other racial groups, while Asian Americans report much lower rates of parenthood and having dependent children (Grant et al., 2011). Additional research on transgender parenthood within a broader cross-section of racialized and ethnic communities would provide useful information about intersections between race, ethnicity, and parenthood.

State-level estimates of transgender adults in the USA show vast differences between states. Hawaii has the largest estimated transgender population (0.8%), while North Dakota has the smallest (0.3%) (Flores et al., 2016). With limited data on trans families, it is difficult to pinpoint where these families live and if/how location differs significantly from family patterns in the general population. The only study to explore choices of residency (with considerations of population density, neighborhood type, and community) among trans parents comes from a sample of LGBTQ-led households in Australia and New Zealand in which the authors explore perceptions

of social connectedness depending on region type (e.g., rural, regional, metropolitan) (Power et al., 2014). Trans individuals only comprise one percent ($n = 7$) of this sample, so it is difficult to discern any patterns or differences among only trans-parent families. Sixty percent of the sample lived in a regional or rural area compared to 40% in an inner metropolitan area, contradicting the assumption that most LGBTQ individuals reside in inner city areas. Their findings demonstrate that LGBTQ families living in inner metropolitan areas tended to have fewer children than those living in regional or rural spaces. Given the small sample sizes of transgender participants in this and many other studies, additional research should be conducted to better understand residential patterns of transgender-parent families. Doing so may reveal the constellation of considerations these families must make when determining where they will live (e.g., cost of living, proximity to extended family members, and/or family of choice). One of these considerations, of course, is just how welcoming and safe various neighborhoods and geographic spaces will be for transgender-parent families.

## Social Perceptions and Discrimination

An unfortunately common occurrence across research literatures is to lump trans-parent families into analyses of LGBQ-parent families. While this may be helpful in distinguishing the issues that "nontraditional" families face, as a group, certain experiences and challenges may be unique to trans individuals and their families. Thus, this literature may inadvertently minimize or erase trans and trans family experience. Further, this also contributes to the enormous misunderstanding of trans identity and conflates gender and sexual identities. This may also skew the general public's perception of trans individuals and trans families. Such misunderstanding and lack of awareness may then further contribute to transphobic assumptions and stereotypes, such as the notion that the children of trans parents may be more likely to be gender or sexually non-normative or fluid themselves and that this is problematic per se. There is also a critical need for increased awareness of policy issues affecting transgender individuals specifically, not only LGBQ-identified people (Cahill & Tobias, 2006).

Media coverage has also tended to present only a partial picture of trans parents and families. In 2008, Thomas Beatie became known as the "first pregnant man" (Beatie, 2008). As the media framed and sensationalized his story, it caused a great deal of public controversy, some of which persists today. In 2015, Caitlyn Jenner—a medal-winning former Olympian and reality television star—announced to the media that she was transgender, becoming a hot topic of conversation as cameras followed and documented various aspects of her transition. Jenner's children were all adults at the time that she came out as transgender and began her public transition. Public controversy was intensified by the fact of Jenner's outspoken Republican political affiliation, challenging the myth that all transgender people must be politically liberal rather than conservative. While expanding visibility of transgender parents and trans parent families may usher in broader public awareness and acceptance of transgender individuals and their families, media reports may also offer incomplete and stigmatizing portrayals as well, further contributing to misunderstanding and transphobia.

At the family level, we know that trans parents and families may struggle in the public eye. Some qualitative interview data on the adaptation of trans-parent families indicate that trans parents may want to have discussions with their children about bullying and parental pronouns, names, and parental designators (e.g., "mom" or "dad") used in public spaces in order to protect them from discrimination and violence (Dierckx & Platero, 2018; Petit, Julien, & Chamberland, 2017). Because trans identity is perceived as non-normative or deviant, trans-parent families must often consider ways to safely navigate across different social spheres.

In general, transgender people report facing greater discrimination, have fewer legal rights and protections, and often experience greater pathologization than their cisgender peers in the LGBQ community (Levi & Monnin-Browder, 2012; Pyne et al., 2015). Transgender parents report struggling with discrimination both within their families and outside their families as well. For example, some cisgender partners of transgender people have used their partner's experience of being trans as grounds to build cases against them during divorce and in determining both visitation and custodial arrangements (Dierckx et al., 2017; Stotzer et al., 2014). In an online qualitative survey of 50 trans families, many parents reported transphobic bullying and discrimination experienced by both themselves and family members—including children, particularly within the context of schools (Haines, Ajayi, & Boyd, 2014). Similarly, a comparison of survey data from both trans parents and nonparents revealed that both groups experienced similar levels of transphobia, and most participants reported having been bullied for being trans (Pyne et al., 2015).

Being transgender may also be disqualifying for some prospective parents (as a matter of either policy or de facto discrimination) when it comes to registrations of births and legal adoptions (Cahill & Tobias, 2006; Pyne et al., 2015; Sabatello, 2011; Stotzer et al., 2014). Highlighting the intersectional impacts of discrimination, there is also evidence that court interventions are more frequently experienced by transgender parents of color (Haines et al., 2014). Researchers note the particular forms that transphobia may take involve not only overt discriminatory acts but acts of implicit bias as well—such as failing to consider that transgender individuals may be or wish to become parents (Pyne et al., 2015). It is in this context of transphobia and discrimination that transgender people and their families must "come out" to others, often at considerable personal and familial risk.

## Coming Out

Coming out is the process of actively disclosing one's sexual and/or gender identity that falls outside of societal expectations of heterosexuality and a strict binary gender system. Because binary and normative assumptions of gender and sexual identities have been adopted into mainstream society, anyone who does not "fit" these social constructions is designated as an "other." While coming out is often depicted as a one-time experience or linear process, it is instead a lifelong and iterative process that often involves continuous self-reflection as well as conversations with family, friends, employers, and disclosures to bureaucratic systems and individuals who serve as social gatekeepers to regulated social institutions (Dziengel, 2015).

Some of the most extensive work on the process of coming out as transgender comes from Lev's (2004) book, *Transgender Emergence*, in which she outlines six stages of the "emergence process" that clinicians may observe in counseling and supporting transgender individuals. These stages are awareness, seeking information/reaching out, disclosure to significant others, exploration of identity and transition, exploring transition and body modification, and integration and pride. Further, because these stages are a guide and "not meant to 'label' people, define transgender maturity, or limit anyone to these experiences," acknowledging how each individual's own unique experiences and standpoint may shape and influence this developmental coming-out process is a crucial part of adequately addressing the needs of transgender individuals and their families (Lev, 2004, p. 234). This finding is reiterated in more recent clinical works in which case studies of trans individuals point to the need for individualized therapy and purposeful empowerment through this complex process of transitioning (Dworkin & Pope, 2012).

"Family emergence" is yet another dimension of coming out in which family members of the trans individual experience their own developmental process (Lev, 2004). Again, this trajectory is not necessarily linear and typically requires much adaptation and the acquisition of new knowledge about transgender identities. The family emergence model contains four stages: discovery and disclosure, turmoil, negotiation, and finding balance. There is a wide range of scenarios and responses that family members may experience after a trans parent comes out (e.g.,

shock, feeling overwhelmed, anger, and grief). Echoing these observations, other studies also address gender transition as not only an individual process but a family process as well (Dierckx et al., 2017; Dierckx & Platero, 2018; Haines et al., 2014; Veldorale-Griffin & Darling, 2016). For example, while some cis partners of trans individuals described their partner's transition as "selfish," others acted as a main source of support throughout this process (Dierckx & Platero, 2018). Families also showed great concern for trans people's parental roles and how dynamics within the family may be altered in the context of transition. Boundary ambiguity through a parent's gender transition may temporarily negatively impact family functioning and interpersonal interactions (Veldorale-Griffin & Darling, 2016). However, these potential or actual family changes in the context of a trans parent's transition were not always perceived as undesirable, with some individuals citing positive experiences and outcomes throughout the process (Dierckx & Platero, 2018). Notably, one study concluded that "the transition experience was also a means for both the family as a whole and for each individual to become more resilient" (Dierckx et al., 2017, p. 408).

Although initial reactions to a family member's coming out and transition may be negative, research is varied as to the long-term effects/impact of coming out on family relationships. Some research suggests that coming out can help to better family relationships and foster more support. For example, in a study of 6456 transgender and gender-nonconforming persons, 61% of trans individuals reported a slow improvement in family relationships after coming out, suggesting that the passage of time may be an important factor for acceptance (Grant et al., 2011). Coming out to "key members" of one's family (identified as father and partner) may also be related to better quality of these relationships and, subsequently, better well-being for the trans individual (Erich, Tittsworth, Dykes, & Cabuses, 2008). This finding is particularly important as key family members may have the ability to help other members who are struggling to cope with the transition. For instance, acceptance or non-acceptance of a trans parent's identity by cisgender family members (such as co-parents or grandparents) can influence subsequent responses from their children (Dierckx et al., 2017). This finding is evidence of how crucial the support of just one family member may be after coming out, particularly for trans individuals who had children pre-transition. This is also evidence that "those individuals, who have at least one parent or a close family member often find just enough love and support to make it through unimaginable hardships associated with a harsh, transphobic society" (Israel, 2005, p. 58).

On the other hand, some findings indicate higher rates of parental conflict between cis and trans partners and conflict between trans parents and children after coming out. For example, nearly half of National Transgender Discrimination Survey respondents experienced relationship termination with a spouse or partner following coming out, and 30% of respondents had children who chose to discontinue their relationship (Grant et al., 2011). Also, while children of trans parents show signs of normal development (see section on "Family Functioning and Child Outcomes" for a review of child development outcomes), they do report marital conflict between parents as a common problem (Freedman, Tasker, & di Ceglie, 2002). A few qualitative studies have also demonstrated conflict as a recurring theme between partners, some resulting in divorce or separation (Haines et al., 2014; Hines, 2006; Pyne, 2012). There may also be differences in partner and child acceptance that are related to a trans person's gender. Notably, trans women tend to report higher rates of rejection from both partners and children due, in part, to social censure and stigmatization of what is perceived as male femininity (Grant et al., 2011). Furthermore, racial and ethnic minorities, those with lower socioeconomic status, and less educated individuals appear to experience more rejection within the family and to fare worse in court custody cases (Grant et al., 2011).

While the process of coming out may be a time of significant strain for many individuals, coming out to one's children may be a particularly challenging experience with many complex nuances. Having children prior to transitioning could prolong the amount of time taken to initiate transitioning and may even stop individuals from transitioning entirely (Church, O'Shea, & Lucey, 2014). Research on trans parents who had children pre-transition suggests that there is a complex process of negotiation that happens between the trans parent and child. This process usually involves the discussion of how the relationship can be maintained or redefined in such a way that is comfortable for both parties. Researchers note that some children opt to use a name other than "mom" or "dad" to refer to their parent, such as a gender-neutral pronoun (such as "they") or an agreed-upon nickname for the trans parent (Dierckx et al., 2017; Dierckx & Platero, 2018; Hines, 2006). Many factors may go into decisions about which parental designators will be used, including whether children were born before or after a parent's transition and negotiations with children and other members of the family (Petit et al., 2017).

Ultimately, family recognition and acceptance of a trans family member's gender identity is imperative to being able to effectively face social stigma and transphobia both individually and as a family system (Dierckx & Platero, 2018). The coming-out process is made easier for children and parents alike by maintenance of familiar routines, open communication, and asking and answering questions without judgment. These strategies serve as protective factors and foster resilience in families (Dierckx et al., 2017). Importantly, children's rejection of trans parents may not be as widespread as once thought as a recent qualitative study of both trans parents and their adult children demonstrated mostly positive or neutral responses to the parent's transition and disclosure (Veldorale-Griffin, 2014).

## Family Functioning

In a meta-analysis of studies focusing on transgender parenting, the vast majority of transgender parents reported that their relationships with their children were generally positive, and this was particularly so following either transition or coming out (Stotzer et al., 2014). Positive family dynamics in transgender families, particularly in the context of a parent's gender transition, seem highly dependent on the degree to which open communication is encouraged and the relationship between co-parents is amicable (Dierckx et al., 2017; Israel, 2005; Pyne et al., 2015). Having positive social and community support, along with buffers against societal stigma and discrimination, is also critical (Dierckx et al., 2017). Indeed, some research addresses the development of family resilience in the context of transgender parenthood, noting the possibility that families and their members may become stronger and more capable of adaptive responses to internal and external stressors following the experience of going through a parent's gender transition (Dierckx et al., 2017).

Challenges to family functioning, when they do occur in transgender-parent families, are sometimes connected to fears about or experiences with transphobic social discrimination and bullying (Haines et al., 2014). Tensions or aggression between co-parents may constitute another potential source of family dysfunction. Some cisgender partners (or ex-partners) of transgender people, who began their relationships prior to a partner's transition, may feel that they were targets of deception or that years of their lives were wasted or a lie (Haines et al., 2014; Pfeffer & Castañeda, 2018).

High levels of conflict may exist between trans individuals and their partners after transition, likely due to the shifting gender dynamics and relational norms (Haines et al., 2014). This can lead to increased stress for both partners and some trans individuals feeling discriminated against by their own family. In a study of cis women partners of trans men, feminist-identified cis women partners employed individualist and free will discourse when describing gender-normative divisions of household labor and emotion work (Pfeffer, 2010). For example, many cis women asserted that they simply chose to do more of the laundry or dishes because they liked to do them or because they were better at doing laundry or dishes than their trans men partners. This suggests that normative gender roles in family labor do not

necessarily disappear in the context of contemporary trans families and conscious desire to construct gender-egalitarian households.

## Marriage and Divorce

Much of the research literature shows unfavorable results for marriage and divorce in transparent families, with reference to widespread transphobia, social stigma, and anti-transgender bias in laws and policies (Cahill & Tobias, 2006; for a more comprehensive overview of trans relationship dissolution and divorce, see Pfeffer & Castañeda, 2018). Until relatively recently, trans people's marriages were often not legally recognized and the same protections that were afforded to cis couples were often denied to trans couples. Even in the context of broader legal recognition of various types of marriage, as Cahill and Tobias (2006) note: "Paths to transgender marriage are susceptible to legal challenge. Transgender people… must therefore live with the fear that… their relationship will not be recognized-an uncertainty that other married couples do not confront" (p. 68).

Benefits of legal partner recognition are plentiful in the USA and legal recognition of transgender spouses and families is critical for their well-being and access to regulated social resources (Cahill & Tobias, 2006). These benefits include the ability to provide care for a loved one in the event of an emergency, access to health insurance coverage, survivorship and inheritance rights, and the emotional and physical health that accompanies formal recognition of familial relationships. Continuing legal and social policy challenges with regard to gender identity and rights for LGBTQ people and their partners and families has rendered recent legal gains and recognition for these communities uncertain under the Trump administration (Cahill, Wang, & Jenkins, 2019).

## Child Outcomes

Another common manifestation of transphobia and heterosexism is the frequent questioning of the "fitness" of LGBTQ individuals to create families and raise children. This longstanding debate among researchers has resulted in numerous studies on the children of lesbian and gay parents and, now, on trans parents and children. As noted by Clarke and Demetriou (2016), some scholars have questioned the appropriateness of a researcher focus on trans families, noting that this focus often serves to further pathologize the trans community and promote the idea that trans people are ill-suited for parenting by allowing for the possibility that LGBTQ parents are in some way unfit as a potential research outcome (also see Clarke, 2002). However, other social scientists disagree with this assessment, stating that it is important to acknowledge cisnormative and transphobic stereotypes and myths and to actively challenge such narratives (Pfeffer, 2017; Ryan, 2009).

Literature on trans parents has shown overwhelmingly positive trends in child outcomes and general well-being. Most findings indicate that children raised by trans parents do not differ substantially, on a developmental level, from those raised by cisgender parents (Chiland, Clouet, Golse, Guinot, & Wolf, 2013; Freedman et al., 2002; Green, 1978, 1998). In fact, it appears that most children of trans parents demonstrate typical development on multiple dimensions, including both sexual and gender identity and physical, mental, and emotional development (Chiland et al., 2013; Freedman et al., 2002; Green, 1978, 1998). It is important to note, however, that much of this research is cross-sectional and retrospective.

The first cited work on the outcomes of children with trans parents comes from Green's (1978, 1998) reports on 37 children raised by homosexual or "transsexual" parents. While many variables may play a role in child development, "these children...developed a typical sexual identity, including heterosexual orientation" (Green, 1978, p. 696). In a study of the children of trans parents who were referred to a clinic focusing on gender identity disorder (GID), 17 out of 18 children in the sample showed no clinical features of GID, and of the two children old enough to indicate sexual preference, both were

heterosexual (Freedman et al., 2002). Additionally, children of trans parents show signs of typical development across many dimensions (not only measures of sexual and gender identity), including measures of healthy attachment, psychomotor development, speech and language skills, and positive body image (Chiland et al., 2013).

Still, age differences are likely to exist in adjustment to a parent's coming out, as younger children typically fare better than older children and teenagers (Israel, 2005). After surveying a small sample of therapists who worked with trans patients, White and Ettner (2004) found that a child's younger age at the time of parent's transition served as a protective factor in most cases (see White & Ettner [2007] and Pyne et al. [2015] for similar findings).

Further, in a study of adult children of LGBTQ parents, children normalized their parent's identity in everyday conversation and were characterized as quite socially aware (Clarke & Demetriou, 2016). This prompted them to openly challenge transphobic/homophobic and heterosexist narratives about their trans parent and family. As far as internal pressures to promote healthy development in their children, a common theme among trans parents and their partners is the concern they share for their child's well-being (Haines et al., 2014). This includes concern about the stigma and bullying their children may experience because of widespread cultural transphobia and anti-trans bias. Despite these challenges, trans parents frequently report positive relationships with their children (Church et al., 2014). Future research would benefit from more focused inclusion of the voices and perspectives of children of trans parents.

## The Impact of Transition on Family Systems, Identities, and Social Roles

In earlier eras, parents who struggled with their gender identity may have felt compelled to leave their families, viewing the realization of their need to transition and maintaining their existing family connections as antithetical (Israel, 2005).

Contemporary shifts in LGBTQ politics and awareness, however, mean that more and more people are transitioning within the context of their families (Hines, 2006) and working to balance their own and their family's needs (Haines et al., 2014). Institutional transphobia, however, continues to present challenges to trans-parent families and their members. Researchers report that, due to greater societal comfort with female masculinity than with male effeminacy, parental transitions may be more challenging when the parent transitioning is a trans woman than when they are a trans man (Dierckx et al., 2017). There are also particular aspects of trans embodiment and bodily transitions that may be associated with heightened institutional transphobia. For example, trans men who are pregnant and/or who chestfeed may face considerable isolation given social stigma connected to gender-liminal embodiments (MacDonald, 2016; MacDonald et al., 2016; Riggs, 2013; Ryan, 2009).

Because families constitute a system, when a parent transitions, the family and each of its individual members may be said to be transitioning along with their transgender family member (Dierckx et al., 2017; Haines et al., 2014; Hines, 2006). As such, the role of social support for families in which a parent is transitioning is particularly critical (Veldorale-Griffin & Darling, 2016). Veldorale-Griffin and Darling (2016) found that the factors most responsible for determining family functioning are ambiguous boundaries, having a sense of coherence, and stigma. Moreover, in this research drawing upon family stress theory, having a sense of coherence was protective against stigma in the context of family functioning.

Research on transgender parents often focuses on the impact of transition on family member identities, social roles, and dynamics (Haines et al., 2014). A parent's gender transition tends to affect children differently depending on their age and developmental stage, with younger children handling a parent's gender transition more easily than older children and teenagers often having a particularly difficult time with a parent's gender transition (Dierckx et al., 2017; Israel, 2005; Pyne et al., 2015). Some research points to the

importance of understanding a parent's gender transition as an ongoing individual and family systems process rather than an isolated event (Dierckx et al., 2017). Challenges may arise within the family if the desire to be "out" about a parent's transgender identity or transition process is not shared equally across family members or if some family members are ready to be "out" earlier than other family members (Hines, 2006). Further, some children experience greater struggle over a parent's transition than others and duration of time since transition is not always neatly associated with a reduction in these struggles (Tabor, 2018). Most research on transgender parenting has been derived from accounts of transgender people or their partners; accounts from their children are much less common, presenting an area ripe for further empirical investigation (Dierckx et al., 2017; see chapter "The "Second Generation:" LGBTQ Youth with LGBTQ Parents"; Tabor, 2018; Veldorale-Griffin, 2014).

Research suggests that there are a number of key factors associated with positive family system outcomes in the context of a transgender parent's gender transition. These include open communication among family members; receiving positive social support and acceptance for one's family; engaging reflectively on the meaning of transition in family members' own lives and for their family as a unit; maintaining relative behavioral consistency and parental roles within the home; transitioning gradually over time rather than within a short time period; maintaining beloved family recreational activities throughout transition; and co-parents maintaining an amicable relationship throughout transition (Dierckx et al., 2017).

Researchers have addressed transgender parents' sometimes paradoxical experiences of their social roles conflicting with one another. For example, parental status constitutes a relatively privileged and socially normative social role, while transgender status is often assumed to be one's primary (yet socially counternormative and disadvantaged) social role (Haines et al., 2014). Naming practices within families offer particularly salient examples of how a transgender parent's transition interfaces with social and family roles. Consider, for example, how an individual's gender transition may be accompanied not only by a shift in pronouns and name but by a shift in familial membership role as well—from husband to wife, wife to husband, mother to father, and father to mother (Hines, 2006). Research documenting children's struggles with a trans parent's transitions note that this shift in parental role is generally more challenging than shifts in that parent's name or pronouns (Tabor, 2018).

Some trans people report that family members' difficulty reconciling what they view to be discordant social roles (e.g., "I have accepted that my child is a trans man but I cannot accept his desire to give birth to a child given that that is a woman's role") may contribute to trans people's inability or decision not to pursue certain parenting possibilities (von Doussa, Power, & Riggs, 2015). Research in this area sometimes reveals researcher biases in which, despite participants' stated and established naming around social roles (e.g., trans women describing themselves as "mother"), researchers fail to accurately take up this language when describing these familial social roles and, instead, misgender their participants (e.g., describing trans women who are mothers as "fathers"; for an example, see Faccio, Bordin, & Cipolletta, 2013).

One of the areas that may be impacted for family members in the instance of a parent's gender transition is in the perceived or actual sexual orientations of partners and co-parents (Hines, 2006). Some previously heterosexually identified or perceived partners report being socially perceived as sisters as a trans woman partner transitions. Some previously lesbian-identified couples, upon a trans man partner's transition, report being misperceived by others as mother and son. These social misrecognition processes (Pfeffer, 2014) may have impacts that extend beyond partners as well. Having parents who are socially perceived in ways that may be very dissimilar from their actual social roles and relationships within the family may be quite jarring for children, who often find themselves in the position of correcting (or failing to correct) these social misrecognition processes. It is also common for transgender

individuals to experience sexual orientation fluidity or shift during transition and for partners of transgender people to reconsider their own sexual orientation in the context of a partner's shifting gender identity (Israel, 2005; Pfeffer, 2017). All of these potential reconfigurations of gender and sexual identity may impact how family members, their relationships, and the family unit understand one another and are understood (and accepted, or not) by the world outside the family.

## Trans-parent Family Strengths

While much research (earlier work in particular) addresses transgender families from a potential deficits and dysfunction framework, researchers have also highlighted the potentially positive aspects of transgender-parent families—their resilience; family members' development of more fluid gender norms and ideologies; and mutual care, support, and social advocacy (Hines, 2006; Pyne et al., 2015). Despite the wide array of challenges and stressors that may affect trans families, these events may indeed strengthen and foster resilience and acceptance among individual family members and family systems. For example, not only did the adult children in one study challenge homophobic and transphobic social contexts, but they also expressed the importance of living authentically and embracing one's identity (Clarke & Demetriou, 2016). Further, family resilience is often an outcome of a parent's gender transition, and this includes positive changes at both the family and individual levels (Dierckx et al., 2017). These positive changes may include becoming more open-minded and learning to question the binary gender system. Some research on lesbian and gay parents suggests similar findings for instilling more tolerance and acceptance in children (Augustine, Aveldanes, & Pfeffer, 2017). Future research should be conducted on the development of resilience in trans families, including critical approaches toward the concept of resilience that raise caution against overly sunny portrayals of the scars that form from repeated engagement with transphobic social norms and systems.

While most of the literature has not explicitly studied communication in trans-parent families, numerous studies have pointed to the importance of open and honest communication in maintaining healthy relationships. This is particularly true at the initial stages of coming out and the commencement of transitioning. Healthy communication, including positive use of humor, can be a protective factor that may reduce family tensions and increase adaptive coping, particularly for children (Dierckx et al., 2017). Open and honest communication can entail a number of strategies, such as the ability to ask questions, negotiate linguistic changes, and discuss how to deal with external pressures and safeguards that may be needed in public settings (Dierckx et al., 2017; Dierckx & Platero, 2018; Hines, 2006; Petit et al., 2017).

A recurrent concern appearing across the literature is the emphasis on ensuring safety in public spaces due to possible experiences of stigma and transphobia. For instance, parental designations may change depending on whether family members are interacting in a private or public setting (Petit et al., 2017). Parents may have to explicitly clarify rules on when and where it is deemed safe for children to use certain designations or terms (e.g., "mommy" and "daddy"). This indicates that these discussions may be a critical aspect of communication processes and social safety strategies in trans families, similar to "code-switching" practices that occur among other types of marginalized families and their members (Huynh, Nguyen, & Benet-Martínez, 2011).

Even though open communication is an aspiration or goal shared by many families, trans parents—as with all parents—also have a right to privacy. This suggests a need for families to strike a balance between being open and maintaining respect for the privacy of the person who is transitioning. Because coming out and transitioning is a very personal process and may also be a time of great anxiety, this privacy could be a crucial way for trans individuals to advocate for themselves. While many children do best when able to openly communicate with their transitioning parent, trans parents may wish to keep certain aspects of their transition private, such as the details of a surgical transition (Dierckx et al., 2017). Thus, transition-related disclosure practices remain an integral component of communication that trans families and their members must negotiate for the benefit of both individual members and the family system. Some families may benefit from the involvement of clinical professionals to facilitate these conversations as well as to convey tips and strategies for creating or maintaining healthy boundaries and communication.

## Clinical Practice and Transgender Parents and Families

While clinical services directed toward transgender people and their families often focus on transition, coming out, and other directly gender-identity-related issues, it is important to understand that these concerns do not constitute the entirety of why transgender people and their families may seek professional counseling and social services. For example, Stotzer et al. (2014) note that other services of interest include those related to childcare, connecting with other parents for support, and family-planning resources. Further, clinical practice has too often focused on transgender people in isolation rather than fully embedded in social context and relationships—within families, workplaces, and communities (Lev, 2004). One of the necessary contexts to address is the fact that many transgender families may face economic struggles and un- or underemployment of its trans member(s), making access to clinical and therapeutic services particularly challenging (Veldorale-Griffin & Darling, 2016).

An additional challenge to understanding transgender-parent families through the lens of clinical practice is that, until relatively recently, practitioner training and literature have tended to address transgender-parent families either marginally, in stigmatizing ways, or not at all (Lev, 2004; see chapter "Clinical Work with LGBTQ Parents and Prospective Parents"). According to reports, some clinicians in the past even went so far as to advise that transgender people give up their custodial and parental rights if they intend to pursue gender transition (Pyne et al., 2015). Innovations in clinical practice with transgender people and their family have occurred over the past several decades, and this more affirmative approach to counseling practice with trans people and their families has also been accompanied by an expanding literature featuring narratives from trans families and their members as well as guidance on how to provide ethical and competent therapeutic services for these communities (e.g., Dworkin & Pope, 2012; Goldberg & Allen, 2013; Howey & Samuels, 2000; Hubbard & Whitley, 2012; Kalmus & Kalmus, 2017; Lev, 2004).

Of course, providing ethical and competent care requires expanding far beyond the minimum base criteria of being welcoming and affirming; competent care today must be aware of (and responsive to) the actual needs of trans people and their families, as revealed through research and empirical evidence, and equipped to provide tools and skills to address the challenges they face (Goldberg & Allen, 2013). Research focusing on factors associated with positive family functioning suggests that clinicians would do well to focus on addressing boundary and social role ambiguity in the context of families with a transitioning parent, particularly focusing on family member feelings of grief or loss surrounding another family member's transition (Veldorale-Griffin & Darling, 2016).

## Family Theory, Limitations of Existing Research, and Directions for Future Research

In recent years, there has been an upsurge of empirical research on trans families; however, there is still much left to be explored. In this chapter, we have reported on literature spanning across a number of theoretical traditions. For example, contributions to the literature on transgender-parent families discussed in this chapter have drawn upon and expanded: family resilience theory, family stress theory, family sys-

tems theory, feminist theory, critical theory, and stage theory. This is a remarkable cross-section of both traditional and more contemporary strands of theory that speaks to the diffusion and diversity of scholarship on transgender-parent families across multiple fields, disciplines, and areas of practice.

Despite these promising trends, there remains much work left to do. As noted previously, increased efforts to collect data on gender identity would help researchers to produce a more comprehensive picture of what trans families look like and the general demographic makeup of trans parents specifically. The General Social Survey will soon begin using a two-step method for assessing research participants' current gender identity and the sex to which they were assigned at birth (Smith, Davern, Freese, & Morgan, 2019). This is exciting news for researchers studying families.

Collecting this information in a large-scale, nationally representative survey will allow researchers to learn much more about transgender respondents and their families than was previously possible. Current findings suggest that trans family outcomes may differ by other relevant demographics such as race/ethnicity, cohort, socioeconomic status, and gender. While it has been difficult to understand how intersecting identities impact trans families and their outcomes, gathering more comprehensive data on trans identities will enable further investigation of these important questions.

Further, much of the current literature utilizes qualitative methods with relatively small and non-diverse samples. Future research should focus on obtaining samples across a broader cross-section of geographic regions, socioeconomic status, and racial/ethnic groups. Qualitative research surely provides in-depth interview data and detailed understanding of the nuances of specific aspects of some trans families. Because trans parents are a unique subset of the larger transgender population and may be faced with distinct interpersonal and systemic strengths and challenges (Pyne et al., 2015), the lack of larger sample sizes is not surprising. However, with the creation of transgender population estimates and parameters, along with the advent of large-scale and nationally representative surveys including two-step questions addressing participants' sex assigned at birth and current gender identity, quantitative research may be able to provide information about trans families and their members that is more broadly representative.

In much of the existing literature, lesbian, gay, bisexual, and transgender individuals are often lumped together without acknowledging that experiences of parenting may be substantially different for members of each of these groups. While society has become more accepting of lesbian and gay parents, awareness and acceptance or transgender parents have been much more halting. Because transgender identity is still largely misunderstood and pathologized by the general public, this extends into views on parenting. In the future, researchers should be mindful of these issues and focus on more balanced recruitment (and perhaps oversampling) of transgender individuals in these studies. Further, we need more research on the various and diverse configurations of transgender-parent families themselves; far too often, research has focused on largely White, highly educated, middle-class samples.

Care should also be taken to research the experiences not only of self-identified transgender parents but of gender-nonconforming parents as well, a group that may face particular scrutiny given social discomfort with gender ambiguity and liminality. Children may face intrusive questions, from other children or even adults, about a trans parent's gender or social role in their lives due to others' unfamiliarity or discomfort with gender nonbinaries (e.g., not understanding parental roles other than "mom" or "dad" or demanding to know if a parent is a "boy/man" or "girl/woman"). If we consider that research interviews are always interventional, it may be useful to ask cisgender parents and their children to reflect on their understandings of transgender and gender-nonbinary individuals and families in their lives and communities.

Doing so may provoke contemplation and engagement that stimulates consideration of additional gender possibilities or of the absence of particular forms of individual and family diversity in their communities or personal awareness. It also begins to shift the burden for eradicating transphobia and ignorance around transgender issues from those most personally affected and targeted by it to those most likely to engage in and perpetuate it. Longitudinal research on trans-parent families, and on the experiences of children in trans-parent families, is also sorely needed. As trans-parent families continue to grow in number and visibility, researchers will continuously need to examine their own assumptions and to ground their findings in the shifting social contexts shaping these families and their members.

---

# References

Augustine, J. M., Aveldanes, J. M., & Pfeffer, C. A. (2017). Are the parents alright? Time in self-care in same-sex and different-sex two-parent families with children. *Population Review, 56,* 49–77. https://doi.org/10.1353/prv.2017.0007

Beatie, T. (2008). *Labor of love: The story of one man's extraordinary pregnancy.* New York, NY: Avalon.

Biblarz, T. J., & Savci, E. (2010). Lesbian, gay, bisexual, and transgender families. *Journal of Marriage and Family, 72,* 480–497. https://doi.org/10.1111/j.1741-3737.2010.00714.x

Cahill, S., & Tobias, S. (2006). *Policy issues affecting lesbian, gay, bisexual, and transgender families.* Ann Arbor, MI: University of Michigan Press.

Cahill, S., Wang, T., & Jenkins, B. (2019). *Trump Administration continued to advance discriminatory policies and practices against LGBT people and people living with HIV in 2018.* Boston, MA: The Fenway Institute.

Chiland, C., Clouet, A.-M., Golse, B., Guinot, M., & Wolf, J. P. (2013). A new type of family: A 12-year follow-up exploratory study of their children. *Neuropsychiatrie de l' Adolescence, 61,* 365–370. https://doi.org/10.1016/j.neurenf.2013.07.001

Church, H. A., O'Shea, D., & Lucey, J. V. (2014). Parent-child relationships in gender identity disorder. *Irish Journal of Medical Science, 183,* 277–281. https://doi.org/10.1007/s11845-013-1003-1

Clarke, V. (2002). Sameness and difference in research on lesbian parenting. *Journal of Community & Applied Social Psychology, 12,* 210–222. https://doi.org/10.1002/casp.673

Clarke, V., & Demetriou, E. (2016). 'Not a big deal'? Exploring the accounts of adult children of lesbian, gay and trans parents. *Psychology & Sexuality, 7,* 131–148. https://doi.org/10.1080/19419899.2015.1110195

Crissman, H. P., Berger, M. B., Graham, L. F., & Dalton, V. K. (2017). Transgender demographics: A household probability sample of US adults, 2014. *American Journal of Public Health, 107*, 213–215. https://doi.org/10.2105/AJPH.2016.303571

dickey, l. m., Ducheny, K. M., & Ehrbar, R. D. (2016). Family creation options for transgender and gender nonconforming people. *Psychology of Sexual Orientation and Gender Diversity, 3*, 173–179. https://doi.org/10.1037/sgd0000178

Dierckx, M., Mortelmans, D., Motmans, J., & T'Sjoen, G. (2017). Resilience in families in transition: What happens when a parent is transgender? *Family Relations, 66*, 399–411. https://doi.org/10.1111/fare.12282

Dierckx, M., & Platero, R. L. (2018). The meaning of trans* in a family context. *Critical Social Policy, 38*, 79–98. https://doi.org/10.1177/0261018317731953

Dworkin, S. H., & Pope, M. (Eds.). (2012). *Casebook for counseling lesbian, gay, bisexual, and transgender persons and their families*. Alexandria, VA: American Counseling Association.

Dziengel, L. (2015). A be/coming-out model: Assessing factors of resilience and ambiguity. *Journal of Gay & Lesbian Social Services, 27*, 302–325. https://doi.org/10.1080/10538720.2015.1053656

Ellis, S. A., Wojnar, D. M., & Pettinato, M. (2014). Conception, pregnancy, and birth experiences of male and gender variant gestational parents: It's how we could have a family. *Journal of Midwifery and Women's Health, 60*, 62–69. https://doi.org/10.1111/jmwh.12213

Erich, S., Tittsworth, J., Dykes, J., & Cabuses, C. (2008). Family relationships and their correlations with transsexual well-being. *Journal of GLBT Family Studies, 4*, 419–432. https://doi.org/10.1080/15504280802126141

Faccio, E., Bordin, E., & Cipolletta, S. (2013). Transsexual parenthood and new role assumptions. *Culture, Health, & Sexuality, 15*, 1055–1070. https://doi.org/10.1080/13691058.2013.806676

Flores, A. R., Herman, J. L., Gates, G. J., & Brown, T. N. T. (2016). *How many adults identify as transgender in the United States?* Los Angeles, CA: The Williams Institute.

Freedman, D., Tasker, F., & di Ceglie, D. (2002). Children and adolescents with transsexual parents referred to a specialist gender identity development service: A brief report of key developmental features. *Clinical Child Psychology and Psychiatry, 7*, 423–432. https://doi.org/10.1177/1359104502007003009

Goldberg, A. E., & Allen, K. R. (Eds.). (2013). *LGBT-parent families: Innovations in research and implications for practice*. New York, NY: Springer.

Grant, J. M., Mottet, L. A., Tanis, J., Harrison, J., Herman, J. L., & Keisling, M. (2011). *Injustice at every turn: A report of the National Transgender Discrimination Survey*. Washington, DC: National Center for Transgender Equality and National Gay and Lesbian Task Force.

Green, R. (1978). Sexual identity of 37 children raised by homosexual or transsexual parents. *The American Journal of Psychiatry, 135*, 692–697. https://doi.org/10.1176/ajp.135.6.692

Green, R. (1998). Transsexuals' children. *International Journal of Transgenderism, 2*, https://www.acthe.fr/upload/1445876170-green-r-1998-transsexuals-s-children.pdf

Haines, B. A., Ajayi, A. A., & Boyd, H. (2014). Making trans parents visible: Intersectionality of trans and parenting identities. *Feminism & Psychology, 24*, 238–247. https://doi.org/10.1177/0959353514526219

Hines, S. (2006). Intimate transitions: Transgender practices of partnering and parenting. *Sociology, 40*, 353–371. https://doi.org/10.1177/0038038506062037

Howey, N., & Samuels, E. (2000). *Out of the ordinary: Essays on growing up with gay, lesbian, and transgender parents*. New York, NY: Stonewall Inn Editions.

Hubbard, E. A., & Whitley, C. T. (Eds.). (2012). *Trans-kin: A guide for families and friends of transgender people*. Boulder, CO: Boulder Press.

Huynh, Q.-L., Nguyen, A.-M. T. D., & Benet-Martínez, V. (2011). Bicultural identity integration. In S. J. Schwartz, K. Luyckx, & V. L. Vignoles (Eds.), *Handbook of identity theory and research* (pp. 827–842). New York, NY: Springer.

Israel, G. E. (2005). Translove. *Journal of GLBT Family Studies, 1*, 53–67. https://doi.org/10.1300/J461v01n01_05

James-Abra, S., Tarasoff, L. A., green, d., Epstein, R., Anderson, S., Marvel, S., … Ross, L. E. (2015). Trans people's experiences with assisted reproduction services: A qualitative study. *Human Reproduction, 30*, 1365–1374. https://doi.org/10.1093/humrep/dev087

Kalmus, S., & Kalmus, C. (Eds.). (2017). *Queer families: An LGBTQ+ true stories anthology*. Lanesborough, MA: Qommunity LLC.

Lev, A. I. (2004). *Transgender emergence: Therapeutic guidelines for working with gender-variant people and their families*. New York, NY: Haworth Clinical Practice Press.

Levi, J. L., & Monnin-Browder, E. E. (Eds.). (2012). *Transgender family law: A guide to effective advocacy*. Bloomington, IN: AuthorHouse.

Light, A. D., Obedin-Maliver, J., Sevelius, J. M., & Kerns, J. L. (2014). Transgender men who experienced pregnancy after female-to-male gender transitioning. *Obstetrics and Gynecology, 124*, 1120–1127. https://doi.org/10.1097/AOG.0000000000000540

Macdonald, T. (2016). *Where's the mother? Stories from a transgender dad*. Dugald, MB: Trans Canada Press.

MacDonald, T., Noel-Weiss, J., West, D., Walks, M., Biener, M. L., Kibbe, A., & Myler, E. (2016). Transmasculine individuals' experiences with lactation, chestfeeding, and gender identity: A qualitative study. *BMC Pregnancy and Childbirth, 16*, 106–122. https://doi.org/10.1186/s12884-016-0907-y

Mamo, L., & Alston-Stepnitz, E. (2015). Queer intimacies and structural inequalities: New directions in stratified reproduction. *Journal of Family Issues, 36*, 519–540. https://doi.org/10.1177/0192513X14563796

Meier, S. C., & Labuski, C. M. (2013). The demographics of the transgender population. In A. Baumle (Ed.), *International handbook on the demography of sexuality* (pp. 289–327). New York, NY: Springer.

More, S. D. (1998). The pregnant man—An oxymoron? *Journal of Gender Studies, 7*, 319–328. https://doi.org /10.1080/09589236.1998.9960725

Murphy, T. F. (2010). The ethics of helping transgender men and women have children. *Perspectives in Biology and Medicine, 53*, 46–60. https://doi.org/10.1353/ pbm.0.0138

Murphy, T. F. (2012). The ethics of fertility preservation in transgender body modifications. *Bioethical Inquiry, 9*, 311–316. https://doi.org/10.1007/s11673-012-9378-7

Murphy, T. F. (2015). Assisted gestation and transgender women. *Bioethics, 29*, 389–397. https://doi. org/10.1111/bioe.12132

Obedin-Maliver, J., & Makadon, H. J. (2016). Transgender men and pregnancy. *Obstetric Medicine, 9*, 4–8. https://doi.org/10.1177/1753495X15612658

Petit, M.-P., Julien, D., & Chamberland, L. (2017). Negotiating parental designations among trans parents' families: An ecological model of parental identity. *Psychology of Sexual Orientation and Gender Diversity, 4*, 282–295. https://doi.org/10.1037/sgd0000231

Pfeffer, C. A. (2010). "Women's work"? Women partners of transgender men doing housework and emotion work. *Journal of Marriage and Family, 72*, 165–183. https://doi.org/10.1111/j.1741-3737.2009.00690.x

Pfeffer, C. A. (2014). "I don't like passing as a straight woman.": Queer negotiations of identity and social group membership. *American Journal of Sociology, 120*, 1–44. https://doi.org/10.1086/677197

Pfeffer, C. A. (2017). *Queering families: The postmodern partnerships of cisgender women and transgender men*. New York, NY: Oxford University Press.

Pfeffer, C. A., & Castañeda, N. N. (2018). Trans and gender variant individuals and couples: Risk factors for relationship dissatisfaction, conflict, and divorce. In A. E. Goldberg & A. Romero (Eds.), *LGBTQ divorce and relationship dissolution: Psychological and legal perspectives and implications for practice* (pp. 287–311). New York, NY: Oxford University Press.

Power, J., Brown, R., Schofield, M. J., Pitts, M., McNair, R., Perlesz, A., & Bickerdike, A. (2014). Social connectedness among lesbian, gay, bisexual, and transgender parents living in metropolitan and regional and rural areas of Australia and New Zealand. *Journal of Community Psychology, 42*, 869–889. https://doi. org/10.1186/1471-2458-10-115

Pyne, J. (2012). *Transforming family: Trans parents and their struggles, strategies, and strengths*. Toronto, ON: LGBTQ Network, Sherbourne Health Clinic.

Pyne, J., Bauer, J., & Bradley, K. (2015). Transphobia and other stressors impacting trans parents. *Journal of GLBT Family Studies, 11*, 107–126. https://doi.org/10 .1080/1550428X.2014.941127

Riggs, D. W. (2013). Transgender men's self-representations of bearing children post-transition. In F. J. Green & M. Friedman (Eds.), *Chasing rainbows: Exploring gender fluid parenting practices* (pp. 62–71). Toronto, ON: Demeter Press.

Ryan, M. (2009). Beyond Thomas Beatie: Trans men and the new parenthood. In R. Epstein (Ed.), *Who's your daddy? And other writings on queer parenting* (pp. 139–150). Toronto, ON: Sumach Press.

Sabatello, M. (2011). Advancing transgender family rights through science: A proposal for an alternative framework. *Human Rights Quarterly, 33*, 43–75. https://www.jstor.org/stable/23015980

Smith, T. W., Davern, M., Freese, J., & Morgan, S. L. (2019). *General Social Surveys, 1972–2018.* [machine-readable data file]. Principal Investigator, T. W. Smith; Co-Principal Investigators, M. Davern, J. Freese, & S. L. Morgan, NORC ed. Chicago, IL: NORC at the University of Chicago.

Stotzer, R. L., Herman, J. L., & Hasenbush, A. (2014). *Transgender parenting: A review of existing research.* Los Angeles, CA: The Williams Institute.

Tabor, J. (2018). Mom, dad, or somewhere in between: Role-relational ambiguity and children of transgender parents. *Journal of Marriage and Family.* https://doi. org/10.1111/jomf.12537

Tornello, S. L., & Bos, H. (2017). Parenting intentions among transgender individuals. *LGBT Health, 4*, 115–120. https://doi.org/10.1089/lgbt.2016.0153

Veldorale-Griffin, A. (2014). Transgender parents and their adult children's experiences of disclosure and transition. *Journal of GLBT Family Studies, 10*, 475–501. https://doi.org/10.1080/1550428X.2013.866063

Veldorale-Griffin, A., & Darling, C. A. (2016). Adaptation to parental gender transition: Stress and resilience among transgender parents. *Archives of Sexual Behavior, 45*, 607–617. https://doi.org/10.1007/ s10508-015-0657-3

von Doussa, H., Power, J., & Riggs, D. (2015). Imagining parenthood: The possibilities and experiences of parenthood among transgender people. *Culture, Health and Sexuality, 17*, 1119–1131. https://doi.org/10.1080 /13691058.2015.1042919

White, T., & Ettner, R. (2004). Disclosure, risks and protective factors for children whose parents are undergoing a gender transition. *Journal of Gay & Lesbian Psychotherapy, 8*, 129–145. https://doi.org/10.1080/1 9359705.2004.9962371

White, T., & Ettner, R. (2007). Adaptation and adjustment in children of transsexual parents. *European Child and Adolescent Psychiatry, 16*, 215–221. https://doi. org/10.1007/s00787-006-0591-y

Wierckx, K., Van Caenegem, E., Pennings, G., Elaut, E., Dedecker, D., Van De Peer, F., … T'Sjoen, G. (2012). Reproductive wish in transsexual men. *Human Reproduction, 27*, 483–487. https://doi.org/10.1093/ humrep/der406

# Religion in the Lives of LGBTQ-Parent Families

Katie L. Acosta

## LGBTQ Individuals and Religion

Many individuals raised in religious communities are taught that same-sex desire is a sin for which they must seek forgiveness. These teachings can create identity conflict in the lives of LGBTQ youth. In a keynote address at the American Humanist Association, Gavin Grimm, a transgender teenager who sued his school system for the right to use the boys' bathroom, shared his personal struggle growing up in a deeply religious, Southern Baptist family. Despite his best efforts to connect with religious doctrine, Gavin was alienated, traumatized, and, at times, suicidal (Grimm, 2018). Gavin's negative experiences are consistent with Pew Research Center data on religious affiliations and opinions on LGBTQ rights. Pew data revealed that 69% of White evangelicals believe that transgender people should be required to use the restroom consistent with the sex assigned to them at birth and 77% believe that employers should not be required to provide wedding services to same-sex couples (Pew Research Center, 2017). However, not all religiously affiliated individuals share these beliefs. For instance, only 50% of Catholics believe that transgender people should use the

restroom consistent with the sex assigned to them at birth, and even fewer Jews (24%) share this belief (Pew Research Center, 2017).

Regardless of religious affiliation, for those who are raised with negative messages about same-sex desire and/or gender nonconformity, reconciling the conflict between religious and sexual identities can be a lifelong journey. In a study of 174 LGB youth between the ages of 14 and 24, Page, Lindahl, and Malik (2013) found that participating in unsupportive religious systems is associated with internalized homophobia and difficulty accepting sexual identity. One study of Christian, gay, Puerto Rican youth found respondents often left religion in young adulthood but retained a belief in God's love for them (Fankhanel, 2010). Another study of gays and lesbians who attended a Catholic college found that students who created bonds with others who shared their religious and sexual identities were successful at achieving identity integration (Wedow, Schnabel, Wedow, & Konieczny, 2017). However, students who did not create bonds with like others rejected either their religious or sexual identities or became disillusioned with both.

Individuals who are unable to resolve the tensions between their sexual and religious identities may find this conflict adversely affects their mental health in adulthood. One study found that highly religious Latino men who reported sex with men and cisgender and transgender women held high levels of homonegativity and antigay

K. L. Acosta (✉)
Georgia State University, Langdale Hall,
Atlanta, GA, USA
e-mail: kacosta@gsu.edu

sentiment (Severson, Muñoz-Laboy, & Kaufman, 2014). These men attended church regularly but harbored internalized homophobia, which limited their self-acceptance. Another study found that the homonegative religious messages that young Black men who have sex with men received ultimately impacted their ability to develop healthy sexual relationships in adulthood (Quinn & Dickson-Gomez, 2016).

In a study of individuals between the ages of 21 and 30 who experienced non-affirming religious upbringings in either Protestant or Pentecostal churches, Ganzevoort, Van der Laan, and Olsman (2011) found that some chose between their sexual and religious identities; others allowed both identities to coexist in a mutually exclusive, parallel manner, and still others found ways of integrating both identities. Importantly, Ganzevoort et al. (2011) found that the path one takes to reconcile the conflict between religion and sexuality need not be permanent. Individuals may fluctuate across the different coping mechanisms at different points in their lives.

While much of the existing research has found that LGBTQ individuals separate their religious lives from their lives as sexual beings, identity integration may better describe how these individuals resolved this conflict at other points in their lives. In adulthood, individuals who are successful at reconciling their sexual identities with religious teachings adopt a variety of strategies. One study of Orthodox Jews and conservative Christians found that respondents reinterpreted scripture by questioning the authority of its authors, the scriptural translation, or the literal meaning of the text itself (Etengoff & Rodriguez, 2017). As an alternative, some critiqued other believers for applying a literal interpretation of scripture to only select passages which are non-affirming and promote homophobia.

The above-cited scholarship on LGBTQ individuals and religion has relied on stigma management theories (Quinn & Dickson-Gomez, 2016; Wedow et al., 2017). This work has considered stigma stemming from homonegativity within religious spaces and its impact on LGBTQ individuals' mental health. Interestingly, research

has also considered how religion can play an essential role in helping LGBTQ individuals cope with stigma from other social institutions (Battle & DeFreece, 2014; Gattis, Woodford, & Han, 2014). This theoretical inquiry often adopts an intersectional approach allowing scholars to consider how race and sexuality complicate people of color's experiences with religion. The racial solidarity that many LGBTQ people of color receive from their faith communities is coupled with the possible alienation on account of their sexual orientation.

Aware of the trauma that religion has caused many LGBTQ individuals, some religious traditions have intentionally set out to offer a more inclusive environment. In the next section, I offer a historical background of the approaches that religious denominations have taken to foster inclusivity of LGBTQ individuals. This is followed by an overview of research on public attitudes toward LGBTQ-parent families, a section on what motivates LGBTQ parents to seek out religion, and another on gender-nonconforming individuals' experiences in religious spaces. I conclude this chapter with some suggestions for future research and implications for practice.

## Religious Denomination's Approaches to LGBTQ Inclusion

In the United States, several religious faith traditions have prioritized inclusivity and full participation for LGBTQ individuals. The United Church of Christ (UCC) has a long history of LGBTQ inclusivity, dating back to the 1970s when they began ordaining gay leaders. In 1985, the UCC began actively encouraging its congregations to welcome LGBTQ individuals and developed an open and affirming program to guide interested congregations in this process (Pettis, 2004). In 2003, The UCC passed a resolution in support of transgender persons (United Church of Christ, 2003), and in 2006, they passed a resolution in support of same-sex marriages (Norris, 2005). The UCC's support of same-sex marriages caused divisions among some churches, ultimately leading to more than 70 churches leaving the denomination. Still, the UCC maintained its role as a leader in advocating for LGBTQ rights. In 2011, the UCC went on to pass a resolution in support of LGBTQ parents' right to adopt and raise children (Rudolph, 2011).

The Episcopal Church has also had a long history of welcoming LGBTQ individuals. For much of the 1970s and 1980s, the Episcopal Church officially rejected homosexuality but refused to discipline individual churches that took a more inclusive approach (Hill & Watson, 2006). Since the 1970s, bishops have been ordaining gays and lesbians into the priesthood, despite the Episcopal Church's official refusal of this practice. Ellen Marie Barrett, for instance, an out lesbian and avid spokesperson for gay and lesbian rights, was ordained into the priesthood in 1977. Before her, Carter Heyward was one of the first women ever ordained in 1974. She later came out as a lesbian in 1980. These practices reflected the larger division among Episcopalian leadership on same-sex relationships and the issue of ordaining gay and lesbian priests. In 2000, the Episcopal Church passed legislation allowing individual churches to offer blessings to same-sex committed relationships. In 2003, the Episcopal Church received much publicity for ordaining V. Gene Robinson, its first openly gay bishop. In 2018, at its General Convention, the Episcopal Church allows all priests to perform same-sex marriage rites. Christian Century. 15 Aug 2018.

The Metropolitan Community Church (MCC) emerged from its inception as a home for LGBTQ individuals. It has grown to include congregations in more than 20 countries and remains a majority LGBTQ congregation. Some MCC members have found the church offered a space where their sexual and religious identities were salient simultaneously (Rodriguez & Ouellette, 2000). Still, some LGBTQ people have found the religious teachings of the MCC—that centers God's love and acceptance of LGBTQ peoples— compromise some of the religious teachings from their faiths of origin. For instance, in a study on religious experiences among LGBTQ Christians, Hickey and Grafsky (2017) quoted a participant, Liz, as saying:

I've found with some groups that are kind of gay Christian groups, the focus is "we are gay." I want to have gay friends who are Christian, but if we meet together I want to talk about Jesus, about the Bible, about what we can do in the community. I don't want to talk about the fact that we are gay, about how gay people are oppressed. Not because I don't believe it is an issue, but because it is not what I want to be doing at church. (p. 90)

At its inception, MCC's focus on reaffirming God's love for LGBTQ people was essential given the emotional trauma that LGBTQ individuals had endured from other religious traditions. However, in some MCCs the message did not grow beyond affirming God's love even as its followers became more confident in God's love for them (Hartman, 1996). This led some LGBTQ individuals to instead seek to grow in their faith with other religious traditions that focused more on scripture.

Some branches of Judaism have also made efforts toward the inclusion of LGBTQ individuals. There are four branches of Judaism: Orthodox, Conservative, Reform, and Reconstructionist. The latter two have been the most inclusive of LGBTQ individuals in their families. The Reform movement has the longest history of supporting LGBTQ Jews with LGBTQ Reform Synagogues dating back to the early 1970s. The newest branch of Judaism, the Reconstructionist, has fully integrated LGBTQ members and their families (Barrow, 2016).

These traditions, and others, have intentionally made efforts to help LGBTQ individuals maintain or develop a religious identity. Still, other religious faiths have taken a different approach. For instance, The Church of Jesus Christ of Latter-day Saints has had a long tradition of opposing LGBTQ-parent families. After the *Obergefell v. Hodges* (6th Cir., 2015) decision in the United States, the Church of Jesus Christ clarified its position on LGBTQ families. The Church declared those who experience same-sex attraction (a term Latter-day Saints use to differentiate those who experience but do not act on same-sex desires from those who adopt a LGBQ identity) could participate fully in all church rituals and hold leadership positions as long as they abstained from sexual relations with someone of the same sex, same-sex marriage, or raising children within LGBTQ families. Those unable to abstain from these practices face the possibility of excommunication which would sever their ties to eternal salvation (Nielson, 2016).

We know very little about the experiences of LGBTQ parents who desire to raise their children in faith traditions with varying levels of inclusion. This absence is important because research suggests that becoming parents often motivates those who have left religious spaces in adolescence or young adulthood to return (Gurrentz, 2017). Moreover, research suggests that religious return is particularly important for single parents who may be most in need of the fellowship and community religious spaces offer (Uecker, Mayrl, & Stroope, 2016). Next, I explore how religiosity shapes public attitudes on LGBT parent families.

## Public Attitudes of LGBTQ-Parent Families

LGBTQ-parent families' involvement in organized religion may be contingent upon the validation they experience from congregation members. However, congregants' perceptions of LGBTQ-parent families are contingent in part on their perceptions of what makes people non-heterosexual. In a mixed-method study that offers a nuanced account of the public's opinions on who constitutes a family, Powell, Bolzendahl, Geist, and Steelman (2010) found that people who believe sexual orientation is outside of one's control (i.e., that some people are gay, lesbian, or bisexual because God made them that way) are more likely to see a lesbian couple raising children together as a legitimate family than are those who attribute sexual orientation to environmental or individual factors that are within their control. Powell et al. did not offer data on the public's perceptions of other LGBTQ-parent families which are not led by lesbian parents, but other studies suggest people's perceptions of LGBTQ-parent families vary based on their level of religiosity, how these families are formed, and who leads these families. In a study of Catholics' per-

ceptions of same-sex parents, Gross, Vecho, Gratton, D'Amore, and Green (2018) found a hierarchy in their support based primarily on the method these couples use to expand their families. Gross et al.'s respondents viewed same-sex, two-parent families formed after adoption more favorably than those formed via surrogacy or single adoptions. Catholics' views on assisted reproductive technologies fall in the middle of this hierarchy. Gross and colleagues were not able to address why Catholics held a hierarchy of favorability of same-sex parent families, but it is plausible that they viewed same-sex parents who adopt children more favorably because they associated this practice as consistent with their religious humanitarian values, whereas these same Catholics may have viewed assisted reproductive technology as selfish or inconsistent with their humanitarian values.

Whitehead (2018) also conducted a study on Catholic's perceptions of same-sex parents, which distinguished between the religious beliefs and behaviors of Catholic individuals. Whitehead found those who attended church services regularly, prayed often, and viewed the Bible as the literal word of God were more likely to harbor negative attitudes toward same-sex parents, whereas those Catholics who viewed the Bible as a book of fables were most accepting of same-sex parents.

It is unclear how much religious individuals' support for same-sex parents translates into their intentional efforts to create an inclusive space for LGBTQ-parent families in their religious communities. Next, I review the existing research on this topic.

## Tolerance and Silence in Religious Spaces

Despite the examples of some religious institutions prioritizing affirmation for LGBTQ-parent families, many religious institutions have adopted an approach of tolerance or silence rather than one of affirmation. Some religious spaces have promoted the tolerant approach by welcoming LGBTQ individuals as members but not allowing them to participate in leadership roles (Froese, 2016; Wedow et al., 2017). Rather than offering affirmation and validation of LGBTQ individuals and their families, the tolerant approach expects LGBTQ individuals to worship among other believers while also minimizing their potential influence on the rest of the congregation. While the intent of this approach has been to foster an environment of tolerance, it is also a form of alienation. Rostosky, Otis, Riggle, Kelly, and Brodnicki (2008), for example, conducted a qualitative study of how same-sex couples incorporate religiosity into their relationships and found that gay, lesbian, and bisexual couples sought a place where they could worship together and where their active involvement would be welcomed. Allowing LGB individuals to serve in leadership roles is essential to their sense of acceptance. For them, tolerance is not enough.

The Church of Jesus Christ of Latter-day Saints is one example of a religious tradition that limits the participation of LGBTQ-parent families. Supporters pointed to the Church of Jesus Christs' intentional efforts to teach their members, through trainings and ministry, about the unique struggles that LGBTQ Mormons face and about their obligation, as Latter-day Saints, to treat these individuals with love, compassion, and sensitivity (Nielson, 2017). LGBTQ individuals and families who have remained connected with the Church of Jesus Christ have found solace in the belief that God wants them to remain in the Church so that they can offer support for other LDS families who are negatively affected by the Church's position on LGBTQ individuals and their families. Interactions with LGBTQ individuals who have remained a part of the Church of Jesus Christ may prove instrumental in helping LDS parents with LGBTQ offspring in gaining a better understanding of and acceptance for their children and their children's partners (Nielson, 2017). Research has suggested that while very few LGBTQ individuals raised in the Church of Jesus Christ were met with unconditional affirmation from their parents after coming out, those who did reported affirming family members had prior contact (as neighbors or coworkers) with other LGBTQ individuals

(Mattingly, Galligher, Dehlin, Crowell, & Bradshaw, 2016). Comparatively, those who were met with hostility or familial avoidance reported their parents had little information about or past connections with other LGBTQ people (Mattingly et al., 2016).

In my research study based on 42 interviews with sexually nonconforming Latinas, I found respondents wanted to maintain a fulfilling relationship with their higher power while also being loved within their religious spaces as lesbian, bisexual, or queer individuals (Acosta, 2013). While most of the study respondents were not parents, many intended to become parents and craved a religious environment that would nurture that intended family. They wanted authenticity within religious spaces where people would see and validate their families and love them unconditionally (Acosta, 2013). They recognized the limitations of the church's acceptance of them but nonetheless accommodated the church's limitations (Acosta, 2013). My work suggested that LBQ Latinas were confident in God's love for them and sought a religious community where their relationship with God and their families could be fortified and empowered. Unfortunately, my respondents were mostly unsuccessful in finding such a religious space, and those who remained committed to their religions of origin mostly settled for environments that were tolerant of their families rather than environments where their families were celebrated.

For LGBTQ-parent families of color, participating in one's religious institutions of origin is often about remaining connected to racial/ethnic community, culture, and historic roots. Some families experience their participation in these tolerant but not affirming religious spaces as radical acts. In a reflective chapter on religion and marriage equality, sociologist Mignon Moore (2018) wrote about her family's experience participating in her church of origin—the church that her grandparents helped found and where her uncle was pastor. The church is part of a Black Pentecostal tradition that rejects homosexuality and does not believe same-sex families are God's will. Of participating in this space, Moore wrote:

I believe the visible participation of our little LGBT parent family in this storefront Holiness church in Queens, New York, is radical, even revolutionary behavior. Every time, I walk through those doors I am making myself vulnerable while I silently bring my full self to the altar. (p. 77)

Moore's account foregrounds her participation in this church as resistance but perhaps not affirmation.

Moore (2011) addresses the tension between tolerant and affirming religious spaces in greater depth in her empirical work. Moore conducted participant observation, focus groups, a mail-in survey with 100 respondents, and in-depth interviews with 58 Black, gay mothers and/or their partners. Moore found that Black gay mothers gravitated toward churches that were either tolerant of or remained silent about homosexuality. They rationalized their continued involvement in these religious spaces by asserting that they were God's children, even if their same-sex relationships were sinful. While these spaces were not openly accepting of their families, Moore noted that gay Black mothers preferred them, because, unlike gay-affirming churches, churches tolerant of or silent about same-sex relationships offered them the scripture, religious doctrine, and worship experience that they had grown accustomed to.

Christian traditions that take a silent approach to their LGBTQ members are not hostile but rather practice tacit avoidance. While the silent approach is more commonly associated with predominantly heterosexual congregations, these practices also occur in predominantly LGBTQ congregations. For instance, McQueeney (2009) conducted participant observation and interviews with members from two Southern Protestant churches. In Faith Church, a small predominantly Black working-class, mostly lesbian congregation, McQueeny found that Black lesbians attended services with their partners but did not openly name their same-sex relationships out of respect for their church communities. Instead, they minimized their sexuality by separating their sexual and religious identities. Faith Church's pastor, McQueeny noted, emphasized the congregations' Christian identity over their sexual iden-

tities, viewing the latter as secondary to their relationship with God. This, McQueeny argued, was a strategy used to legitimate Faith Church within the larger Protestant denomination.

While many LGBTQ-parent families are content with religious spaces that are tolerant of or silent on their sexualities, there are important limitations to these spaces. For instance, research has suggested that some LGBTQ parents wanted to participate in religious communities in part so that their children could potentially meet other LGBTQ-parent families (Holman & Oswald, 2011). For these parents, the visibility of other LGBTQ-parent families in affirming religious spaces was crucial to fostering their sense of belonging. When LGBTQ-parent families and individuals are not visible within their religious congregations, others may not be aware of their presence, which leaves their needs for connection unmet. In an oral history project entitled *Black. Queer. Southern. Women.*, E. Patrick Johnson (2018) captured how one Black woman experienced this limitation. Vanessa, an active member of a United Methodist Church in the Austin, Texas area, noted:

[T]here's some people that even though it's a downtown church, it's a progressive church, they're still not out. Those of us who are, we're small in number and so it makes it hard. I mean my future wife might be sitting in the next pew and I don't even know it. (p. 214)

One advantage to gay-affirming religious spaces is that, unlike in silent or tolerant religious spaces, members are more likely to be out to their fellow believers.

## What Attracts LGBTQ-Parent Families to Religion?

Regardless of whether religious spaces are gay affirming, tolerant, or silent of LGBTQ families, there has not been much research on their experiences in religious spaces. Research has found that for heterosexual and single individuals, religious return is often prompted by their becoming parents (Gurrentz, 2017; Uecker et al., 2016). Still, scholars are only beginning to explore if raising children have the same or similar impact on religious return for LGBTQ parents, despite their often complex histories with religion in adolescence and young adulthood.

Rostosky, Abreu, Mahoney, and Riggle (2017) found LGBTQ parents utilized religion and spiritual teachings to instill the values of respect, reciprocity, and kindness in their children. The respondents in this study felt compelled to ensure that their children were exposed to a religious foundation so that they would have the opportunity to engage in religious family traditions and to develop a sense of belonging to a community. Nonetheless, these parents were also open with their children about the limitations of religious institutions and helped them critique the flaws in organized religion (Rostosky et al., 2017). Gregory Maguire, a father and children's book author, who was interviewed for an article in *Commonweal* magazine illustrates Rostosky et al.'s findings well. He notes:

> I must share with my children my faith, its dramatic promise and possibilities, its murky history and contradictions, the guidance it can lend, and the challenges it must pose. Andy and I will tell them—when they're old enough –about the courage it took to adopt them in this climate, about the heartache the church from above can sometimes provoke, and the help that the church from below sometimes can provide. (p. 22)

Consistent with this father's explanation, Rostosky et al. found that LGBTQ parents encouraged their children to take a critical approach to their religious involvement. Parents used religious teachings to open a dialogue with their children and ultimately encouraged the children to make their own decisions about the role that religiosity would play in their lives.

McQueeney (2009), who conducted participant observation at two Protestant churches in the South, described one church, Unity, as gay-affirming with a predominantly White middle-class heterosexual congregation. McQueeney found that White lesbian mothers at Unity Church emphasized their role as middle-class parents in monogamous relationships to liken themselves to heterosexual congregants. McQueeney argued their performance of motherhood was motivated by a desire to normalize themselves as good Christians. Interestingly, McQueeny did not observe this performance of motherhood in the other predominantly Black working-class church where she conducted participant observation. Lesbian mothers at Faith Church, unlike those at Unity Church, were single mothers to children conceived in previous heterosexual relationships. Suggesting their different paths to motherhood evoked distinct performances, McQueeny concluded that not all motherhood signaled being a good Christian—only motherhood that occurred within monogamous, committed, intact partnerships that were not formed after a prior relationship dissolution.

Some LGBTQ parents who wanted their children to have a strong religious foundation but were no longer active participants in a religious institution allowed their children to attend religious services with others. Tuthill (2016) conducted interviews with Latina lesbian mothers who were raised in the Catholic Church and were vocal about the hypocrisy that they had encountered there and refuted the priest's authority to banish them to eternal condemnation. These mothers reported not attending church frequently but encouraged their children's regular attendance with grandparents, so that the children might establish a religious routine (Tuthill, 2016). While these mothers refused to attend Catholic Church services regularly, they did engage in prayer rituals, which they saw as an aspect of their spirituality and as nostalgic of their own childhoods. Tuthill found that Latina lesbian mothers were not invested in their children identifying as Catholics in adulthood and instead prioritized their children maintaining a relationship with God regardless of if they ultimately became active in a church in adulthood. These mothers were comfortable in asserting their own religious identities in part because of the religious encouragement they offered their children. This finding echoes previous research on heterosexual mothers, where Gallagher (2007) found that children were a religious resource for mothers and that mothers pointed to their fostering of religiosity among their children as a key practice of their religious identity.

For some LGBTQ-parented families, religious rituals can play an important role in helping to validate LGBTQ-parented families (see chapter "LGBTQ-Parent Families in Community Context"). Participation in religious family traditions can be the primary connection that LGBTQ parents preserve with religious institutions (Oswald, 2001). Oswald, Goldberg, Kuvalanka, and Clausell (2008) conducted a survey of LGBT individuals ($N = 527$) who resided in 38 counties in the state of Illinois and found that same-sex couples who were also parents were more likely to have had commitment ceremonies. Oswald et al. further found that those who had commitment ceremonies were more likely to report religion being an important part of their daily life. Still, only 28% of Oswald et al.'s respondents reported belonging to a supportive congregation, and most respondents in their sample reported not belonging to a congregation at all, suggesting that for some, perhaps religious rituals are an individual pursuit rather than one done within a religious community.

Still, religious ceremonies when performed publicly are an important way to legitimize LGBTQ-parent families, particularly when other institutions do not. One study of gay men who became parents through adoption noted that fathers reported gaining more acceptance and visibility within their churches after becoming parents (Goldberg, 2012). One father attributed the feeling of greater acceptance to their child's baptism within the church. Importantly, some fathers in Goldberg's study did not welcome the additional visibility they gained within their churches. At least one father reported feeling uncomfortable with his increased visibility, noting that since becoming parents, he and his partner no longer blended in with the rest of the congregation. For this dad, attending worship services with only his partner allowed others to see them as individuals, but bringing their child to worship services made them visible to other congregants as a family. This father feared that their families' heightened visibility in the church had become politicized.

Other research on the importance of religious ceremonies for LGBTQ-parent families suggests that the incentives for participating may be about more than a desire for visibility and acceptance. In my research on LBQ Latina parents, one family did not feel safe disclosing their same-sex relationship to the Catholic priest but still arranged to baptize their daughter in the church, because they believed it was necessary for ridding their child of her original sin (Acosta, 2013). For this family, visibility was not the primary goal of the baptism. Rather, they wanted to ensure their daughter did not start her life precluded from heaven after death.

Outside of Catholicism, parents' motivations for participation in public religious rituals can also be about more than visibility. Within Orthodox Judaism in Israel which is the least inclusive branch to LGBTQ congregants, LGB parents find ways to preserve their participation. One ethnographic study of 65 Israeli LGB parents found that even within Orthodox Judaism, bisexual, gay, and lesbian parents still sought access to birth and/or conversion ceremonies for their children, even if they rejected the belief that their children could not legitimately claim a Jewish identity without a conversion ceremony (Lustenberger, 2014). LGB parents, Lustenberger noted, were willing to lie about their relationships to gain access to these ceremonies, because having an Orthodox conversion offered their children future opportunities that they would otherwise be precluded from such as religious permission to marry in Israel. Further, given that Jews have been historically persecuted on account of their religious beliefs, some may feel a sense of responsibility to preserve Judaism in theirs and their children's lives (Barrow & Kuvalanka, 2011). Barrow and Kuvalanka conducted interviews with ten lesbian and bisexual Jewish mothers and found some respondents believed being part of a marginalized religion made it easier for them to accept their identities as sexual minorities. This led to their more seamless identity integration. Barrow and Kuvalanka's respondents also pointed to rabbis as being essential for setting the tone for inclusivity in their synagogues.

In addition to the diverse motivating factors that lead LGBTQ-parent families to remain connected to religious institutions, it is important to consider how children raised in these homes describe their religious involvement. Lytle, Foley, and Aster (2013) found that adult children with one or more gay or lesbian parents reported decreasing their religious participation as they got older. Lytle et al. found adult children became skillful in separating religious doctrine from God and, like their parents, focused on God's love for them despite the lack of acceptance they experienced in the church. They adhered to religious values, but they distanced themselves from organized religion. COLAGE, an organization that offers support and connection to children with LGBTQ parents, produces a newsletter periodically throughout the year featuring youth contributors. In one newsletter, 17-year-old Adam Brown shared his thoughts on religion:

> I have found that spirituality need not be part of a mainstream religion, or even within a group, I believe that faith must be discovered and that the proper faith, and spiritual path will comfort them and make them feel safe, not alienate or make them feel like they need to change. (p. 3)

Adam, much like the children of LGBTQ parents in Lytle et al.'s research, found ways to keep the aspects of religion he deemed useful without being encumbered by the aspects he found harmful. The children of LGBTQ parents share this sentiment in common with those of heterosexual parents. One quantitative study, comparing adult children of same-sex and heterosexual parents, suggested that, much like children raised by heterosexual parents, those raised by same-sex parents recognized the importance of both religion and spirituality and maintained the beliefs they were raised with in adulthood (Richards, Rothblum, Beauchaine, & Balsam, 2017). However, unlike children raised by heterosexual parents, Richards et al. found that most participants with same-sex parents were raised outside of organized religion and, thus, continued to practice spirituality outside of this institution in adulthood. Much like Adam Brown, adult children of same-sex parents recognized that they could be spiritually fulfilled without having to engage in organized religion.

Much like the research on LGBTQ individuals, research on LGBTQ-parent families and reli-gion is informed by several interrelated theoretical approaches: symbolic interactionism, stigma management, identity conflict, and social exchange (Barrow & Kuvalanka, 2011; Fankhanel, 2010; Quinn & Dickson-Gomez, 2016). Given the historical trauma that religious institutions have inflicted on LGBTQ individuals, research has explored the benefits that LGBTQ individuals and families can gain from religion to counteract previous rejection. Largely, this research suggests that LGBTQ-parent families are motivated to participate in religious rituals and ceremonies not out of a desire to assimilate but out of desire for legitimacy, belonging, and access to practices deemed culturally significant. Still, the warm reception one receives from others within a religious space is central to LGBTQ-parent families' continued participation (Barrow & Kuvalanka, 2011). Positive social interactions with religious leaders and fellow congregants differentiate LGBTQ-parent families who actively participate in organized religion from those who instead practice spirituality in their homes. In other words, the benefits that LGBTQ-parent families garner from religious institutions derive from how others receive them in religious spaces, more so than from the doctrine that guides a specific denomination.

## Gender (Non)conformity in Religious Spaces

Regardless of whether religious spaces are tolerant, silent, or affirming, LGBTQ-parent families may struggle to feel welcomed if they are gender nonconforming. For instance, McQueeney (2009) observed in one gay affirming predominantly Black, working-class, lesbian Southern Protestant church that congregants were willing to challenge biblical literalism with regard to same-sex relationships while simultaneously reifying biblical literalism with regard to gender expectations of dress and demeanor. Congregants promoted conventional masculinities for gay men and encouraged ideologies that equated masculinity with leadership. McQueeny attributed this finding to religious leaders' need to affirm their legitimacy within a larger Black, heterosexual, Christian denomination. Even within lesbian relationships, McQueeny found that members promoted gendered, patriarchal, butch-femme relationships. Thus, even though this congregation was supportive of same-sex relationships, it remained inflexible to the subversion of gender roles and gender nonconformity.

While gender conformity remains an important value within many religious traditions, some gender-nonconforming individuals can and do find belonging within these religious spaces. For instance, Johnson's (2008) work chronicled the oral histories of Black, gay men in the South and shed light on their experience in religious spaces. Johnson found that his participants grew up seeing the meaningful roles that effeminate men played in the church choir and viewed religious spaces as socially acceptable venues where flamboyance and drama could be used to serve God.

There is no body of research on gender-nonconforming individuals' relationships with family and religion in adulthood. Still, transgender and/or nonbinary people are becoming more visible within their religious denominations. The UCC, for example, has voiced support for transgender laypersons and clergy (United Church of Christ, 2003). Further, the Reconstructionist branch of Judaism has welcomed transgender rabbis and has developed programs focused on the inclusion of transgender members (Barrow, 2016).

## Directions for Future Research

As this chapter illustrates, the existing research on LGBTQ-parent families and religion has focused largely on Christian faiths and, to a lesser extent, Judaism. The author is not aware of research on LGBTQ-parent families' experiences in religious faiths with smaller congregations in the United States, such as Islam or Buddhism. This absence may be significant as smaller religious faiths may foster greater acceptance for diverse family structures. At least one study, deYoung, Emerson, Yancey, and Kim (2003), has found smaller religious congregations to be more

racially integrated. deYoung et al. conducted participant observation in monoracial and multiracial congregations and found that non-Christian religions in the United States with smaller faith traditions had significantly more racially diverse congregations than did Christian denominations. deYoung et al. rationalized that, unlike Christian faith traditions, Buddhism and Islamic faith traditions could not offer enough worship options for congregants which resulted in more racially integrated services. In contrast, religious traditions with congregations large enough to sustain a plethora of worship opportunities on any given day ultimately became more racially segregated. It is plausible that the same structural limitations that promote racial diversity in Buddhism and Islamic traditions may have a similar effect on family diversity. Buddhism has been largely silent around same-sex relationships. Still, some Buddhist traditions have taken a family-centered approach in their teachings, encouraging long-term, monogamous relationships while also not prescribing that these unions be heterosexual (Yip, 2010b). This religious landscape could potentially foster a community open to family diversity and merits further inquiry.

More work is needed to explore the experiences of LGBTQ Muslims raising children within Islamic faiths. While many predominately Muslim countries have criminalized homosexuality, research suggests Muslim gay men have found ways to remain connected to their religious beliefs (Kamrudin, 2018; Yip, 2010a). One study conducted in the United Kingdom with 17 mostly gay, cisgender Muslim men found that respondents minimized the salience of their sexual identities in order to connect with their religious communities (Yip, 2010a). Other respondents believed strongly that their sexuality and the marginality that emerged from it was a gift from God and fueled their religious conviction. These individuals believed the tensions between their sexual and religious identities furthered their investment in their spiritual journeys. Yip (2010a) found that cisgender gay men did not feel comfortable worshipping in most mosques preferring the safety of their homes. Recognizing the discomfort some LGBTQ Muslims experienced in mosques, a nongovernmental organization in Cape Town, South Africa, created an alternative (Kamrudin, 2018). The People's Mosque is an affirming space for LGBTQ Muslims that does not separate people by gender and seeks to be inclusive of sexual and gender diversity. Given that The People's Mosque is in its infancy, it remains unclear if it will become a worship space that is inclusive of LGBTQ-parent families. It is possible that The People's Mosque will ultimately function in a manner similar to The Metropolitan Community Church in the United States. Such spaces certainly have a place among believers. However, these spaces are limited in their ability to unite believers of diverse sexual orientations and family forms, instead becoming an option that insulates LGBTQ individuals and their families from heterosexual believers.

## Implications for Practice

The existing research on LGBTQ-parent families and religion suggests that many families rely on religion to provide a moral anchor for them and their children but also for building a community of like others. As more religious traditions take steps to make their worship spaces affirming of LGBTQ-parent families, an emphasis should be placed on fostering opportunities for their integration and community building. While some LGBTQ-parent families may choose to attend gay-affirming churches, research suggests that LGBTQ people of color struggle with this option, because they experience religious spaces like The Metropolitan Community Church as diluting religious teachings and focusing primarily on sexuality (Acosta, 2013; Moore, 2011). Some LGBTQ people of color remain grounded in their religions of origin, in part because doing so preserves their connection to their racial/ethnic communities. Irrespective of whether LGBTQ-parent families find religious homes that are affirming, silent, or tolerant, they remain grounded in the belief that God loves them even when the institution is not accepting of them. They work to make sure their children develop a strong understanding of God's love for them, and

they use religion to help cultivate their children's moral compass. It is essential that religious leaders understand these motivations to best serve these communities.

Recently, the United Methodist Church voted to preserve the denomination's bans on same-sex marriage and ordaining LGBTQ clergy rather than allowing local churches to develop their own practices on these divisive issues. Religious traditions like the United Methodist Church that are currently divided on their stance on LGBTQ individuals can learn from how other denominations (e.g., the Episcopal Church and the United Church of Christ) have reconciled these differences and unified their congregations. It is also important that religious leaders recognize that public divisions within religious denominations leave many LGBTQ individuals and their families skeptical of organized religion. Congregations that desire to open up their spaces for LGBTQ-parent families will have to go the length of repairing the distrust created by these contemporary happenings.

Clinicians who seek to treat LGBTQ individuals and their families should recognize that irrespective of the trauma many of them have experienced in religious spaces, many also remain invested in religiosity. Healing efforts should focus on promoting not only self-acceptance but also reintegration in religious spaces.

## References

Acosta, K. L. (2013). *Amigas y amantes: Sexually nonconforming Latinas negotiate family*. New Brunswick, NJ: Rutgers.

Barrow, K. (2016). Jewish LGBTQ people. In A. E. Goldberg (Ed.), *The Sage encyclopedia of LGBTQ studies, volume 2* (pp. 627–630). Los Angeles, CA: Sage.

Barrow, K. M., & Kuvalanka, K. (2011). To be Jewish and lesbian: An exploration of religion, sexual identity, and familial relationships. *Journal of GLBT Family Studies, 7*, 470–492. https://doi.org/10.1080/1550428X.2011.623980

Battle, J., & DeFreece, A. (2014). The impact of community involvement, religion, and spirituality on happiness and health among a National sample of Black lesbians.

*Women, Gender, and Families of Color, 2*(1), 1–31. https://doi.org/10.5406/womgenfamcol.2.1.0001

Christian Century. (2018). Episcoal Church allows all priests to perform same-sex marriage rites. *Christian Century.* 15 Aug 2018.

deYoung, C. P., Emerson, M. O., Yancey, G., & Kim, K. C. (2003). *United by faith.* London, UK: Oxford University Press.

Etengoff, C., & Rodriguez, E. M. (2017). Gay men's and their religiously conservative family allies' scriptural engagement. *Psychology of Religion and Spirituality, 9*, 423–436. https://doi.org/10.1037/rel0000087

Fankhanel, E. H. (2010). The identity development and coming out process of gay youth in Puerto Rico. *Journal of LGBT Youth, 7*, 262–283. https://doi.org/10.1080/19361653.2010.489330

Froese, V. (2016). Compassionate but not affirming: Interview with John Neufeld. *Ministry Compass, 45*, 209–216. Retrieved from http://www.directionjournal.org/45/2/compassionate-but-not-affirming.html

Gallagher, S. K. (2007). Children as religious resources: The role of children in the social re-formation of class, culture, and religious identity. *Journal for the Scientific Study of Religion, 46*, 169–183. https://doi.org/10.1111/j.1468-5906.2007.00349.x

Ganzevoort, R. R., Van der Laan, M., & Olsman, E. (2011). Growing up gay and religious: Conflict, dialogue, and religious identity strategies. *Mental Health, Religion, and Culture, 12*(4), 21–48. https://doi.org/10.1300/J056v12n04_02.

Gattis, M. N., Woodford, M. R., & Han, Y. (2014). Discrimination and depressive symptoms among sexual minority youth: Is gay-affirming religious affiliation a protective factor? *Archives of Sexual Behavior, 43*(8), 1589–1599. https://doi.org/10.1007/s10508-014-0342-y

Goldberg, A. E. (2012). *Gay dads: Transitions to adoptive fatherhood.* New York, NY: NYU Press.

Grimm, G. (2018, November-December). About a boy: My transition from religion and the trauma it inflicts. *The Humanist.* Retrieved from https://thehumanist.com

Gross, M., Vecho, O., Gratton, E., D'Amore, S., & Green, R.-J. (2018). Religious affiliation, religiosity, and attitudes toward same-sex parenting. *Journal of GLBT Family Studies, 14*, 238–259. https://doi.org/10.1080/1550428X.2017.1326016

Gurrentz, B. T. (2017). Family formation and close social ties within religious congregations. *Journal of Marriage and Family, 79*, 1125–1143. https://doi.org/10.1111/jomf.12398

Hartman, K. (1996). *Congregations in conflict: The battle over homosexuality.* New York, NY: Rutgers.

Hickey, K. A., & Grafsky, E. L. (2017). Family relationships and religious identities of GLBQ Christians. *Journal of GLBT Family Studies, 13*, 76–96. https://doi.org/10.1080/1550428X.2015.1129660

Hill, H., & Watson, J. (2006). In Christ there is no gay or straight. Homosexuality and the Episcopal Church. *Anglican and Episcopal History, 75*(1), 37–68.

Holman, E. G., & Oswald, R. F. (2011). Nonmetropolitan GLBTQ parents: When and where does their sexuality matter? *Journal of GLBT Family Studies, 7*, 436–456. https://doi.org/10.1080/1550428X.2011.623937

Johnson, E. P. (2008). *Sweet tea: Black gay men of the South.* Durham, NC: University of North Carolina Press.

Johnson, E. P. (2018). *Black. Queer. Southern. Women. An oral history.* Durham, NC: University of North Carolina Press.

Kamrudin, A. (2018). Bringing queer into Muslim spaces: Community-based pedagogy in Cape Town. *Journal of Feminist Studies in Religion, 34*(1), 143–148. https://doi.org/10.2979/jfemistudreli.34.1.22

Lustenberger, S. (2014). Questions of belonging: Same-sex parenthood and Judaism in transformation. *Sexualities, 17*(5/6), 529–545. https://doi.org/10.1177/1363460714526117.

Lytle, M. C., Foley, P. F., & Aster, A. M. (2013). Adult children of gay and lesbian parents: Religion and the parent-child relationship. *The Counseling Psychologist, 41*, 530–567. https://doi.org/10.1177/0011000012449658

Mattingly, M. S., Galligher, R. V., Dehlin, J. P., Crowell, K. A., & Bradshaw, W. S. (2016). A mixed methods analysis of the family support experiences of GLBQ Latter Day Saints. *Journal of GLBT Family Studies, 12*, 386–409. https://doi.org/10.1080/1550428X.2015.1085345

McQueeney, K. (2009). 'We are God's children, y'all:' Race, gender, and sexuality in lesbian- and gay-affirming congregations. *Social Problems, 56*(1), 151–173. https://doi.org/10.1525/sp.2008.56.1.151

Moore, M. R. (2011). *Invisible families: Gay identities, relationships, and motherhood among Black women.* Berkeley, CA: University of California Press.

Moore, M. R. (2018). Reflections on marriage equality as a vehicle for LGBTQ political transformation. In M. Yarborough, A. Jones, & J. N. DeFilippis (Eds.), *Queer families and relationships after marriage equality* (pp. 73–79). New York, NY: Routledge.

Nielson, E. (2016). Inclusivity in the latter-days: Gay Mormons. *Mental Health, Religion & Culture, 19*(7), 752–768. https://doi.org/10.1080/13674676.2016.1277987

Nielson, E. (2017). When a child comes out in the latter-days: An exploratory case study of Mormon parents. *Mental Health, Religion & Culture, 20*, 260–276. https://doi.org/10.1080/13674676.2017.1350942

Norris, M. (2005, August). United Church of Christ endorses marriage equality. *Lesbian News.* Retrieved from https://www.lesbiannews.com/

Obergefell v. Hodges, 576 U.S. (6th Cir., 2015).

Oswald, R. F. (2001). Religion, family, and ritual: The production of gay, lesbian, bisexual and transgender outsiders-within. *Review of Religious Research, 43*, 39–50. https://doi.org/10.2307/3512242

Oswald, R. F., Goldberg, A., Kuvalanka, K., & Clausell, E. (2008). Structural and moral commitment among same-sex couples: Relationship duration, religiosity, and parental status. *Journal of Family Psychology, 22*(3), 411–419. https://doi.org/10.1037/0893-3200.22.3.411

Page, M. J. L., Lindahl, K. M., & Malik, N. M. (2013). The role of religion and stress in sexual identity and mental health among lesbian, gay, and bisexual youth. *Journal of Research on Adolescence, 23*, 665–677. https://doi.org/10.1111/jora.12025

Pew Research Center. (2017). *Where the public stands on religious liberty vs. nondiscrimination*. Retrieved from http://www.pewforum.org/2016/09/28/where-the-public-stands-on-religious-liberty-vs-nondiscrimination/

Pettis, R. M. (2004). United Church of Christ/Congregationalism. *glbtq*. Retrieved from http://www.glbtq.com

Powell, B., Bolzendahl, C., Geist, C., & Steelman, L. C. (2010). *Counted out: Same-sex relations and American's definitions of family*. New York, NY: Russell Sage Foundation.

Quinn, K., & Dickson-Gomez, J. (2016). Homonegativity, religiosity, and the intersecting identities of young Black men who have sex with men. *AIDS and Behavior, 20*(1), 51–64. https://doi.org/10.1007/s10461-015-1200-1

Richards, M. A., Rothblum, E. D., Beauchaine, T. P., & Balsam, K. F. (2017). Adult children of same-sex and heterosexual couples: Demographic 'thriving. *Journal of GLBT Family Studies, 13*(1), 1–15. https://doi.org/10.1080/1550428X.2016.1164648

Rodriguez, E. M., & Ouellette, S. C. (2000). Gay and lesbian Christians: Homosexual and religious identity integration in the members and participants of a gay-positive church. *Journal for the Scientific Study of Religion, 39*, 333–347. https://doi.org/10.1111/0021-8294.00028

Rostosky, S. S., Otis, M. D., Riggle, E. D. B., Kelly, S., & Brodnicki, C. (2008). An exploration of lived religion in same-sex couples from Judeo-Christian traditions. *Family Process, 47*, 389–403. https://doi.org/10.1111/j.1545-5300.2008.00260.x

Rostosky, S. S., Abreu, R. L., Mahoney, A., & Riggle, E. D. B. (2017). A qualitative study of parenting and religiosity/spirituality in LGBTQ families. *Psychology of Religion and Spirituality, 9*(4), 437–455. https://doi.org/10.1037/rel000077.

Rudolph, D. (2011, July 13). Church supports rights of LGBT parents and their children. *Windy City Times*. Retrieved from http://www.windycitymediagroup.com/

Severson, N., Muñoz-Laboy, M., & Kaufman, R. (2014). 'At times, I feel like I'm sinning': The paradoxical role of non-lesbian, gay, bisexual and transgender-affirming religion in the lives of behaviourally-bisexual Latino men. *Culture, Health & Sexuality, 16*, 136–148. https://doi.org/10.1080/13691058.2013.843722

Tuthill, Z. (2016). Negotiating religiosity and sexual identity among Hispanic lesbian mothers. *Journal of Homosexuality, 63*, 1194–1210. https://doi.org/10.1080/00918369.2016.1151691

Uecker, J. E., Mayrl, D., & Stroope, S. (2016). Family formation and returning to institutional religion in young adulthood. *Journal for the Scientific Study of Religion, 55*(2), 384–406. https://doi.org/10.1111/jssr.12271

United Church of Christ. (2003). *Affirming the participation and ministry of transgender people within the United Church of Christ and supporting their civil and human rights* [PDF file]. Retrieved from http://uccfiles.com/pdf/2003-AFFIRMING-THE-PARTICIPATION-AND-MINISTRY-OF-TRANSGENDER-PEOPLE-WITHIN-THE-UNITED-CHURCH-OF-CHRIST-AND-SUPPORTING-THEIR-CIVIL-AND-HUMAN-RIGHTS.pdf

Wedow, R., Schnabel, L., Wedow, L. K. D., & Konieczny, M. E. (2017). 'I'm gay and I'm Catholic': Negotiating two complex identities at a Catholic university. *Sociology of Religion: A Quarterly Review, 78*, 289–317. https://doi.org/10.1093/socrel/srx028.

Whitehead, A. (2018). Homosexuality, religion and the family: The effects of religion on Americans' appraisals of the parenting abilities of same-sex couples. *Journal of Homosexuality, 65*(1): 41–65.https://doi.org/10.1080/00918369.2017.1310550

Yip, A. K. T. (with Khalid, A.). (2010a). Looking for Allah: Spiritual quests of queer Muslims. In K. Browne, S. R. Munt, & A. K. T. Yip (Eds.), *Queer spiritual spaces: Sexuality and sacred places* (pp. 65–80). Farnham, UK: Ashgate.

Yip, A. K. T. (with Smith, S.). (2010b). Queerness and Sangha: Exploring Buddhist lives. In K. Browne, S. R. Munt, & A. K. T. Yip (Eds.), *Queer spiritual spaces: Sexuality and sacred places* (pp. 81–114). Farnham, UK: Ashgate.

# LGBTQ-Parent Immigrant Families: We're Here, We're Queer, We're Invisible

Nadine Nakamura

In 2018, I was invited to be part of a conference panel on LGBTQ families. The facilitator asked us to speak about an experience of discrimination we had encountered related to being part of an LGBTQ family. I was asked to speak first, and I talked about the role that discriminatory immigration policies played in my family formation. My wife and I are a same-sex binational couple, and she had been in the USA on a variety of visas for many years. We did not see a way to a green card for her since, at the time, we could not obtain it through marriage. Thus, she interviewed for a job in Canada and, when she got the job, was able to sponsor me (a US citizen) as her common law spouse. I had just received my PhD, and this move to another country meant putting my career on hold or at least off track for the foreseeable future. We decided that we could not have any serious conversations about having children until we could sort out our immigration challenges. Mentally and emotionally, it felt like there were too many balls in the air and too much uncertainty. We lived in Canada for 4 years before she was able to serendipitously return to the USA through an intercompany transfer, which eventually led to her green card. Once she got her green card, we started talking in earnest about building our future family and took the necessary steps

less than a year later. After conveying that experience, the facilitator turned to me and said, "Okay, so can you tell us about an experience of discrimination? What about in school? Do your kids ever get asked questions about having two moms?" I was taken aback because I had just shared what, to me, was the most impactful form of discrimination that affected whether, when, how, and if my wife and I were even going to become parents. My experience did not fit the assumed narrative of what LGBTQ-parent families experience, and therefore it was dismissed as a valid experience of discrimination.

In considering LGBTQ-parent families, it is necessary to approach the topic with an intersectional lens. Intersectionality theory was originally conceptualized to consider the experiences of Black women who faced oppression based on both race and gender (Crenshaw, 1989). Intersectionality recognizes "how multiple social identities such as race, gender, sexual orientation, SES, and disability intersect at the micro level of individual experience to reflect interlocking systems of privilege and oppression (i.e., racism, sexism, heterosexism, classism) at the macro social-structural level" (Bowleg, 2012, p. 1267). Intersectionality asserts that lives cannot be explained by taking into account single categories (e.g., gender, race, and socioeconomic status), that lived realities are shaped by different factors and social dynamics operating together, that people can experience privilege and

N. Nakamura (✉)
Department of Psychology, University of La Verne, La Verne, CA, USA
e-mail: nnakamura@laverne.edu

© Springer Nature Switzerland AG 2020
A. E. Goldberg, K. R. Allen (eds.), *LGBTQ-Parent Families*,
https://doi.org/10.1007/978-3-030-35610-1_14

oppression simultaneously, and that it depends on what situation or specific context they are in (Hankivsky, 2014).

Unfortunately, the vast majority of the psychological literature on immigration assumes that immigrants are cisgender and heterosexual (Nakamura, Kassan, & Suehn, 2017; Nakamura & Pope, 2013) and LGBTQ immigrant families are nowhere to be found in the literature. By not considering LGBTQ immigrant families, scholars overlook the systems of oppression, such as racism, xenophobia, heterosexism, and transphobia that may be impacting these families. Since there is no research base to draw from, this chapter relies on an inadequate additive model to describe this understudied group's experiences and highlights the need for intersectional research. This chapter first provides a brief overview of how immigrant populations to the USA have changed over time as a result of immigration policy. Next, the literature on LGBTQ immigrants is reviewed. Since there is little mention of LGBTQ-parent immigrant families in the psychological literature, relevant themes from the broader immigrant family literature are presented. Finally, research on LGBTQ immigrant families without children is reviewed with mention of LGBTQ-parent immigrant families where appropriate. Recommendations for future research and implications for practice are provided.

## Immigrants

Immigration has been part of the fabric of the USA from its inception. Today, immigrants account for 13.9% of the US population (Radford & Budiman, 2018). Of those, the majority (76%) are in the country legally, with 44% as naturalized US citizens, 27% as permanent residents, and 5% as temporary residents, while 24% of all immigrants are undocumented. Laws and policies shape who has had access to immigration and citizenship and have historically excluded non-European and LGBTQ immigrants.

Before 1965, US immigration policy explicitly favored immigrants from Europe (American Psychological Association, 2012). Many previous laws and policies, such as the Chinese Exclusion Act of 1882, banned immigrants from non-European countries from immigrating to the USA. For example, in 1960, 84% of immigrants came from Canada and Europe, with the remainder coming from Mexico (6%), South and East Asia (3.8%), the rest of Latin America (3.5%), and other areas (2.7%) (Radford & Budiman, 2018). This meant that the majority of these immigrants could assimilate to US culture and their offspring could claim the identity of "American" without any prefix or adjective to explain their ethnic origin.

Since the 1965 Immigration and Naturalization Act, there has been a shift in where most immigrants to the USA have come from (Radford & Budiman, 2018). In 2016, Europeans and Canadians made up only 13.2% of immigrants, while as of 2018, South and East Asians account for 26.9%, Mexicans account for 26.5%, and other Latin Americans account for 24.5% of the US immigrant population, with 8.9% from other regions (Radford & Budiman, 2018). About 68% of all green cards in 2016 were family based, meaning that a family member sponsored the immigrant (Krogstad & Gonzalez-Barrera, 2018). Unlike immigrants from Europe who became American after a generation by assimilating, the majority of today's immigrants and their offspring are perpetually marked as "foreign" by their racial features. Many immigrants experience discrimination rooted in racism and xenophobia. For example, in a study of 1387 immigrants from Africa, Latin America, and Southeast Asia to the Midwest, 30% reported experiencing discrimination in the past year and race/ethnicity or country of origin were the most frequently cited reasons for discrimination (Tran, Lee, & Burgess, 2010). Perceived discrimination, in turn, has been linked to negative mental health outcomes and substance use among immigrants (Tran et al., 2010; Yip, Gee, & Takeuchi, 2008).

## LGBTQ Immigrants

The USA has a long history of excluding groups from immigration based not only on race and ethnicity but also gender and sexual orientation (Heller, 2009; Howe, 2007; Reynolds, 1980). In 1990, US immigration law changed to no longer deny entry to individuals based solely on their sexual orientation (Rank, 2002). However, other obstacles have made immigration especially difficult for sexual minority individuals. "Family reunification" has been a cornerstone of US immigration since the 1950s when the Immigration and Nationality Act of 1952 began to allow US citizens and permanent residents to sponsor spouses, children, siblings, and parents for immigration (Human Rights Watch/Immigration Equality, 2006). However, same-sex spouses were not considered family under the Defense of Marriage Act (DOMA) (US General Accounting Office, 2004). In June 2013, the US Supreme Court overturned Section 3 of DOMA. Section 3 barred the US federal government from recognizing same-sex couples as married, which denied them over 1000 federal rights of marriage, including immigration rights (US General Accounting Office, 2004). Since DOMA was struck down by the Supreme Court in 2013, same-sex binational couples have the same access to spousal-based immigration that different-sex couples do. However, barriers still exist that are unique to LGBTQ immigrants. For example, in many countries, it is not safe to be openly LGBTQ and same-sex couples may be very private and secretive about their relationship in order to not draw attention to themselves. This can complicate proving the validity of a same-sex couple's relationship to immigration officials, who will expect couples to have evidence to substantiate their relationship (Carron, 2014). Such evidence is essentially a paper trail of the relationship such as photos, letters, joint ownership of property or other joint financial liability, and affidavits from family and friends attesting to knowledge of the relationship. These types of requirements can be a significant barrier for those who are coming from countries that are hostile to LGBTQ people.

There were an estimated 904,000 LGBTQ foreign-born adults in the USA in 2013 (Gates, 2013). Of those, an estimated 70% were documented, while 30% were undocumented (Gates, 2013). Among undocumented LGBTQ immigrants, 71% were Latinx, 15% were Asian Pacific Islander, 8% were White, and 6% were Black. Among documented LGBTQ immigrants, 30% were Latinx and 35% were Asian Pacific Islander. While the estimates on LGBTQ immigrants are likely underreported, it appears that they represent more ethnic diversity and are more likely to be undocumented, younger, and male compared to non-LGBTQ immigrants (Gates, 2013).

LGBTQ immigrants have a variety of reasons for migrating from their countries of origin. One reason that LGBTQ immigrants come to the USA is the desire to live as an "out" LGBTQ person (Bianchi et al., 2007). Carrillo (2004) introduced the concept of sexual migration, which refers to "international relocation that is motivated, directly or indirectly, by the sexuality of those who migrate" (p. 59). Bianchi et al. (2007) conducted qualitative interviews with Brazilian, Colombian, and Dominican immigrant men who have sex with men to understand their motivations for migration and their sexual behavior post-migration. Common reasons given were to improve their economic situation, further their education, join family members, escape political instability, escape homonegativity in their home country, and have more sexual freedom. In a quantitative study, Nieves-Lugo et al. (2019) examined a sample of Brazilian, Colombian, and Dominican immigrant men who have sex with men to understand the relationship between sexual migration and HIV risk. The top five reasons that they endorsed as reasons to migrate to the USA were to improve their financial situation (49%), to affirm their sexual orientation (40%), to study (37%), came with family (not participant's decision) (33%), and came as a tourist but decided to stay (20%).

LGBTQ immigrants may feel that moving to another country will protect their family of origin from stigma (Adames, Chavez-Dueñas, Sharma, & La Roche, 2018). However, this can come at a cost to the LGBTQ immigrant, including separation from social support and family back in their home country. Adames et al. (2018) present a case study of a young, dark-skinned, cisgender, queer man of Afro-Colombian descent who left Colombia because of heterosexism and was greeted in the USA by racism, as well as other forms of discrimination, including heterosexism. LGBTQ immigrants may experience psychological distress from not being able to escape systematic oppression no matter where they go. It can be especially isolating when homophobia occurs within immigrant communities as it can cut LGBTQ immigrants off from a source of support that non-LGBTQ immigrants are able to access.

## LGBTQ Asylum Seekers

While immigrants leave their home countries for a host of reasons such as family reunification or better educational or occupational opportunities in another country, asylum seekers are a type of immigrant who flee their home country for protection in another country. Some LGBTQ people flee their home countries as a result of persecution. The United Nations High Commissioner for Refugees (UNHCR) (2016) defines a refugee or asylee as a person:

> owing to a well-founded fear of being persecuted for reasons of race, religion, nationality, membership of a particular social group or political opinion, is outside the country of his nationality and is unable or, owing to such fear, is unwilling to avail himself the protection of that country. (p. 2)

In 1994, US asylum policy changed to include persecution based on sexual orientation (Rank, 2002). The Department of Homeland Security does not record applicants' sexual orientation or gender identity (McGuirk, Niedzwiecki, Oke, & Volova, 2015). However, the Organization for Refuge, Asylum, and Migration estimates it is about 5% of US asylum claims (UNHCR, 2013). The numbers are likely higher today. For example, Immigration Equality (2019), an LGBTQ immigrant rights organization that handles asylum cases, reports a record caseload due to the worldwide persecution of LGBTQ people. In many countries, including Jamaica, Iran, and

Sudan, LGBTQ people experience persecution, imprisonment, and, in some cases, death sentences based on their sexual orientation or gender identity (International Lesbian, Gay, Bisexual, Trans and Intersex Association [ILGA], 2019). Transgender people may be subjected to forced sterilization or castration, so-called corrective rape, forced sex work, and persecution at the hands of the police throughout the world including Central America and Africa (American Psychological Association, 2019; Bach, 2013; Jagmohan, 2018; Morales, Corbin-Gutierrez, & Wang, 2013; Nakamura & Morales, 2016; Reading & Rubin, 2011). In response to this persecution and violence, LGBTQ people may leave their country of origin to seek asylum.

Compared to their heterosexual, cisgender asylum-seeking counterparts, LGBTQ asylum seekers have experienced higher rates of sexual violence, persecution in childhood, persecution by family members, and suicidal ideation (Hopkinson et al., 2017). Alessi, Kahn, and Chatterji (2015) conducted a study on 26 LGBTQ refugees and asylum seekers in the USA and Canada from countries in Asia, Africa, the Caribbean, Eastern Europe, Latin America, and the Middle East in order to understand their experiences of violence. Participants reported that they had experienced severe verbal, physical, and sexual abuse throughout their youth at home, in school, and in the community with no protections available to them. Notably, participants made a connection between their experiences of abuse and their later depression, anxiety, traumatic stress, and suicidality.

Piwowarczyk, Fernandez, and Sharma (2017) conducted a retrospective chart review of 50 patients self-identified as lesbian, gay, or bisexual who were asylum seekers or refugees seen through a program for survivors of torture between 2009 and 2014. Three-fourths of the participants were from Uganda where homosexuality is criminalized, 74% had been in the USA for less than a year at the time of intake, and the average age of the participants was 30. Almost all (98%) experienced persecution due to their sexual orientation and 84% were survivors of torture (see chapter "LGBTQ-Parent Families in Non-

Western Contexts"). All presented with symptoms of depression and anxiety, and 70% had a diagnosis of post-traumatic stress disorder (PTSD). Persecution by the police, arrest or detention, and history of torture were all significantly associated with a PTSD diagnosis. Three quarters were with a partner in the year prior to fleeing their home country. These relationships often had tragic endings. In six cases, partners disappeared; in three cases, partners were killed; in two cases, partners were detained; and in one case, the partner committed suicide. After fleeing the country, only four of the participants were in contact with their partner, while the remaining were unsuccessful in being able to reach their partners. Some participants had children, but no additional information about this aspect of the participants' life was provided.

Unfortunately, many LGBTQ asylum seekers also experience violence when they arrive in the USA. Gorwin, Taylor, Dunnington, Alshuwaiyer, and Cheney (2017) conducted a study with 45 transgender women asylum seekers from Mexico. All had experienced some type of threat of harm, physical assault, and/or sexual assault while still living in Mexico, most by multiple perpetrators as well as unstable environments and fear for their safety. Participants also experienced verbal and physical assaults in the USA from community members and strangers, employers, significant others, and family members. In addition, they faced unstable living environments, extreme stress related to their undocumented status, and economic insecurity. All of the participants had a PTSD diagnosis and 93% had a diagnosis of depression, highlighting the unique and serious mental health needs of transgender asylum seekers.

Despite their high need for services, LGBTQ immigrants often do not utilize them due to various barriers. In Gorwin et al.'s study (2017), participants reported little or no use of health or social services due to shame, fear of government entities, or language or transportation barriers. Some reported having experienced abuse, including harassment and physical or sexual assault within programs by staff or other members. Those who accessed services often withheld information from providers or did not follow through with treatments. Chavez (2011) conducted a needs assessment of LGBTQ immigrants and refugees in Southern Arizona through interviews with 32 service providers, LGBTQ migrants, and their supporters. Results indicated a lack of formal support services for LGBTQ immigrants and refugees. Barriers to health care included cultural insensitivity, lack of discreet services, and fear of having their legal status revealed. Participants also had a number of concerns related to housing, including challenges with finding and keeping housing, particularly for those who are undocumented and lack of adequate housing resources. Participants also identified legal concerns related to fear of deportation. The need for culturally sensitive services across the board was highlighted as a major need for this population.

Three things are clear from reviewing the literature on LGBTQ immigrants. First, the literature on LGBTQ immigrants is scarce, which makes it difficult to paint an adequate picture of this population. Second, this population is very diverse. Documentation status and reason for coming to the USA vary and have a major impact on the experiences of LGBTQ immigrants. Their language skills, race and ethnicity, gender, socioeconomic status, and family structure are also varied. Third, many LGBTQ immigrants, particularly those who are undocumented or have sought asylum, have experienced a great deal of stress and trauma. More research is necessary in order to have an adequate understanding of the experiences of LGBTQ immigrants. In particular, there is virtually no literature on LGBTQ immigrant families. Therefore, I provide a brief overview of presumably heterosexual, cisgender immigrant families before reviewing the very limited literature on LGBTQ immigrant couples and the literature where there are brief mentions of LGBTQ-parent immigrant families.

## Immigrant Families

Just as LGBTQ families are incredibly diverse, so are immigrant families. Age of immigration, as well as length of time since immigration, makes a huge difference when considering how immigration is experienced (APA, 2012). Recent immigrants will have different challenges than those who have been living in the USA for most of their lives. Some immigrants will have come to the USA for educational or financial opportunities, while others will have come to escape violence in their country of origin. When it comes to families, some may have children who are US citizens, while others have children who immigrated with their parents (Menjívar, 2012). Children of immigrants make up 11.9% of the US population (Radford & Budiman, 2018). By 2020, one in three children under the age of 18 is projected to be the child of an immigrant (Mather, 2009).

Acculturation, which is defined as one of "cultural change and adaptation that occurs when individuals with different cultures come into contact" (Gibson, 2001, p. 19), can be stressful as it involves losses of community ties, jobs, customs, and social ties (Falicov, 1998, 2009; García Coll & Magnuson, 1997; Suárez-Orozco & Suárez-Orozco, 2001). It is a multidimensional process of adjustment to a new culture that involves language acculturation, behavioral acculturation, and understanding and possibly adjusting one's cultural and ethnic identity (APA, 2012). The acculturation experience of an immigrant is often influenced by experiences in their country of origin and reasons for immigration, as well as the environment of their receiving country (Gibson, 2001). Those who are fleeing persecution and seeking asylum are likely to have a very different experience with acculturation than those who immigrate for economic reasons, for example. Those who leave their countries as refugees often intend for their stay to be temporary and may be less inclined to put down roots. Whether the immigrant lives in a community with many people from their country of origin can also impact their acculturation process. Acculturative stress can be a byproduct of the acculturation process and can be exacerbated by experiences of discrimination (APA, 2012).

Children tend to have an easier time acculturating, as they are immersed in the new culture through school and have an easier time acquiring a new language. While there are many benefits to acculturation for children, such as being able to speak more than one language and being able to help the family, there can also be challenges. There are often acculturation gaps between parents and their children, where children become translators and cultural brokers for their parents, and this can negatively impact parent-child relationships (APA, 2012). For example, in a qualitative study of 25 Latino parents and adolescents on language brokering by Corona et al. (2012), one participant spoke of her experience as a language broker for her parents saying:

> It is hard. I think what takes a hit is the pecking order in the family. Because you know that link into the world through language and through knowledge and through understand what's going on around you suddenly becomes this child's. That's how it was for me anyway. And um it's a little hard when you're little you want your parents to guide you but that's sort of flips around and you find yourself guiding your parents.

Language brokering can be especially difficult for children when this takes place in medical settings where children may not understand medical terms that they are translating and may worry about not conveying important information correctly.

Whether immigrants are documented or undocumented will have an enormous impact on their experience. Brabeck, Sibley, and Lykes (2016) conducted structured interviews with 178 families with an immigrant parent from Mexico, Central America, and the Dominican Republic and a child (aged 7–10 years) born in the USA; they found that 49% of the participants were undocumented. Undocumented participants had less education, greater poverty, and greater stress during migration, compared to documented participants. Once in the USA, undocumented participants experienced higher job-related stress, lower access to/use of social services, lower social support, greater obstacles to learning English, higher experiences of discrimination, and the fear of discovery and deportation. One of the biggest stressors for undocumented immigrants is the possibility of deportation, which can lead to familial separation.

In 2012 there were an estimated 4.5 million US citizen children in families where one or more of their parents were undocumented (Satinsky et al., 2013). The threat of deportation alone puts children at risk for distress, with parents reporting anxiety in almost half of children and PTSD symptoms in nearly 75% (Satinsky et al., 2013). Fear of deportation contributes to a decrease in accessing public places including school and health and social services (Rodriguez & Hagan, 2004), as well as community events, churches, restaurants, stores, libraries, and parks (Hagan, Rodriguez, & Castro, 2011). Children whose families live under threat of detention or deportation will finish fewer years of school and have challenges focusing on their studies (Satinsky et al., 2013). One example of this comes from an undocumented mother with three sons who, as part of a focus group, said:

> Now, when he is doing his homework I notice that he loses concentration a lot. I've noticed that he is thinking all the time. He is distracted. With his homework, he used to have very good grades. He went down a bit. It is more difficult for him now to concentrate. (Satinsky et al., 2013, p. 16)

This quote demonstrates that children with undocumented parents are impacted by the stress created by the threat of deportation. Poor education can have lifelong impacts on health and occupational outcomes (Satinsky et al., 2013).

In a report on detention and deportation in California, Human Rights Watch (2017) found that 42% of those detained and 47% of those deported were parents to at least one US citizen child. According to Satinsky et al., in 2012 there were an estimated 152,426 US citizen children whose parents had been deported. US immigration law bars the reentry of people who have been deported for up to 10 years (Thronson, 2008). Separation from parents has major impacts on the psychological and physical health of children (Chaudry et al., 2010). Children of detained and deported parents suffer in a myriad of ways. Chaudry et al. (2010) interviewed 87 parents from families that had been impacted by parents being arrested; this led to deportation of a parent in 20 of the 87 families. Data indicated that 6 months or less after arrest, about two-thirds of children had eating and sleeping changes and more than half of children cried more often and were more fearful, and more than a third experienced increases in anxiety, anger, or aggression or were more withdrawn or clingy after a parent's arrest. Many families also experienced loss of income, housing instability, and food insecurity. Partners of deported parents will have a shorter lifespan related to the stress they experience (Satinsky et al., 2013). In this way, we can see how family separation leads to both psychological trauma and economic devastation.

## LGBTQ Immigrant Couples

Given that much of the research on immigrants focuses on families and children, there seems to be an understanding that immigration is intricately connected to the context of families. Therefore, the dearth of accounts of LGBTQ immigrant families' experiences in the psychological literature is striking. While there is a small body of literature on LGBTQ immigrant couples, the focus of this research is on couples, most of whom do not have children.

The little research that has focused on LGBTQ immigrant families has examined the experiences of same-sex binational couples who immigrated to Canada in order to remain with their partners before DOMA was overturned in the USA. Kassan and Nakamura (2013) conducted a qualitative study with 17 such individuals in same-sex binational relationships. These couples were comprised of one partner who was an American citizen and one partner who was a citizen of a different country. While most participants were not parents, those who were had adult children and thus children were not a focus of the research. Results indicated that participants felt forced to immigrate to Canada because the US partner was unable to sponsor their partner for US immigration.

As a result, participants faced challenges related to their careers both during their time in the USA on temporary visas and in Canada due to lack of networks, problems with transferability of credentials, and experiences of discrimination. Nakamura, Kassan, and Suehn (2015) examined the impact that immigrating to Canada had on these 17 participants' relationships. Friendships were often strained as friends did not often fully grasp why immigration to Canada was necessary and did not understand the injustice that same-sex binational couples were experiencing. Familial relationships were also similarly strained with the added element of guilt, worry, and sadness about leaving ill or aging parents behind. Despite the struggles they faced, some participants indicated that the immigration experience brought them closer emotionally to their partners and solidified their commitment. Finally, Nakamura et al. (2017) examined the role of resilience with the same sample. One theme that emerged was the process of building a life in Canada. Some participants approached Canada as a temporary place to live but eventually began to view it as a place that they wanted to settle in for the long term. They also noted a shift as they developed a stronger sense of stability in terms of their careers, sense of home, and social support networks, which impacted their identity.

Nakamura and Tsong (2019) conducted a study on the experiences of same-sex binational couples living in the USA. This quantitative study examined a sample of 183 individuals in same-sex binational relationships who were living in the USA in June 2013 before the Supreme Court overturned DOMA. More than half of the participants (61.2%) were US citizens and 33% had a partner living outside the USA. Participants reported higher levels of perceived stress in comparison to the general population normative data found in previous studies, as well as a severe level of anxiety and the presence of significant depressive symptoms. Perceived stress significantly contributed to both depression and anxiety, while resilience had a moderating and buffering effect on the negative impact perceived stress had on depression. This study suggests that in addition to the minority stress (Meyer, 2003) that all LGBTQ people experience, discriminatory immigration laws added stress on many same-sex binational couples.

## LGBTQ-Parent Immigrant Families

Unfortunately, a review of the psychological literature gives the impression that LGBTQ immigrants do not have children, which is not the case. In 2013, it was estimated that there were 33,500 LGBTQ couples with at least one foreign-born partner who were raising 41,000 children under the age of 18 in the USA (Gates, 2013). This represents 25% of same-sex couples with a foreign spouse or partner who are raising children, which is lower than the 58% of different-sex couples with a foreign spouse or partner who are raising children. These data represent the landscape in the USA before DOMA was overturned, so it is possible that discriminatory immigration laws contributed to the depression in family formation among same-sex binational couples. Post-DOMA data do not exist to be able to draw any definitive conclusions. Same-sex binational couples are also facing institutional discrimination regarding the recognition of birthright citizenship for children born abroad when they are not biologically related to the US citizen parent (Sacchetti, 2018).

While the immigration literature has explored the issue of familial separation, it has not examined this issue with LGBTQ immigrant families. Nakamura and Morales (2016) conducted a case study with "Scarlett," a Central American transgender woman who sought asylum in the USA after receiving death threats from gang members when she would not agree to sell drugs for them. While her family was not the focus of the interview, she shared that she had been caring for her nieces and nephews—the children of her sister—who had left for the USA before her. When she fled her home country, she left those children, whom she considered her own children at that point, behind. This case raises many questions about what happens to children when their caretakers flee for their lives due to LGBTQ-related persecution. In another example of how

LGBTQ families might be impacted by familial separation, Morales (2013) wrote about Latino LGBTQ immigrants in the USA and mentioned gay men having children in Latin America. However, this was in the context of concealing their gay identity by stating that they have children in order to present as heterosexual. It is not known what becomes of the parent-child relationship when these men immigrate to the USA.

## Future Research Directions

More research on LGBTQ-parent immigrant families is clearly needed in order to examine the unique stressors that these families face in addition to the many other stressors that immigrant families experience. Another unexplored topic related to LGBTQ immigrant families relates to rejection they might experience from their families of origin. The research on LGBTQ family acceptance suggests that many ethnic minority families are accepting of their LGBTQ youth. For example, Kane, Nicoll, Kahn, and Groves (2012) surveyed almost 2000 Latino youth and found that more than half said their families accepted LGBTQ people. However, this report did not address the issue of immigration, so it is unknown how many of the youth surveyed were immigrants themselves or whether acculturation or generation status factored into family acceptance. The lack of information on immigration status is yet another example of LGBTQ immigrants being overlooked.

Another angle that is understudied is immigrant families who have LGBTQ children. Cruz and Perez-Chavez (2017) provide a case example of a Central American gay man who came to the USA when he was 3 years old with his family. He was "outed" by a cousin to his family. While his family did not reject him, they were not completely accepting either. His mother, for example, was very religious and prayed for him to become heterosexual. Despite this, he still spoke to her several times per week. He was married to a man, but his mother did not know this and had not met his husband. This example demonstrates how LGBTQ people negotiate their relationships with their families of origin and with their

spouses/partners and children. Research is needed to understand how LGBTQ-parent immigrant families negotiate acceptance with their families of origin.

## Implications for Practice

The lack of literature on LGBTQ-parent immigrant families highlights how invisible this population is. Invisibility is a form of marginalization and demonstrates that LGBTQ immigrant families are not prioritized, understood, or even considered. There is a great need for research on this population, particularly because LGBTQ immigrants are more likely to be undocumented and are more likely to be people of color compared to their non-LGBTQ counterparts, suggesting that LGBTQ immigrants experience multiple forms of oppression. It is important for clinicians to expand their view of LGBTQ families in order to not inadvertently further marginalize this population, particularly in the therapeutic context. Likewise, it is important for practitioners to not assume that all members of immigrant families are heterosexual. In order to be truly culturally responsive and to not further alienate LGBTQ immigrant clients and their families, therapists must be able to recognize their clients' multiple marginalized identities and how they are impacted by heterosexism, racism, xenophobia, and other systems of oppression (Adames et al., 2018).

## References

Adames, H. Y., Chavez-Dueñas, N. Y., Sharma, S., & La Roche, M. J. (2018). Intersectionality in psychotherapy: The experiences of an AfroLatinx queer immigrant. *Psychotherapy, 55*, 73–79. https://doi.org/10.1037/pst0000152

Alessi, E. J., Kahn, S., & Chatterji, S. (2015). 'The darkest times of my life': Recollections of child abuse among forced migrants persecuted because of their sexual orientation and gender identity. *Child Abuse and Neglect, 51*, 93–105. https://doi.org/10.1016/j.chiabu.2015.10.030.

American Psychological Association [APA]. (2012). *Crossroads: The psychology of immigration in the new century*. Retrieved from https://www.apa.org/images/immigration-report_tcm7-134644.pdf

American Psychological Association [APA]. (2019). *LGBTQ asylum seekers: How clinicians can help.* Retrieved from https://www.apa.org/pi/lgbt/resources/lgbtq-asylum-seekers.pdf

Bach, J. (2013). Assessing transgender asylum claims. *Forced Migration Review, 42*, 34–36.

Bianchi, F. T., Reisen, C. A., Zea, M. C., Poppen, P. J., Shedlin, M., & Montes-Penha, M. (2007). The sexual experiences of Latino men who have sex with men who migrated to a gay epicentre in the U.S.A. *Culture, Health and Sexuality, 9*, 505–518. https://doi.org/10.1080/13691050701243547

Bowleg, L. (2012). The problem with the phrase women and minorities: Intersectionality—An important theoretical framework for public health. *American Journal of Public Health, 102*, 1267–1273. https://doi.org/10.2105/AJPH.2012.300750

Brabeck, K. M., Sibley, E., & Lykes, M. B. (2016). Authorized and unauthorized immigrant parents: The impact of legal vulnerability on family contexts. *Hispanic Journal of Behavioral Sciences, 38*, 3–30. https://doi.org/10.1177/0739986315621741

Carrillo, H. (2004). Sexual migration, cross-cultural sexual encounters, and sexual health. *Sexuality Research & Social Policy, 1*, 58–70. https://doi.org/10.1525/srsp.2004.1.3.58

Carron, A. (2014). Marriage-based immigration for same-sex couples after DOMA: Lingering problems of proof and predjudice. *Northwestern. University Law Review., 109*, 1021–1052

Chaudry, A., Capps, R., Pedroza, J. M., Castaneda, R. M., Santos, R., & Scott, M. M. (2010). *Facing our future: Children in the aftermath of immigration enforcement.* Retrieved from https://www.urban.org/sites/default/files/publication/28331/412020-Facing-Our-Future.PDF

Chavez, K. R. (2011). Identifying the needs of LGBTQ immigrants and refugees in Southern Arizona. *Journal of Homosexuality, 58*, 189–218. https://doi.org/10.1080/00918369.2011.540175

Corona, R., Stevens, L. F., Halfond, R. W., Shaffer, C. M., Reid-Quiñones, K., & Gonzalez, T. (2012). A qualitative analysis of what Latino parents and adolescents think and feel about language brokering. *Journal of Child and Family Studies, 21*, 788–798. https://doi.org/10.1007/s10826-011-9536-2

Crenshaw, K. (1989). Demarginalizing the intersection of race and sex: A Black feminist critique of antidiscrimination doctrine, feminist theory and antiracist politics. *The University of Chicago Legal Forum, 140*, 139–167.

Cruz, X., & Perez-Chavez, J. G. (2017). Queer Latinxs coming out: The dance between family love and authenticity. *Latina/o Psychology Today, 4*(2), 15–18.

Falicov, C. J. (1998). The cultural meaning of family triangles. In M. McGoldrick (Ed.), *Re- visioning family therapy: Race, culture, and gender in clinical practice* (pp. 37–49). New York, NY: Guilford Press.

Falicov, C. J. (2009). Religion and spiritual traditions in immigrant families: Significance for Latino health and mental health. In F. Walsh (Ed.), *Spiritual resources in family therapy* (pp. 156–173). New York, NY: Guilford Press.

García Coll, C., & Magnuson, K. (1997). The psychological experience of immigration: A developmental perspective. In A. Booth, A. C. Crouter, & N. Landale (Eds.), *Immigration and the family* (pp. 91–132). Mahwah, NJ: Erlbaum.

Gates, G. J. (2013). *LGBT adult immigrants in the United States.* Retrieved from https://williamsinstitute.law.ucla.edu/wp-content/uploads/LGBTImmigrants-Gates-Mar-2013.pdf

Gibson, M. A. (2001). Immigrant adaptation and patterns of acculturation. *Human Development, 44*, 19–23. https://doi.org/10.1159/000057037

Gorwin, M., Taylor, E. L., Dunnington, J., Alshuwaiyer, G., & Cheney, M. K. (2017). Needs of a silent minority: Mexican transgender asylum seekers. *Health Promotion Practice, 18*, 332–340. https://doi.org/10.1177/1524839917692750

Hagan, J. M., Rodriguez, N., & Castro, B. (2011). Social effects of mass deportations by the United States government, 2000–10. *Ethnic and Racial Studies, 34*, 1374–1391. https://doi.org/10.1080/01419870.2011.575233

Hankivsky, O. (2014). *Intersectionality 101.* The Institute for Intersectionality Research & Policy, Simon Fraser University, 1–34. Retrieved from https://www.researchgate.net/profile/Olena_Hankivsky/publication/279293665_Intersectionality_101/links/56c35bda08ae602342508c7f/Intersectionality-101.pdf

Heller, P. (2009). Challenges facing LGBT asylum-seekers: The role of social work in correcting oppressive immigration processes. *Journal of Gay & Lesbian Social Services, 21*, 294–308. https://doi.org/10.1080/10538720902772246

Hopkinson, R. A., Keatley, E., Glaeser, E., Erickson-Schroth, L., Fattal, O., & Sullivan, M. N. (2017). Persecution experiences and mental health of LGBT asylum seekers. *Journal of Homosexuality, 64*, 1650–1666. https://doi.org/10.1080/00918369.2016.1253392

Howe, C. (2007). Sexual borderlands: Lesbian and gay migration, human rights, and the metropolitan community church. *Sexuality Research and Social Policy, 4*, 88–106. https://doi.org/10.1215/9780822391166-003

Human Rights Watch. (2017). *"I still need you": The detention and deportation of Californian parents.* Retrieved from https://www.hrw.org/report/2017/05/15/i-still-need-you/detention-and-deportation-californian-parents

Human Rights Watch/Immigration Equality. (2006). *Family, unvalued discrimination, denial, and the fate of binational same-sex couples under U.S. law.* Retrieved from https://www.hrw.org/sites/default/files/reports/FamilyUnvalued.pdf

Immigration Equality. (2019). *Legal services.* Retrieved from https://www.immigrationequality.org/our-work/#legal-services

International Lesbian, Gay, Bisexual, Trans and Intersex Association [ILGA]. (2019). *State-sponsored homophobia 2019*. Retrieved from https://ilga.org/downloads/ILGA_State_Sponsored_Homophobia_2019.pdf

Jagmohan, K. (2018). *Trans women bemoan violence, corrective rape at #TotalShutdown*. Retrieved from https://www.iol.co.za/sunday-tribune/news/watch-trans-women-bemoan-violence-corrective-rape-at-to-talshutdown-16350493

Kane, R., Nicoll, A. E., Kahn, E., & Groves, S. (2012). *Supporting and caring for our Latino LGBT youth*. Retrieved from https://assets2.hrc.org/files/assets/resources/LatinoYouthReport-FINAL.pdf?_ga=2.65718316.366525342.1555720823-1074057717.1555720823

Kassan, A., & Nakamura, N. (2013). "This was my only option": Career transitions of same- sex binational couples immigrating to Canada. *Journal of LGBT Issues in Counseling, 7*, 154–171. https://doi.org/10.1080/15538605.2013.785466

Krogstad, J. M., & Gonzalez-Barrera, A. (2018). *Key facts about U.S. immigration policies and proposed changes*. Retrieved from http://www.pewresearch.org/fact-tank/2018/02/26/key-facts-about-u-s-immigration-policies-and-proposed-changes/

Mather, M. (2009). *Children in immigrant families chart new path*. Washington, DC: Population Reference Bureau. Retrieved from http://www.prb.org/pdf09/immigrantchildren.pdf

McGuirk, S., Niedzwiecki, M., Oke, T., & Volova, A. (2015). *Stronger together, a guide to supporting LGBT asylum seekers*. Washington, DC: LGBT Freedom and Asylum Network.

Menjívar, C. (2012). Transnational parenting and immigration law: Central Americans in the United States. *Journal of Ethnic and Migration Studies, 38*, 301–322. https://doi.org/10.1080/1369183X.2011.646423

Meyer, I. H. (2003). Prejudice, social stress, and mental health in lesbian, gay, and bisexual populations: Conceptual issues and research evidence. *Psychological Bulletin, 129*, 674–697. https://doi.org/10.1037/0033-2909.129.5.674

Morales, A., Corbin-Gutierrez, E. E., & Wang, S. C. (2013). Latino, immigrant, and gay: A qualitative study about their adaptation and transitions. *Journal of LGBT Issues in Counseling, 7*, 125–142. https://doi.org/10.1080/15538605.2013.785380

Morales, E. (2013). Latino lesbian, gay, bisexual, and transgender immigrants in the United States. *Journal of LGBT Issues in Counseling, 7*, 172–184. https://doi.org/10.1080/15538605.2013.785467

Nakamura, N., Kassan, A., & Suehn, M. (2015). Immigrants in same-sex binational relationships under DOMA. *Psychology of Sexual Orientation and Gender Diversity, 2*, 12–21. https://doi.org/10.1037/sgd0000089

Nakamura, N., Kassan, A., & Suehn, M. (2017). Resilience and migration: The experiences of same-sex binational couples in Canada. *Journal of Gay & Lesbian Social Services, 29*, 201–219. https://doi.org/10.1080/10538720.2017.1298489

Nakamura, N., & Morales, A. (2016). The criminalization of transgender immigrants. In R. Furman, A. Ackerman, & G. Lamphear (Eds.), *The immigrant other: Lived experiences in a transnational world* (pp. 48–61). New York, NY: Columbia University Press.

Nakamura, N., & Pope, M. (2013). Borders and margins: Giving voice to lesbian, gay, bisexual, and transgender immigrant experiences. *Journal of LGBT Issues in Counseling, 7*, 122–124. https://doi.org/10.1080/15538605.2013.785235

Nakamura, N., & Tsong, Y. (2019). Perceived stress, psychological functioning, and resilience among individuals in same-sex binational relationships. *Psychology of Sexual Orientation and Gender Diversity, 6*, 175–181. https://doi.org/10.1037/sgd0000318

Nieves-Lugo, K., Barnett, A., Pinho, V., Reisen, C., Poppen, P., & Zea, M. C. (2019). Sexual migration and HIV Risk in a Sample of Brazilian, Colombian and Dominican immigrant MSM living in New York City. *Journal of Immigrant and Minority Health, 21*, 115–122. https://doi.org/10.1007/s10903-018-0716-7

Piwowarczyk, L., Fernandez, P., & Sharma, A. (2017). Seeking asylum: Challenges faced by the LGB community. *Journal of Immigrant Minority Health, 19*, 723–732. https://doi.org/10.1007/s10903-016-0363-9

Radford, J., & Budiman, A. (2018). *Facts on U.S. immigrants, 2016: Statistical portrait of the foreign-born population in the United States*. Retrieved from http://www.pewhispanic.org/2018/09/14/facts-on-u-s-immigrants/#fb-key-charts-top

Rank, L. (2002). Gays and lesbians in the U.S. immigration process. *Peace Review, 14*, 373–377. https://doi.org/10.1080/1040265022000039141

Reading, R., & Rubin, L. R. (2011). Advocacy and empowerment: Group therapy for LGBT asylum seekers. *Traumatology, 17*, 86–98. https://doi.org/10.1177/1534765610395622

Reynolds, W. T. (1980). The immigration and nationality act and the rights of homosexual aliens. *Journal of Homosexuality, 5*, 79–87. https://doi.org/10.1300/J082v05n01_07

Rodriguez, N., & Hagan, J. (2004). Fractured families and communities: Effects of immigration reform in Texas, Mexico and El Salvador. *Latino Studies, 2*, 328–351. https://doi.org/10.1057/palgrave.lst.8600094

Satinsky, S., Hu, A., Heller, J., & Farhang, L. (2013). *Family unity, family health: How family-focused immigration reform will mean better health for children and families*. Oakland, CA: Human Impact Partners.

Sacchetti, M. (2018, January 22). In lawsuits, same-sex couples say U.S. wrongly denied their children citizenship. *The Washington Post*. Retrieved from https://www.washingtonpost.com/local/immigration/in-lawsuits-same-sex-couples-say-us-wrongly-denied-their-children-citizenship/2018/01/22/1c83c98a-fd34-11e7-8f66-2df0b94bb98a_story.html?utm_term=.9ab120254f77

Suárez-Orozco, C., & Suárez-Orozco, M. (2001). *Children of immigration*. Cambridge, MA: Harvard University Press.

Thronson, D. B. (2008). Custody and contradictions: Exploring immigration law as federal family in the context of child custody. *Hasting Law Journal, 59*, 453–513.

Tran, A. G. T. T., Lee, R. M., & Burgess, D. J. (2010). Perceived discrimination and substance use in Hispanic/Latino, African-born Black, and Southeast Asian immigrants. *Cultural Diversity and Ethnic Minority Psychology, 16*, 226–236. https://doi.org/10.1037/a0016344

U.S. General Accounting Office. (2004). *Defense of Marriage Act: Update to prior report (GAO-04-353R)*. Washington, D.C.: Author. Retrieved from http://www.gao.gov/new.items/d04353r.pdf

United Nations High Commissioner for Refugees [UNHCR]. (2016). *UNHCR's views on asylum claims based on sexual orientation and/or gender identity using international law to support claims from LGBTI individuals seeking protection in the U.S.* Retrieved from https://www.unhcr.org/5829e36f4.pdf

Yip, T., Gee, G. C., & Takeuchi, D. T. (2008). Racial discrimination and psychological distress: The impact of ethnic identity and age among immigrant and United States-born Asian adults. *Developmental Psychology, 44*, 787–800. https://doi.org/10.1037/0012-1649.44.3.787

# The "Second Generation:" LGBTQ Youth with LGBTQ Parents

Katherine A. Kuvalanka and Cat Munroe

The term "second generation" or "second gen" has been used to refer to "gay children of gay parents" for more than 25 years (Kirby, 1998). This term was coined by Dan Cherubin, a gay man with a lesbian mother, who founded a group for individuals like himself in the early 1990s and named it "Second Generation" (COLAGE, 2013). Such an act was deemed radical and even dangerous at the time—the 1980s and 1990s—when the social science literature on gay and lesbian parenting was in its infancy and the struggle for adoption and marriage equality rights was just getting underway. Gay and lesbian parents were fighting for custody of their children, desperately pushing back against their homophobic critics and trying to convince family court judges that gay and lesbian parents raise "normal" and "healthy" children—and, incidentally, "normal" and "healthy" meant "heterosexual" and "cisgender" (Garner, 2004). As legal fights for gay family rights unfolded, members of the second generation—i.e., now defined as lesbian, gay, bisexual, transgender, and queer (LGBTQ) individuals with LGBTQ parents (COLAGE, 2013)—were sometimes pushed into the LGBTQ "family closet" for fear that highlighting their existence would detract from these efforts. Cherubin, who received some horrified reactions from gay and lesbian parents when he spoke out about himself as second gen, understood and explained this fear when he said to the *New York Times* in 1998: "People are afraid of losing their kids" (Kirby, 1998).

Meanwhile, Cherubin and others were working to push open the LGBTQ family closet door to shed light on the experiences and support needs of the second generation. In the late 1990s, COLAGE (https://www.colage.org/)—the grassroots, community network of support for individuals with LGBTQ parents—partnered with Cherubin and has been providing community and support for "Second Genners" ever since. In 2004, Abigail Garner highlighted firsthand accounts from second gen youth and young adults in her pioneering, popular press book, *Families Like Mine: Children of Gay Parents Tell It Like It Is*, prompting calls in the social science literature (Goldberg, 2007; Mooney-Somers, 2006) for investigations into their experiences. Kuvalanka and Goldberg (2009) provided the first analysis in the social science literature that focused exclusively on second generation individuals, pulling from two larger studies of adults with LGB parents. Based upon their qualitative interviews, both Garner (2004) and Kuvalanka and Goldberg (2009) described potential

K. A. Kuvalanka (✉)
Department of Family Science and Social Work,
Miami University, Oxford, OH, USA
e-mail: kuvalaka@miamioh.edu

C. Munroe
University of California, San Francisco,
San Francisco, CA, USA
e-mail: cat.munroe@ucsf.edu

© Springer Nature Switzerland AG 2020
A. E. Goldberg, K. R. Allen (eds.), *LGBTQ-Parent Families*,
https://doi.org/10.1007/978-3-030-35610-1_15

advantages and challenges that second genners have experienced against the contextual backdrop of societal heterosexism and cisgenderism. The findings of Garner (2004) and Kuvalanka and Goldberg (2009), however, are limited by the relative homogeneity of their samples; most of their second gen research participants were well-educated, White, cisgender females with lesbian or bisexual mothers who grew up in the United States. The following quote from Garner (2004) reminds us of the diversity and variety of experiences among the second generation yet to be fully explored:

> A lesbian daughter of politically active lesbian mothers…will have a different second generation experience than a daughter raised by a closeted gay dad. Another family could include a transgender child and a gay dad. Another might have a bisexual mother with more than one queer son. Although "second generation" is an umbrella term for all LGBT kids with LGBT parents, there is no definitive second generation family experience that represents them all. (p. 179)

In the past decade, more research on the experiences of second gen individuals has emerged, such as a study focused exclusively on transgender and gender-diverse children with LGBQ parents (Kuvalanka, Allen, Munroe, Goldberg, & Weiner, 2018). Indeed, family scholars continue to have a role to play in moving the conversation about second gen youth beyond the simplistic and, often, homophobic debate about whether or not "gay parents raise gay kids"—we have a responsibility to articulate the richness and diversity in experiences among this population with the aim of learning more about the second generation and their families, to improve understanding and, ideally, acceptance of all families.

## Purpose of Current Chapter and Theoretical Underpinnings

In this chapter, we summarize what has been learned about second generation youth and adults in the popular press and social science literatures from Garner (2004) and Kuvalanka and Goldberg (2009) until now. We also draw from the first author's qualitative data with 30 second gen indi-

viduals to share previously unpublished findings, thereby extending what is known about the second generation by gleaning new insights from our participants' reflections upon their own lives and experiences. We provide nuance to previously articulated themes regarding the benefits and challenges experienced by second generation individuals; for example, we share how some participants described their LGBTQ parents as overcoming or bridging the "queer generation gap" described by Garner (2004) in relation to the generational divide between parents' and second genners' queer experience. We also share participants' diverse—and sometimes conflicted—reactions when asked what they think of use of the term *second generation* to describe themselves.

Our theoretical grounding is rooted firmly in a social constructionist perspective. That is, we view gender, sexual orientation, and family as socially and materially constructed (see Oswald, Blume, & Marks, 2005). Both biological (Hines, 2004) and social (Kitzinger, 1987) processes, as well as broader historical, cultural, and ideological contexts (Crotty, 1998; Schwandt, 2000), are deemed to be important influences on how individuals understand, experience, and assign labels to their gender and sexual orientation identities. Some second gen individuals may ultimately come to identify as LGBTQ due to shared genetics with their LGBTQ parent or due to their familial environment that allowed for gender and sexual identity exploration without fear of censure (Kuvalanka & Goldberg, 2009). Family context—as well as social interactions and cultural norms that celebrate or condemn queer persons and families—may uniquely influence second generation individuals' gender and sexual orientation identity formation (e.g., making coming out easier or harder) compared to LGBTQ individuals with heterosexual and cisgender parents (Kuvalanka & Goldberg, 2009).

We also consider a model of hegemonic heteronormativity recently put forth by Allen and Mendez (2018), which extended Oswald et al.'s (2005) theoretical model. Incorporating and building upon aspects of queer, feminist, intersectionality, and life course theories, Allen and

Mendez call upon family scholars to more explicitly and intentionally consider and interrogate how cisnormativity (in relation to gender), homonormativity (in relation to sexuality), and mononormativity (in relation to family) operate within spheres of contextual influence, such as race, class, ability, ethnicity, and nationality, over time. As such, Allen and Mendez suggest ways to expand our theorizing about second generation individuals' experiences, complementing suggestions for future research provided in Kuvalanka (2013), as well as in this chapter—namely, to extend utilization and application of social constructionist, intersectionality, and life course theories in future analyses.

## Increasing Second Gen Diversity in Published Research

In light of these theoretical underpinnings, we begin by describing the demographics of published study samples involving second gen participants and then follow with a summary of those studies' findings. Given the diversity of second generation individuals (Garner, 2004), more published studies mean more opportunities to better understand the diversity of this population's experiences. We begin with Garner (2004) and Kuvalanka and Goldberg (2009), which represent the two primary sources of data on the second generation and then proceed chronologically.

Garner (2004) did not explicitly say how many of the 50 adults she interviewed for her book identified as LGBTQ, but she devoted an entire chapter, "Second Generation: Queer Kids of LGBT Parents," to sharing their perspectives and experiences. Her participants were "in their 20s and 30s" (p. 8). Presumably, most participants were White, although demographics in regard to race and ethnicity were not provided. Most of the participants were born into the context of a heterosexual marriage, and then one or both of their parents later came out. Many participants were living in one of three cities—Minneapolis, New York, or San Francisco—but others lived throughout the United States, such

as Florida, Hawaii, Mississippi, Texas, and Washington, DC.

Kuvalanka and Goldberg (2009) drew their sample of 18 second generation participants (ages 18–35 years old; $M = 23.2$ years) from two separate larger studies involving adults with LGB parents. Eleven of the eighteen identified as female, three as male, three as genderqueer, and one as gender-ambiguous. Seven of the participants identified as bisexual, five as queer, three as gay, one as lesbian, one as mildly bisexual, and one as tranny-dyke. All but one of the participants were White; one participant was Chicano and White. In regard to education, all but one had attended at least some college. Most ($n = 16$) had lesbian mothers, one participant had a bisexual mother, and one had a lesbian mother and a bisexual mother. Most participants ($n = 13$) were born into the context of a heterosexual union and had mothers who later came out; three were born via donor insemination to two lesbian/bisexual mothers; two were born to unpartnered lesbian mothers. All but one participant (from the United Kingdom) grew up in the United States (six in the Northeast, six in the West, three in the South, and two in the Midwest).

A handful of works since Garner (2004) and Kuvalanka and Goldberg (2009) have explicitly discussed their inclusion of second generation participants in their larger samples of mostly heterosexual and cisgender individuals with LGBTQ parents. In their longitudinal study of planned lesbian mother families, who were recruited prior to having children, Gartrell, Bos, and Goldberg (2011) reported on the sexual orientations and sexual behavior of 78 adolescents (39 girls and 39 boys, 17 years old), whose lesbian mothers had been out as lesbians for the children's entire lives. All of the children were conceived via donor insemination. Approximately 87% of the adolescents identified their race/ethnicity as White, 4% as Latina/o, 3% as African American, 3% as Asian/Pacific Islander, 1% as Armenian, 1% as Lebanese, and 1% as Native American. In regard to their sexual orientations and behavior, more of the girls (19%) self-identified in the bisexual spectrum of the Kinsey Scale than the boys

(3%), while more of the boys (5%) self-identified as predominantly to exclusively homosexual than the girls (0%). Relatedly, the girls were significantly more likely to have ever engaged in same-sex sexual behavior compared to age- and gender-matched adolescents from a national probability sample, but the boys were not. Gartrell et al. (2011) referred to previous evidence (e.g., Diamond, 2007) of the fluidity of sexual orientation development and expression in general, and especially among women, to help explain the differences observed between the girls and boys in their sample.

One study explored the role that LGBTQ parents' involvement in the LGBTQ community plays in the lives of second gen youth when investigating how 42 young adults with LGBTQ parents navigated queer communities as adults (Goldberg, Kinkler, Richardson, & Downing, 2012). Of the 42 participants (ages 18–29 years), 33 identified as female, 8 as male, and 1 as genderqueer. Five identified as queer, two as gay, two as bisexual, and one as lesbian, and the rest as heterosexual. In regard to race/ethnicity, three participants identified as Hispanic/Latin American, two as multiracial, one as African American, and the rest (>85%) as White. All but one of the participants had attended at least some college. The family contexts in which participants grew up varied, with roughly half being raised by LGBQ parents from birth and half being born to (seemingly heterosexual) parents who later came out.

More recently, DiBennardo and Saguy (2018) investigated how 28 adults (ages 21–32 years)—all with at least one sexual minority (i.e., LGBQ) parent—negotiated the stigma they experienced related to their parents' stigmatized identity over time. The sample included 15 women, 12 men, and 1 person with a nonbinary gender identity. In terms of race, 14 participants identified as White, "eight responded that they racially identified as Jewish," and 4 identified as "mixed raced, ambiguous, or other" (p. 294). All participants had attended at least some college. Eleven of the twenty-eight participants were second generation in that they identified their sexual orientation as lesbian, gay, bisexual, or queer.

A recent anthology of stories by *queerspawn*—an intentionally controversial and political term coined by Stefan Lynch, the first Director of COLAGE, to refer to individuals with LGBTQ parents—was edited by Epstein-Fine and Zook (2018) and titled *Spawning Generations: Rants and Reflections on Growing Up with LGBTQ+ Parents.* Epstein and Zook, queerspawn themselves, sought out voices for their collection that would "span generations—from kids, teenagers, and young, middle-aged, and older adults" (p. 10). Although some of the contributors did identify as LGBTQ, a number of the authors in the anthology did not indicate their sexual orientation or gender identity; whether authors felt the information simply was not relevant, or whether their choice not to share their own sexual orientation or gender identity was an act of resisting others' curiosity and scrutiny of their identity, is unknown.

Finally, we describe a sample of 30 second gen young adults (ages 18–35 years; $M = 25.5$) from the first author's unpublished dataset (Kuvalanka, 2019). Most (70%; $n = 21$) of the participants identified as White; four identified as bi- or multiracial (African American and White; Black and White; Black/Native American and White; Native, Chicano, and White), three as White-Jewish, and two as Black or African American. The majority (57%; $n = 17$) identified as female, while eight identified as transgender or nonbinary (e.g., "transgenderqueer-fluid," "male-bodied/genderqueer"), and five as male. Just over half ($n = 16$) reported their sexual orientation as queer, while five identified as gay, three as bisexual, two as lesbian, and four used unique labels, including "gayqueer-homo" and "queer questioning." The majority (70%; $n = 21$) had one or more lesbian mothers, three had bisexual fathers, two had a mother they described as "butch-dyke," one described their mother as "queer/gay," one had a "female-to-male transsexual" parent, and one had a "male-to-female transgender" parent. Finally, all 30 participants grew up in the United States: 11 in the Northeast, 7 in the South, 7 in the West, and 5 in the Midwest.

While early second gen research (Garner, 2004) highlighted potential differences among second generation individuals and their parents in regard to gender, sexual orientation, and degree of "outness," increasingly diverse samples and theoretical lenses draw attention to other influential factors, such as race and geographical context—and the potential interplay between contextual and demographic factors. For example, it is not difficult to imagine that a White, queer woman who grew up on the West Coast with her bisexual and lesbian mothers had a somewhat different second generation experience than a White, queer FTM transgender man who grew up with a straight FTM transsexual parent in the Midwest. Indeed, the myriad of experiences and perspectives of second gen individuals have only begun to be represented in the social science literature.

## Expanding Understanding of Diverse Second Generation Experiences

One universal commonality in the lives of second gen individuals has been the presence of hetero sexism and cisgenderism—sources of adversity that shaped their experiences and their understandings of themselves and their families. One participant from Kuvalanka's (2019) dataset said: "I think that our experience growing up and existing in the world is that much richer…and more difficult as well…It's outside of the norm and outside of people's expectations and, in some cases, outside of what people find acceptable." As this participant alludes to, in addition to the potential challenges facing the second generation, there are also potential benefits to having LGBTQ parents when one also identifies as LGBTQ.

## Potential Advantages of Being Second Gen

Both Garner's (2004) and Kuvalanka and Goldberg's (2009) research revealed that having LGBTQ parents when one identifies as LGBTQ may be beneficial. Some participants, for exam-

ple, felt they had a less arduous coming out process than they otherwise might have had if their parents had been heterosexual. Some of Kuvalanka and Goldberg's (2009) participants said that they were able to discover their own LGBTQ identities sooner, in that having a non-heterosexual parent allowed them to explore and question their sexual or gender identities at a younger age, facilitating their own self-discovery. Participants from both studies believed that having LGBTQ parents had given them broader conceptualizations of the sexual orientation and gender identity options available to them. Many of them also did not worry about rejection upon disclosure of their identities to their LGBTQ parents. As one White gay man with a lesbian mother explained: "I didn't have that added fear of rejection from my mother, because no matter what, it was always like, there's no way she can reject me" (Kuvalanka & Goldberg, 2009, p. 912). Perhaps parental LGBTQ identity, support, and acceptance have the potential to counteract societal heterosexism and cisgenderism for some second gen youth, fostering self-acceptance, leading them to construct their own LGBTQ identities as normal and acceptable (Garner, 2004; Kuvalanka & Goldberg, 2009).

**Benefits of Early Socialization into LGBTQ Identities and Communities** Later studies built upon these findings of potential advantages. Gartrell et al. (2011), for example, noted that the adolescents in their sample were "born into families headed by mothers who were completely open about their lesbian orientation and active participants in the lesbian community" (p. 1205). Echoing prior scholars (Biblarz & Stacey, 2010; Garner, 2004; Kuvalanka & Goldberg, 2009; Stacey & Biblarz, 2001), they posited that "perhaps this type of family environment made it more comfortable for adolescent girls with same-sex attractions to explore intimate relationships with their peers" (p. 1205). DiBennardo and Saguy (2018) reported that one of their second gen queer participants felt that having LGBQ parents provided an early connection to the LGBQ community—a tie that she found beneficial as she formed her own queer identity. Similarly, Goldberg et al.' (2012) findings revealed differences between their second generation and heterosexual participants, in that the latter felt excluded from queer communities as adults: "For individuals who, in addition to having LGBQ parents, also identified as LGBTQ, such exclusionary practices were less salient since their legitimacy in LGBTQ communities was not questioned" (p. 81). These studies provide evidence that intergenerational LGBTQ socialization, including the fostering of connections to queer communities, is a topic worthy of further investigation for its benefits to second gen individuals in particular (Garner, 2004).

Indeed, some participants in Kuvalanka's (2019) dataset of 30 second gen young adults spoke about the benefits of having early ties and connections to LGBTQ communities, culture, and history via their parents. In doing so, they provided evidence for Garner's (2004) assertion that second generation youth may benefit from having "out" and "proud" LGBTQ parents who can serve as positive role models, having a strong connection to the LGBTQ community from a young age, and having a deep understanding of LGBTQ history and culture. One of Kuvalanka's (2019) participants, who identified as a biracial queer female, had a bisexual father who died of HIV/AIDS when she was a child. She felt that her early, close connections to the queer community profoundly shaped her experiences: "I grew up during the AIDS epidemic, you know, in the queer community...and I don't know other people who have a comparison to that."

As Garner notes, "LGBT parents...have the opportunity to pass on a priceless gift to their second gen children: pride in discovering their authentic selves" (p. 192). This unique advantage became evident for one of Kuvalanka's (2019) participants, who was biracial and genderqueer with White lesbian mothers. Upon entering college, the participant observed their LGBTQ peers with heterosexual and cisgender parents lamenting a lack of LGBTQ socialization.

This participant drew parallels between LGBTQ community socialization and race socialization in families:

> I think that there's a couple of issues that second generations bring forward that are really significant. I definitely really see this in the comparison of my experience of race and sexual orientation. This parallel became really visible to me, being both a second genner and being a person of color raised by White parents. I went to college and got involved in queer groups, and...no one had this sense of intergenerational queerness or queer history or connection with other generations of queer people. And people would often kind of highlight this difference between sexual orientation and race being, like, "People of color grow up in families of color, and they get to talk about racism, and they get strategies for dealing with racism in how they grow up, and queer people don't get that." And it was really big for me that second gen queer people do!...Second genners have this kind of familial background of queerness...especially for the people who grow up with queer parents, there's this sense of queer awareness and collective queer culture and queer history from a very young age. And it's very interesting to see queer communities I'm in lament the lack of that, and kind of be like, "Wait, some of us do have that!" But that is really significant and special and valuable and important to kind of have this opportunity to tap into queer culture maybe a decade or more before all of your peers, because, you know, most people have to wait until they come out as queer before they start experiencing queer culture, but second genners tend to get the opportunity to experience queer culture long before they come out as queer.

As such, this participant alludes to the protective role that early socialization into LGBTQ culture and intergenerational transmission of LGBTQ history and identity can have for LGBTQ individuals, as they are confronted with heteronormativity and cisnormativity in society—similar to the role that race socialization plays for children of color, preparing them for the impacts of racism.

That said, the diversity of second generation experiences in regard to early socialization into LGBTQ communities was evident in participants' stories from Kuvalanka's (2019) dataset. Some felt much more a part of LGBTQ communities than their parents ever were, while other participants wished that they had been exposed to more LGBTQ people when they were younger. One White queer female participant whose lesbian mom did not come out until the participant was an adult spoke about how her own coming out would have been easier if she had such socialization when she was younger. Even though her mother and father were open-minded, she was without "a model of what it even means to come out." She explained: "We did not have a queer politic as a family…there was no language, and there was no images, and there was no models for any of it."

**Bonding Over Queer Identities and Experiences** For the second gen individuals in Kuvalanka's (2019) dataset who did have out queer parents, some spoke in terms of feeling a special "bond" with their LGBTQ parent because of their shared LGBTQ identity—a concept that can be viewed as a potential protective advantage for second generation individuals. One participant referred to a sense of "camaraderie," while a queer bisexual woman with a lesbian mother and gay father said that she felt a "solidarity" with her non-heterosexual parents. A White gay male participant described his relationship with his lesbian mother as a special connection due to their shared experiences, something that LGBTQ individuals with non-LGBTQ parents (and LGBTQ parents with non-LGBTQ children) likely do not share:

> We're able to relate on a level that other LGBT people may not be able to if they have straight parents or straight children…I feel like I have that kind of connection with my mother, in terms of, I don't always have to explain things to her. She just kind of knows…I think it's just the implicit understanding…I think there's just that underlying sense of a shared experience that I feel as a second generation.

Kuvalanka's (2019) participants' narratives also raise questions about how this special connection or bond plays out in the context of other familial relationships. In some cases, participants noticed that their non-LGBTQ siblings were missing out on this special connection. Speaking to this, a White gay male participant with a lesbian mother

noted: "It creates this interesting bond that I know my sister doesn't share with my mom, because my sister's straight." In addition to serving a protective function, such a special "insider" connection between first and second generation LGBTQ family members may have the potential to cause tension or friction in second gen individuals' relationships with other family members; such tensions (or lack thereof) could be explored in future research.

## Potential Challenges

Participants in Garner's (2004) and Kuvalanka and Goldberg's (2009) research described challenges they faced as second gen youth. Some said they felt pressure from their LGBTQ parents and others to be heterosexual and gender-conforming—so much so that some delayed coming out as LGBTQ due to fears of fulfilling critics' assertions that "gay parents raise gay kids." Some felt annoyed with, or disempowered by, the assumption that their sexual or gender identities were necessarily related to their parents being LGBTQ. One White queer woman elaborated:

> That's something that's really been pushed on me—like, "You're like this because of your mom," which feels, like, really disempowering in a lot of ways. And I think that is probably the thing that has hurt the most … just this feeling of like, my claim to my identity is being taken away. (Kuvalanka & Goldberg, 2009, p. 911)

Some of Kuvalanka and Goldberg's (2009) participants also said that they initially did not want to be or had concerns about being LGBTQ, after witnessing the homophobic prejudice and discrimination that their parents had endured. Second generation youth are often aware of the heterosexism and cisgenderism their parents have faced (Mooney-Somers, 2006) and likely realize that they could face similar struggles. Such realizations may cause ambivalence or fear about coming out to others, evidence that having a LGBTQ parent is not guaranteed protection against the influence of societal heterosexism and cisgenderism.

**Pressure, Scrutiny, and Disempower-ment** Later writings echoed the findings of Garner (2004) and Kuvalanka and Goldberg (2009). Some of DiBennardo and Saguy's (2018) second gen participants feared that their own sexual orientation identities would validate others' assumptions that their parents caused them to LGBQ. Some felt that their parents' LGBQ identities constrained their own in that they felt pressure to be straight or that their sexual identity was "overshadowed" by that of their parents, giving participants less authenticity with others in the LGBQ community. These challenges were also evident in the essays in Epstein-Fine and Zook's (2018) anthology. Many of the contributors spoke to the constant curiosity others would express about their sexual orientation upon learning that one or both of their parents were queer. One woman described her experience responding to such questions by LGBTQ prospective parents in the years prior to her own coming out:

> It's not that the queer parents would have rejected me if I were queer, but I was the projection of their hope; I was the practically-perfect-in-every-way daughter who proved that queer people can raise children and they can turn out all right…I had to give these prospective parents…hope that they would not fuck up their future children and that their queerness was a gift, something of which their children would be fiercely proud. (pp. 80–81)

The words of the second gen persons in Epstein-Fine and Zook's (2018) anthology further demonstrate that there is no single experience of having queer parents or being second gen. Many described an ambivalence regarding disclosure of their parents' queer identities due to others' reactions and the associated questions that typically followed, as described above, and situated this ambivalence in the time they came of age—often, in the 1980s and 1990s, at a time of particularly intense cultural stigmatization of queer identities and parenthood. One third-generation (i.e., at least one parent and grandparent were LGBTQ) queer woman writing for Epstein-Fine and Zook's queerspawn anthology described the following:

> It takes a lot of work to open up about my origin story knowing that there is a history and context to our reality that goes undefined in these rapid-fire question interrogations…as queer people, we are expected to either discuss family matters that are both personal and political to educate our neighbours, friends, and colleagues on command, or to remain silent and private as not to upset anyone or make them feel too uncomfortable. (p. 172)

Such testimonials underscore the stigmatization of queer identities and families and the ways that second gen queer people worked to either avoid or challenge that stigma.

**LGBTQ Parents as Inhibitors of Second Gen Identity Development** Perhaps counterintuitively, several of Kuvalanka and Goldberg's (2009) participants reported that they did not turn to their lesbian/bisexual mothers for support when exploring and discovering their sexual and gender identities. Sons of lesbian/bisexual mothers, especially, tended to tap other sources of support. Some sons may have been hesitant to turn to their mothers because of perceptions that aspects of gay male culture (e.g., pornography) may clash with lesbian political leanings (Jensen, 2004). Some mothers' internalized homophobia and shame also seemed to inhibit open discussions about sexual orientation identities. Further, timing of parents' and children's coming out can be a crucial factor in how or if second gen youth look to their LGBTQ parents for support (see chapter "LGBTQ Siblings and Family of Origin Relationships"). Garner (2004) noted that not all second generation individuals come out to a parent who is openly LGBTQ: "Sometimes a parent comes out *after* the child, rather than the other way around" (p. 184). Although it might be assumed that most LGBTQ parents serve as lifelong LGBTQ role models for their children, a parent's disclosure of a non-heterosexual or gender-nonconforming identity might happen later in life—perhaps during a child's questioning of their own identity or even after a child has already come out as LGBTQ. Thus, the timing of a parent's coming out is likely to have an influence on second generation youth's exposure to queer identities and communities and, subsequently, on their LGBTQ identity formation. Having "out and proud" parents from a young age might encourage second gen youth to more readily accept their own queer identities. Having parents come out during their children's adolescence, however, when these youth may be questioning their own identities and also trying to establish independence from their parents, could perhaps cause some youth to postpone their own LGBTQ identity formation.

Several participants in Kuvalanka's (2019) dataset, whose parents came out later in life, spoke to this theme. One White queer female participant's mother came out when the participant was a teenager; prior to the mother discovering her own lesbian identity, the mother was unhappy and ended up having an affair with a woman while still married to the participant's father. This family turmoil was happening as the participant was beginning to figure out her own sexual orientation—thus, she felt that her own coming out was negatively impacted: "I think that…had I been in a happy and healthy home environment that I probably would have come out earlier and actually been out." Furthermore, this participant felt that she might have turned to her mother for support had her mother not been going through her own period of sexual identity discovery:

> It felt a little weird for me to be going through the same thing my mom was going through, like, figuring out sexuality, and so I didn't want to talk to her about it. And so I think the idea of talking about sexuality with somebody who knew something about being bisexual or queer, I think that would have been something I might have considered…but I didn't feel like my mom necessarily had that knowledge at that point, because she had just come out. And…I almost didn't want to take away her new, exciting thing that was going on in her life. I didn't want her to have to deal with me. 'Cause you, you know, it's like she was stuck in this like rut of unhappiness for so long, and then all of a sudden figured out what was wrong…And so…I didn't want to share that journey with her at all, and I also wanted her to just like be unencumbered by me.

This participant wanted her journey to be distinct from her mother's for herself and for her mother.

Additionally, a "queer generation gap" (Garner, 2004, p. 181)—differences in social norms and experiences between the first and second queer generations—also seemed to be a barrier to LGBTQ youth turning to their LGBTQ parents for support or to their parents providing support. Participants of both Garner (2004) and Kuvalanka and Goldberg (2009) cited disagreements between themselves and their parents about how out to be in their communities and also utilized different language (e.g., *queer* as opposed to *lesbian* or *gay*) to describe their own identities. Further, some participants with nonbinary gender identities in Kuvalanka and Goldberg's study said that their cisgender lesbian/bisexual mothers had difficulty comprehending non-cisgender identities.

**Broadening Understanding of the "Queer Generation Gap"** Goldberg et al. (2012) findings extend understanding of the queer generation gap—a divide that second gen individuals may widen in order to gain a sense of independence. The researchers categorized participants' connections to LGBTQ communities as children and then identified trajectories in terms of how those connections changed or were maintained over time; seven of the ten second gen participants described weak connections to queer communities as children that later grew to become strong connections as adults. For some of these participants, their parents came out later in life, which may explain some of the weak connections during childhood. But the authors also posited that perhaps these participants retrospectively perceived their childhood connections to LGBTQ communities as weak and their present connections as stronger given their sexual orientation identities—and that, for some of these second gen adults, creating distinctions between their own and their parents' connections to LGBTQ communities was important. According to the authors:

> They may…wish to emphasize their personal feelings of agency in creating a unique type of community engagement that extends beyond the kinds of community involvement that their parents forged when they were children. For example, 24-year-old Kate explained that her lesbian mother's LGBTQ community was significantly different from her own: "They're more conservative in

their social openness than I and my friends are. Also, they socialize at different venues. I go to gay clubs; my mom goes to church." For Kate and others, it was important to make a distinction between the LGBTQ communities to which their parents belonged and those they called their own. (p. 79)

Second gen participants from Kuvalanka's (2019) dataset, like those in other studies, spoke to this generation gap. Yet their narratives extend this discussion by providing examples of how their parents had worked to bridge the gap over time. For example, a Jewish queer female participant with a butch dyke mother (and a genderqueer sibling) spoke to the effort put forth by her mother:

My mom is very much of her generation, but she's also really dynamic and has learned a lot over the course of my lifetime and really learned from and with us about queerness and about politics. And I don't know very many people who are queerspawn whose parents…get anything about trans stuff or who are actually totally cool and fine and happy about their kids being trans, you know, 'cause of all that generational stuff of dykes who are like, "Why aren't you just a butch?" So, our mom has really, you know, it took work for her, and she was interested and willing to do that work, because she's got a dynamic kind of engagement with identity and the world, so that's something that I'm really, really grateful for.

As this participant and others alluded to, it is not only the first generation that teaches the second generation about LGBTQ issues and culture— teaching and learning happens in the other direction as well. A White queer female participant explained how she expanded her lesbian mother's and her mother's partner's understandings of gender and gender identity in particular:

[I] have had really interesting conversations with mom and [my mom's partner] and have really helped them shift and open and widen their view of gender and [how they talk] about identity…As I started to date folks who were trans and/or masculine identified, I think it pushed a lot of their buttons to think differently and more broadly about gender.

As in previous analyses (Kuvalanka & Goldberg, 2009), Kuvalanka's (2019) nonbinary participants discussed their parents' lack of knowledge about trans identities. Notably, a White genderqueer participant with lesbian mothers was also

hesitant to come out to their parents about being in a polyamorous relationship. This hesitation was due to the perceived queer generation gap that existed between the participant and their parents that had played a role in the mothers not being supportive of the participant's trans identity and which the participant assumed extended to their relationship orientation—although those perceptions eventually improved:

[My parents] are heavily influenced by second-wave feminism…They [don't]…have much awareness of trans issues or even bi issues…And for me, I spend almost all my time in queer spaces that are critically thinking about gender and attraction. So it definitely does feel like a difference when I spend time in the same circles that my parents spend time in—like, it's a different queer community. And, you know, I grew up in it, so it is very much my home, but it's also, like, not the same kind of safe space, the same kind of community… And…a lot of times they just dismissed the parts of my version of queerness that were very, very important to me…[But] they've definitely become more supportive. I think it's been three years now, they've gotten really good about using the right pronouns and acknowledging the important parts of my identity and having a better understanding of what's going on for me…[But] I spent a couple of years afraid to come out to them as poly because, like, they're having enough difficulty with the whole trans thing…[But] they just totally completely accepted the whole poly thing right off the bat…As far as, like, being a poly family unit, my parents totally are accepting of that and always try…and make sure that both [of my partners] are feeling included and welcomed into the family, and that's been really great.

In one fell swoop, this participant speaks to actual and anticipated resistance from within their own family when challenging cisnormativity, homonormativity, and mononormativity (Allen & Mendez, 2018). For this participant and their parents, the queer generation gap narrowed over time, allowing for the second generation to feel more accepted, understood, and pleasantly surprised by the first.

**The Complexity of Family Acceptance** Early analyses (Garner, 2004; Kuvalanka & Goldberg, 2009) discussed the reactions of LGBTQ parents upon learning that their children were also LGBTQ. Some second gen individuals reported that they knew their LGBTQ parents would accept them, while others were disappointed with how their LGBTQ parents responded. Those less-than-positive reactions included parents voicing fears about potential discrimination their children might face or worries that others would "blame" the parents for their children's LGBTQ identity.

Interviews from Kuvalanka's (2019) dataset also reflected a diversity of experiences in regard to familial reactions, revealing the potential complexity of family acceptance. Second generation individuals often must navigate coming out to multiple people in their families and, thus, may be confronted with various reactions from different family members. For example, a queer and genderqueer participant of color, who was adopted by two lesbian mothers, shared the mothers' differing reactions to learning that their child was queer before they knew their child was nonbinary:

> I told them that I had a girlfriend…my mom was kind of just like, "Okay," and then was like, "Well, don't jump to conclusions in assuming your gay." I'm like, "Okay, it sounds pretty gay to me, but okay [Participant laughs]." And my other mom was just kind of like, she took it well and…she always asked about my girlfriend…but my other mom like never ever mentioned my girlfriend…so that was a little difficult.

This participant demonstrated how familial acceptance is a complex concept in that LGBTQ individuals may have varying degrees of it in their families—even among the first generation.

Family members' reasons for having positive, negative, or ambivalent reactions to the coming out of a second generation individual can vary as well. A White gay male participant shared his lesbian mother's reaction, as well as his straight father's and stepmother's differing responses:

> [My mom] wasn't…as happy as I would have expected. I think she was surprised…I think she initially felt…I don't want to say felt sorry for me, but she knew first-hand some of the crap I was going to have to deal with…but I mean, she was very open and accepting…I told my dad at a later time…and he was pretty accepting—I think more accepting than I was expecting…And then I told my stepmother…and she just, like, blew a gasket.

> Like, she was just so disappointed and crying and…was like, "I'll never have grandkids." (Kuvalanka, 2019)

Thus, this participant was confronted with a range of reactions that were unexpected and that were also borne from different concerns, including fear for the child and (presumed to be) dashed future plans.

For second generation individuals from divorced families where parents came out after having children, non-LGBTQ parents may be struggling emotionally with a former spouse's coming out. By extension, these non-LGBTQ parents might have a difficult time untangling their ex-spouses' and their children's coming out. A White bisexual female participant shared how she and her gay father came out to one another on the same night and also her mother's negative response:

> So me and him had this conversation one night over dinner where he told me—he was like, "Take it or leave it, love me for who I am, or whatever you want to do"…and I was like, "Well, Dad, me and you are more alike than we thought." [laughs] So, then I told him about me being bisexual, and he was thrilled, and he was like, "Yay, I'm not alone"…[My mother] is not very accepting of it…I think she's in denial. She doesn't want anyone in her family to be gay. She doesn't want my dad to be gay, she doesn't want me to be bisexual. (Kuvalanka, 2019)

When considering sources of support for second generation individuals, the potential complexity of family structures and relationships, as well as variations in beliefs and attitudes, must be recognized.

Important to note is that family members' attitudes toward second gen individuals and their LGBTQ identities can change over time. Illustrating this from Kuvalanka's (2019) dataset, a White gay male participant, with a gay father who came out when the participant was 17 years old, described how his straight mother's response to her son being gay improved over time:

> Mom did not receive it as well, so I had to deal with that. Dad obviously received it well, because he identifies that way…[but] mom cried, she was very upset, went to the psychologist to see, like, what was wrong with me…[She's] more come to

grips with it now, knows who I'm dating—like, she's been to dinner with a boyfriend of mine.

Thus, initial familial reactions can morph over time into more accepting attitudes and behaviors. That said, family scientists should continue to draw attention to the various challenges that second generation youth may face stemming from the myriad familial contexts in which they exist.

## Sexual Minority Mothers of Transgender and Gender-Diverse Children

We turn now to sharing findings from a subset of data from the first author's longitudinal study of 49 families with transgender and gender-diverse (i.e., trans) youth (Kuvalanka et al., 2018). This research focused on eight White, sexual minority mothers of trans children (ages 6–11 years; $M = 7.9$ years) living in the United States and the ways in which participants' sexual minority identities affected their acceptance of and response to their trans child. Seven of the eight mothers identified as female, and one identified as gender fluid. Four of the eight mothers identified as bisexual, three as lesbian, and one as bi-/pansexual; we refer to these sexual minority mothers collectively as "queer." At the time of data collection, three of the participants were single mothers; five were involved in intimate relationships (three were involved with women; two were involved with men). All eight had at least attended some college; four had bachelor's degrees, and two had graduate degrees. In regard to the children's demographics, six were assigned male at birth; two were assigned female. Six of the children identified as a gender other than the one they had been assigned at birth and had fully socially transitioned. Six of the eight children were White, and two were Latina/o and White. Although Kuvalanka et al.'s (2018) work did not address the perspectives of the second generation children themselves, the perspectives and experiences of the parents interviewed were thematically similar to prior research on second gen individuals (Garner, 2004; Kuvalanka & Goldberg, 2009).

Several of the sexual minority parents in Kuvalanka et al.'s (2018) study described their queer identities as conferring both a set of benefits and unique challenges as they worked to parent their trans children. Several described a personal acceptance of gender nonconformity, as well as prior exposure to trans individuals in the context of the LGBTQ community, which enabled them to be accepting of their child's gender presentation from an early stage in the child's development. Parents described a personal understanding of "being different," which instilled in them the knowledge that providing support to their child regarding gender identity and expression was crucial. Simultaneously, parents also described their own experience of being queer and marginalized as increasing their anxiety for their children's safety; at times, parents described this anxiety as resulting in a temporary effort to police or discourage their children's gender expression. In addition, parents described social pressure to have cisgender, heterosexual children, in order to demonstrate the legitimacy of queer parenthood. These concerns dovetail with previous findings that some second gen individuals experienced internalized heterosexist stigma resulting in felt pressure not to confirm a stereotype that queer parents have queer children. At times, internalized heterosexism was observed in sexual minority mothers who dissuaded their trans children from coming out. Reminiscent of reports from Kuvalanka and Goldberg's (2009) trans and nonbinary participants, most of the mothers were not initially aware of or educated about non-cisgender identities, highlighting the differences and, perhaps, tensions and historical rifts within LGBTQ communities (Dickey, 2016). Indeed, "identifying as a sexual minority does not equate to understanding, or being comfortable with, trans people or trans issues" (Kuvalanka et al., 2018, p. 82).

## Reactions to the Term "Second Generation"

Before we conclude this chapter, we (the authors of this chapter) felt it was important to take a step back to find out what LGBTQ individuals with LGBTQ parents might think about the label, "second generation," that has been ascribed to them. We drew from the first author's dataset of 30 LGBTQ young adults with LGBTQ parents (Kuvalanka, 2019) to learn how these participants felt about the term.

Several of the participants shared ambivalence about the label "second gen." Although some said that the term conjured a feeling of kinship with other queer individuals who also had queer parents—a White queer female participant with a bisexual mother said, "When I found out about [the term], I was really excited to know that I wasn't the only one, and that there's an identity for it"—this was often described alongside a desire to separate one's self and identity from that of their parents. These concerns were tied to a dislike of the assumption that they are queer "because of" their parents, a desire to have their own identity and sense of belonging to the queer community separate from that of their parents, and discomfort with assumptions being made about their identity due to their second generation status. The extent to which these concerns reflected a desire for individual identity vs. resistance to stigma—i.e., cultural assumptions that queer parents raise queer children and that somehow represents failure or inability to parent "correctly"—is unclear. In addition, several participants were uncomfortable with the term because of concerns that "second generation" implies a genetic component to queer identity and anxiety that identification of such a gene could lead to attempted genocide of queer-identified persons. This underscores the anxiety held not only by queer persons broadly, who chronically face stigma and stigmatizing experiences, but by second generation queer persons specifically, as though their existence creates risk or vulnerability for the queer community.

Of note is that one participant, a biracial queer female participant whose father was bisexual, did not feel "strongly attached to" the second generation label but liked it, "because it acknowledges that there's history." She went on to argue that the term should be opened up to more LGBTQ people who have been influenced by "queer elders." She explained:

> I know folks who don't have any queer parents but had a queer uncle, or their mom's best gay friend, who was a huge source of support or influence in acceptance of their own queerness, who would just as excitedly accept the term "second gen," and I think deserve it.

Thus, this participant challenges us to reconsider the boundaries of LGBTQ family concepts—namely, the primacy of parents in children's lives—by suggesting that the second generation circle be widened to include even more queer experiences and stories.

## Implications for Practice

Clinicians and other family professionals should not dismiss the concerns of LGBTQ individuals with LGBTQ parents that their openness about their identities—and even the claiming of the "second generation" label—could bring harm to their families. Despite the US Supreme Court's marriage equality decision in 2015, LGBTQ individuals continue to experience institutionalized discrimination, and LGBTQ-parent families and the second generation in particular continue to be the focus of anti-LGBTQ scrutiny. Family professionals have a responsibility to advocate for social justice on the part of participants and clients and to push back against harmful anti-LGBTQ policies and rhetoric. That said, the worries and fears of the second generation are shaped by historical time and place; the visibility of and threats to LGBTQ individuals and families are different today than they were for LGBTQ youth with LGBTQ parents growing up two and three decades ago. Thus, the needs and strengths of this population are not only diverse, given the diversity of individual demographics, but also dynamic relative to larger societal changes over time.

In summary, second gen individuals may benefit from certain advantages of which family professionals should make themselves aware. Early exposure to LGBTQ identities and communities may facilitate and foster the development of second gen individuals' sexual and gender identities (relatively) free from heteronormative and cisnormative shame and fear. Further, early LGBTQ community socialization may also serve a protective function; that is, queer socialization can be likened to that of race socialization in that it may instill pride in young people and prepare them for and buffer against the negative impact of societal discrimination. Opportunities for second gen youth to learn about queer culture and to participate in LGBTQ cultural events, such as Pride Parades, could lessen the negative impact of societal heterosexism and cisgenderism. Given that geographic locale will determine the number and type of such opportunities, clinicians living in areas with fewer resources might work to ensure that second gen youth at the very least have access to books and films that depict LGBTQ individuals and history. Some second gen individuals might also feel a special bond with their LGBTQ parents, deepening emotional and psychological closeness between parent and child, as well as with the LGBTQ community, which may translate into easier transitions into and stronger connections to LGBTQ communities as an adult.

Second gen individuals might also face certain challenges. In this chapter, we illustrated how many of these challenges, such as feeling pressure to be heterosexual or cisgender, stem from societal heterosexism and cisgenderism. Internalized heterosexism and cisgenderism can lead LGBTQ parents to react less-than-positively to their children's coming out. Parents who are concerned for their children's safety may effectively inhibit their children's sexual orientation and gender development and expression. Family professionals can help parents weigh the costs of such actions both in the short and long term and help guide them toward more supportive behaviors regarding their children. Further, the timing of a parents' coming out can have a stifling impact on second gen youth, especially if both the parent's and the adolescent's identity development and disclosure occur around the same time. Second gen individuals may also experience a queer generation gap between themselves and their parents, which can reflect generational differences and changes in queer communities

and culture over time. The sheer diversity of sexual and gender identity labels that exist today are exponentially larger than in years past—thus, first and second generation individuals may not share the same language to discuss what it means to be LGBTQ, which can lead to misconceptions and disconnection. Indeed, first and second gen individuals may not have all that much in common, especially if, for example, a parent is cisgender and a child is not. Our research revealed, however, the potential for flexibility and growth among both the first and second generations, who can learn from each other, which may foster their resilience as a family. Knowledgeable clinicians can help negotiate conversations and learning between the first and second generations, helping each to gain a greater understanding of the other.

In this chapter, we also highlighted the vast diversity that exists among this population in terms of, for example, familial structure, parent-child LGBTQ identity combinations, timing of parental out, and familial reactions to and acceptance of second generation individuals' sexual orientation and gender identities. Clinicians working with this population should not make assumptions about the influence that an LGBTQ parent may have had on a second gen individual, their response to that individual (e.g., in terms of their coming out), the connection the second gen individual had to queer communities or culture during childhood, or even the feelings that a LGBTQ individual with LGBTQ parents might have about the *second generation* label. They should also be aware that degrees and sources of acceptance and support can vary for second generation individuals—and that family members' attitudes, understanding, and support can change over time.

## Directions for Future Research

Future research on the second generation needs to continue to expand the diversity of samples so that they eventually reflect the actual diversity that exists among this population. Despite making strides in the past decade in this regard, such as the representation of trans and nonbinary individuals with LGBTQ parents and the inclusion of individuals who were raised by out LGBTQ parents from very young ages, most of our research is still focused on White, highly educated individuals with lesbian mothers. As evidenced by the review of research in this chapter, as a field we are making progress toward greater inclusivity—yet, work remains to be done. For example, little is known about working-class second generation individuals or about LGBTQ individuals with transgender parents. Further, given that research participants from majority racial groups seldom spontaneously reflect upon how their racial identity has impacted their experiences— and researchers rarely prompt them to do so— future research should intentionally set out to address such questions (Allen & Mendez, 2018). We concur with Epstein-Fine and Zook (2018), who reflected upon how historical forms of privilege shaped their own volume, and lament those "whose histories do and do not get told" (p. 9). Indeed, there are gaps and shortcomings that persist in the social science literature on second generation individuals. Yet, we also acknowledge that strides have been made and opportunities abound and are ripe for LGBTQ scholars to expand our understanding of LGBTQ families in general and second gen individuals in particular—a population that will undoubtedly keep pushing the family field forward.

## References

Allen, S. H., & Mendez, S. N. (2018). Hegemonic heteronormativity: Toward a new era of queer family theory. *Journal of Family Theory & Review, 10*, 70–86. https://doi.org/10.1111/jftr.12241

Biblarz, T. J., & Stacey, J. (2010). How does the gender of the parents matter? *Journal of Marriage and Family, 72*, 3–22. https://doi.org/10.1111/j.1741-3737.2009.00678.x

COLAGE. (2013). *2nd Gen FAQ—For LGBTQ folks with LGBTQ parents*. Retrieved from: https://www.colage.org/2nd-gen-faq-for-lgbtq-folks-with-lgbtq-parents/

Crotty, M. (1998). *The foundations of social research: Meaning and perspective in the research process*. London, UK: Sage.

Diamond, L. M. (2007). A dynamical systems approach to the development and expression of female same-sex sexuality. *Perspectives on Psychological Science, 2*, 142–161. https://doi.org/10.1111/j.1745-6916.2007.00034.x

DiBennardo, R., & Saguy, A. (2018). How children of LGBQ parents negotiate courtesy stigma over the life course. *Journal of International Women's Studies, 19*, 290–304. Retrieved from: https://vc.bridgew.edu/jiws/vol19/iss6/19

Dickey, L. M. (2016). Transgender inclusion in the LGBTQ rights movement. In A. E. Goldberg (Ed.), *The SAGE encyclopedia of LGBTQ studies* (pp. 1223–1226). Thousand Oaks, CA: Sage.

Epstein-Fine, S., & Zook, M. (2018). *Spawning generations: Rant and reflections on growing up with LGBTQ+ parents*. Bradford, ON: Demeter Press.

Garner, A. (2004). *Families like mine: Children of gay parents tell it like it is*. New York, NY: Harper Collins.

Gartrell, N. K., Bos, H. M. W., & Goldberg, N. G. (2011). Adolescents of the U.S. national longitudinal lesbian family study: Sexual orientation, sexual behavior, and sexual risk exposure. *Archives of Sexual Behavior, 40*, 1199–1209. https://doi.org/10.1007/s10508-010-9692-2

Goldberg, A. E. (2007). Talking about family: Disclosure practices of adults raised by lesbian, gay, and bisexual parents. *Journal of Family Issues, 28*, 100–131. https://doi.org/10.1177/0192513X06293606

Goldberg, A. E., Kinkler, L. A., Richardson, H. B., & Downing, J. B. (2012). On the border: Young adults with LGBQ parents navigate LGBTQ communities. *Journal of Counseling Psychology, 59*, 71–85. https://doi.org/10.1037/a0024516

Hines, M. (2004). *Brain gender*. New York, NY: Oxford University Press.

Jensen, R. (2004). Homecoming: The relevance of radical feminism for gay men. *Journal of Homosexuality, 47*, 75–81. https://doi.org/10.1300/J082v47n03_05

Kirby, D. (1998, June 7). The second generation. *The New York Times*. Retrieved from: http://query.nytimes.com/gst/fullpage.html?res=950CE1D91E3BF934A35755C0A96E958260

Kitzinger, C. (1987). *The social construction of lesbianism*. London, UK: Sage.

Kuvalanka, K., & Goldberg, A. (2009). "Second generation" voices: Queer youth with lesbian/bisexual mothers. *Journal of Youth and Adolescence, 38*, 904–919. https://doi.org/10.1007/s10964-008-9327-2

Kuvalanka, K. A. (2013). The "second generation:" LGBTQ children of LGBTQ parents. In A. E. Goldberg & K. R. Allen (Eds.), *LGBT-parent families: Innovations in research and implications for practice* (pp. 163–175). New York, NY: Springer.

Kuvalanka, K. A. (2019). *Interviews with 30 second generation adults* (Unpublished raw data).

Kuvalanka, K. A., Allen, S. H., Munroe, C., Goldberg, A. E., & Weiner, J. L. (2018). The experiences of sexual minority mothers with trans* children. *Family Relations, 67*, 70–87. https://doi.org/10.1111/fare.12226

Mooney-Somers, J. (2006). What might the voices of the second generation tell us? *Lesbian & Gay Psychology Review, 7,* 66–69.

Oswald, R. F., Blume, L. B., & Marks, S. (2005). Decentering heteronormativity: A model for family studies. In V. L. Bengtson, A. C. Acock, K. R. Allen, P. Dilworth-Anderson, & D. M. Klein (Eds.), *Sourcebook of family theory & research* (pp. 143–154). Thousand Oaks, CA: Sage.

Schwandt, T. (2000). Three epistemological stances for qualitative inquiry: Interpretivism, hermeneutics, and social constructionism. In N. K. Denzin & Y. S. Lincoln (Eds.), *Handbook of qualitative research* (2nd ed., pp. 189–214). Thousand Oaks, CA: Sage.

Stacey, J., & Biblarz, T. (2001). (How) does the sexual orientation of parents matter? *American Sociological Review, 66,* 159–183. https://doi.org/10.2307/2657413

# LGBTQ Siblings and Family of Origin Relationships

Katie M. Barrow and Katherine R. Allen

LGBTQ-parent families exist as part of larger family networks where they actively participate in their roles as children, siblings, aunts or uncles, cousins, partners/spouses, parents, and grandparents. Immediate and extended family networks can influence processes as far ranging as identity formation and disclosure processes, to parenting decisions and later life care. Studying family relationships that exist beyond the spousal or parent-child relationship, which tend to be the focus of research and practice, improves our understanding of the embeddedness of family ties across time (Bertone & Pallotta-Chiarolli, 2014; Connidis, 2007).

How LGBTQ individuals, such as siblings, relate to members of their family beyond the intragenerational tie of partners and intergenerational tie of parent-child is an understudied yet exciting topic ripe for research. That is, when family members are included in research, it is usually at the intersection of LGBTQ individuals' romantic relationships and/or parenting processes. The dichotomy between a seemingly heteronormative family of origin and the creation of queer families draws attention to the tension that may arise between LGBTQ individuals and their family members (Bertone & Pallotta-Chiarolli, 2014). As LGBTQ individuals move throughout their life course, how they negotiate these tensions within their families of origin is vital to our understanding of how family members shape each other's lives.

The sibling relationship is one of the main relationships associated with the family of origin. Research is now emerging on the experiences of siblings in the lives of LGBTQ individuals and families. In this chapter, we examine the emerging scholarship on the various ways that siblings operate as friend, confidant, surrogate or donor parent, caretaker, distant relative, and adversary. Attention to race, ethnicity, gender, gender identity, sexual orientation, and social class further reveals distinct opportunities for those working with LGBTQ families to redefine—and purposefully utilize—sibling roles and relationships.

The chapter begins with an overview on current and promising theoretical frameworks used to discuss LGBTQ individuals and their relationships with siblings and family networks. We draw on a variety of theories embedded in scholarship often focused broadly on LGBTQ-parent families but with limited attention to the sibling relationships within these families. Next, we discuss sibling relationships as part of the broader family of origin. Then, we highlight the myriad of ways that siblings interact with and rely on one another

K. M. Barrow (✉)
School of Human Ecology, Louisiana Tech University, Ruston, LA, USA
e-mail: kbarrow@latech.edu

K. R. Allen
Department of Human Development and Family Science, Virginia Tech, Blacksburg, VA, USA
e-mail: kallen@vt.edu

© Springer Nature Switzerland AG 2020
A. E. Goldberg, K. R. Allen (eds.), *LGBTQ-Parent Families*,
https://doi.org/10.1007/978-3-030-35610-1_16

across the life course. We end the chapter with implications for practice and further research, offering remarks on the future of this understudied area and its invaluable contributions to LGBTQ family research.

## Theoretical Insights

Several theoretical frameworks have shed light on the family relationships of LGBTQ individuals, including life course perspective (Orel & Fruhauf, 2013), symbolic interaction (Glass & Few-Demo, 2013), family stress theory (Willoughby, Doty, & Malik, 2008; Willoughby, Malik, & Lindahl, 2006), systems theory (Heatherington & Lavner, 2008; Scherrer, Kazyak, & Schmitz, 2015), feminist perspectives (Glass & Few-Demo, 2013), queer theories (Catalpa & McGuire, 2018; Kuvalanka & Goldberg, 2009), social constructionism (Kuvalanka & Goldberg, 2009; Vinjamuri, 2015), ambiguous loss (Catalpa & McGuire, 2018; McGuire, Catalpa, Lacey, & Kuvalanka, 2016), and minority stress (Oswald, Cutherbertson, Lazarevic, & Goldberg, 2010). In the following sections, we expound upon select theories that have contributed to literatures on both adult sibling relationships and LGBTQ family relationships and highlight a promising new theory on transfamily relationships (McGuire, Kuvalanka, Catalpa, & Toomey, 2016).

A compelling theoretical framework that cuts across literatures on adult sibling relationships as well as LGBTQ relationships is a life course perspective. Life course theory emphasizes the importance of life stages, transitions, and trajectories and how they are linked across family members (Allen & Henderson, 2017; Walker, Allen, & Connidis, 2005). An LGBTQ sibling deciding to adopt a child will most likely create a ripple effect throughout the family, signifying the effect of linked lives. While the concepts of *LGBTQ individual* and *parent* pose a contradictory and unexpected transition for some families, the expectation that most people will parent (and thus produce grandchildren for their parents) signals a transition into a new role of grandparent or

aunt/uncle. Additionally, timing of events can be in unison or out-of-synch insofar as siblings who become parents at about the same time, for example, may forge connections around this similar life experience. As one gay father surmised, about becoming closer to his siblings, who also had children: "We talk a lot more. We have more in common." (Bergman, Rubio, Green, & Padron, 2010, p. 216).

Family systems theory is another framework found in both the adult sibling literature and the LGBTQ relationships literature. This approach posits that family processes can be best understood when taking into account the entire family system, acknowledging that relationships occur at various subsystems (e.g., parent-child, sibling) and suprasystems. As Whitchurch and Constantine (1993) explain, a suprasystem is larger than the immediate family system and can be explored in relation to families of origin and extended kin networks, as well as within racial-ethnic communities.

The desire for the family to remain stable and in a state of equilibrium can help explain why family members are resistant to a child or sibling coming out. This could further illuminate coalitions that arise between individuals who are out and the family members who know and/or are accepting or rejecting (Heatherington & Lavner, 2008). For example, one Taiwanese mother in Brainer's (2017) study of gender and sexually nonconforming people and their Taiwanese families had been trying for the last 12 years—since her child was in middle school—to change her transmasculine daughter's gender identity. Persistent traditional, cultural notions of gender, sexuality, and family—as well as the larger societal impact of being the parent of a gender-nonconforming child—forced this Taiwanese mother to tirelessly work toward maintaining a sense of balance in the family. A coalition arose in which mother, transmasculine daughter, and heterosexual son worked to keep the father from knowing the daughter's gender-nonncomforming identity. A separate coalition also arose between siblings during middle childhood and adolescence, as evident by this quote from Skye, the transmasculine child:

[My mom] started picking on my dressing and all that…I think at that time I was in her room, and Tim [Skye's older brother] was also there, and he supported me. Tim said, "I don't think there's anything wrong with the [shirt]. Why do you make a big deal out of such a small thing?" And my mom said, "Ask your sister if she's a freak." (p. 932)

Moreover, the desire by those working with LGBTQ families to move away from a "family binary [that] privileges biological and legal ties as 'genuine' family" (Oswald, Blume, & Marks, 2005, p. 146) is rooted in feminist, queer, and social constructivist lenses. Sibling relationships transcend bio-legal constraints and can be defined in a variety of ways, such as through a sibling's marriage (i.e., brother- or sister-in-law), parent's cohabitating relationship (i.e., quasi-sibling; Weisner, 1989), or those formed through foster care. Continual changes in family structure can cause stepsiblings and half siblings to enter and exit the family system well throughout adulthood (Spitze & Trent, 2018; White, 1998), which begs the question, *who counts as a sibling?* Perhaps the more important question is how individuals define their sibling and family relationships. In a study of 14 LGBQ youth, Grafsky, Hickey, Nguyen, and Wall (2018) considered the role of stepfamilies in decisions surrounding the coming out process. In referencing her stepmom, who legally adopted her, one youth stated: "She's not my [mom]; she's not even a friend" (p. 155), while another youth imagined her stepsiblings as part of her immediate family. Indeed, Goldberg and Allen's (2013) work examining how young adults in LGB-parent families navigate parental break-ups and stepfamily formation further stresses the need for individuals to adopt expansive notions of sibships (i.e., sibling relationships) that incorporate context and flexible definitions reflecting the complexity of LGBTQ family life. A 17-year-old woman with two mothers, who separated when she was six, had this to say when asked about her sibships:

I was adopted. . . .My mom got a sperm donor, so my sister is biologically one of my mother's children, and then I was adopted when I was two-and-a half. . . .Both my parents got divorced and remar-

ried [when] I was in first grade. . . .They're both currently remarried and each of my new parents had children from previous relationships, so in total I gained four stepsisters and stepbrothers. (p. 540)

The further application of an intersectional framework (Few-Demo, 2014) sharpens a focus on historical and contextual interlocking systems of oppression and how race, ethnicity, gender, sexual orientation, and social class interact to influence how LGBTQ individuals and families engage their family networks. LGBTQ individuals and families from multiracial and multinational backgrounds, in particular, utilize extended family and fictive kin networks, in African American (Glass & Few-Demo, 2013; Moore, 2011), Latinx (Swendener & Woodell, 2017), and Asian (Merighi & Grimes, 2000; Ocampo, 2014) families. Moore's (2011) ethnographic study on Black lesbian women in New York City illustrates gender, race, and social class intersecting to shape family circumstances. A prevailing theme in the story of Jackie, one of Moore's participants, is survival for her immediate and extended family as she navigates parent and sibling drug addictions, financial instability, and custody arrangements. At certain times, Jackie was responsible for parenting her siblings before eventually assuming responsibility for her siblings' children. Although she faced deafening backlash as a single lesbian mother adopting her nephew, she reiterated: "That's my nephew. That's my blood." (p. 136). Moore stipulates that for the women in her study, "tradition of kinship care and tightly woven interfamilial relationships…dictated their course toward parenthood more strongly than innate or intense personal desires to mother" (p. 141), reflecting a perceived social responsibility to parenthood.

Finally, transfamily theory, an emergent theory developed by McGuire, Kuvalanka, et al. (2016), focuses on cisnormativity and gender binaries, critiquing the presumed existence of only two genders and that physical sex equates to gender. Transfamily theory emphasizes the unique processes related to learning that a sibling is transgender and the shift in identity that accompanies this knowledge, for example, from a brother to a sister (Kuvalanka, Allen, Munroe, Goldberg, & Weiner, 2017). In a study of five mothers with transgender children, Kuvalanka, Wiener, and Mahan (2014) acknowledge that siblings can be "affected by the social transition and may undergo important transformations as they travel on this 'journey' with their transgender siblings and families" (p. 369). Gender, in particular, is ubiquitous in organizing sibling and family interaction, and a transfamily theory holds promise for understanding how a change in this defining sibling structure influences the meaning imbued in sibling relationships.

## Broader LGBTQ Family Networks as a Context for Sibling Relationships

Envisioning LGBTQ-parent families as part of broader family systems, such as their families of origin and extended kin networks, affords a multilayered perspective on the enduring ties of family life and the intersecting roles of immediate and extended family members—including siblings—in different family contexts. Research incorporating the immediate and extended family networks of LGBTQ individuals and families tends to cluster around management of a sexual or gender minority status and coming out processes, which are typically situated in a Western perspective (Jhang, 2018), the acknowledgment and inclusion of LGBTQ partners by family members, and support before, during, and after the transition to parenthood. Despite the scarcity of literature on LGBTQ sibling relationships, we suggest that these relationships may play an important role during each of these family processes. For this reason, we briefly review this related literature in order to shed light on the diversity of family networks and sibling ties.

Several relational and contextual factors influence identity management and the decision to disclose an LGBTQ status in a family system. For racial-ethnic minority individuals, an LGBTQ identity overlaps with identities nested in race, ethnicity, and culture. A qualitative inquiry into the lives of 57 African-, European-,

Mexican-, and Vietnamese-American young adult gay men underscores the unique challenges faced by young gay people of color (Merighi & Grimes, 2000). A 24-year-old Mexican-American gay male captures the complexity of identifying as a gay man situated in extended family networks and broader cultural expectations:

> I just felt like I was going to be a bad son by [coming out]….By saying that I'm gay, I might have a negative effect in the family in terms of how others might view the family, not just me….I have so many nieces and nephews. I was concerned about how they would be viewed, especially in our hometown of Mexico…how would my relatives treat my family? I would never feel good if my family would be mistreated and seen as a bad family or an immoral family only because I'm gay. (p. 35–36)

Findings from Merighi and Grimes (2000) call attention to the reality that some families live in a family closet. The family closet is created based on the heteronormative expectations of family and social networks, directly reflecting a family's sense of who they can or cannot come out to (Švab & Kuhar, 2014). Indeed, a focus on multicultural contexts underscores the linked lives of LGBTQ individuals with immediate and extended families, drawing attention to the centrality of family and perceived role of culture in disclosure processes.

How family networks recognize and include LGBTQ partnerships is another burgeoning area of scholarship that reveals important considerations for LGBTQ families. Employing an integrated symbolic interactionist and Black feminist theory framework, Glass and Few-Demo (2013) interviewed 11 Black lesbian couples about their family of origin and extended family experiences, noting that all but one couple had children. Couples in their study received mixed reactions from families with regard to social support, yet findings show flexible pathways by which immediate and extended kin demonstrate support to sexual and gender minority families. Specifically, the positioning of Black lesbian partners as fictive kin allowed extended families to envision partners as family members who share in cultural events and celebrations. Fictive kin are unrelated via bio-legal definitions yet occupy roles and duties in the extended family that may accompany a "relabeling" (Glass & Few-Demo, 2013, p. 721) such as "sis" or "sister." The importance of fictive kin has been observed in Black families, as historic race-based discrimination and current structural barriers (e.g., poverty, incarceration) have prompted their creation and preservation as a means for survival (Allen, Blieszner, & Roberto, 2011; Glass & Few-Demo, 2013; Taylor, Chatters, Woodward, & Brown, 2013).

In addition, the family of origin fulfills vital roles in the journey to and through LGBTQ parenthood. Research has largely focused on the negative experience of LGBTQ individuals and couples within their family of origin, including the lack of support received from parents, siblings, and other family members when articulating parenting desires (Brown, Smalling, Groza, & Ryan, 2009; von Doussa, Power, & Riggs, 2015). Some LGBTQ individuals are met with contradictory responses, as family members show acceptance of a sexual or gender minority status yet view queer parenting as in direct opposition to traditional, cisnormative notions of family and parenting (Brown et al., 2009; Goldberg, 2012). Other LGBTQ individuals report an increased closeness with families of origin across the journey to parenthood (Bergman et al., 2010). A qualitative investigation examining 35 predominantly White gay couples' motivations for pursuing parenthood found that one-third of men described a positive experience growing up in a close family (Goldberg, Downing, & Moyer, 2012). For these men, the enduring interconnection of their own family ties demonstrated a family process of closeness that they hoped to reproduce with their own children. And still for some, they hoped to augment this closeness through biological connection. Indeed, research on decision-making processes of LGBTQ parents choosing parenthood (e.g., through surrogacy, donor insemination, or adoption) indicates a preference by some individuals for a biogenetic connection with future children (Goldberg & Scheib, 2015; Karpman, Ruppel, & Torres, 2018; Nebeling Petersen, 2018). Several explanations support the desire for biological relatedness, and a salient theme in this literature underscores the

significance of a shared race and cultural heritage by both the LGBTQ couple and their families. As one Iranian lesbian couple mentioned when interviewed about their family formation process: "For actually both my family and Maana's family. . .I think Iranians culturally care a lot more about genetics [and] biology" (Karpman et al., 2018, p. 124). Indeed, some findings point to biological relatedness as a way to strengthen the family of origin ties (Nebeling Petersen, 2018) while simultaneously causing nongenetically related family members to have difficulty recognizing the child as a member of the family (see chapter "Gay Men and Surrogacy"). In concluding our examination of the broader networks of LGBTQ families as the major context for experiencing relationships among siblings, we now return to the influential ways in which LGBTQ families are shaped by their sibships.

## LGBTQ Families and Sibling Relationships

Sibling relationships tend to be the longest-lasting familial relationship, influential from early childhood through later life (e.g., Walker et al., 2005; Whiteman, McHale, & Soli, 2011). For LGBTQ individuals, sibships prove vital during the development and maintenance of a sexual or gender minority status, as coming out can yield exciting and challenging opportunities for relating to one another (Gorman-Murray, 2008). When contemplating future family formations, LGBTQ youth profess a commitment to include their siblings during this phase of life (Merighi & Grimes, 2000), and research shows that LGBTQ individuals and couples deciding on parenthood do indeed rely on their siblings in unique ways (Karpman et al., 2018). Akin to heterosexual sibships, sibships in which one or more individual is LGBTQ tend to experience ebbs and flows across the life course. For example, scholars have begun turning their attention to the role of LGBTQ siblings in midlife and late life, such as their capacity to serve as caregivers (Cohen & Murray, 2006), and in doing so underline the enduring interconnections of sibships. The purposeful inclusion of sibships as a unit of analysis in LGBTQ family research, however, remains rare, as does the inclusion of LGBTQ sibships in sibling and family of origin research. As such, the following section outlines key areas in both literatures where an overlap has been established.

## Coming Out to Siblings

Much research has been dedicated to understanding the dynamic process of revealing (or not revealing) an LGBTQ identity, relationship, and family. "Coming out" has traditionally been told through a White, androcentric, middle-class lens that overlooks interlocking, systemic forms of oppression (Brooks, 2016; Moore, 2011) and may not apply to the experiences of collectivistic cultures (Jhang, 2018). Terms such as "coming in" (Moore, 2011), "staying in" (Brooks, 2016), and "scaffolding" (Jhang, 2018) have been coined to better capture diverse coming out experiences. Scholars have also highlighted the ongoing process of coming out whereby LGBTQ individuals must repeatedly come out to the same people, come out to different people and in different contexts, and make ongoing decisions regarding if and how to reveal an LGBTQ identity (Denes & Afifi, 2014; McLean, 2008).

When individuals choose to self-disclose to family members, it is usually first to a mother figure (Carnelley, Hepper, Hicks, & Turner, 2011; Scherrer et al., 2015), although a growing number of studies indicate that siblings are often the recipient of a first disclosure (Barrow & Allen, 2019; Grafsky et al., 2018; Reczek, 2016; Salvati, Pistella, Ioverno, Laghi, & Baiocco, 2018; Toomey & Richardson, 2009). Given the presumed egalitarian nature of sibships—as opposed to the hierarchal parent-child relationship—disclosing to a sibling may be viewed as less threatening and serve a wider purpose of gauging how the larger family system might react. Individuals may also share a close bond with their sibling and find meaning in ensuring they are aware of a sexual or gender minority identity. If the sibling reacts positively, they may be further used as a source of support when eventually coming out to

other family members. A study of 40 Filipino and Latino gay young men found that siblings provided support when coming out to immigrant parents, offering to stand up for their sibling and challenge heteronormative expectations:

> My mom was crying when I first told her I had a boyfriend. My dad yelled at me about who was gonna pass along our family name. My sister yelled at them to shut up, "I'll just hyphenate my last name if that makes you happy!" (Ocampo, 2014, p. 169)

Siblings may also act as shields for one another. First described by Jhang (2018) in a study of 28 LGB Taiwanese individuals and their family relationships, shields were formed when the issues of other siblings (e.g., academic probation, substance abuse) diverted parental attention away from the sexual orientation of the LGB sibling. Some sibling issues may be transitory (e.g., parental dissatisfaction with a sibling's single status), while others might be a persistent distractor (e.g., addiction).

Further, siblings often occupy dual roles in the family system and may act as a source of support for an LGBTQ sibling as well as for parents. Ocampo (2014) signals the inherent stress associated with acting in the mediator role yet underscores its significance in bridging the family, as best articulated when one heterosexual sibling "felt it was worth it when she saw her parents finally become open not only to their gay children, but also their children's partners" (p. 170). For other families, acceptance is nonexistent, and heterosexual siblings may reside in a perpetual state of being stuck in the middle. A case study of a Romani family living in Belgium showed that after their father became violent toward their gay brother, two siblings intervened and years later their brother occasionally "asks [them] to say hello to his father for him" (Haxhe, Cerezo, Bergfeld, & Walloch, 2018, p. 413). This situation represents the triangulation of heterosexual siblings in order to maintain indirect communication with another member of the family, which can be activated by the LGBTQ sibling, heterosexual sibling, or parent.

A unique finding to emerge in the literature on coming out and LGBTQ sibling relationships is the impact of coming out in a family when a sibling has already disclosed a sexual or gender minority identity (Barrow, 2016). In a study by Barrow and Allen (2019), 15 young adults reflected on their experiences formulating an LGBTQ identity and their perceptions of being the second sibling (and second child) to disclose a nonheterosexual identity. Participants were concerned about how their family would react to having yet another LGBTQ child, and a subset were concerned they would be perceived as merely copying or imitating their sibling, as seen in this quote from Maggie: "I am not simply following my brother, obviously, but [I've wondered] if it's something that won't cross people's minds." Overall, participants spoke with love and affection for their LGBTQ sibling and articulated a strong sense of camaraderie and mutual understanding due to sharing a minority identity, as illustrated by Sofia: "[We] unite under the banner of being sexual minorities. We both view love as the same: It's love, no matter who you are. That's what we share." In light of a shared understanding, many siblings went on to lean on each other during the coming out process to parents, other siblings, and extended family. They learned more about themselves and their identities through observing what their sibling went through, which shed light on gender biases surrounding sexual orientation (e.g., being a gay man versus a lesbian, or being "butch" versus "femme") as well as stigmas faced by bisexual and transgender individuals in their own families and the larger LGBTQ community.

## Creating and Sustaining Families

Previously we discussed the concept of a family closet by which families of origin must navigate the process of revealing a child or sibling's sexual or gender minority status. Alternatively, parenthood precipitates a rearranging of the closet (Bergstrom-Lynch, 2012). Significant transitions along the life course, such as committing to a partner or having a child, may serve as a touchstone for siblings to reconnect or reaffirm their support for one another. While limited research

describes the role of heterosexual siblings in commitment ceremonies and wedding rituals (Badgett, 2011; Reczek, 2016), several studies elucidate the various roles of sibships across the journey to and through parenthood.

A critical life event such as the birth of a child by a heterosexual sibling can bring siblings together or increase distance, depending on the nature of the sibship (Jenkins, 2008). For some heterosexual siblings, their concern over or flatout disagreement of a sexual or gender minority status leads them to minimize or eliminate contact between their children and LGBTQ sibling, highlighting the ambivalence of family of origin relationships experienced by many (Reczek, 2016). The existence of LGBTQ families contrasts with their values and stokes fear that a sexual or gender minority status is contagious (Jenkins, 2008). Many heterosexual and nonheterosexual siblings, however, are actively engaged in their role as aunt or uncle to their LGBTQ sibling's children (see chapter "Race and Ethnicity in the Lives of LGBTQ Parents and Their Children: Perspectives from and Beyond North America"; Grafsky et al., 2018).

Receiving support from siblings positively influences the creation of LGBTQ families. In a qualitative study exploring transgender adults' attitudes toward parenthood, Tom, a transman, felt encouraged to pursue parenthood after his sister characterized him as "someone who'd be good with kids" (von Doussa et al., 2015, p. 1126). In some cases, individuals demonstrate support for the parenting desires of their LGBTQ siblings by serving as a donor parent and/or a surrogate. This provocative way of "doing family" uniquely positions the sibling relationship as a space where LGBTQ families can concurrently sustain and actively challenge heteronormative assumptions of family creation. A desire by some parents for their children to resemble them (Dempsey, 2013; Nebeling Petersen, 2018) reinforces the centrality of biogenetic ties and, for queer families of color, is situated within overlapping identities on the margins of race, ethnicity, and culture. Queer parents of color may seek a shared racial-ethnic minority identity with their child and are critical of a "color-blind" approach that deemphasizes cultural connections by adoption agencies and those who pursue adoption, viewing this as a barrier to transracial adoptions (Karpman et al., 2018). Moreover, the use of siblings in the creation of LGBTQ-parent families further challenges standard notions of family formation and family structure. For example, Karpman et al. (2018), who investigated the family formation process of queer couples of color, describe one of their participant families like this: "Shannon, who identified as half-Filipina and half-White, was married to a White woman. Her wife carried their child, and they used Shannon's brother as their donor" (p. 127). Lastly, for some LGBTQ siblings, they are the only child in the family who can or wants to have children, causing excitement among parents because they may be seen as their parents' only hope for grandchildren (Goldberg, 2012). In these situations, their decision to raise a child can be met with sibling support (e.g., a brother who does not desire to have children is excited to be an uncle) or may be met with discontentment (e.g., a sister who is struggling with fertility issues may harbor resentment).

## Sibling Ties in Midlife and Later Life

Taking into account the historical context of mid- and later-life LGBTQ sibships, themes of homophobia, transphobia, and ostracization are likely to be present. These siblings did not come-of-age during *Obergefell v. Hodges* or the Black Lives Matter movement or at a time when the word "transgender" was widely used. This cohort came-of-age in the context of the cultural revolution for gay liberation that was marked by the Stonewall Riots of June 1969, a time when homosexuality was still illegal and deemed a mental illness. In the 1980s and 1990s, LGBTQ older adults witnessed the illness and death of their friends during the AIDS crisis, and legislation such as Don't Ask, Don't Tell and the Defense of Marriage Act were signed into law. Older LGBTQ cohorts experienced a much more deeply entrenched heteronormative, gender, and racial bias that operated at every level of government

and within families, schools, and communities. Although these discriminatory attitudes and practices still exist across a multitude of personal and political contexts, they are becoming less tolerated by younger generations (Pew Research Center, 2019).

Very little attention has been paid to LGBTQ sibling relationships in later life, with the exception of Connidis (2007, 2010) who has used case studies to reveal the value of sibling and family of origin ties for older gay men and lesbians. When research areas are understudied, the use of finely grained methodological strategies, such as memoir (Connidis, 2012) and personal narrative (Allen, 2019), open the door to new ways of considering unexamined family ties, such as sibling relationships in adulthood. In her personal narrative of the dissolution of her previous lesbian relationship and the loss of contact with her ex-partner's biological son, Allen interviewed her brother and his husband for their perspectives on the break-up. Allen's brother-in-law was the donor of her lost son. In this analysis, the three members of the sibling subset—a biological sister, a biological brother, and a brother-in-law—revealed their divergent perspectives about marriage, parenthood, and relational dissolution in their extended family, thereby shedding new light on both hardship and recovery of family ties over the life course.

Social support networks are frequently cited as vital to the overall health and well-being of LGBTQ older adults; however, these networks rarely include a sibling or other family member (Fredriksen-Goldsen, Kim, Shiu, Goldsen, & Emlet, 2015). Instrumental (e.g., grocery shopping) and emotional support are twice as likely to arise from informal support networks and families of choice as opposed to families of origin (Brennan-Ing, Seidel, Larson, & Karpiak, 2014). Previous research illuminates how partners, friends, neighbors, and community members (e.g., pastor) lend support and buffer the risk of becoming isolated (Czaja et al., 2016). For transgender adults in particular, though, the lack of formal and informal support might be the cause of higher reports of depression, unemployment, and low income (Hoy-Ellis & Fredriksen-

Goldsen, 2017). Further, some LGBTQ older adults have never revealed their identity to family members. In a study assessing healthcare of 124 Hispanic and non-Hispanic LGBT adults ages 50–89, one participant mused: "To what extent do [we] feel comfortable being out with these providers if [we are LGBT]? Many of us have not even disclosed this to our siblings!" (Czaja et al., 2016, p. 1108). Considering the lifelong heterosexism experienced by LGBTQ adults, many older individuals maintain secrecy within the confines of sibling and family relationships (Orel, 2017). One study of LG older adults noted that of the individuals who were out—and subsequently rejected by family members—some may have never received familial recognition or acceptance until a partner's death (Barrett, Whyte, Lyons, Crameri, & Comfort, 2015).

Notwithstanding, the family of origin can also promote a sense of belonging for LGBTQ adults, especially as they perform their roles as sibling, aunt/uncle, and child (Orel, 2017). Older LGBTQ adults undertake caregiver roles for their siblings as well as for their parents (Cohen & Murray, 2006). These duties usually fall along gender lines, reflecting the structural confines of gender in sibships that designate women as natural caretakers. Additionally, apart from the typical roles that siblings tend to enact throughout their lives, a few studies have showcased the idiosyncrasies of sibships in midlife and late life. One such study acknowledged the presence of siblings in aiding the connectivity of intergenerational relationships between LG children, their partners, and the family of origin during the downsizing and clearing out of the family home (Reczek, 2014). Another study demonstrated sibling support during midlife via the inclusion of LGB partners in family rituals, with one participant reflecting on feeling especially included when his partner's siblings became outraged over the possibility he might not bring his "[coveted] homemade caramels and jellies" to the Christmas celebration (Oswald & Masciadrelli, 2008, p. 1065). When being inclusive of LGBTQ partners, the seemingly ordinary processes that siblings reenact at various points in midlife and late life become flashpoints of acceptance within the sibling and family relationships.

## Practical Implications and Future Research Directions

Across broadening family networks that increasingly utilize sibling relationships, LGBTQ families are showcasing creative ways of doing family. Considering how the lives of siblings and their families intersect with age, clinicians, practitioners, educators, and scholars should recognize the value of intentionally including siblings in their work. Sibling relationships, as the longest lasting of all family ties, are often contentious and ambivalent, but they are also reservoirs of potential support that individuals may tap into at different points in the life course.

The importance of and reliance on family networks during single parenthood has been well-documented in the literature across all racial-ethnic groups. However, this work has been done almost exclusively on heterosexual single parents, raising the question what about LGBTQ single parenthood? As research denotes, LGBTQ individuals look to their siblings as donors or surrogates, thus upholding yet resisting heteronormative ideals of how families ought to look. What role do siblings and family networks play in the lives of single parents? How might perceived family closeness impact an LGBTQ person's decision to enter into single parenthood?

An area for future research to address is the difficult topic of aggression, bullying, and violence that sometimes occurs in sibling relationships (Martinez & McDonald, 2016; McDonald & Martinez, 2016). We tend to shy away from these painful, often misunderstood topics, and yet now that a multitude of research on LGBTQ families is emerging, we are in a position to delve deeper into the invisible aspects of family relationships. Given what research on sibling relationships has uncovered about sibling rivalry, violence, and parental tendencies to minimize its impact (McDonald & Martinez, 2016), how might aggression and violence in childhood or adolescence affect the sibling relationship in midlife and late life? More importantly, when we factor in that one or more siblings might be navigating a sexual or gender minority status, how does this impact sibling aggression?

Investigating how sibships and the family of origin shape the lives of LGBTQ families can yield insight into the multilayered roles of sibling and parents in navigating various family processes, such as coming out. When a sibling comes out, coalitions may form and alliances shift. Emergent research has illustrated the concept of sibling shielding (Jhang, 2018) and mediation (Barrow & Allen, 2019) in the process of coming out. Future research could closely examine reorganizations in family alliances, as well as investigate the presence or absence of expectations related to heteronormative ideas of the family. Clinicians and practitioners working with LGBTQ individuals, couples, and family members can help unmask and bring into the open these invisible alliances (and any presumptive heteronormative assumptions) in the family of origin as a way to improve family relationships and family communication processes. Siblings continue to show support in a variety of ways, and when family practitioners purposely center this unique family relationship in practice and in research, we deepen our understanding of sibships and the family of origin in the lives of LGBTQ families.

# References

Allen, K. R. (2019). Family, loss, and change: Navigating family breakup before the advent of legal marriage and divorce. In A. E. Goldberg & A. Romero (Eds.), *LGBTQ divorce and relationship dissolution: Psychological and legal perspectives and implications for practice* (pp. 221–232). New York, NY: Oxford University Press.

Allen, K. R., Blieszner, R., & Roberto, K. A. (2011). Perspectives on extended family and fictive kin in the later years: Strategies and meanings of kin reinterpretation. *Journal of Family Issues, 32*, 1156–1177. https://doi.org/10.1177/0192513X11404335

Allen, K. R., & Henderson, A. C. (2017). *Family theories: Foundations and applications*. Malden, MA: Wiley.

Badgett, M. V. L. (2011). Social inclusion and the value of marriage equality in Massachusetts and the Netherlands. *Journal of Social Issues, 67*, 316–334. https://doi.org/10.1111/j.1540-4560.2011.01700.x

Barrett, C., Whyte, C., Lyons, A., Crameri, P., & Comfort, J. (2015). Social connection, relationships and older lesbian and gay people. *Sexual & Relationship Therapy, 30*, 131–142. https://doi.org/10.1080/14681994.2014.963983

Barrow, K. M. (2016). Relationship with siblings, youth. In A. E. Goldberg (Ed.), *The Sage encyclopedia of LGBTQ studies* (pp. 936–939). Thousand Oaks, CA: Sage.

Barrow, K. M., & Allen, K. R. (2019). *Coming out as the second LGBTQ sibling: Perceptions of a shared family identity*. Manuscript submitted for publication.

Bergman, K., Rubio, R. J., Green, R. J., & Padron, E. (2010). Gay men who become fathers via surrogacy: The transition to parenthood. *Journal of GLBT Family Studies, 6*, 111–141. https://doi.org/10.1080/15504281003704942

Bergstrom-Lynch, C. A. (2012). How children rearrange the closet: Disclosure practices of gay, lesbian, and bisexual prospective parents. *Journal of GLBT Family Studies, 8*, 173–195. https://doi.org/10.1080/1550428X.2011.623929

Bertone, C., & Pallotta-Chiarolli, M. (2014). Putting families of origin into the queer picture: Introducing this special issue. *Journal of GLBT Family Studies, 10*, 1–14. https://doi.org/10.1080/1550428X.2013.857494

Brainer, A. (2017). Mothering gender and sexually nonconforming children in Taiwan. *Journal of Family Issues, 38*, 921–947. https://doi.org/10.1177/0192513X15598549

Brennan-Ing, M., Seidel, L., Larson, B., & Karpiak, S. E. (2014). Social care networks and older LGBT adults: Challenges for the future. *Journal of Homosexuality, 61*, 21–52. https://doi.org/10.1080/00918369.2013.835235

Brooks, S. (2016). Staying in the hood: Black lesbian and transgender women and identity management in North Philadelphia. *Journal of Homosexuality, 63*, 1573–1593. https://doi.org/10.1080/00918369.2016.1158008

Brown, S., Smalling, S., Groza, V., & Ryan, S. (2009). The experiences of gay men and lesbians in becoming and being adoptive parents. *Adoption Quarterly, 12*, 229–246. https://doi.org/10.1080/10926750903313294

Carnelley, K. B., Hepper, E. G., Hicks, C., & Turner, W. (2011). Perceived parental reactions to coming out, attachment, and romantic relationship views. *Attachment & Human Development, 13*, 217–236. https://doi.org/10.1080/14616734.2011.563828

Catalpa, J. M., & McGuire, J. K. (2018). Family boundary ambiguity among transgender youth. *Family Relations, 67*, 88–103. https://doi.org/10.1111/fare.12304

Cohen, H. J., & Murray, Y. (2006). Older lesbian and gay caregivers: Caring for families of choice and caring for families of origin. *Journal of Human Behavior in the Social Environment, 14*, 275–298. https://doi.org/10.1300/J137v14n01_14

Connidis, I. A. (2007). Negotiating inequality among adult siblings: Two case studies. *Journal of Marriage and Family, 69*, 482–499. https://doi.org/10.1111/j.1741-3737.2007.00378.x

Connidis, I. A. (2010). *Family ties and aging* (2nd ed.). Los Angeles, CA: Pine Forge Press.

Connidis, I. A. (2012). Interview and memoir: Complementary narratives on the family ties of gay adults. *Journal of Family Theory & Review, 4,* 105–121. https://doi.org/10.1111/j.1756-2589.2012.00127.x

Czaja, S. J., Sabbag, S., Lee, C. C., Schulz, R., Lang, S., Vlahovic, T., … Thurston, C. (2016). Concerns about aging and caregiving among middle-aged and older lesbian and gay adults. *Aging & Mental Health, 20,* 1107–1118. https://doi.org/10.1080/13607863.2015.1072795

Dempsey, D. (2013). Surrogacy, gay male couples and the significance of biogenetic paternity. *New Genetics and Society, 32,* 37–53. https://doi.org/10.1080/14636778.2012.735859

Denes, A., & Afifi, T. D. (2014). Coming out again: Exploring GLBQ individuals' communication with their parents after the first coming out. *Journal of GLBT Family Studies, 10,* 298–325. https://doi.org/10.1080/1550428X.2013.838150

Few-Demo, A. L. (2014). Intersectionality as the "new" critical approach in feminist family studies: Evolving racial/ethnic feminisms and critical race theories. *Journal of Family Theory & Review, 6,* 169–183. https://doi.org/10.1111/jftr.12039

Fredriksen-Goldsen, K. I., Kim, H.-J., Shiu, C., Goldsen, J., & Emlet, C. A. (2015). Successful aging among LGBT older adults: Physical and mental health-related quality of life by age group. *The Gerontologist, 55,* 154–168. https://doi.org/10.1093/geront/gnu081

Glass, V. Q., & Few-Demo, A. L. (2013). Complexities of informal social support arrangements for black lesbian couples. *Family Relations, 62,* 714–726. https://doi.org/10.1111/fare.12036

Goldberg, A. E. (2010). *Lesbian and gay parents and their children: Research on the family life cycle.* Washington, DC: American Psychological Association.

Goldberg, A. E. (2012). *Gay dads: Transitions to adoptive parenthood.* New York, NY: New York University Press.

Goldberg, A. E., & Allen, K. R. (2013). Same-sex relationship dissolution and LGB stepfamily formation: Perspectives of young adults with LGB parents. *Family Relations, 62,* 529–544. https://doi.org/10.1111/fare.12024

Goldberg, A. E., Downing, J. B., & Moyer, A. M. (2012). Why parenthood, and why now? Gay men's motivations for pursuing parenthood. *Family Relations, 61,* 157–174. https://doi.org/10.1111/j.1741-3729.2011.00687.x

Goldberg, A. E., & Scheib, J. E. (2015). Why donor insemination and not adoption? Narratives of female-partnered and single mothers. *Family Relations, 64,* 726–742. https://doi.org/10.1111/fare.12162

Gorman-Murray, A. (2008). Queering the family home: Narratives from gay, lesbian and bisexual youth coming out in supportive family homes in Australia. *Gender, Place & Culture: A Journal of Feminist Geography, 15,* 31–44. https://doi.org/10.1080/09663690701817501

Grafsky, E. L., Hickey, K., Nguyen, H. N., & Wall, J. D. (2018). Youth disclosure of sexual orientation to siblings and extended family. *Family Relations, 67,* 147–160. https://doi.org/10.1111/fare.12299

Haxhe, S., Cerezo, A., Bergfeld, J., & Walloch, J. C. (2018). Siblings and the coming-out process: A comparative case study. *Journal of Homosexuality, 65,* 407–426. https://doi.org/10.1080/00918369.2017.1321349

Heatherington, L., & Lavner, J. A. (2008). Coming to terms with coming out: Review and recommendations for family systems-focused research. *Journal of Family Psychology, 22,* 329–343. https://doi.org/10.1037/0893-3200.22.3.329

Hoy-Ellis, C. P., & Fredriksen-Goldsen, K. I. (2017). Depression among transgender older adults: General and minority stress. *American Journal of Community Psychology, 59,* 295–305. https://doi.org/10.1002/ajcp.12138

Jenkins, D. A. (2008). Changing family dynamics: A sibling comes out. *Journal of GLBT Family Studies, 4,* 1–16. https://doi.org/10.1080/15504280802084365

Jhang, J. (2018). Scaffolding in family relationships: A grounded theory of coming out to family. *Family Relations, 67,* 161–175. https://doi.org/10.1111/fare.12302

Karpman, H. E., Ruppel, E. H., & Torres, M. (2018). "It wasn't feasible for us": Queer women of color navigating family formation. *Family Relations, 67,* 118–131. https://doi.org/10.1111/fare.12303

Kuvalanka, K. A., Allen, S. H., Munroe, C., Goldberg, A. E., & Weiner, J. (2017). The experiences of sexual minority mothers with trans* children. *Family Relations, 6,* 70–87. https://doi.org/10.1111/fare.12226

Kuvalanka, K. A., & Goldberg, A. E. (2009). "Second generation" voices: Queer youth with lesbian/bisexual mothers. *Journal of Youth and Adolescence, 38,* 904–919. https://doi.org/10.1007/s10964-008-9327-2

Kuvalanka, K. A., Wiener, J. L., & Mahan, D. (2014). Child, family, and community transformations: Findings from interviews with mothers of transgender girls. *Journal of GLBT Family Studies, 10,* 354–379. https://doi.org/10.1080/1550428X.2013.834529

Martinez, K., & McDonald, C. (2016). By the hands of our brothers: An exploration of sibling to sibling aggression for victimized heterosexual and sexual minority women. *Journal of GLBT Family Studies, 12,* 242–256. https://doi.org/10.1080/1550428X.2015.1041069

McDonald, C., & Martinez, K. (2016). Parental and others' responses to physical sibling violence: A descriptive analysis of victims' retrospective accounts. *Journal of Family Violence, 31,* 401–410. https://doi.org/10.1007/s10896-015-9766-y

McGuire, J. K., Catalpa, J. M., Lacey, V., & Kuvalanka, K. A. (2016). Ambiguous loss as a framework for interpreting gender transitions in families. *Journal of Family Theory & Review, 8,* 373–385. https://doi.org/10.1111/jftr.12159

McGuire, J. K., Kuvalanka, K. A., Catalpa, J. M., & Toomey, R. B. (2016). Transfamily theory: How the presence of trans* family members informs gender development in families. *Journal of Family Theory & Review, 8*, 60–73. https://doi.org/10.1111/jftr.12125

McLean, K. (2008). "Coming out, again": Boundaries, identities and spaces of belonging. *Australian Geographer, 39*, 303–313. https://doi.org/10.1080/00049180802270507

Merighi, J. R., & Grimes, M. D. (2000). Coming out to families in a multicultural context. *Families in Society, 81*, 32–41. https://doi.org/10.1606/1044-3894.1090

Moore, M. R. (2011). *Invisible families: Gay identities, relationships, and motherhood among black women.* Berkeley, CA: University of California Press.

Nebeling Petersen, M. (2018). Becoming gay fathers through transnational commercial surrogacy. *Journal of Family Issues, 39*, 693–719. https://doi.org/10.1177/0192513X16676859

Ocampo, A. C. (2014). The gay second generation: Sexual identity and family relations of Filipino and Latino gay men. *Journal of Ethnic & Migration Studies, 40*, 155–173. https://doi.org/10.1080/1369183X.2013.849567

Orel, N. A. (2017). Families and support systems of LGBT elders. *Annual Review of Gerontology & Geriatrics, 37*, 89–109. https://doi.org/10.1891/0198-8794.37.89

Orel, N. A., & Fruhauf, C. A. (2013). Lesbian, gay, bisexual, and transgender grandparents. In A. E. Goldberg & K. R. Allen (Eds.), *LGBT-parent families: Innovations in research and implications for practice* (pp. 177–192). New York, NY: Springer.

Oswald, R. F., Blume, L. B., & Marks, S. R. (2005). Decentering heteronormativity: A model for family studies. In V. Bengtson, A. Acock, K. Allen, P. Dilworth-Anderson, & D. Klein (Eds.), *Sourcebook of family theory & research* (pp. 143–165). Thousand Oaks, CA: Sage.

Oswald, R. F., Cutherbertson, C., Lazarevic, V., & Goldberg, A. E. (2010). New developments in the field: Measuring community climate. *Journal of GLBT Family Studies, 6*, 214–228. https://doi.org/10.1080/15504281003709230

Oswald, R. F., & Masciadrelli, B. P. (2008). Generative ritual among nonmetropolitan lesbians and gay men: Promoting social inclusion. *Journal of Marriage & Family, 70*, 1060–1073. https://doi.org/10.1111/j.1741-3737.2008.00546.x

Pew Research Center. (2019). *Attitudes on same-sex marriage.* Retrieved from https://www.pewforum.org/fact-sheet/changing-attitudes-on-gay-marriage/

Reczek, C. (2016). Ambivalence in gay and lesbian family relationships. *Journal of Marriage & Family, 78*, 644–659. https://doi.org/10.1111/jomf.12308

Reczek, C. (2014). The intergenerational relationships of gay men and lesbian women. *Journals of Gerontology Series B: Psychological Sciences & Social Sciences, 69*, 909–919. https://doi.org/10.1093/geronb/gbu042

Salvati, M., Pistella, J., Ioverno, S., Laghi, F., & Baiocco, R. (2018). Coming out to siblings and internalized sexual stigma: The moderating role of gender in a sample of Italian participants. *Journal of GLBT Family Studies, 14*, 405–424. https://doi.org/10.1080/1550428X.2017.1369916

Scherrer, K. S., Kazyak, E., & Schmitz, R. (2015). Getting "bi" in the family: Bisexual people's disclosure experiences. *Journal of Marriage & Family, 77*, 680–696. https://doi.org/10.1111/jomf.12190

Spitze, G. D., & Trent, K. (2018). Changes in individual sibling relationships in response to life events. *Journal of Family Issues, 39*, 503–526. https://doi.org/10.1177/0192513X16653431

Švab, A., & Kuhar, R. (2014). The transparent and family closets: Gay men and lesbians and their families of origin. *Journal of GLBT Family Studies, 10*, 15–35. https://doi.org/10.1080/1550428X.2014.857553

Swendener, A., & Woodell, B. (2017). Predictors of family support and well-being among Black and Latina/o sexual minorities. *Journal of GLBT Family Studies, 13*, 357–379. https://doi.org/10.1080/1550428X.2016.1257400

Taylor, R. J., Chatters, L. M., Woodward, A. T., & Brown, E. (2013). Racial and ethnic differences in extended family, friendship, fictive kin, and congregational informal support networks. *Family Relations, 62*, 609–624. https://doi.org/10.1111/fare.12030

Toomey, R. B., & Richardson, R. A. (2009). Perceived sibling relationships of sexual minority youth. *Journal of Homosexuality, 56*, 849–860. https://doi.org/10.1080/00918360903187812

Vinjamuri, M. (2015). Reminders of heteronormativity: Gay adoptive fathers navigating uninvited social interactions. *Family Relations, 64*, 263–277. https://doi.org/10.1111/fare.12118

von Doussa, H., Power, J., & Riggs, D. (2015). Imagining parenthood: The possibilities and experiences of parenthood among transgender people. *Culture, Health and Sexuality, 17*, 1119–1131. https://doi.org/10.1080/13691058.2015.1042919

Walker, A. J., Allen, K. R., & Connidis, I. A. (2005). Theorizing and studying sibling ties in adulthood. In V. Bengtson, A. Acock, K. Allen, P. Dilworth-Anderson, & D. Klein (Eds.), *Sourcebook of family theory & research* (pp. 167–190). Thousand Oaks, CA: Sage.

Weisner, T. S. (1989). Comparing sibling relationships across cultures. In P. G. Zokow (Ed.), *Sibling interactions across cultures* (pp. 11–25). New York, NY: Springer.

Whitchurch, G. G., & Constantine, L. L. (1993). Systems theory. In P. G. Boss, W. J. Doherty, R. LaRossa, W. R. Schumm, & S. K. Steinmetz (Eds.), *Sourcebook of family theories and methods: A contextual approach* (pp. 325–355). New York, NY: Plenum.

White, L. (1998). Who's counting? Quasi-facts and step-families in reports of number of siblings. *Journal of Marriage and Family, 60*, 725–733. Retrieved from https://www.jstor.org/stable/353541

Whiteman, S., McHale, S., & Soli, A. (2011). Theoretical perspectives on sibling relationships. *Journal of*

*Family Theory & Review, 3*, 124–139. https://doi.org/10.1111/j.1756-2589.2011.00087.x

Willoughby, B. L. B., Doty, N. D., & Malik, N. M. (2008). Parental reactions to their child's sexual orientation disclosure: A family stress perspective. *Parenting, 8*, 70–91. https://doi.org/10.1080/15295190701830680

Willoughby, B. L. B., Malik, N. M., & Lindahl, K. M. (2006). Parental reactions to their sons' sexual orientation disclosures: The roles of family cohesion, adaptability, and parenting style. *Psychology of Men & Masculinity, 7*, 14–26. https://doi.org/10.1037/1524-9220.7.1.14

# LGBTQ Parents and the Workplace

Ann Hergatt Huffman, Nicholas A. Smith, and Satoris S. Howes

Few would dispute that parenting is hard, and perhaps harder today than in the past (Mikolajczak, Brianda, Avalosse, & Roskam, 2018). Moreover, being a working parent brings additional complexities, with working parents experiencing greater levels of physical and emotional fatigue than non-working parents (Ilies, Huth, Ryan, & Dimotakis, 2015). Indeed, work-family conflict, which occurs when work and family demands clash (Greenhaus & Beutell, 1985), is positively related to the number of children one has and negatively related to the age of one's youngest child living at home (Byron, 2005). Add to this an LGBTQ status and the intricacies of being a working parent become more complex, and far less researched.

In this chapter, we explore the workplace experiences of LGBTQ parents. We start by presenting policies that have the potential to uniquely impact LGBTQ working parents. Following this, we provide an overview of contemporary theoretical perspectives that have been used to help understand workplace experiences of LGBTQ parents as well as critical theories that we believe pose the greatest possibility for advancement as they incorporate a more nuanced understanding of LGBTQ working parents. We then summarize the literature that has incorporated the various theoretical approaches to empirically explore the workplace experiences of LGBTQ parents. Finally, we provide implications for practice and recommendations for future research. In the spirit of Bronfenbrenner's (1979) larger systems perspective, we provide suggestions at the individual, organizational, and national levels.

## Workplace Policies Impacting LGBTQ Parents

National and state laws and policies likely play a large role in the work and family experiences of employees (Den Dulk & Peper, 2016). For example, important issues such as healthcare for oneself and one's family are less relevant in countries that provide free or universal healthcare compared to countries in which similar

A. H. Huffman (✉)
Psychological Sciences and WA Franke College of Business, Northern Arizona University, Flagstaff, AZ, USA
e-mail: ann.huffman@nau.edu

N. A. Smith
Oregon Institute of Occupational Health Sciences, Oregon Health & Science University, Portland, OR, USA
e-mail: smitnich@ohsu.edu

S. S. Howes
College of Business, Oregon State University, Bend, OR, USA
e-mail: satoris.howes@osucascades.edu

© Springer Nature Switzerland AG 2020
A. E. Goldberg, K. R. Allen (eds.), *LGBTQ-Parent Families*,
https://doi.org/10.1007/978-3-030-35610-1_17

healthcare program are nonexistent. Although many laws and policies may impact LGBTQ individuals generally, and LGBTQ employees more specifically (e.g., discrimination), we limit our focus on laws/policies that are most germane to LGBTQ employees' experiences as *parents*, including family/parental leave and family medical coverage.

## Family/Parental Leave

Depending on the country, the amount of time allowed for family leave varies substantially. For example, whereas employees in the United States of America (USA) are not guaranteed any maternal leave, employees in Austria, Germany, the Netherlands, Norway, and Singapore get 100% wage replacement for an established period of time (for those countries, 14 to 146 weeks; Earle, Mokomane, & Heymann, 2011). The pattern is similar for paternal leave.

LGBTQ employees who are citizens of countries with paid leave will experience fewer issues related to getting time off for adoption or caring for sick child(ren) than LGBTQ employees who are citizens of countries without paid leave. Since the law in such countries surrounding paid leave allows all parents time for parental responsibilities, sexual or gender orientation status is less relevant to paid parental leave. However, in countries without mandatory paid leave, decisions about whether or not to grant parental leave is at the organization's discretion. Interestingly, Goldberg (2010) reports that biological lesbian mothers may have more access to parental leave compared to nonbiological mothers. Worthy of mention is the point that LGBQ couples adopt at higher rates than different-sex couples (i.e., different-sex couples have nonbiological children—step or adopted—at a rate of 4% compared to same-sex couples' rate of 21%; Lofquist, 2011). This is notable because adoption benefits are not as common as traditional parental birth leave (Hara & Hegewisch, 2013). In turn, many LGBTQ parents who adopt their children may face limited or no formal parental leave.

## Family Medical Coverage

Healthcare, which also varies considerably by country, is another important benefit for employed parents. The majority of all developed countries have either free (78%) or universal (59%) healthcare (STC, 2018). Unlike most other countries, most health benefits in the USA are not government sponsored and often are the responsibility of employers (see Ridic, Gleason, & Ridic, 2012). As of 2018, organizations in the USA with more than 50 employees are required to provide health coverage or must pay a penalty. A limitation in this system is that health coverage is quite variable such that not all conditions or treatments are covered by all insurers.

In countries that have free or universal healthcare, there should be few issues for LGBTQ employed parents since the national medical care would presumably cover the employee, partner, and children, regardless of one's sexual or gender orientation. LGBTQ employed parents without free or universal healthcare, however, will likely experience additional stress. Countries without a national healthcare system, such as the USA and Mexico (the only two OECD countries without universal health coverage; OECD, 2014), depend on private health insurers, often through one's employer. The USA is a notable example of this type of system whereby health insurance is secured through one's employer, through purchasing one's own insurance, or for certain groups (aged/disabled, economically disadvantaged) through the government (Ridic et al., 2012). This becomes relevant for LGBTQ individuals who may not have access to a company's health insurance, who may have to take additional steps to prove eligibility for insurance compared to married heterosexual parents, who may experience additional tax burdens when obtaining coverage for domestic partners, or when only legally married partners are eligible for healthcare coverage and the couple's union is not legally recognized (see Potter & Allen, 2016). As parents, this could be further complicated if only one parent is afforded legal guardianship over a child, and that parent becomes unemployed and therefore the child's health insurance coverage is at risk (or is at risk of becoming prohibitively costly).

In summary, some stark differences in work-life experiences, especially medical and leave issues, exist at the national or country level. Yet we would be naïve to suggest that these policies by themselves affect an LGBTQ employed parent's workplace experience. There are transgender employed parents in Germany, for example, who would state their work-life interface is very stressful. Conversely, there are lesbian employed parents in the USA who would say they have very positive work-life experiences. In the following section, we provide an overview of theoretical perspectives that have been used to help understand workplace experiences of LGBTQ parents as well as theories that pose the greatest possibility for advancement in this area.

## Theoretical Foundation

We next provide a brief review of contemporary theoretical perspectives that researchers have used to help understand workplace experiences of LGBTQ parents, including role theory, stigma theory, and minority stress theory. Worthy of note is that we provide only a short summary of these perspectives; readers interested in a more comprehensive discussion of these theoretical orientations along with implications for LGBTQ workers are encouraged to see King, Huffman, and Peddie (2013). Following this overview, we provide a glimpse into critical theories going forward for understanding LGBTQ parents in the workforce. While the contemporary theories still have utility for future scholars, particularly given the paucity of research that remains regarding LGBTQ employed parents, we present additional critical theories that pose perhaps the greatest possibility for the advancement of research on the workplace experiences of LGBTQ parents, as they incorporate a more nuanced understanding of the target sample. Specifically, we discuss transformative perspectives, feminism, and queer theory.

## Contemporary Theoretical Perspectives: A Nod to the Past

**Role theory** The first theoretical perspective that can help better understand work-family experiences for LGBTQ individuals is role theory (Katz & Kahn, 1978). This theory posits that individuals hold multiple roles at any given time, and each of these roles are associated with particular expectations that may create conflict when they contradict or interfere with one another. While most individuals simultaneously engage in multiple roles that may create stress (e.g., employee, spouse, parent), LGBTQ parents may have more complicated role fulfillment and potential for problems than other employees in that they may occupy multiple roles perceived by others as conflicting (e.g., gender roles). As such, LGBTQ parents may experience additional stressors compared to non-LGBTQ parents. A sub-theory within role theory is gender role theory. Gender roles refer to an individual's attitudinal identification with a particular gendered role (such as the need for a woman to fulfill domestic duties and for a man to serve as the main breadwinner), or the degree to which one complies with expectations that exist for one particular gender role versus another (Larsen & Long, 1988). Although gender roles in the past were rigid and associated with negative consequences when individuals violated them, role expectations have become more fluid with society becoming more accepting of crossover in traditional gender role stereotypes (de Visser, 2009).

Nevertheless, gender roles impact how LGBTQ parents are perceived at work, and correspondingly how they behave at work. For example, Hennekam and Ladge (2017) argued that sexuality is a key component of one's gender role and pregnancy adds an interesting component to how individuals perceive others in the workplace. When a lesbian woman is pregnant, it might elicit two different reactions from coworkers. The state of pregnancy might lead coworkers to see her as more feminine, and therefore closer to their expected gender role, which may increase their comfort with this worker. Conversely, the idea of a pregnant lesbian might lead some coworkers to have conflicting thoughts about the person's gender role (i.e., they are fulfilling a role that is not the norm), therefore leading the coworkers to feel less comfortable with their lesbian coworker.

**Stigma theory** Also relevant to LGBTQ employed parents is stigma theory (Goffman, 1963), which suggests that social meanings are constructed around attributes of an individual, some of which are deeply discrediting. These discredited attributes are related to negative stereotypes (Jones et al., 1984) and may result in negative treatment for those who possess—or are thought to possess—the stigmatized attribute (Major & O'Brien, 2005). As both sexual and gender minority statuses are stigmatized, LGBTQ parents may choose to conceal their sexual identity, gender identity, or parental status, which has important implications with regard to their physical and psychosocial well-being (Ragins, 2008) and access to available resources.

Pregnancy in the workplace, regardless of sexual orientation or identity, can be considered a stigmatized state (Jones, 2017). Thus, pregnant lesbian women potentially have multiple stigmas in the workplace: being a woman, being pregnant, and being a lesbian. Additionally, Hennekam and Ladge (2017) utilized stigma theory to understand the management of multiple stigmatized identities for pregnant lesbian employees, finding that an organization's diversity climate strongly influenced pregnancy disclosure decisions and the ease with which one's maternal identity was claimed among both biological and nonbiological mothers. Similarly, Sawyer, Thoroughgood, and Ladge (2017) used stigma theory to illustrate a unique stressor that LGBTQ employees experience in the workplace. They suggest that LGBTQ employees with a family have a unique family stigma that leads to stigma-based work-family conflict. To cope with this stigma, the LGBTQ employee uses different family-related identity behaviors (e.g., suppression of family information),

which leads to additional strain above and beyond the typical outcomes related to work-family conflict. These strains (e.g., depersonalization, denial of family dignity, and hypervigilance) in turn increase the likelihood of deleterious work-family outcomes such as physical distress and negative work outcomes.

**Minority stress theory** Related to stigma theory is minority stress theory (Meyer, 1995), which suggests that members of a stigmatized group experience additional stressors beyond those that nonminority group members experience, which may lead to negative health outcomes. These additional stressors are categorized as either distal (e.g., discrimination) or proximal (e.g., engaging in identity management) stressors. As LGBTQ parents are a minority within the LGBTQ community, they may experience additional stressors both compared to their non-LGBTQ peers, and also compared to LGBTQ individuals who are not parents.

Researchers have used minority stress theory in several studies to examine sexual minority parents, although not specifically *working* parents. For example, Goldberg and Smith (2014) examined same-sex parents in schools and investigated whether openness in an educational setting would affect their engagement in school events and other school-related outcomes. They found that indeed, perceptions of stigma were related to key outcomes such as satisfaction with the school. In a later exploratory study that examined health outcomes of same-sex couple parents, Goldberg, Smith, McCormick, and Overstreet (2019) used minority stress theory as a framework to help understand how unique minority stressors operate for sexual minority parents. Their study revealed that sexual minority status was related to health outcomes, although the nature of effects differed for lesbian mothers and gay fathers. Although neither of these studies examined working parents, their findings do provide evidence that minority stress is a unique stressor for LGBTQ parents.

## Critical Theoretical Perspectives: A Glimpse to the Future

**Transformative perspectives** Transformative frameworks (Mertens, 2010) are based on the assumptions that knowledge (and science) is value laden and that research should be conducted with an agenda to enact positive political change against social oppression. Methodologically, research drawing upon transformative frameworks may be qualitative, quantitative, or mixed methods, depending upon the underlying philosophical assumptions. Oftentimes the research is conducted "with" rather than "on" participants, such as in participatory action research (Kemmis & Wilkinson, 1998). We believe that participatory action research is particularly advantageous when considering inquiry regarding work-family issues for LGBTQ parents as LGBTQ individuals have been historically taken advantage of by the scientific community and this technique empowers oppressed individuals to bring about practical change in a collaborative fashion as it actively involves participants in the research process.

**Feminism** Feminism—a lens with which to examine particular questions (Fox-Keller, 1985)—brings gender to the foreground and seeks to end gender disparities (see Lather, 1991). Williams (2010) has directly considered work-family issues from a feminist perspective, arguing that the workplace is structured around traditional gender roles and gendered assumptions:

> As long as good jobs are designed around men's bodies and men's traditional life patterns, mothers will remain marginalized. As long as mothers remain marginalized, women will not approach equality—and a society that marginalizes its mothers impoverishes its children... .In the past thirty years, it has become abundantly clear that reshaping the work-family debate will require changes both in the ways we think about gender and in the ways we think about class. (p. 281)

Similar critiques exist in reference to organizational theory and structures in reference to sexism and sexual harassment (Hassard & Parker,

1993). Importantly, scholars in this space realize that gender does not occur in a vacuum, and thus often draw on an intersectional feminist perspective—considering the ways that other characteristics such as race, class, and sexuality intersect with gender (e.g., Few-Demo, 2014; Mahler, Chaudhuri, & Patil, 2015). By putting gender front and center and considering the gendered nature of the workplace along with the division of the public and the private (e.g., paid work vs. domestic work; Williams, 2010), we argue that it is possible to gain a deeper understanding of LGBTQ parent's work-family experiences.

**Queer theory** Queer theory (Foucault, 1978) seeks to examine categories (such as sexuality and gender) and how power is distributed among these categories (Watson, 2005). Queer theory is deconstructionist in nature (e.g., challenges the idea that identity is "singular, fixed or normal" [Watson, 2005, p. 38], rejects gender and sexuality binaries, assumes gender and sexual fluidity) and emphasizes performativity (i.e., gender and sexuality are performed by gestures, movements, and clothing; Butler, 2004). Power and the concept of "normal" is produced both situationally and discursively, and all can potentially position—or be positioned—as powerful or normal (Watson, 2005). For example, the "private" can be made "public" through performativity, and heteronormativity need not be considered "normal" (see Berlant & Warner, 1998). From this perspective, it is possible to challenge dominant narratives and understandings of sexuality and gender, which, Nestle, Howell, and Wilkins (2002) argued, could have a profound impact on gaining equality for all people.

In the family field, authors have leveraged queer theory to discuss methodological and theoretical advancements and review prior work (e.g., Acosta, 2018; Fish & Russell, 2018). For example, Acosta (2018) discussed how heteronormative assumptions of family structures and configurations can be challenged as a queer perspective allows for an "infinity [of] possibilities... including (but not limited to) those consisting of same-sex, transgender, or polyamorous families" (p. 409). Importantly, a queer perspective on family examines the manner in which people actively are engaged in "doing family," rather than being a passive recipient of the institution of family (Oswald, Blume, & Marks, 2005); for example, LGBTQ individuals may construct families of choice (Weeks, Heaphy, & Donovan, 2001). Considering family as a verb is particularly useful as doing so expands the idea of family from a socially constructed institution and allows for increased fluidity and ambiguity (Stiles, 2002; Weeks et al., 2001). Queer intersectional scholarship, discussed next, expands on this notion by further considering how the intersection of sexuality, race, gender, class, etc., forms reality (see Acosta, 2013, 2018). As such, this perspective could illuminate work-family research by considering the ways in which LGBTQ parents construct the role of "parent" and the idea of "family."

**Intersectionality** Although much can be gained by considering LGBTQ work-family issues from the theoretical perspectives described above, adopting an intersectionality perspective continues to be of extreme importance. Intersectionality is a lens that draws upon feminist and critical race theories (Crenshaw, 1991) and explores the experience of individuals while considering their multiple social identities. An intersectionality perspective rejects that group memberships can be added together to predict particular types of treatment, and rather asserts the multiple lived identities are intertwined and form unique experiences (Simien, 2007). Indeed, for example, experiences of transgender employees report unique experiences compared not only to hetero "normal" colleagues, but also to their lesbian, gay, and bisexual colleagues (Sawyer, Thoroughgood, & Webster, 2016). Of note, scholars have recognized the importance of taking an intersectional perspective and considering the unique lived experiences of LGBTQ parents of differing identity categories such as age, class, ethnicity, gender, race, sexuality, etc. (e.g., Acosta, 2013, 2018; Allen & Jaramillo-Sierra, 2015; Few-Demo, 2014; King et al., 2013; Mahler et al., 2015; Moore, 2011). For example, Acosta's (2013) work explores the

experiences of LGBTQ Latinx parents, and Moore (2011) considers race, family formation, and motherhood among Black gay women. We believe that this perspective is important for work-family scholarship and practice as the lived experiences of individuals with multiple stigmatized identities may be unique and it is possible that the theoretical and empirical work to this point may not fully encompass the experiences of such individuals.

## Workplace Experiences of LGBTQ Parents

Although in recent years there has been interest in the positive interaction between work and family, much of the work-family research has focused on work-family conflict. Work-family conflict is defined by Greenhaus and Beutell (1985) as "a form of interrole conflict in which the role pressures from the work and family domains are mutually incompatible in some respect" (p. 77). Meta-analytical reviews have revealed some common themes related to employees' experiences with the work and family domains. First, whereas parental status is a key demographic predictor of work-family conflict, sex and marital status are less influential (Byron, 2005). In terms of situational predictors, role stress and role involvement have both been tied to work-family conflict. Second, there is evidence that work-family conflict leads to decreased job satisfaction, life satisfaction, marital satisfaction, and both physical and psychological health (Allen, Herst, Bruck, & Sutton, 2000). Finally, research that has examined strategies to attenuate work-family conflict have included dependent care, flexibility, supervisor support, and informal organizational support (Allen, 2013), with the latter two having the strongest effects.

The aforementioned work-family findings have been predominantly determined by research on heterosexual two-parent families with biological children, with very little research on LGBTQ parent families. Moreover, in the first edition of this chapter (King et al., 2013), there were only four identified studies on LGBTQ parents in the workplace, and these studies focused on LGBTQ parents (Goldberg & Sayer, 2006; Mercier, 2007; O'Ryan & McFarland, 2010; Tuten & August, 2006). We are only just beginning to see an increase in workplace research that extends the definition of family to include trans and queer parent families.

We are aware of only a single published study that has examined work-related issues of transgender working parents (Pyne, Bauer, & Bradley, 2015). In particular, the focus of this survey study was to examine stressors that transgender parents in Ontario, Canada, were experiencing. With regard to workplace stressors, 28% of transgender parents reported being turned down from a job, and 6% reported being fired from a job due to their transgender identity or gender expression. Thus, transgender working parents may have more perceived and actual job insecurity than do their colleagues. Importantly, to our knowledge, no study has explicitly considered genderqueer or nonbinary parents' workplace experiences. Thus, our focus in the following section is on the few work related studies that have examined LGBTQ parents.

Recent research on work-family issues of LGBTQ employed parents has revealed three emerging themes: transition to parenthood, support and resources, and role management. Worthy of note is that some sub-differences exist within the larger group of LGBTQ employed parents and some studies focused exclusively on one subgroup so findings may not generalize to others. Accordingly, we first review each theme, and then discuss potential subgroup differences.

## Transition to Parenthood

Transitioning to parenthood can be stressful for any new parent (Vismara et al., 2016) and necessitate changes for employees. While there are certainly similarities between LGBQ[1] employ-

ees and their non-LGBQ counterparts, there also appears to be some clear differences. Hennekam and Ladge (2017), for example, found that lesbian women in the Netherlands experienced the transition to motherhood differentially depending on the phase of their pregnancy, whether they were the biological or the nonbiological mother, and the degree to which they were out about their sexual orientation at work. Specifically, nonbiological mothers had a different experience than biological mothers, and the women's experiences differed depending on the stage of the mothering phase. In line with gender theory, stigma theory, and minority stress theory, during the earlier stages (e.g., during pregnancy), nonbiological mothers had more advantages because they manifested fewer stigmatized roles (being a woman was the only visual stigmatized role). However, over time including after the child's birth, nonbiological mothers were treated differently because they were not seen as "real" mothers (see Hayman, Wilkes, Jackson, & Halcomb, 2013).

Transitioning to parenthood is also significant for working gay fathers. Bergman, Rubio, Green, and Padrón's (2010) study on gay fathers (via surrogacy) in the USA and found that most of their sample experienced occupational changes after becoming fathers, including extended leaves of absence, changing to part-time work, changing work schedules, working later at night, sleeping less, or switching to a job with less work hours or travel. Fathers who described their workplaces more positively discussed increased communication with coworkers. These fathers noted their family structure was more legitimized after having children, they had more to talk about with coworkers, and they felt like they had more in common with bosses who were also parents (see Goldberg, 2012, and Richardson, Moyer, & Goldberg, 2012, for similar findings).

## Support and Resources

Support and resources are important factors in managing work-family conflict (Byron, 2005).

---

[1]Note that we are purposeful with our acronym of LGBQ (vs. LGBTQ or LGBT) given the focus of the research studies we examined.

It has been consistently shown that employed parents are going to be the most successful, and the most satisfied with their job, if they have some type of support mechanisms to help them manage their work and family demands. Although there has been little research on support mechanisms of LGBTQ employed parents, Mercier (2007) found in a sample of American lesbian parents that most of their work-family experiences were similar to heterosexual parents' experiences. This was true for the four major themes that emerged from interviews (instrument support, interpersonal support, integration of work and family, and strategies for balancing work and family). Despite the similarities, some differences emerged, including lesbian parents reporting significantly fewer partner benefits (e.g., health insurance, flexible spending accounts) than heterosexual mothers.

## Role Management

The process of establishing rules and expectations of an individual embodies the concept of role management. With regard to work-life issues of employed partners, role management refers to the process that a couple goes through to establish what each individual will be expected to do as an employee and as a family member. In a different-sex couple, and in line with gender role theory, this role management process is usually influenced by gender norms such that women find themselves more likely to have more caregiving responsibilities and men are usually more likely to take a larger role in supporting the family financially (Diekman & Goodfriend, 2006). In a relationship that does not have these traditional gender cues (e.g., that of a same-sex couple), there are fewer preconceived gender roles that determine the tasks of each individual in the couple, leaving their work and family roles open for consideration. Yet this also creates a need for some type of decision-making process to help the couple establish specific roles.

This becomes even more relevant when individuals in a same-sex couple becomes parents.

Role management is intertwined with the division of labor that is established by the couple. In a study on American heterosexual, gay, and lesbian parents who were adopting a child, Goldberg, Smith, and Perry-Jenkins (2012) found that lesbian and male gay parents were more likely to share the division of labor than heterosexual parents. Yet their findings also revealed that for all groups, differences in pay and work hours affected the division of labor for feminine tasks (e.g., laundry) but not for child care. Furthermore, Goldberg (2013) noted that same-sex couples interpret their division of labor as uniquely defined by their same-sex relational status, and not imitative of heterosexual couples. Similarly, in a sample of same-sex and heterosexual parents in New Zealand and Australia, Perlesz et al. (2010) found that same-sex partners were more likely to have a greater level of egalitarianism in their division of labor of household tasks. The authors noted that lesbian parents were more likely to negotiate a strategy so that both parents had an opportunity to both work and to care for their child(ren). Rawsthorne and Costello (2010) found similar results in a sample of Australian lesbian parents. They further found that de-stabilizing of scripts related to gender roles decreased family stress and conflict.

Another issue is how to manage these roles in a way that is comfortable to both members of the couple, despite having roles that may be unacceptable to coworkers. Sawyer et al. (2017) introduced the concept of stigma-based work-family conflict, a type of conflict in which an LGBTQ employee may feel that their family identity is stigmatized since it does not represent the traditional definition of family. In their study of American LGBTQ parents, Sawyer et al. found that LGBTQ parents were less likely to have typical roles or behaviors associated with being a parent (e.g., displaying child's art, discussing family events) due to reactions they anticipated from coworkers.

## Subgroup Differences

It should be noted that most of the studies have focused on lesbian women and gay men, with only a few on bisexual parents, and to our knowledge no studies that examined queer identified parents in the workplace.[2] One US study found that gay male dual-earner parents reported more anxiety than did lesbian women dual-earner parents (Goldberg & Smith, 2013). The authors proposed that these differences could be because others' perceptions of gay men as parents might be more negative due to the stereotypes that men are less nurturing as parents and that gay men are less fit as parents (see Goldberg & Smith, 2009 for similar findings).

Although bisexual parents are the largest group of sexual minority parents (approximately 64%; Goldberg, Gartrell, & Gates, 2014), it is interesting that few studies have examined bisexual parents, and even fewer have examined bisexual parents and workplace issues. In a qualitative study, Bartelt, Bowling, Dodge, and Bostwick (2017) found that American parents who are bisexual are concerned about finding or keeping a job and about negative impacts of their bisexuality on their career and earnings. For these parents, the concern extends beyond their own well-being to concerns about being able to provide for their children and have a stable household. Interestingly, these parents also mentioned feeling a bond with the larger LGBTQ community but feeling that the commu-

nity did not accept them. Thus, for bisexual parents, legitimizing their identity and providing social support appear particularly important.

## Practical Implications and Future Research Recommendations

Although few studies have examined LGBTQ working parents, they have provided an initial framework for understanding this population. Moreover, considerable work on work-life issues and LGBTQ issues provides additional insight on their work and family experiences. Based on these literatures, and the aforementioned theoretical perspectives, we provide implications and recommendations relevant for both practitioners and researchers.

## Implications and Strategies for Workplace Change

Role management emerged as an important issue for LGBTQ employed parents. O'Ryan and McFarland's (2010) research on gay and lesbian dual-career couples provides insight into how gay and lesbian couples can manage their work and family roles to be successful as parents, partners, and employees. Although their research was not focused on LGBTQ *parents*, their findings could benefit LGBTQ employed parents. Specifically, they found that three strategies help LGBTQ dual-earners be successful: planfulness, creating positive social networks, and shifting from marginalization to consolidation and integration. We argue that these same strategies would be useful for LGBTQ employed parents. Planfulness describes the need for the individual to use decision-making and strategizing "to maneuver through the social milieu of the workplace" and to use introductions "to develop a social network" (O'Ryan & McFarland, p. 74). Parenting opens one's social network, yet in the workplace the employee is dealing with unknowns related to acceptance. The LGBTQ parent might need to go through this process in a thoughtful manner to ensure that newly developed

---

[2]We wish to emphasize that the term "queer" has multiple meanings and is used by some members of the LGBT community as an overarching inclusive term (i.e., to refer to those who are either not heterosexual or not cisgender). Queer has been used to refer to sexual orientations that reject or go beyond the gender binary and also to refer to one's own gender identity (i.e., "genderqueer," which may also refer to those who identify as gender nonbinary, agender, or gender nonconforming). For some, queer has sociopolitical meanings and is strongly tied to schools of thought such as queer theory. In such cases, queer can refer to the deconstruction or rejection of heteronormative assumptions about gender and sexuality and seeks to claim space in society. As such, we take an inclusive approach throughout the chapter.

social networks are ones that will be status affirming and provide a positive sense of duality (i.e., moving easily from work and family). O'Ryan and McFarland found that when LGBTQ couples "teamed up" to gain strength to belong in the workplace environment, they shifted from marginalization to consolidation and integration. As parents who may be struggling to adjust to new roles and potential increased stigma, such strategizing with the intent of building a support system and establishing resources can only help. Additionally, the role of coworkers acting as allies may be of key importance at the individual level. Although not work-life specific, prior research examining the experience of transgender workers demonstrated that having their gender identity affirmed by others (relational authenticity) explained why gender transition was related to positive workplace outcomes (Martinez, Sawyer, Thoroughgood, Ruggs, & Smith, 2017). Further, sexual orientation minorities have expressed the importance of allies engaging in supportive behaviors in the workplace (see Martinez, Hebl, Smith, & Sabat, 2017). As such, the powerful role that affirming allies play cannot be underestimated.

Scholars have also proposed ways in which career counselors may specifically aid LGBTQ employees. Perrone (2005), for example, noted that the extra challenges experienced by same-sex, dual-earner couples likely requires counselors who are able to help such couples prepare for potential economic difficulties (e.g., due to potential nonexistent insurance coverage for same-sex couples), identify work environments where discrimination is less likely to occur, and engage in frank discussions about types of employment discrimination and relevant laws and employment policies that may impact them and their unique situations. Perrone also noted the need to consider challenges related to social connectedness or stressors related to custodial rights with regard to LGBTQ parents and stepparents, as such stressors can greatly impact the employed parent/stepparent's work-family interface.

Although individual-level considerations are important, change must also occur at the organiza-

tional and national level. In terms of the organization, the structure of the workplace needs to be designed so that it is inclusive and accepting to all employees, regardless of sexual orientation, gender identity, or parental status. Organizations must ensure that LGBTQ parents receive support—and are comfortable asking for support—from different workplace entities. This is specifically important since support and resources emerged as a theme of particular importance to LGBTQ parents in the workplace. Huffman, Watrous-Rodriguez, and King (2008) found that supervisor, coworker, and organizational support were all important for LGBTQ employees and were related to unique outcomes. Not only do supportive workplaces affect factors such as retention, they also provide an environment in which employees are more likely to feel safe using the organization's programs (Kim & Faerman, 2013). Perceptions of support come from both a family-friendly organizational culture and from formalized family-friendly policies (e.g., flex-time; Lu, Kao, Chang, Wu, & Cooper, 2011).

At the national level, all countries need to reexamine their policies that affect LGBTQ employees who are parents. This spans policies and laws related to family, sexual and gender minorities, and the workplace in general. To ensure that LGBTQ employed parents are treated fairly and have opportunities as both parents and employees, change needs to start at the top. Although there are some countries in which the need for change is straightforward (e.g., USA; laws to protect the rights of LGB employees), all countries must revisit their policies to ensure they are truly inclusive to sexual and gender minorities, and the policies have the intended effects. Again, although the Netherlands, for example, has quite generous leave and healthcare programs, LGBTQ employed parents in the Netherlands still experience challenges that are not experienced by their heterosexual, cisgender counterparts (Hennekam & Ladge, 2017). Thus, we applaud progressive policies, but if there continues to be differences for LGBTQ parents in the workplace, even those countries and their policies need to be re-examined.

## Recommendations for Future Research

Compared to heterosexual and cisgender parents, LGBTQ employed parents are more likely to be in dual-career relationships and share many of the challenges of dual-career employees who are not a sexual minority status (O'Ryan & McFarland, 2010). Research should examine the additional role of dual-earner status for LGBTQ parents. In addition, the dual-career literature has examined gender differences of the couples using dyadic analysis. A study by ten Brummelhuis, Haar, and van der Lippe (2010) found that the cross-over experiences between spouses differed by gender, with time and energy deficits crossing from men to women, and distress crossing from women to men. It would be interesting to see how these processes worked for same-sex couples, or if the gender norms were similar for same-sex couples such that lesbian mothers experienced more distress, and gay fathers experienced more feelings of time/energy deficit. This could be problematic if both individuals within the couple encounter the same stressor or experience couple-level minority stress (LeBlanc, Frost, & Wight, 2015). These shared experiences of stress could create a larger, harder to manage level of stress, or it could be beneficial if it provides the couple with a shared understanding of their work-life stressors. Research has shown that division of labor is less of an issue for lesbian and gay parents (Goldberg, 2013; Goldberg et al., 2012) suggesting that their status might provide some benefits related to stressors associated with being in a dual-career relationship.

Although there has been a noticeable increase in research on LGBTQ workplace and parenting issues over the past 5 years, there continues to be a dearth of research on the intersection of the two, namely LGBTQ parents in the workplace. Within this realm, it appears that the work-family literature is built upon heteronormative assumptions (such as the way in which "family" is defined; e.g., Agars & French, 2017; King et al., 2013), thus "organiz[ing] and privilege[ing] heterosexuality by infusing it into organizational cultures, systems, and struc-

tures"; Sawyer et al., 2017, p. 24). It is clear that organizations at all levels (e.g., employers, countries), as well as researchers, need to define family in a more inclusive manner. We argue that family should be described in such a way that is inclusive of key characteristics (e.g., formation: origin vs. chosen families; structure; demographic characteristics; configuration: extended, polyamorous; etc.), although we are hesitant to place restrictions on the ways in which "family" should be defined. Rather, we argue that considering family as a verb (see Stiles, 2002) is particularly useful as doing so allows for a deeper consideration of the many varied ways in which people "do family." Although this more fluid definition of family may not be easily integrated into organizational (or federal) policies, there is much that could be learned not only about families with LGBTQ members, but also about families in general. As Benkov (1995) eloquently stated in reference to lesbian-parented families:

> I came to see my subjects not as families on the margin to be compared to a central norm, but rather, as people on the cutting edge of a key social shift, from whom there was much to be learned about the meaning of family and about the nature of social change. (p. 58)

Additionally, we argue that researchers and practitioners should carefully attend to and deeply consider the language that they employ when discussing work-family issues. It has been argued that "we do not only use language, it uses us. Language is recursive: it provides the categories in which we think" (Hare-Mustin, 1994, p. 22). Further, though we included queer as one of the subgroups within our umbrella of sexual and gender minorities, we were not able to find much research on the experiences of employed queer parents. Moving forward, researchers should make a particular effort to bring the unique experiences of these individuals to light.

Similarly, there needs to be more research on bisexual parents in the workplace. This lack of research is disheartening since not only are they the largest of the subgroups (Gates, 2011), and the most likely to be parents (Goldberg et al., 2014), but they also report more negative experiences (see chapter "What Do We Now Know About Bisexual Parenting? A Continuing Call for Research"). Arena and Jones (2017), for example, argue that bisexual individuals have unique experiences and more negative health and well-being outcomes compared to LG individuals. In their research, they found that bisexual employees were less likely to be open about their sexual orientation in the workplace. Researchers need to do a better job to ensure that this group's work-family experiences are understood.

Finally, one area that remains missing in the LGBTQ work-family literature is intersectionality (Crenshaw, 1991). Scarce research in this area has examined other minority status groups (e.g., people of color). This is important as members of multiple minority groups may experience additional forms of stigmatization and oppression (e.g., "multiple jeopardy"). Thus, in line with King et al.'s (2013) recommendations, it remains particularly important to consider the unique lived experiences of LGBTQ parents of differing identity categories (e.g., age, class, ethnicity, gender, race, sexuality).

## Conclusion

This chapter examined the workplace experiences of LGBTQ parents from micro through macro lenses. We identified three major themes concerning LGBTQ employed parents—transition to parenthood, support and resources, and role management. We discussed several theories that help explain these issues, and introduced some alternative worldviews that we believe could contribute to the understanding of work-family experiences of LGBTQ employed parents. Finally, we stress that each of these subgroups L – G – B – T – Q, although they share some commonalities, have unique characteristics and therefore must examined both as a group and also individually. It is our hope that this chapter will benefit researchers, clinicians, and anyone interested in bettering the lives of LGBTQ employed parents and will serve as a springboard from

which to enact positive change. As Williams (2010) noted:

> Cultural problems require cultural solutions—which begin with flights of the imagination. Then comes the hard work. Everything looks perfect from far away; it is much harder to come down and develop effective strategies for social, political, organizational—and personal—change. Let's begin. (p. 282)

## References

Acosta, K. L. (2013). Amigas y Amantes: Sexually non-conforming latinas negotiate family. New Brunswick, NJ: Rutgers University Press

Acosta, K. L. (2018). Queering family scholarship: Theorizing from the borderlands. *Journal of Family Theory & Review, 10*, 406–418. https://doi.org/10.1111/jftr.12263

Agars, M. D., & French, K. A. (2017). Considering underrepresented populations in work and family research. In T. D. Allen & L. T. Eby (Eds.), *The Oxford handbook of work and family* (pp. 362–375). New York, NY: Oxford University Press.

Allen, K. R., & Jaramillo-Sierra, A. L. (2015). Feminist theory and research on family relationships: Pluralism and complexity. *Sex Roles: A Journal of Research, 73*, 93–99. https://doi.org/10.1007/s11199-015-0527-4

Allen, T. (2013). Some future directions for work-family research in a global world. In S. Poelmans, J. H. Greenhaus, & M. L. H. Maestro (Eds.), *Expanding the boundaries of work-family research: A vision for the future* (pp. 333–347). London, UK: Palgrave Macmillan UK.

Allen, T. D., Herst, D. E. L., Bruck, C. S., & Sutton, M. (2000). Consequences associated with work-to-family conflict: A review and agenda for future research. *Journal of Occupational Health Psychology, 5*, 278–308. https://doi.org/10.1037/1076-8998.5.2.278

Arena, D. F., & Jones, K. P. (2017). To "B" or not to "B": Assessing the disclosure dilemma of bisexual individuals at work. *Journal of Vocational Behavior, 103*, 86–98. https://doi.org/10.1016/j.jvb.2017.08.009

Bartelt, E., Bowling, J., Dodge, B., & Bostwick, W. (2017). Bisexual identity in the context of parenthood: An exploratory qualitative study of self-identified bisexual parents in the United States. *Journal of Bisexuality, 17*, 378–399. https://doi.org/10.1080/15299716.2017.1384947

Benkov, L. (1995). Lesbian and gay parents: From margin to center. *Journal of Feminist Family Therapy, 7*, 49–64. https://doi.org/10.1300/J086v07n01_06

Bergman, K., Rubio, R. J., Green, R. J., & Padrón, E. (2010). Gay men who become fathers via surrogacy: The transition to parenthood. *Journal of GLBT Family Studies, 6*, 111–141. https://doi.org/10.1080/15504281003704942

Berlant, L., & Warner, M. (1998). Sex in public. *Critical Inquiry, 24*, 547–566. https://doi.org/10.1086/448884

Bronfenbrenner, U. (1979). *The ecology of human development: Experiments by nature and design.* Cambridge, MA: Harvard University Press.

Butler, J. (2004). *Undoing gender.* New York, NY: Routledge.

Byron, K. (2005). A meta-analytic review of work–family conflict and its antecedents. *Journal of Vocational Behavior, 67*, 169–198. https://doi.org/10.1016/j.jvb.2004.08.009

Charmaz, K. (2014). *Constructing grounded theory* (2nd ed.). Thousand Oaks, CA: Sage.

Crenshaw, K. (1991). Mapping the margins: Intersectionality, identity politics, and violence against women of color. *Stanford Law Review, 43*, 1241–1299. https://doi.org/10.2307/1229039

Den Dulk, L., & Peper, B. (2016). The impact of national policies on work-family experiences. In T. D. Allen & L. T. Eby (Eds.), *The Oxford handbook of work and family* (pp. 300–314). Oxford, UK: Oxford University Press.

de Visser, R. O. (2009). "I'm not a very manly man": Qualitative insights into young men's masculine subjectivity. *Men and Masculinities, 11*, 367–371. https://doi.org/10.1177/1097184X07313357

Diekman, A. B., & Goodfriend, W. (2006). Rolling with the changes. A role congruity perspective on gender norms. *Psychology of Women Quarterly, 30*, 369–383. https://doi.org/10.1111/j.1471-6402.2006.00312.x

Earle, A., Mokomane, Z., & Heymann, J. (2011). International perspectives on work-family policies: Lessons from the world's most competitive economies. *The Future of Children, 21*, 191–210. https://doi.org/10.1353/foc.2011.0014

Few-Demo, A. L. (2014). Intersectionality as the "new" critical approach in feminist family studies: Evolving racial/ethnic feminisms and critical race theories. *Journal of Family Theory & Review, 6*, 169–183. https://doi.org/10.1111/jftr.12039

Fish, J. N., & Russell, S. T. (2018). Queering methodologies to understand queer families. *Family Relations, 67*, 12–25. https://doi.org/10.1111/fare.12297

Foucault, M. (1978). *The history of sexuality.* New York, NY: Pantheon Books.

Fox-Keller, E. (1985). *Reflections on gender and science.* New Haven, CT: Yale University Press.

Gates, G. J. (2011). *How many people are lesbian, gay, bisexual, and transgender.* The Williams Institute. http://williamsinstitute.law.ucla.edu/wp-content/uploads/Gates-How-Many-People-LGBT-Apr-2011.pdf

Goffman, E. (1963). *Stigma: Notes on the management of spoiled identity.* Englewood Cliffs, NJ: Prentice Hall.

Goldberg, A. E. (2010). The transition to adoptive parenthood. In T. W. Miller (Ed.), *Handbook of stressful transitions across the life span* (pp. 165–184). New York, NY: Springer.

Goldberg, A. E. (2012). *Gay dads: Transitions to adoptive fatherhood.* New York, NY: NYU Press.

Goldberg, A. E. (2013). "Doing" and "undoing" gender: The meaning and division of housework in same-sex couples. *Journal of Family Theory & Review, 5*, 85–104. https://doi.org/10.1111/jftr.12009

Goldberg, A. E., Gartrell, N. K., & Gates, G. (2014). *Research report on LGB-parent families.* Los Angeles, CA: The Williams Institute, UCLA School of Law. Retrieved from The Williams Institute website: https://williamsinstitute.law.ucla.edu/wp-content/uploads/lgb-parent-families-july-2014.pdf

Goldberg, A. E., & Sayer, A. G. (2006). Lesbian couples' relationship quality across the transition to parenthood. *Journal of Marriage and Family, 68*, 87–100. https://doi.org/10.1111/j.1741-3737.2006.00235.x

Goldberg, A. E., & Smith, J. Z. (2009). Perceived parenting skill across the transition to adoptive parenthood among lesbian, gay, and heterosexual couples. *Journal of Family Psychology, 23*, 861–870. https://doi.org/10.1037/a0017009

Goldberg, A. E., & Smith, J. Z. (2011). Stigma, social context, and mental health: Lesbian and gay couples across the transition to adoptive parenthood. *Journal of Counseling Psychology, 58*, 139–150. https://doi.org/10.1037/a0021684

Goldberg, A. E., & Smith, J. Z. (2013). Work conditions and mental health in lesbian and gay dual-earner parents. *Family Relations, 62*, 727–740. https://doi.org/10.1111/fare.12042

Goldberg, A. E., & Smith, J. Z. (2014). Perceptions of stigma and self-reported school engagement in same sex couples with young children. *Psychology of Sexual Orientation and Gender Diversity, 1*(3), 202–212. https://doi.org/10.1037/sgd0000052

Goldberg, A. E., Smith, J. Z., McCormick, N. M., & Overstreet, N. M. (2019). Health behaviors and outcomes of parents in same-sex couples: An exploratory study. *Psychology of Sexual Orientation and Gender Diversity, 6*, 318. https://doi.org/10.1037/sgd0000330

Goldberg, A. E., Smith, J. Z., & Perry-Jenkins, M. (2012). The division of labor in lesbian, gay, and heterosexual new adoptive parents. *Journal of Marriage and Family, 74*, 812–828. https://doi.org/10.1111/j.1741-3737.2012.00992.x

Greenhaus, J. H., & Beutell, N. J. (1985). Sources of conflict between work and family roles. *Academy of Management Review, 10*, 76–88. https://doi.org/10.2307/258214

Hara, Y., & Hegewisch, A. (2013). *Maternity, paternity, and adoption leave in the United States.* Institute for Women's Policy Research. Retrieved from https://iwpr.org/wp-content/uploads/wpallimport/files/iwpr-export/publications/A143%20Updated%202013.pdf

Hare-Mustin, R. T. (1994). Discourses in the mirrored room: A postmodern analysis of therapy. *Family Process, 33*, 19–36. https://doi.org/10.1111/j.1545-5300.1994.00019.x

Hassard, J., & Parker, M. (Eds.). (1993). *Postmodernism and organizations.* Thousand Oaks, CA: Sage.

Hayman, B., Wilkes, L., Jackson, D., & Halcomb, E. (2013). *De Novo* lesbian families: Legitimizing the other mother. *Journal of GLBT Family Studies, 9*, 273–287. https://doi.org/10.1080/1550428X.2013.781909

Hennekam, S. A. M., & Ladge, J. J. (2017). When lesbians become mothers: Identity validation and the role of diversity climate. *Journal of Vocational Behavior, 103*, 40–55. https://doi.org/10.1016/j.jvb.2017.08.006

Huffman, A. H., Watrous-Rodriguez, K., & King, E. (2008). Supporting a diverse workforce: What type of support is most meaningful for lesbian and gay employees? *Human Resource Management, 47*, 237–253. https://doi.org/10.1002/hrm.20210

Ilies, R., Huth, M., Ryan, A. M., & Dimotakis, N. (2015). Explaining the links between workload, distress, and work–family conflict among school employees: Physical, cognitive, and emotional fatigue. *Journal of Educational Psychology, 107*, 1136–1149. https://doi.org/10.1037/edu0000029

Jones, K. P. (2017). To tell or not to tell? Examining the role of discrimination in the pregnancy disclosure process at work. *Journal of Occupational Health Psychology, 22*, 239–250. https://doi.org/10.1037/ocp0000030

Jones, E. E., Farina, A., Hastorf, A. H., Markus, H., Miller, D. T., & Scott, R. A. (1984). *Social stigma: The psychology of marked relationships*. New York, NY: W. H. Freeman.

Katz, D., & Kahn, R. L. (1978). *The social psychology of organizations*. Hoboken, NJ: Wiley.

Kemmis, S., & Wilkinson, M. (1998). Participatory action research and the study of practice. In B. Atweh, S. Kemmis, & P. Weeks (Eds.), *Action research in practice: Partnership for social justice in education* (pp. 21–36). New York, NY: Routledge.

Kim, J. S., & Faerman, S. R. (2013). Exploring the relationship between culture and family-friendly programs (FFPs) in the Republic of Korea. *European Management Journal, 31*, 505–521. https://doi.org/10.1016/j.emj.2013.04.012

King, E., Huffman, A., & Peddie, C. (2013). LGBT parents and the workplace. In A. E. Goldberg & K. R. Allen (Eds.), *LGBT-parent families: Possibilities for new research and implications for practice* (pp. 225–237). New York, NY: Springer.

Larsen, K. S., & Long, E. (1988). Attitudes toward sex-roles: Traditional or egalitarian? *Sex Roles, 19*, 1–12. https://doi.org/10.1007/bf00292459

Lather, P. (1991). *Getting smart: Feminist research and pedagogy with/in the post-modern*. New York, NY: Routledge.

LeBlanc, A. J., Frost, D. M., & Wight, R. G. (2015). Minority stress and stress proliferation among same-sex and other marginalized couples. *Journal of Marriage and Family, 77*, 40–59. https://doi.org/10.1111/jomf.12160

Lofquist, D. (2011). Same-sex couple households. *American Community Survey Briefs, 10*(3), 1–4. Retrieved from https://www2.census.gov/library/publications/2011/acs/acsbr10-03.pdf

Lu, L., Kao, S.-F., Chang, T.-T., Wu, H.-P., & Cooper, C. L. (2011). Work/family demands, work flexibility, work/family conflict, and their consequences at work: A national probability sample in Taiwan. *International Perspectives in Psychology: Research, Practice, Consultation, 1*(S), 68–81. https://doi.org/10.1037/2157-3883.1.s.68

Mahler, S. J., Chaudhuri, M., & Patil, V. (2015). Scaling intersectionality: Advancing feminist analysis of transnational families. *Sex Roles, 73*, 100–112. https://doi.org/10.1007/s11199-015-0506-9

Major, B., & O'Brien, L. T. (2005). The social psychology of stigma. *Annual Review of Psychology, 56*, 393–421. https://doi.org/10.1146/annurev.psych.56.091103.070137

Martinez, L. R., Hebl, M. R., Smith, N. A., & Sabat, I. E. (2017). Standing up and speaking out against prejudice toward gay men in the workplace. *Journal of Vocational Behavior, 103*, 71–85. https://doi.org/10.1016/j.jvb.2017.08.001

Martinez, L. R., Sawyer, K. B., Thoroughgood, C. N., Ruggs, E. N., & Smith, N. A. (2017). The importance of being "me": The relation between authentic identity expression and transgender employees' work-related attitudes and experiences. *Journal of Applied Psychology, 102*, 215–226. https://doi.org/10.1037/apl0000168

Mercier, L. R. (2007). Lesbian parents and work: Stressors and supports for the work-family interface. *Journal of Gay & Lesbian Social Services, 19*, 25–47. https://doi.org/10.1080/10538720802131675

Mertens, D. M. (2010). Transformative mixed methods research. *Qualitative Inquiry, 16*, 469–474. https://doi.org/10.1177/1077800410364612

Meyer, I. (1995). Minority stress and mental health in gay men. *Journal of Health Sciences and Social Behavior, 36*, 38–56. https://doi.org/10.2307/2137286

Mikolajczak, M., Brianda, M. E., Avalosse, H., & Roskam, I. (2018). Consequences of parental burnout: Its specific effect on child neglect and violence. *Child Abuse & Neglect, 80*, 134–145. https://doi.org/10.1016/j.chiabu.2018.03.025

Moore, M. R. (2011). *Invisible families: Gay identities, relationships, and motherhood among Black women*. Berkeley, CA: University of California Press.

Nestle, J., Howell, C., & Wilkins, R. (Eds.). (2002). *Genderqueer: Voices from beyond the sexual binary*. Los Angeles, CA: Alyson Books.

OECD. (2014). *Society at a glance 2014: OECD social indicators*. OECD Publishing. https://doi.org/10.1787/soc_glance-2014-en

O'Ryan, L. W., & McFarland, W. P. (2010). A phenomenological exploration of the experiences of dual-career lesbian and gay couples. *Journal of Counseling & Development, 88*, 71–79. https://doi.org/10.1002/j.1556-6678.2010.tb00153.x

Oswald, R. F., Blume, L. B., & Marks, S. R. (2005). Decentering heteronormativity: A model for family studies. In V. L. Bengtson, A. C. Acock, K. R. Allen, P. Dilworth-Anderson, & D. M. Klein (Eds.),

*Sourcebook of family theory & research* (pp. 143–165). Thousand Oaks, CA: Sage Publications.

Oswald, R. F., Kuvalanka, K. A., Blume, L. B., & Berkowitz, D. (2009). Queering "the family". In S. A. Lloyd, A. L. Few, & K. R. Allen (Eds.), *Handbook of feminist family studies* (pp. 43–55). Thousand Oaks, CA: Sage.

Perlesz, A., Power, J., Brown, R., McNair, R., Schofield, M., Pitts, M., … Bickerdike, A. (2010). Organising work and home in same-sex parented families: Findings from the work love play study. *Australian and New Zealand Journal of Family Therapy, 31*, 374–391. https://doi.org/10.1375/anft.31.4.374

Perrone, K. M. (2005). Work-family interface for same-sex, dual-earner couples: Implications for counselors. *Career Development Quarterly, 53*, 317–324. https://doi.org/10.1002/j.2161-0045.2005.tb00662.x

Pyne, J., Bauer, G., & Bradley, K. (2015). Transphobia and other stressors impacting trans parents. *Journal of GLBT Family Studies, 11*, 107–126. https://doi.org/10.1080/1550428X.2014.941127

Potter, E. C., & Allen, K. R. (2016). Agency and access: How gay fathers secure health insurance for their families. *Journal of GLBT Family Studies, 12*, 300–317. https://doi.org/10.1080/1550428X.2015.1071678

Ragins, B. R. (2008). Disclosure disconnects: Antecedents and consequences of disclosing invisible stigmas across life domains. *Academy of Management Review, 33*, 194–215. https://doi.org/10.5465/amr.2008.27752724

Rawsthorne, M., & Costello, M. (2010). Cleaning the sink: Exploring the experiences of Australian lesbian parents reconciling work/family responsibilities. *Community, Work & Family, 13*, 189–204. https://doi.org/10.1080/13668800903259777

Richardson, H. B., Moyer, A. M., & Goldberg, A. E. (2012). "You try to be Superman and youdon't have to be": Gay adoptive fathers' challenges and tensions in balancing work and family. *Fathering, 10*, 314–336. https://doi.org/10.3149/fth.1003.314

Ridic, G., Gleason, S., & Ridic, O. (2012). Comparisons of health care systems in the United States, Germany and Canada. *Materia Socio-Medica, 24*, 112–120. https://doi.org/10.5455/msm.2012.24.112-120

Sawyer, K., Thoroughgood, C., & Ladge, J. (2017). Invisible families, invisible conflicts: Examining the added layer of work-family conflict for employees with LGB families. *Journal of Vocational Behavior, 103*, 23–39. https://doi.org/10.1016/j.jvb.2017.08.004

Sawyer, K., Thoroughgood, C., & Webster, J. (2016). Queering the gender binary: Understanding transgender workplace experiences. In T. Köllen (Ed.), *Sexual orientation and transgender issues in organizations: Global perspectives on LGBT workforce diversity* (pp. 21–42). New York, NY: Springer.

Schwandt, T. A. (2000). Three epistemological stances for qualitative inquiry: Interpretivism, hermeneutics, and social constructionism. In N. K. Denzin & Y. S. Lincoln (Eds.), *Handbook of qualitative research* (pp. 189–213). Thousand Oaks, CA: Sage.

Simien, E. M. (2007). Doing intersectionality research: From conceptual issues to practical examples. *Politics & Gender, 3*, 264–271. https://doi.org/10.1017/S1743923X07000086

STC. (2018). *The 2018 STC health index* [Data file]. Retrieved from http://globalresidenceindex.com/hnwi-index/health-index/

Stiles, S. (2002). Family as a verb. In D. Denborough (Ed.), *Queer counselling and narrative practice* (pp. 15–10). Adelaide, AU: Dulwich Centre Publications.

ten Brummelhuis, L. L., Haar, J. M., & van der Lippe, T. (2010). Crossover of distress due to work and family demands in dual-earner couples: A dyadic analysis. *Work and Stress, 24*, 324–341. https://doi.org/10.1080/02678373.2010.533553

Tuten, T. L., & August, R. A. (2006). Work-family conflict: A study of lesbian mothers. *Women in Management Review, 21*, 578–597. https://doi.org/10.1108/09649420610692525

Vismara, L., Rollè, L., Agostini, F., Sechi, C., Fenaroli, V., Molgora, S., … Tambelli, R. (2016). Perinatal parenting stress, anxiety, and depression outcomes in first-time mothers and fathers: A 3- to 6-months postpartum follow-up study. *Frontiers in Psychology, 7*, 1–10. https://doi.org/10.3389/fpsyg.2016.00938

Watson, K. (2005). Queer theory. *Group Analysis, 38*, 67–81. https://doi.org/10.1177/0533316405049369

Weeks, J., Heaphy, B., & Donovan, C. (2001). *Same sex intimacies: Families of choice and other life experiments*. London, UK: Routledge.

Williams, J. C. (2010). *Reshaping the work-family debate: Why men and class matter*. Cambridge, MA: Harvard University Press.

# LGBTQ-Parent Families and Schools

Abbie E. Goldberg and Eliza Byard

Children are influenced by multiple contexts, including their families and schools. Research on children with lesbian, gay, bisexual, trans, and queer (LGBTQ) parents has primarily focused on their experiences in the context of their families, with little attention to their experiences in the school context. The lack of research on the family-school interface of LGBTQ-parent families is troubling, in that these families are vulnerable to marginalization and stigma in their broader communities and society at large, which likely extend to the school environment (Goldberg, 2010). Further, because strong family-school collaborations are linked to more positive educational outcomes in children (Beveridge, 2005; Fedewa & Clark, 2009), it is essential to understand and ultimately eradicate such experiences of marginalization, which have the potential to undermine LGBTQ-parent families' full engagement in school life.

This chapter reviews research on children with LGBTQ parents, with particular attention to those domains that are most relevant to teachers, administrators, and other school personnel. Thus, we review research on the academic achievement, social functioning, and bullying of children with LGBTQ parents. We also address research on LGBTQ parents themselves, including their experiences selecting and interacting with their children's schools—as well as the positive consequences for families of inhabiting an inclusive school environment. We end with practical recommendations for educators and practitioners who may encounter LGBTQ-parent families in their work, and who wish to create as inclusive environment as possible for these families.

It is important to provide a key caveat about the cultural context of the studies that are reviewed. The majority of studies on LGBTQ-parent families and schools have been conducted in the USA or Western Europe (e.g., the UK: Nixon, 2011; and Australia: Lindsay et al., 2006; Power et al., 2014); less is known regarding the experiences of LGBTQ-parent families and schools in non-Western contexts. Contemporary knowledge about LGBTQ-parent families has developed primarily in a Euro-Americanized cultural context, which represents a fairly monocultural perspective on these families (Lubbe, 2013; Moore & Stambolis-Ruhstorfer, 2013). The diversity and complexity of same-sex practices in various cultures, and the norms, values, and laws that surround them, inevitably influence the experiences and treatment of LGBTQ-parent families in society and in the educational setting specifically. Thus, it is important to recognize the

A. E. Goldberg (✉)
Department of Psychology, Clark University, Worcester, MA, USA
e-mail: agoldberg@clarku.edu

E. Byard
GLSEN: The Gay, Lesbian & Straight Education Network, New York, NY, USA
e-mail: Eliza.Byard@glsen.org

© Springer Nature Switzerland AG 2020
A. E. Goldberg, K. R. Allen (eds.), *LGBTQ-Parent Families*,
https://doi.org/10.1007/978-3-030-35610-1_18

cultural specificity of the work that we review here, and the need for work on LGBTQ-parent families and schools in non-Western contexts—which will ultimately expand, nuance, and deepen what we know about LGBTQ-parent families and schools.

Another caveat is that most of this research has focused on children raised by two mothers or two fathers—that is, same-sex parent families—with little attention to the actual sexual identities (gay, lesbian, bisexual, queer) of parents. In this chapter, the term lesbian-parent family is used interchangeably with two-mother or female same-sex parent family. When bisexual, trans, or queer identified parents are explicitly identified as included in a particular study, we note this. No research that we know of has explored school-related dynamics of trans parents, although we address this in a final section on future research as well as in our guidelines to educators and families.

Of note is that feminist, minority stress, and ecological theories dominate much of the research on LGBTQ-parent families in the past decade (see van Eeden-Moorefield, Few-Demo, Benson, Bible, & Lummer, 2018), which is an advancement over prior decades' overreliance on more deficit-based approaches (see Farr, Tasker, & Goldberg, 2017), yet more intersectional approaches are needed (van Eeden-Moorefield et al., 2018). Purposeful and explicit attention to intersectionality may illuminate important ways in which class, race, sexual orientation, and geographic location intersect to shape parents', and children's, schooling experiences (Goldberg, Allen, Black, Frost, & Manley, 2018; Power et al., 2014).

## Academic and Social Functioning of Children of LGBTQ Parents

Non-heterosexualities have long been stigmatized in society, and, by extension, both the capacity and deservingness of LGBTQ parents have been scrutinized, with the expectation that children raised by such parents will suffer emotionally and socially. In turn, research has frequently focused on whether the psychological outcomes of children raised in same-sex parent families differ from those of children raised in different-sex parent parents—reflecting a more heteronormative paradigm wherein LGBTQ-parent families are compared to the "gold standard" or "norm" of heterosexual-parent families (see Farr et al., 2017). This research tends to find few differences in such outcomes as a function of family structure (see Goldberg, Gartrell, & Gates, 2014). Children in same-sex parent families show similar psychological adjustment to their counterparts in heterosexual-parent families, and do not differ in terms of self-esteem, rates of emotional/behavioral problems, and overall well-being (Goldberg et al., 2014). Further, more recent research—which, reflecting the movement of the field to encompass more strengths-based frameworks, wherein LGBTQ-parent families are studied in their own right, without comparison to a "gold standard"—has found that youth raised by LGBTQ parents often view themselves as being especially tolerant and compassionate toward marginalized individuals as a function of their growing up experience (Cody, Farr, McRoy, Ayers-Lopez, & Ledesma, 2017; Goldberg, 2007).

## Academic Achievement

Although far less studied than psychological adjustment, some work has focused on school-related experiences and outcomes of children in same-sex parent families, including academic achievement and educational progress, in relation to children in different-sex parent families. Some of this work has used nationally representative data; this work indicates that children with same-sex parents do not appear to suffer in terms of their academic and educational outcomes (Potter, 2012; Rosenfeld, 2010; Wainright, Russell, & Patterson, 2004). Using the US Census data, Rosenfeld (2010) found that growing up in same-sex parent families did not disrupt or delay progression through elementary school. Wainright et al. (2004) also used nationally representative data and found that family structure (growing up in a same-sex parent family versus a different-sex parent family) was not associated with school outcomes for adolescents; rather, family process factors (e.g., closeness to parents) were significant predictors of academic adjustment. Using data from the Early Childhood Longitudinal Study-Kindergarten cohort, Potter (2012) found that children in same-sex parent families had lower math achievement scores than their peers in married, two-biological parent households; however, once the number of family transitions was taken into account, there were no differences between the two groups of children.

Other studies utilizing nonrepresentative data (e.g., Gartrell & Bos, 2010; Gartrell, Bos, Peyser, Deck, & Rodas, 2012) have also found that adolescents with same-sex parents do not show compromised academic achievement. In a sample of 17-year-old adolescents raised by lesbian mothers from birth, Gartrell et al. (2012) found that the teens had higher than average academic performance, with overall grades typically falling in the A− to B+ range. Further, 90% of teens hoped to attend a 4-year college, and 50% of the sample expected to enter a career that required additional post-baccalaureate training, suggesting high educational aspirations. Notably, these data are not from a representative sample; most of the families lived in progressive areas of the USA, such as San Francisco. More work is needed that examines the educational and professional aspirations of children with sexual minority parents who reside in rural and/or politically conservative regions of the USA, as well as in non-Western contexts.

## Social Functioning

Another domain that is relevant to educators is the social functioning of children with LGBTQ parents—that is, their ability to interact and form relationships with others. Schools and classrooms serve as key socializing contexts where children learn not only facts and figures but also how to navigate friendships and resolve peer conflicts (Cemalcilar, 2010; Grusec & Hastings, 2006). Despite concerns that children

of same-sex parents would show deficiencies in social skills and peer relationships—due to their "atypical" family form, their parents' sexual orientation, and/or the absence of a male/female parent in the home—research indicates that the social functioning of children with same-sex parents is similar to that of children with different-sex parents (see Goldberg et al., 2014, for a review). For example, using a nonrepresentative sample of intentional lesbian-mother households, Gartrell, Deck, Rodas, Peyser, and Banks (2005) found that parents' ratings of their 10-year-old children's social skills were in the normal range, as compared to national age and gender norms; further, 81% of children were described as relating well to their peers. Golombok et al. (2003) used a representative community sample in the UK to examine 7-year-olds' perceptions of peer relations. The authors found no evidence that children of lesbian mothers viewed their peer relationships more negatively than children of heterosexual parents. Thus, children in same-sex parent families do not appear to show deficiencies in social competence, and seem to have positive relationships with peers.

Some studies have also examined the social functioning (e.g., peer relationships) of teenagers with LGBTQ parents. Wainright and Patterson (2008) used data from a large national sample of adolescents and found that according to both self and peer reports, adolescents with female same-sex parents and adolescents with heterosexual parents did not differ in the quality of their peer relationships; rather, adolescents whose parents described closer relationships with them reported having more friends and having higher quality peer relationships. Thus, family process was again more significant than family structure in predicting children's outcomes.

## Peer Stigma, Teasing, and Bullying

Based on the research described thus far, the social abilities of children with LGBTQ parents do not appear to differ appreciably from that of children with heterosexual parents. However, these studies do not address the question of whether, in the larger school context, these children may be more likely to be teased. Indeed, these children may have good social skills and close friends but may still be more likely to be teased (e.g., due to their parents' sexual orientation or family structure).

Some studies have examined teasing and bullying experiences, specifically, in school-aged children. Using a nonrepresentative sample, Vanfraussen, Ponjaert-Kristoffersen, and Brewaeys (2002) compared school-aged children from intentional lesbian-mother households with children from heterosexual-parent families in Belgium and found no differences in the rates of teasing between the two groups. Children in both groups reported being laughed at, excluded, and called names. Clothing, physical appearance (height, hair, etc.) and intelligence (being "too" smart or being "stupid") were among the reported reasons for teasing in both groups. Family-related reasons for teasing were mentioned only by children from lesbian-mother families, a quarter of whom reported having been teased about having two mothers, having a lesbian mother, not having a father, or being gay themselves. Thus, children from different family types experienced the same amount of teasing, but reasons for the teasing differed across family forms.

Other studies have focused on bullying in adolescents with same-sex parents. Using data from a school-based survey, Rivers, Poteat, and Noret (2008) found that adolescents (aged 12–16) raised in families led by female same-sex couples were no more likely to be victimized than adolescents raised in families led by heterosexual couples. MacCallum and Golombok (2004) utilized a nonrepresentative sample of 12-year-old children in the UK from lesbian-mother families, single heterosexual-mother families, and heterosexual two-parent families and found no differences among the groups in terms of mothers' worries about children's relationships at school or children's self-reported experiences of bullying.

Some research suggests greater frequencies of teasing and bullying than the above studies describe. GLSEN conducted a 2008 study of over 500 LGBTQ-parent families' experiences in education found that 40% of the 154 students surveyed reported being verbally harassed in school because of their family (Kosciw & Diaz, 2008). Further, although the vast majority of the students identified as heterosexual, 38% of students reported being verbally harassed at school because of their real or perceived sexual orientation (i.e., they were assumed to be gay because their parents were gay) (Kosciw & Diaz, 2008). Similarly, Fairtlough (2008) found that about half of young adults with LGBTQ parents recall having heard homophobic comments or experienced homophobic abuse (verbal or physical) from peers at school during their youth.

There is some evidence that the children of LGBTQ parents may be particularly likely to experience teasing at certain developmental stages. In their longitudinal study of children raised in intentional lesbian-mother families, Gartrell et al. (2000) found that 18% of mothers reported that their 5-year-old children had experienced some type of homophobia from peers or teachers. By age 10, almost half of children in the sample had reportedly experienced some form of homophobia (e.g., teasing; Gartrell et al., 2005), suggesting that as children grow older, they may come into contact with teasing and discrimination on a more frequent basis.

Welsh (2011) conducted a small qualitative study of 14 adolescents with lesbian and gay parents and found that half of participants described middle school as the most difficult time in their lives, in part because of the heteronormative attitudes and teasing they encountered in their peer group. Similarly, Cody et al. (2017) studied 24 youth (mean age = 16 years) adopted via foster care by LG parents and found that youth sometimes reported teasing by peers at school—but often remarked that teasing was worse when they were younger, e.g., in middle school. Likewise, retrospective reports by adults raised by LG parents suggests that most recalled their social experiences as becoming more positive across the life course and reported less stigma and more benefits related to their family structure in adulthood than in earlier developmental periods (Lick, Patterson, & Schmidt, 2013).

Some research (e.g., Casper & Schultz, 1999; Goldberg, Allen, et al., 2018; Kosciw & Diaz, 2008; Lindsay et al., 2006) suggests that middle- and upper-middle-class LGB parents may be at an advantage with regard to protecting their children from bullying. Their socioeconomic and professional status may enhance their ability to choose places to live that are safe from sexual orientation-related discrimination and to send their children to school where harassment related to their family structure is unlikely to occur (Casper & Schultz, 1999; Goldberg, Allen, et al., 2018). Indeed, a study of lesbian and gay adoptive-parent families in the USA found that parents with more resources often elected to live in urban areas and/or send their children to private schools—both of which seemed to be more gay-affirming settings in which their children were less likely to encounter stigma or victimization (Goldberg, Allen, et al., 2018). And, a study of LGBTQ parents in Australia found that parents in rural/suburban areas were more likely to report that their child had experienced bullying or discrimination related to their parents' sexual orientation at school than parents in major urban areas (Power et al., 2014).

Of note, however, is that class and geographic privilege inevitably protects White LGBTQ-parent families more than LGBTQ-parent families of color, or multiracial families, who face discrimination based on both their sexuality and race, in a variety of different contexts (Croteau, Talbot, Lance, & Evans, 2002). Children of color with LGBTQ parents—particularly White parents—may face marginalization in the peer setting based on the multiple ways that they are "different" (Farr, Crain, Oakley, Cashen, & Garber, 2016; Gianino, Goldberg, & Lewis, 2009). Recognizing this, parents may specifically seek out social settings where their children are not the only children of color (e.g., churches or afterschool programs), as well as those where they are not the only children with LGBTQ parents (e.g., LGBTQ parenting groups) (Goldberg, Frost, Manley, & Black, 2018; Goldberg, Sweeney, Black, & Moyer, 2016).

**Consequences of peer stigma, teasing, and bullying** Peer stigma and teasing have in turn been linked to compromised well-being in children of lesbian and gay parents (Bos & van Balen, 2008; Farr, Oakley, & Ollen, 2016; Gartrell et al., 2005). Bos and van Balen (2008) interviewed 8–12-year-old children in planned lesbian-mother families in the Netherlands and found that children who perceived greater stigmatization by peers experienced lower well-being (although, in general, children reported low levels of stigma), with findings differing by gender: Girls who perceived greater stigma reported lower self-esteem, whereas boys who perceived greater stigma were rated as more hyperactive by parents. In a study of 10-year-old children in intentional lesbian-mother families, Gartrell et al. (2005) found that experiencing homophobia was associated with more emotional/behavioral problems, although on average, these children did not experience more problems that would be expected in the general population. Farr, Oakley, and Ollen (2016) studied lesbian and gay parents of 8-year-olds and found that although only 8% of parents reported that their child had been teased or bullied for having LG parents, these children had more behavioral difficulties, according to parent and teacher reports.

Significantly, supportive aspects of the school setting can buffer the negative impact of homophobic teasing on well-being among children with LGBTQ parents. Bos, Gartrell, Peyser, and van Balen (2008) found that although homophobia had a negative impact on children's well-being overall, attending schools with LGBTQ curricula served as a buffer against the negative impact of homophobia. Bos and Gartrell (2010) found that when these children were 17, experiencing homophobia was also associated with higher levels of problem behavior. Yet parent-relationships served as a buffer against the negative impact of perceived stigmatization, such that adolescents who had positive relationships with their lesbian mothers showed resilience in response to homophobic stigmatization. And, in a study of adolescents with lesbian mothers in

Canada, Vyncke, Julien, Jouvin, and Jodoin (2014) found that higher levels of school support for LGBTQ people (e.g., having a club for LGBTQ youth; LGBTQ topics included in the curriculum; LGBTQ-inclusive school paperwork) moderated the association between adolescents' experiences of heterosexism and internalizing problems. These findings, taken together, suggest that the broader school context, as well as what happens within families, may have important implications for children's emotional and behavioral well-being, even offsetting the negative impact of peer stigma and bullying.

Beyond well-being, peer stigmatization may have negative consequences for educational outcomes as well. Findings from the 2008 GLSEN survey indicated that students with LGBTQ parents who reported high levels of harassment at school were much more likely to report that they missed classes or entire days of school because of feeling unsafe (Kosciw & Diaz, 2008). Thus, in addition to directly impacting adolescents' psychosocial well-being, being bullied may have indirect effects on academic achievement and educational outcomes (i.e., youth who stay home because of fear or anxiety may fall behind in school and fail to advance academically). More research is needed to examine the long-term effects of early harassment and mistreatment on educational outcomes, particularly in contexts where school advancement is already threatened (e.g., poor and/or violent neighborhoods; poor-performing school districts).

**Factors that reduce peer stigma, teasing, and bullying** It is important to understand what factors—e.g., at the school level—may reduce the likelihood that children of LGBTQ parents are the recipients of peer stigma and bullying. The GLSEN survey found that although only 35% of students with LGBT parents reported that their school's anti-bullying/harassment policy dealt explicitly with sexual orientation and/or gender identity/expression, those whose schools had LGBTQ-inclusive anti-bullying policies reported fewer negative experiences at school, especially in regard to teacher and peer mistreatment related to their parents' sexual orientation (Kosciw &

Diaz, 2008). The survey also found that relatively few parents (10%) were aware of school personnel having received training on LGBT issues; yet, parents who did report awareness of such trainings were less likely than other parents to report that their children had been bullied at school (Kosciw & Diaz, 2008). These findings suggest that policies and trainings may represent important ways to reduce the incidence of LGBTQ-related stigma at school. Given that many teachers do not receive any training or education on the topic of sexual diversity and/or lesbian-/gay-parent families (Kintner-Duffy, Vardell, Lower, & Cassidy, 2012), systematic inclusion of these topics in teacher training and educational programs should be a priority.

More research is needed to explore how other school practices—such as the presence of GSAs (Gay-Straight Alliances)—may reduce the incidence or negative impact of bullying for children of LGBTQ parents. The presence of and involvement in GSAs may have positive consequences for the well-being of LGBTQ youth, in some cases buffering the negative effect of anti-gay victimization on mental health (Ioverno, Belser, Baiocco, Grossman, & Russell, 2016; Toomey, Ryan, Diaz, & Russell, 2011). Youth in schools with GSAs report lower substance use, less truancy, lower victimization, and safer climates than youth in schools without GSAs (Russell & Horne, 2017). GSAs and similar programs may have the effect of changing the school climate to be more affirming of LGBTQ youth—as well as youth with LGBTQ parents.

## School Experiences of LGBTQ Parents

Much of the existing research on the experiences and perspectives of LGBTQ parents has focused their mental health, relationship quality, parenting skills, and parent-child relations. This research has found few differences in these domains as compared to heterosexual parents (see Goldberg et al., 2014). For example, rates of mental health problems and levels of parenting stress do not appear to differ as a function of parent sexual orientation (Goldberg et al., 2014). Relatively little research has examined LGBTQ parents' experiences in school settings, despite evidence that they experience concerns related to how they, and their children, will be received by teachers, school administrators, and other school personnel (Casper & Schultz, 1999; Goldberg, Allen, et al., 2018; Kosciw & Diaz, 2008; Lindsay et al., 2006). Parents' experiences with school selection, and their perceptions of exclusion versus integration in the school environment, have received some attention in the literature; these domains will be addressed.

## Parenting Concerns and School Selection

Research on LGBTQ parents' experiences interfacing with the school system suggests that parents are often aware of the potential for homophobic bullying. For example, when asked about their parenting concerns, LGBTQ parents often state that they worry that their children will be teased or discriminated against because of their (parents') sexual orientation (Goldberg, 2009; Goldberg, Allen, et al., 2018; Johnson & O'Connor, 2002; Lindsay et al., 2006; McDermott, 2011). In turn, they often seek out progressive and diverse schools and communities in an effort to reduce the stigma to which their children are exposed (Casper & Schultz, 1999; Goldberg & Smith, 2014a, 2014b; Kosciw & Diaz, 2008; Mercier & Harold, 2003). The GLSEN study of LGBTQ parents, most of whom had a child in elementary school, found that many parents considered the diversity of the school population (31%), the school's reputation for valuing diversity (22%), the presence of other children with LGBTQ parents at the school (17%), and the school's reputation for being welcoming of LGBT families (17%), in selecting their children's school (Kosciw & Diaz, 2008). Other frequently cited reasons for selecting their children's school were the following: It was the local/neighborhood school (59%), the school's academic reputation (54%), and knowing other

families at the school (29%) (Kosciw & Diaz, 2008). LGBTQ parents of children of color were more likely to choose schools based on the diversity of the school population (43%) than were LGBT parents with a White student (25%), regardless of the race/ethnicity of the parents (about 16% of the families represented had White parent(s) and a child of color, and about 14% of the families represented were comprised of one White and one non-White parent; Kosciw & Diaz, 2008).

The tendency for LGBTQ parents to emphasize diversity in their school selection has been observed in several studies of parents with young children. Although most LGBTQ parents have little control over the schools that their children attend (e.g., due to finances), and ultimately most parents send their children to their local public schools (Kosciw & Diaz, 2008), parents of young children typically do play an active role in selecting early childhood environments for their children (i.e., daycare, preschool, and kindergarten). Gartrell et al. (1999) interviewed 84 lesbian-parent families with toddlers about their plans for child care/preschool and found that 87% of mothers planned to enroll their children in programs that included children and teachers of different social classes, genders, races, ethnicities, and cultures, out of a belief that "exposure to diversity was the most effective method of fortifying their children against homophobia" (p. 367). A study of lesbian, gay, and heterosexual adoptive parents of preschool-aged children found that parents, regardless of sexual orientation, frequently considered educational philosophy and cost in selecting a preschool (i.e., 83% and 58% of the full sample, respectively) (Goldberg & Smith, 2014a). In addition, 61% of lesbians and 65% of gay men considered the gay-friendliness of the school, and 23% of lesbians and 16% of gay men considered the presence of other lesbian-/gay-parent families in their search for a school (Goldberg & Smith, 2014a). Significantly more lesbians and gay men considered the racial diversity of the school, as compared to heterosexuals (55%, 52%, and 29%, respectively). These data, then, are quite consistent with the findings of the GLSEN sample

(Kosciw & Diaz, 2008), which focused primarily on LGBTQ parents of elementary school-aged children.

LGBTQ parents who have adopted transracially demonstrate unique concerns when they are parenting a child of color. Research on lesbian and gay parents of preschoolers (Goldberg, 2014) and kindergarteners (Goldberg, Allen, et al., 2018) suggests that White parents who have adopted transracially often struggle to find a school that is both racially diverse and also LGBTQ friendly (Goldberg, 2014). Some of the parents in this research observed that the urban, racially diverse schools in their areas were typically not the same schools as the gay-friendly schools; rather, the latter tend to be predominantly White. In turn, some parents—particularly lesbian mothers of children of color—juggled concerns for their children's emerging racial identity with concerns that their family structure would be appreciated and respected (Goldberg, 2014; Goldberg, Allen, et al., 2018). When children have special needs (e.g., significant trauma history; learning disabilities), LGBTQ adoptive parents juggle even more considerations in selecting a school for their child, as they strive to access schools with appropriate supports and services (Goldberg, Allen, et al., 2018; Goldberg, Frost, & Black, 2017) and ultimately must downplay race and family structure considerations due to more pressing considerations.

## Advocating for Children

In addition to seeking out more progressive schools, LGBTQ parents may seek to promote a supportive school climate for their children by talking directly to their children's teachers about their family structure (Goldberg, Black, Sweeney, & Moyer, 2017; Lindsay et al., 2006; Mercier & Harold, 2003; Power et al., 2014). The GLSEN survey, for example, found that the LGBTQ parents in their sample often approached their children's schools early on in the school year, in order to lay the foundation for a positive school experience for their child. Forty-eight of parents in the GLSEN study reported having gone to the

school at the beginning of the school year to discuss their family (Kosciw & Diaz, 2008). Parents may also try to promote a more positive school experience for their children by making suggestions to teachers about ways to incorporate awareness of diverse families into the curricula (Goldberg, Black, Sweeney, & Moyer, 2017; Lindsay et al., 2006; Mercier & Harold, 2003). By offering input and suggestions regarding school content and foci, as well as donating resources (e.g., books) to their children's schools, LGBTQ parents often assert themselves as active and concerned school citizens, and also potentially help to create a more inclusive school environment for their families and children (Goldberg, 2014; Goldberg, Black, Sweeney, & Moyer, 2017).

Of course, it is quite possible that teachers and school personnel will not be open to—or may simply not "get"—LGBTQ parents' suggestions and concerns (Goldberg, Frost, & Black, 2017; Lindsay et al., 2006). In turn, parents who provide input into their children's school experiences (including confronting or challenging heterosexist or homophobic practices at school), only to be dismissed or ignored, may ultimately become less engaged with their children's schools. Alternatively, they may actively resist such dismissal, and persist in confronting heterosexism. Or, they may seek out alternative schooling environments for their children. More research is needed to explore how LGBTQ parents respond to and deal with teachers' explicit or implicit refusal to alter their school practices and/or curriculum to be more inclusive and accepting.

Little work has explored the school experiences of parents who identify as bisexual or queer (but see Pallotta-Chiarolli, 2012). This work suggests that bisexual and queer parents face marginalization and invisibility in the school system. Significantly, these parents may experience—or fear experiencing—suspicion and mistrust if they choose to assert their identities (Goldberg, Ross, Manley, & Mohr, 2017). That is, bisexual and queer parents may worry that they will be questioned about the "relevance" of their sexual identity insomuch as they should simply be content to have their sexual identities inferred from their partnership status (e.g., lesbian if partnered with a woman; heterosexual if partnered with a man). Asexual, pansexual, and trans-identified parents who seek to educate teachers about their identities—or who simply come out to teachers—will likely face even greater difficulty (e.g., suspicion, resistance, disregard) due to the unfamiliarity of most teachers with many sexual minority identities—much less non-cisgender gender identities.

## Experiences in Schools: Exclusion, Integration, and Involvement

Some research has examined LGBTQ parents' experiences with teachers, school personnel, and other parents. This research suggests that, like their children, LGBTQ parents may encounter exclusion and stigma. The GLSEN survey, for example, found that more than half (53%) of parents reported various forms of exclusion from their children's school communities (e.g., being excluded or prevented from fully participating in school activities and events, being excluded by school policies and procedures) (Kosciw & Diaz, 2008). Further, 26% of LGBT parents reported being mistreated by other parents (e.g., being stared at, whispered about, or ignored). Likewise, a study of lesbian and gay adoptive parents of preschoolers found that about one-third of parents reported that they had faced school-related challenges or difficulties, which were often, but not always, related to their sexual orientation (Goldberg, 2014). A common theme identified by parents was feeling "different" at the school (e.g., not being treated equal to other parents; not knowing other adoptive or same-sex parents at the school), and some parents also reported feeling that teachers displayed a lack of sensitivity or experience with diverse families (e.g., teachers used the phrase "mom and dad" or asserted that they were "color blind").

Perceptions of mistreatment, especially by other parents, may have implications for parents' school involvement: In the GLSEN survey, parents who reported more exclusion and mistreatment at school were less likely to be involved in volunteering at their children's schools (Kosciw

& Diaz, 2008). Likewise, a study of lesbian and gay parents with preschool-aged children found that parents who reported higher levels of exclusion by other parents were less involved in their children's schools (Goldberg & Smith, 2014b). Lesbian and gay parents who tended not to socialize with other parents were also less involved (Goldberg & Smith, 2014b).

It is important to note, however, that studies show very high levels of school involvement overall by LGBTQ parents (Goldberg & Smith, 2014b; Kosciw & Diaz, 2008). For example, 94% of the parents in the GLSEN sample reported that they had attended a parent-teacher conference or back-to-school evening, and two-thirds of parents had volunteered at their children's schools (Kosciw & Diaz, 2008). Research with lesbian, gay, and heterosexual parents of kindergarteners found that parents were generally at least somewhat involved with their children's school, although how parents conceptualized their involvement varied (Goldberg, Black, Manley, & Frost, 2017). For example, some were involved primarily through making donations to the school (e.g., books and snacks—typically because their work schedule did not allow them to volunteer), whereas others volunteered in classrooms or on school committees. Gay male couples and heterosexual couples more often described differential involvement, whereby one partner (the woman in heterosexual couples) was more involved at school than the other. In lesbian couples, both women tended to be fairly involved—perhaps in part due to gendered norms surrounding school volunteering. Benefits of involvement included reduced likelihood of marginalization—among lesbian and gay parents in particular—and influencing the school to create change (Goldberg, Black, Manley, & Frost, 2017).

Thus, anticipating potential exclusion and mistreatment, LGBTQ parents may be especially invested in having a voice in their children's schools. This tendency, however, may be more pronounced for middle-class parents than working-class parents—in part because of greater barriers to school involvement in the latter group. Nixon (2011) conducted a qualitative study of working-class lesbian mothers in the UK and found that negative experiences of school (based on both class and sexuality), trepidation about their ability to help their children with their schoolwork (based on their own personal experiences of "failure" at school), and a sense of being "out of place" at their children's schools, were all identified as barriers to being more involved with their children's schools—including volunteering, talking to teachers about their families, and meeting with school personnel in the event of a problem (e.g., bullying). In addition to social class, geographic location may also impact parents' school experiences. Indeed, Power et al.'s (2014) study of LGBTQ parents found that parents were less likely to be "out" about their sexual orientation at their children's schools in rural and suburban areas than major metropolitan areas. Insomuch as outness is related to parent-school relationships (Fedewa & Clark, 2009), it is possible that parents who were not out were also less likely to be involved.

Parents' involvement matters for children. For example, strong parent-school collaborations are consistently related to more positive academic outcomes for children (Beveridge, 2005; Jeynes, 2007). Among lesbian and gay parents of young adopted children, higher levels of school involvement (e.g., volunteering; attending school events; visiting their child's classroom) and fewer conflicts with teachers during their children's preschool years were associated with lower levels of child internalizing (e.g., depression, anxiety) problems in kindergarten (Goldberg & Smith, 2017). Also, parents who reported higher levels of acceptance by other parents in preschool tended to report lower levels of internalizing and externalizing (i.e., behavior) problems in their children in kindergarten (Goldberg & Smith, 2017).

## Future Research Directions

More research is clearly needed on how social class, race, and other key social structures shape feelings of inclusion and school involvement. For

example, White LGBTQ parents who are parenting children of color may feel out of place if their children are attending schools that are predominantly White, as well as if their children are attending schools where there are few White parents or families. Indeed, multiracial and/or adoptive families may struggle in finding a school community that reflects their families in meaningful ways and, in turn, that feels truly accepting. More research is also needed that explicitly interrogates the experience of bisexual and queer parents, as well as even less often studied sexual minorities—such as pansexual and asexual parents. Such parents may encounter particular struggles in relation to schools—for example, they may want to counter bisexual erasure and binegativity in schools (Elia, 2010), but be uncertain of how to do so, and may be apprehensive of the potential consequences.

Research on trans parents' experiences interfacing with schools is also needed. Indeed, although some research has begun to explore the experiences of trans parents (see chapter "Transgender-Parent Families"), no work that we know of has explicitly addressed their experiences navigating child care or school environments. Of note, however, is that in their study of lesbian and gay parents' school involvement, Goldberg, Black, Manley, and Frost (2017) observed that one source of perceived exclusion for parents was gender expression. That is, lesbian parents who presented less traditionally "femininely" (i.e., more masculine, more "butch," more androgynously) described a unique form of marginalization by other parents, whereby they did not feel included or understood.

More research on how the academic and social experiences of youth raised by LGBTQ parents varies according to neighborhood and community climate, as well as state-level policies, is needed. Youth with LGBTQ parents who live in poor and/or violent neighborhoods, for example, may face unique challenges to their academic success and advancement—for example, due to the intersection of underperforming school districts and inadequate community resources (both general and LGBTQ specific). More work is also needed on the transition to college for youth with LGBTQ parents; indeed, of interest is how these youth seek and adapt to diverse college communities and the extent to which they are "out" about their families in these new academic and social environments (see Goldberg, Kinkler, Richardson, & Downing, 2011).

## Recommendations for Practice

### Educators and Practitioners

By creating a more LGBTQ-inclusive environment, schools can attract and retain LGBTQ-parent families, who are, in many cases, inclined to be engaged and active members of the school community. In recent years, the professional world of K–12 education has evolved significantly toward greater inclusiveness of LGBTQ people—parents and students alike. For example, the National Parent Teacher Association (PTA) has passed numerous resolutions regarding LGBTQ families and students, a particularly important development given the resistance that LGBTQ parents often face from other parents (National PTA, 2018).

There are many ways that schools can create more inclusive environments that support LGBTQ-parent families. First, at a broad level, schools must critically examine and seek to decenter heteronormativity in every domain. For example, forms that parents and prospective parents complete should have spaces for "parent 1" and "parent 2" rather than "mother" and "father," and might even provide spaces for a third and fourth parent, to accommodate more complex families of all kinds. Likewise, schools should consider whether there are LGBTQ people on staff, among their school personnel and administration, and actively seek out LGBTQ people for teaching and leadership positions. Further, schools can create a more welcoming atmosphere for all types of families by ensuring that the artwork and photographs on their website and in their hallways and classrooms represent a diverse range of families. Schools should also provide professional development trainings or workshops

for teachers and other school personnel to support them in working effectively with diverse families, including LGBTQ parents.

Within the classroom, teachers can be more inclusive by employing a wide range of curricular resources (e.g., see www.glsen.org). In addition to including books about and examples of LGBTQ-parent families in their classrooms, teachers and schools can celebrate LGBT events (e.g., Coming Out Day, LGBT History Month) and sponsor supportive student clubs (e.g., GSAs). Such efforts, taken together, may significantly improve the climate for LGBTQ youth as well as youth with LGBTQ parents (see chapter "Reflectivity, Reactivity, and Reinventing: Themes from the Pedagogical Literature on LGBTQ-Parent Families in the Classroom and Communities").

### Policy and School Culture

School personnel who are in charge of making school policy should ensure that their non-discrimination policies are inclusive of sexual orientation and gender identity/expression and that they have adopted policies that support equal access to school facilities for transgender people. They should also ensure that their anti-bullying policies cover harassment and mistreatment related to sexual orientation and gender identity/expression. These and other policies will help to communicate and in turn create a supportive school climate for LGB parents and their children. (Model laws and policies can be found at: https://www.glsen.org/article/model-laws-policies.)

In addition to adopting formal policies that are LGBTQ-inclusive and affirming, schools should ensure that all events discussing school culture and expectations for building community within the school walls are explicit about the intention to make LGBT parents and their children feel welcome. Such communications are most effective when they are clearly and consistently made to the entire school community, including other parents, and are articulated as an extension of the core values and educational mission of the school.

## LGBTQ-Parent Families

LGBTQ parents should seek as much information as possible from and about any schools that they are considering for their children, in terms of the school's policies, atmosphere, and curriculum regarding LGBTQ-parent families. LGBTQ parents of young children should consider speaking to their children's teachers regarding their family structure, as well helping their children's teachers with language to describe their families. Parents may also wish to tell their children's teachers how they would like them to address and respond to other children's questions regarding their families—for example, taking a proactive, preemptive approach (Goldberg, 2014)—not one that builds "resilience in the child per se [but one that]…attempt[s] to build resilience into the environment in which the child [is] immersed" (Crouch, McNair, & Waters, 2017, pp. 2209). LGBTQ parents of older children may take a more collaborative approach with their children, whereby they allow their children to take the lead in sharing any relevant information or concerns, or obtain their children's input about what they wish their parents to share—indeed, older youth tend to be more strategic and choiceful regarding whether and when to share that they have LGBTQ parents (Cody et al., 2017; Gianino et al., 2009). Children themselves should seek to identify supportive and affirming teachers and spaces in the school community; if such spaces are not readily available, they should seek outside support (e.g., via COLAGE, an organization for children with LGBTQ parents: see www.colage.org).

## References

Beveridge, S. (2005). *Children, families, and schools: Developing partnerships for inclusive education.* London, UK: Routledge Falmer.

Bos, H., & Gartrell, N. (2010). Adolescents of the USA National Longitudinal Family Study: Can family characteristics counteract the negative effects of stigmatization? *Family Process, 49*, 559–572. https://doi.org/10.1111/j.1545-5300.2010.01340.x

Bos, H. M., Gartrell, N. K., Peyser, H., & van Balen, F. (2008). The USA National Longitudinal Lesbian Family Study (NLLFS): Homophobia,

psychological adjustment, and protective factors. *Journal of Lesbian Studies, 12*, 455–471. https://doi.org/10.1080/10894160802278630

Bos, H. M. W., & van Balen, F. (2008). Children in planned lesbian families: Stigmatization, psychological adjustment, and protective factors. *Culture, Health, & Sexuality, 10*, 221–236. https://doi.org/10.1080/13691050701601702

Casper, V., & Schultz, S. (1999). *Gay parents/straight schools: Building communication and trust.* New York, NY: Teachers College Press.

Cemalcilar, Z. (2010). Schools as socialisation contexts: Understanding the impact of school climate factors on students sense of school belonging. *Applied Psychology: An International Review, 59*, 243–272. https://doi.org/10.1111/j.1464-0597.2009.00389.x

Cody, P. A., Farr, R. H., McRoy, R. G., Ayers-Lopez, S. J., & Ledesma, K. J. (2017). Youth perspectives on being adopted from foster care by lesbian and gay parents: Implications for families and adoption professionals. *Adoption Quarterly, 20*, 98–118. https://doi.org/10.1080/10926755.2016.1200702

Croteau, J. M., Talbot, D. M., Lance, T. S., & Evans, N. J. (2002). A qualitative study of the interplay between privilege and oppression. *Journal of Multicultural Counseling and Development, 24*, 239–258. https://doi.org/10.1002/j.2161-1912.2002.tb00522.x

Crouch, S., McNair, R., & Waters, E. (2017). Parent perspectives on child health and well-being in same-sex families: Heteronormative conflict and resilience building. *Journal of Child and Family Studies, 26*, 2202–2214. https://doi.org/10.1007/s10826-017-0796-3

Elia, J. P. (2010). Bisexuality and school culture: School as a prime site for bi-intervention. *Journal of Bisexuality, 10*, 452–471. https://doi.org/10.1080/15299716.2010.521060

Fairtlough, A. (2008). Growing up with a lesbian or gay parent: Young people's perspectives. *Health & Social Care in the Community, 16*, 521–528. https://doi.org/10.1111/j.1365-2524.2008.00774.x

Farr, R., Crain, E., Oakley, M., Cashen, K., & Garber, K. (2016). Microaggressions, feelings of difference, and resilience among adopted children with sexual minority parents. *Journal of Youth and Adolescence, 45*, 85–104. https://doi.org/10.1007/s10964-015-0353-6

Farr, R., Oakley, M., & Ollen, W. (2016). School experiences of young children and their lesbian and gay adoptive parents. *Psychology of Sexual Orientation & Gender Diversity, 3*, 442–447. https://doi.org/10.1037/sgd0000187

Farr, R., Tasker, F., & Goldberg, A. E. (2017). Theory in highly cited studies of sexual minority parent families: Variations and implications. *Journal of Homosexuality, 64*, 1143–1179. https://doi.org/10.1080/00918369.2016.1242336

Fedewa, A. L., & Clark, T. P. (2009). Parent practices and home-school partnerships: A differential effect for children with same-sex coupled parents? *Journal of GLBT Family Studies, 5*, 312–339. https://doi.org/10.1080/15504280903263736

Gartrell, N., Banks, A., Hamilton, J., Reed, N., Bishop, H., & Rodas, C. (1999). The National Lesbian Family Study: 2. Interviews with mothers of toddlers. *American Journal of Orthopsychiatry, 69*, 362–369. https://doi.org/10.1037/h0080410

Gartrell, N., Banks, A., Reed, N., Hamilton, J., Rodas, C., & Deck, A. (2000). The National Lesbian Family Study: 3. Interviews with mothers of five-year-olds. *American Journal of Orthopsychiatry, 70*, 542–548. https://doi.org/10.1037/h0087823

Gartrell, N., & Bos, H. (2010). US National Longitudinal Lesbian Family Study: Psychological adjustment of 17-year-old adolescents. *Pediatrics, 126*, 28–36. https://doi.org/10.1542/peds.2009-3153

Gartrell, N., Bos, H. M., Peyser, H., Deck, A., & Rodas, C. (2012). Adolescents with lesbian mothers describe their own lives. *Journal of Homosexuality, 59*, 1211–1229. https://doi.org/10.1080/00918369.2012.720499

Gartrell, N., Deck, A., Rodas, C., Peyser, H., & Banks, A. (2005). The National Lesbian Family Study: 4. Interviews with the 10-year-old children. *American Journal of Orthopsychiatry, 75*, 518–524. https://doi.org/10.1037/0002-9432.75.4.518

Gianino, M., Goldberg, A. E., & Lewis, T. (2009). Family outings: Disclosure practices among adopted youth with gay and lesbian parents. *Adoption Quarterly, 12*, 205–228. https://doi.org/10.1080/10926750903313344

Goldberg, A. E. (2007). (How) does it make a difference?: Perspectives of adults with lesbian, gay, and bisexual parents. *American Journal of Orthopsychiatry, 77*, 550–562. https://doi.org/10.1037/0002-9432.77.4.550

Goldberg, A. E. (2009). Heterosexual, lesbian, and gay preadoptive couples' preferences about child gender. *Sex Roles, 61*, 55–71. https://doi.org/10.1007/s11199-009-9598-4

Goldberg, A. E. (2010). *Lesbian and gay parents and their children: Research on the family life cycle*. Washington, DC: American Psychological Association.

Goldberg, A. E. (2014). Lesbian, gay, and heterosexual adoptive parents' experiences in preschool environments. *Early Childhood Research Quarterly, 29*, 669–681. https://doi.org/10.1016/j.ecresq.2014.07.008

Goldberg, A. E., Allen, K. R., Black, K., Frost, R., & Manley, M. (2018). "There is no perfect school…": The complexity of school decision-making among lesbian and gay adoptive parents. *Journal of Marriage & Family, 80*, 684. https://doi.org/10.1111/jomf.12478

Goldberg, A. E., Black, K., Manley, M., & Frost, R. (2017). "We told them that we are both really involved parents": Sexual minority and heterosexual adoptive parents' engagement in school communities. *Gender & Education, 29*(5), 614–631. https://doi.org/10.1080/09540253.2017.1296114

Goldberg, A. E., Black, K., Sweeney, K., & Moyer, A. (2017). Lesbian, gay, and heterosexual adoptive parents' perceptions of inclusivity and receptiveness in early childhood education settings. *Journal of Research in Childhood Education, 31*, 141–159. https://doi.org/10.1080/02568543.2016.1244136

Goldberg, A. E., Frost, R., & Black, K. A. (2017). "There is so much to consider": School-related decisions and experiences among families who adopt non-infant children. *Families in Society, 98*, 191–200. https://doi.org/10.1606/1044-3894.2017.98.24

Goldberg, A. E., Frost, R. L., Manley, M. H., & Black, K. A. (2018). Meeting other moms: Lesbian adoptive mothers' relationships with other parents at school and beyond. *Journal of Lesbian Studies, 22*, 67–84. https://doi.org/10.1080/10894160.2016.1278349

Goldberg, A. E., Gartrell, N. K., & Gates, G. J. (2014). *Research report on LGB-parent families*. Los Angeles, CA: UCLA, The Williams Institute.

Goldberg, A. E., Kinkler, L. A., Richardson, H. B., & Downing, J. B. (2011). On the border: Young adults with LGBQ parents navigate LGBTQ communities. *Journal of Counseling Psychology, 59*, 71–85. https://doi.org/10.1037/a0024576

Goldberg, A. E., Ross, L., Manley, M., & Mohr, J. (2017). Male-partnered sexual minority women: Sexual identity disclosure to health care providers during the perinatal period. *Psychology of Sexual Orientation and Gender Diversity, 4*, 105–114. https://doi.org/10.1037/sgd0000215

Goldberg, A. E., & Smith, J. Z. (2014a). Preschool selection considerations and experiences of school mistreatment among lesbian, gay, and heterosexual adoptive parents. *Early Childhood Research Quarterly, 29*, 64–75. https://doi.org/10.1016/j.ecresq.2013.09.006

Goldberg, A. E., & Smith, J. Z. (2014b). Perceptions of stigma and self-reported school engagement in lesbian and gay parents with young children. *Psychology of Sexual Orientation and Gender Diversity, 1*(3), 202–212. https://doi.org/10.1037/sgd0000052

Goldberg, A. E., & Smith, J. Z. (2017). Parent-school relationships and young adopted children's psychological adjustment in lesbian-, gay-, and heterosexual-parent families. *Early Childhood Research Quarterly, 40*, 174–187. https://doi.org/10.1016/j.ecresq.2017.04.001

Goldberg, A. E., Sweeney, K., Black, K., & Moyer, A. (2016). Lesbian, gay, and heterosexual parents' socialization approaches to children's minority statuses. *The Counseling Psychologist, 44*, 267–299. https://doi.org/10.1177/0011000015628055

Golombok, S., Perry, B., Burston, A., Murray, C., Mooney-Somers, J., Stevens, M., & Golding, J. (2003). Children with lesbian parents: A community study. *Developmental Psychology, 39*, 20–33. https://doi.org/10.1037/0012-1649.39.1.20

Grusec, J. E., & Hastings, P. D. (Eds.). (2006). *Handbook of socialization: Theory and research*. New York, NY: Guilford.

Ioverno, S., Belser, A. B., Baiocco, R., Grossman, A. H., & Russell, S. T. (2016). The protective role of gay-straight alliances for lesbian, gay, bisexual, and questioning students: A prospective analysis. *Psychology of Sexual Orientation and Gender Diversity, 3*, 397–406. https://doi.org/10.1037/sgd0000193

Jeynes, W. H. (2007). The relationship between parental involvement and urban secondary school student academic achievement: A meta-analysis. *Urban Education, 42*, 82–110. https://doi.org/10.1177/0042085906293818

Johnson, S. M., & O'Connor, E. (2002). *The gay baby boom: The psychology of gay parenthood*. New York, NY: New York University Press.

Kintner-Duffy, V., Vardell, R., Lower, J., & Cassidy, D. (2012). "The changers and the changed": Preparing early childhood teachers to work with lesbian, gay, bisexual, and transgender families. *Journal of Early Childhood Teacher Education, 33*, 208–223. https://doi.org/10.1080/10901027.2012.705806

Kosciw, J. G., & Diaz, E. M. (2008). *Involved, invisible, ignored: The experiences of lesbian, gay, bisexual, and transgender parents and their children in our nation's K-12 schools*. New York, NY: GLSEN. www.glsen.org/cgi-bin/iowa/all/news/record/2271.html

Lick, D. J., Patterson, C. J., & Schmidt, K. M. (2013). Recalled social experiences and current psychological adjustment among adults reared by gay and lesbian parents. *Journal of GLBT Family Studies, 9*, 230–253. https://doi.org/10.1080/1550428X.2013.781907

Lindsay, J., Perlesz, A., Brown, R., McNair, R., de Vaus, D., & Pitts, M. (2006). Stigma or respect: Lesbian-parented families negotiating school settings. *Sociology, 40*, 1059–1077. https://doi.org/10.1177/0038038506069845

Lubbe, C. (2013). LGBT parents and their children: Non-western research and perspectives. In A. E. Goldberg & K. R. Allen (Eds.), *LGBT-parent families: Innovations in research and implications for practice* (pp. 209–224). New York, NY: Springer.

MacCallum, F., & Golombok, S. (2004). Children raised in fatherless families from infancy: A follow-up of children of lesbian and single heterosexual mothers at early adolescence. *Journal of Child Psychology & Psychiatry, 45*, 1407–1419. https://doi.org/10.1111/j.1469-7610.2004.00324.x

McDermott, E. (2011). The world some have won: Sexuality, class and inequality. *Sexualities, 14*, 63–78. https://doi.org/10.1177/1363460710390566

Mercier, L. R., & Harold, R. D. (2003). At the interface: Lesbian-parent families and their children's schools. *Children & Schools, 25*, 35–47. https://doi.org/10.1093/cs/25.1.35

Moore, M. R., & Stambolis-Ruhstorfer, M. (2013). LGBT sexuality and families at the start of the twenty-first century. *Annual Review of Sociology, 39*, 491–507. https://doi.org/10.1146/annurev-soc-071312-145643

National PTA. (2018). *LGBTQ children and families*. Retrieved from https://www.pta.org/home/run-your-pta/Diversity-Inclusion-Toolkit/supporting-multicultural-membership-growth/Lesbian-Gay-Bisexual-Transgender-and-Queer-Questioning-LGBTQ-Children-and-Families

Nixon, C. A. (2011). Working-class lesbian parents' emotional engagement with their children's education: Intersections of class and sexuality. *Sexualities, 141*, 78–99. https://doi.org/10.1177/1363460710390564

Pallotta-Chiarolli, M. (2012). *Border sexualities, border families in schools*. Langham, MD: Rowman & Littlefield.

Potter, D. (2012). Same-sex parent families and children's academic achievement. *Journal of Marriage & Family, 74*, 556–571. https://doi.org/10.1111/j.1741-3737.2012.00966.x

Power, J., Brown, R., Schofield, M., Pitts, M., McNair, R., Perlesz, A., & Bickerdike, A. (2014). Social connectedness among LGBT parents living in metropolitan and regional and rural areas of Australia and New Zealand. *Journal of Community Psychology, 42*, 869–889. https://doi.org/10.1002/jcop.21658

Rivers, I., Poteat, V. P., & Noret, N. (2008). Victimization, social support, and psychosocial functioning in same-sex and opposite-sex couples in the United States. *Developmental Psychology, 44*, 127–134. https://doi.org/10.1037/0012-1649.44.1.127

Rosenfeld, M. J. (2010). Nontraditional families and childhood progress through school. *Demography, 47*, 755–775. https://doi.org/10.1353/dem.0.0112

Russell, S., & Horne, S. (Eds.). (2017). *Sexual orientation, gender identity, and schooling: The nexus of research practice and policy*. New York, NY: Oxford.

Toomey, R. B., Ryan, C., Diaz, R. M., & Russell, S. T. (2011). High school gay-straight alliances (GSAs) and young adult well-being: An examination of GSA presence, participation, and perceived effectiveness. *Applied Developmental Science, 15*, 175–185. https://doi.org/10.1080/10888691.2011.607378

van Eeden-Moorefield, B., Few-Demo, A. L., Benson, K., Bible, J., & Lummer, S. (2018). A content analysis of LGBT research in top family journals 2000–2015. *Journal of Family Issues, 39*, 1374–1395. https://doi.org/10.1177/0192513X17710284

Vanfraussen, K., Ponjaert-Kristoffersen, I., & Brewaeys, A. (2002). What does it mean for youngsters to grow up in a lesbian family created by means of donor insemination? *Journal of Reproductive and Infant Psychology, 20*, 237–252. https://doi.org/10.1080/0264683021000033165

Vyncke, J., Julien, D., Jouvin, E., & Jodoin, E. (2014). Systemic heterosexism and adjustment among adolescents raised by lesbian mothers. *Canadian Journal of Behavioural Science, 46*, 375–386. https://doi.org/10.1037/a0034663

Wainright, J. L., & Patterson, C. J. (2008). Peer relations among adolescents with female same-sex parents. *Developmental Psychology, 44*, 117–126. https://doi.org/10.1037/0012-1649.44.1.117

Wainright, J., Russell, S., & Patterson, C. (2004). Psychosocial adjustment, school outcomes, and romantic relationships of adolescents with same-sex parents. *Child Development, 75*, 1886–1898. https://doi.org/10.1111/j.1467-8624.2004.00823.x

Welsh, M. G. (2011). Growing up in a same-sex parented family: The adolescent voice of experience. *Journal of GLBT Family Studies, 7*, 49–71. https://doi.org/10.1080/1550428X.2010.537241

# LGBTQ-Parent Families in Community Context

Ramona Faith Oswald, Elizabeth Grace Holman, and Jasmine M. Routon

Lesbian, gay, bisexual, transgender, and queer (LGBTQ) parents and their children live in every US state (Rodriguez & Gaitlin, 2013, using 2010 census data on same-sex partner households). These families are not, however, randomly distributed. Instead, they cluster in residential locations that are less urban (Rodriguez & Gaitlin, 2013). The communities in which LGBTQ-parent families reside vary in their level and type of support. For example, although some LGBTQ parents raise children in the context of urban "gayborhoods," same-sex partner households with children are more prevalent in less urban communities that have more child-rearing amenities, such as good schools and parks, and few LGBTQ-identified resources (Gates, 2013; Gates & Ost, 2004).

These varied contexts have different implications for the lives of LGBTQ parents and their children. Studying the interaction between LGBTQ-parent families and their local communities is still relatively new. Much of the early literature that addressed this interaction utilized adult non-parent samples of sexual minorities, and relevance to LGBTQ-parented families had to be inferred (e.g., McLaren, 2009). However, in the last 5 years, many scholars began incorporating a more community-focused lens in their investigations of LGBTQ-parented families. Studies now show how community climate affects children with LGBTQ parents and how communities can (and have) shifted to reduce the stigmatization of these families (see Oswald & Lazarevic, 2011; Oswald, Routon, McGuire, & Holman, 2018). Despite this progress, much of the available research focuses on sexual minority parents specifically. The need for research on transgender parents will be discussed as a critical future direction.

The purpose of this chapter is to document current knowledge about the communities in which LGBTQ parents live and how the daily lives of LGBTQ-parented families are differentially affected by these residential contexts. We begin by examining the diversity of LGBTQ-parented families and the diversity of communities in which they live. Then we review the literature discussing several key aspects of community climate, including the following contexts: legal, political, religious, workplace, and school. For each setting, we describe the current state of affairs, as well as the effects it has on LGBTQ-parented families. Implications for practice, as well as directions for future research, are

R. F. Oswald (✉) · J. M. Routon
Department of Human Development and Family Studies, University of Illinois at Urbana-Champaign, Urbana, IL, USA
e-mail: roswald@illinois.edu; routon@illinois.edu

E. G. Holman
Human Development and Family Studies Program, Bowling Green State University, Bowling Green, OH, USA
e-mail: eholman@bgsu.edu

© Springer Nature Switzerland AG 2020
A. E. Goldberg, K. R. Allen (eds.), *LGBTQ-Parent Families*,
https://doi.org/10.1007/978-3-030-35610-1_19

discussed. Throughout this chapter, we incorporate key theoretical perspectives including place identity, intersectionality, and minority stress.

## Geographical Diversity of LGBTQ-Parent Families

In this chapter, the term "community" or "residential community" refers to the municipalities or unincorporated places where LGBTQ-parent families live. Residential communities vary by degree of rurality/urbanicity (Economic Research Service, 2019) and are nested within counties and states. Our place-based theoretical approach is distinct from those who define communities as face-to-face or virtual social networks (e.g., Wellman, 2002) because we are concerned with linking LGBTQ-parent families to social conditions that are location specific. Research on LGBTQ-parent families should attend to the complexities of geographical differences, as well as variations in gender, race, class, attachment to place, and family visibility. The use of an intersectional approach (De Reus, Few, & Blume, 2005) moves the field toward an understanding of diversity that arises from the interaction of social structure and individuals' social locations within residential contexts.

Situating LGBTQ-parent families in community context encourages examination of family member attachments to their local communities. Residential place attachment is the sense that one belongs to, and is invested in, where one lives (Altman & Low, 1992). Residential community attachment correlates with greater psychological well-being (McLaren, 2009; McLaren, Jude, & McLachlan, 2008). Oswald and Lazarevic's (2011) study of 77 lesbian mothers living in nonmetropolitan Illinois found that they were more attached to their residential communities when they were in more frequent contact with their families of origin, when there was a local LGBTQ organization, and when the mothers were less religious. These findings imply that place attachment is related to the integration of families of origin with the LGBTQ community. Further, given the prevalence of religiously based anti-

LGBTQ sentiment in the region studied by Oswald and Lazarevic, it may be that less religious mothers are more immune to the effects of local religious hostility. Overall, this study provides evidence that place attachment is affected by aspects of the residential community.

Place attachment may also be affected by how long someone lives in a community. For example, inter-state migration is more common among lesbians and gay men than the general population, and this is associated with higher educational attainment (Baumle, Compton, & Poston, 2009). It follows that more mobile LGBTQ parents and their children may experience lower place attachment, and this may have effects on the quality of their family and community relationships. For instance, a recently re-located lesbian mother in Holman and Oswald's (2013) qualitative research on LGBTQ-parent families in nonmetropolitan contexts reported that she and her family were rejected by local church members, not because they were lesbians with children, but because the congregation did not like outsiders.

Additionally, aspects of identity such as race and gender presentation may impact place attachment. For instance, Holman and Oswald (2013) interviewed a rural lesbian couple where one partner presented as more masculine. They reported being perceived by others as a husband and wife with children. The more feminine partner conducted all checkbook transactions in local businesses so that the more masculine partner would not be asked to produce identification. A different participant in the same study described how the fact that she was a single White mother with an African-American child meant that (a) people assumed she was heterosexual because she did not have a female partner and (b) issues of race were far more salient than sexuality when negotiating public spaces (see Goldberg, 2009). In a case study of one lesbian mother living in rural poverty, the mother maintained a low profile because could not afford to rupture the family ties that aided her economic survival (Mendez, Holman, Oswald, & Izenstark, 2016).

Thus, when examining geographical diversity, researchers must also consider gender, race/

ethnicity, and class differences among LGBTQ-parented families (Goldberg, Gartrell, & Gates, 2014), and how these identities relate to where LGBTQ-parent families live. For example, LGBQ women under the age of 50 are more than twice as likely to be raising children as are GBQ men of the same age (48% vs. 20% respectively, Gates, 2013). Further, although both female and male same-sex partner households reside in similar areas, males seem to prefer locations that might be considered "gay-identified" (e.g., San Francisco) whereas the national distribution of female households is more dispersed (Baumle et al., 2009). Although the inclusion of only self-reported same-sex partner households limits these data, Baumle et al.'s (2009) findings suggest that the location of female households is less segregated by sexual orientation than that of male households. The researchers surmise that this gender difference is due to economic and family considerations: Because female households are more likely to have children while also having lower incomes and female same-sex couples have fewer residential choices and more interest in the child-related amenities, such as playgrounds and good schools, that may be more available outside of gay enclaves (Baumle et al., 2009). One implication of this is that single and partnered sexual minority female-headed families may be less visible as "LGBTQ-parent families" to members of their residential communities; others may perceive them as "mothers" more than as sexual minority women (see Sullivan, 2004). Invisibility may be especially true in residential communities where mothering outside of heterosexual marriage is normative. Gay and bisexual fathers, on the other hand, may be more visible because they are primary caregivers of children and therefore may be read by others as gender transgressive (Berkowitz, 2008). Being seen in this way could lead to gay and bisexual fathers either being over-praised for their father involvement or stigmatized for violating masculinity norms.

Analyses using 2010 Census data have also documented racial differences among same-sex partner households. First, African-American, Hispanic/Latino, and Asian-American same-sex partner households tend to exist in areas with high densities of racially similar households (Kastanis & Wilson, 2014). For example, the largest concentration of Asian Pacific Islander same-sex couples lives in the west, African Americans in the south, Hispanic/Latinos in the southwest, Native American in the mountain states, and Whites in the northeast (Kastanis & Wilson, 2014). This distribution mirrors the racial distribution of the US population overall (Kastanis & Wilson, 2014). Thus sexual minority parents and their children are more likely to be raising their children in racially similar communities. Second, racial minority same-sex partner households are more likely than their White counterparts to include minor children (Kastanis & Wilson, 2014). More research on racial and ethnic minority LGBTQ-parent families is needed (Acosta, 2013; Moore, 2011), and this research should attend to differences related to living within a racial majority or racial minority context (see Mendez, 2014, 2017). The experience, for example, of an African-American lesbian couple raising children in Burlington, Vermont (where 1% of same-sex couples households include at least one African-American partner, and 25% have children; Gates & Ost, 2004) is undoubtedly different than a similar couple raising children in Pine Bluff, Arkansas where the majority of same-sex couples are African American and presumably most are parents (Dang & Frazer, 2005).

There are also social class differences among LGBTQ households that intersect with gender and race. According to analyses using Census 2000 or 2010 data, same-sex partner households stratify by gender, such that male households have higher incomes than female households (O'Connell & Lofquist, 2009). Racial minority parents with a same-sex partner are less educated, less likely to have health insurance, and have a lower median income compared to both White same-sex couples and different-sex couples (Kastanis & Wilson, 2014), and urban households earn more than rural (Albelda, Badgett, Gates, & Schneebaum, 2009). Furthermore, compared to heterosexually married couple households with children, both male and female same-sex partner households with children are more likely to live in poverty (Prokos & Keene, 2010).

## Diversity in Residential Community Climate

In addition to identifying residential and LGBTQ trends related to geographical location and diversity, situating LGBTQ-parent families in community context requires us to theorize the mechanisms that link macro- and micro-systems. For this, we expand upon Meyer's (2003) minority stress theory that identifies minority stress processes (e.g., anti-LGBTQ victimization, expectations of rejection, closeting, internalized homophobia) as the mechanisms through which health disparities (e.g., higher rates of mental health concerns among sexual minorities) occur. In Meyer's model, the link between minority stress processes and outcomes is moderated by social support, coping, and LGBTQ identity salience, integration, and valence. Minority stress processes are made possible by "general environmental circumstances" (p. 678), briefly described as macro-level social inequalities that lead to minority statuses.

We expand upon Meyer's (2003) model by operationalizing general circumstances in the environment as "residential community climate." Community climate is the level of support for sexual minorities within a residential community (Holman, 2016; Oswald, Cuthbertson, Lazarevic, & Goldberg, 2010). This level of support is manifest within both distal and proximal institutions, norms, and social networks. Distal community manifestations of climate include the state and municipal legal codes, political affiliations, economic and social service infrastructure, and religious/moral tone that are prevalent in a community. More proximal indicators of climate include messages of support or rejection within organizational settings (e.g., the workplace, schools, or religious organizations) and social networks. The social climate that is apparent within these institutions, norms, and networks allows or inhibits minority stress processes,

which are theorized to affect the well-being of LGBTQ individuals and their families.

Research provides support for our hypothesis that community climate enables minority stress processes such as perceived stigma. A study from the Netherlands found that sexual minority mothers who reported higher levels of stigmatizing interactions within their communities were more likely to say that they felt they had to defend their position as a mother and were more likely to report that their children had behavior problems (Bos, van Balen, van den Boom, & Sandfort, 2004). In addition to research on perceived stigma, there is a growing body of evidence demonstrating that elements of community climate promote or inhibit the health and well-being of LGBTQ individuals and their families as specified by minority stress theory (Meyer, 2003). Below we briefly describe different elements of community climate—including legal, political, religious, employment, and school climate—and then summarize and evaluate the research showing the outcome effects that climate can have on LGBTQ people and their loved ones. Some of this research uses samples of LGBTQ adults and not specifically parents or their children. We highlight these distinctions throughout so it is evident when we are extrapolating to LGBTQ-parented families.

## Legal Context

**Current Legal Climate** Residential communities vary in the rights and protections that they provide to LGBTQ parents and their families (Oswald & Kuvalanka, 2008). This variation stems from the complex interactions between federal, state, and local law. For example, same-sex marriage is now legal in all 50 states (Obergefell v. Hodges, 2015). This ruling granted access to various pathways toward parenthood that are regulated by marital status. As a result, joint and stepparent adoption are now accessible in all 50 US states for same-sex married couples (Movement Advancement Project [MAP], 2018). Furthermore, US presumptive parentage laws mean that any child born into a married same-sex relationship is the legal child of both parents.

Despite this profound and positive legal shift at the national level, numerous forms of state and local legal inequality remain; there is also evidence of a legal backlash against marriage equality. For instance, 10 states permit state-licensed child welfare agencies to refuse to place foster or adoptive children with LGBTQ people (single or partnered) if doing so conflicts with their personal religious beliefs (Eggert, 2015; MAP, 2018). Also, several US states prohibit surrogacy contracts, leaving LGBTQ individuals who pursue this pathway to parenthood vulnerable to not being recognized as legal parents (Carroll, 2015; Creative Family Connections, 2016; Spivack, 2010). In the case of divorce, custody decisions made in the "best interest of the child" can be discriminatory against sexual minority parents because they depend upon the opinions of court officials who may be biased (Haney-Caron & Heilbrun, 2014; Pearson, 2018).

Furthermore, states differ in whether they allow "non-legal" parents to take leave from work to care for a child (MAP, 2018). Looking at access to housing, vacation accommodations, or borrowing money, in more than half of US states it is legal to deny housing, hotel rooms, and credit to LGBTQ individuals and families (MAP, 2018). There are also inconsistent protections against hate crimes related to sexual orientation and gender identity/expression across the USA (MAP, 2018). Thus, despite the gain of marriage equality, the legal climate for LGBTQ-parent families still varies dramatically in the USA and can affect sexual minority individuals' ability to become parents, to be recognized as legal parents, and to protect their families from discrimination (Kazyak & Woodell, 2016).

**Legal Climate Outcomes** Before the *Obergefell v. Hodges* (2015) decision, longitudinal studies showed that the denial of marriage rights (at the state level) had a deleterious effect on same-sex couples (e.g., Hatzenbuehler, McLaughlin, Keyes, & Hasin, 2010; Rostosky, Riggle, Horne, & Miller, 2009). Additionally, cross-sectional research of individuals in same-sex relationships showed that being in a legally recognized relationship is associated with better psychological adjustment (Riggle, Rostosky, & Horne, 2010), greater relationship commitment, greater social inclusion (Shecter, Tracy, Page, & Luong, 2008), a reduction in perceived stigma (Shapiro, Peterson, & Stewart, 2009), and a greater chance of exercising more than 3 days per week (Goldberg, Smith, McCormick, & Overstreet, 2019).

Now that marriage is accessible to same-sex couples nationwide, scholars are researching how the lives of LGBTQ individuals, including parents, have changed post-*Obergefell v. Hodges* (2015). A cohort study of 279 individuals in same-sex relationships and 266 individuals in different-sex relationships used survey data collected once before, and three time-points after, the 2015 *Obergefell v. Hodges* decision (see Ogolsky, Monk, Rice, & Oswald, 2019). At T1, 43% of respondents lived in a state that banned same-sex marriage (e.g., Georgia), 42% lived in a state where same-sex marriage was under court challenge (e.g., Texas), and 15% lived in a state that recognized same-sex marriage (e.g., Illinois). The average participant in a same-sex relationship was a cisgender lesbian female or gay male, aged 36 years, White, college educated, employed full time, married or in a committed relationship, and cohabiting with their partner of 7 years; 84 participants (31%) had children. The average participant in a different-sex relationship was demographically similar but far more likely to identify as heterosexual, be legally married, and have children. One publication from this study used the full sample to examine how federal, state, and local marriage recognition influences well-being (Ogolsky et al., 2019). Before the ruling, individuals in same-sex relationships had lower levels of reported well-being compared to those in different-sex relationships. After *Obergefell v. Hodges*, individuals in same-sex relationships perceived less stigma than did those in different-sex relationships. Also, their levels of family support increased after the ruling, while support from friends decreased. The researchers controlled for residential location, which suggests that access to federal marriage equality itself had a positive impact on individuals in same-sex relationships over and above any climate changes at the local or state level. The *Obergefell v. Hodges* ruling had no significant effects on individuals in different-sex relationships.

A different analysis using just the 279 individuals in same-sex relationships looked at the impact of national marriage equality on psychological distress and life satisfaction (Ogolsky, Monk, Rice, & Oswald, 2018). Before *Obergefell v. Hodges* (2015), psychological distress positively correlated with levels of internalized homonegativity, isolation, and vicarious trauma (observing anti-LGBTQ things happen to other people); life satisfaction negatively correlated with levels of felt stigma and vicarious trauma. Controlling for participants' residential community, the authors found that there was no average change in psychological adjustment or life satisfaction from before to after the *Obergefell v. Hodges* ruling. However, following this Supreme Court decision, trajectories of psychological distress decreased, and trajectories of life satisfaction increased specifically for individuals who had reported higher levels of minority stress prior to federal marriage equality. Thus, regardless of where same-sex couples were living, this shift in the national legal climate positively affected those who were most vulnerable.

Together, these analyses suggest that gaining the right to marry has reduced minority stress, and increased psychological well-being, for individuals in same-sex couples, many of whom are parents. These gains are especially true for those who were more distressed before the *Obergefell v. Hodges* ruling (see Goldberg & Smith, 2011, for findings that lesbian and gay parents are more sensitive to legal climate when they have more internalized minority stress).

## Political Context

**Current Political Climate** The political climate refers to the prevailing ideologies that reflect conservative or liberal leanings that are prevalent in specific locations and manifested through political attitudes, speech, and behavior such as voting and activism (Oswald et al., 2010). In this chapter, political activism refers to actions, such as public protesting, lobbying, or providing demonstrations that promote and raise awareness about a set of specific issues to advocate for social justice (Martin, 2007). The political and legal climates are inextricably linked given that political ideas and behavior drive changes in the law and changes in the law compel further political activism and may shift attitudes and beliefs. For example, increasing support for same-sex marriage came about through lobbying across the political aisle which contributed to the 2015 *Obergefell v. Hodges* ruling. Indeed, politically conservative individuals are now more likely to accept than reject sexual minority individuals as compared to before the ruling (Pew Research Center, 2017).

Kazyak and Stange (2018) tested the public opinion of LGBTQ issues in Nebraska after the *Obergefell v. Hodges* (2015) decision to see whether there was a public backlash to the decision. Using data from 2013 and 2015 waves of the Nebraska Annual Social Indicators Survey (NASIS), they found a significant increase in support for same-sex marriage over 2 years, even after controlling for political, religious, and demographic characteristics. The authors noted that a negative political backlash regarding *Obergefell v. Hodges* did not occur even among groups who are known to be less supportive of same-sex marriage, such as born-again Christians and Republicans (Kazyak & Stange, 2018).

While evidence shows ample support for same-sex marriage, the *Obergefell v. Hodges* (2015) decision has not translated to support for other critical political issues that affect LGBTQ-parent families and may have spurred a complicated political backlash. For example, Kazyak and Stange (2018) reported that public support for other LGBTQ protective policies (i.e., adoption, employment) did not increase following the *Obergefell v. Hodges* decision. Furthermore, politicians with conservative-leaning sentiments voted to ban gay and lesbian people from adopting and appointed Neil Gorsuch, who dissented against a ruling that requires states to list parents in same-sex couples on birth certificates, to the Supreme Court (Stern, 2017). Also, the Southern Poverty Law Center (SPLC) identified 52 anti-LGBTQ organizations that are disseminating propaganda to make the public fearful of LGBTQ people (Southern Poverty Law Center, 2017). Therefore, the political climate has positively affected LGBTQ-parent families in recent years regarding increased support around marriage equality but may have negatively impacted the progression of other LGBTQ-specific legislation (i.e., parenting rights, adoption) due to political backlash or stalled political activism.

**Political Climate Outcomes** Local, state, and national anti-LGBTQ politics have harmful psychological and social impacts on LGBTQ individuals, including parents (e.g., Rostosky, Riggle, Horne, Denton, & Huellemeier, 2010; Russell & Richards, 2003) and their loved ones (e.g., Arm, Horne, & Leavitt, 2009). Furthermore, studies of LGBTQ people's responses to anti-LGBTQ ballot initiatives have shown that political activism such as organizing and protesting helps LGBTQ individuals and their loved ones feel empowered (e.g., Russell & Richards, 2003; Short, 2007).

Winning marriage equality in 2015 may have toned down the pressing urge of LGBTQ activism temporarily, but anti-LGBTQ events, such as the 2016 Pulse Nightclub Massacre in which one man murdered 49 LGBTQ individuals in less than 1 hour, quickly reenergized political activism and civic engagement (Hanhardt, 2016). The 2016 presidential election spurred volatile regression of LGBTQ equality at the national level, such as the removal of the LGBTQ rights page on the White House website and the reinstatement of a ban on transgender people serving in the military (National Center for Transgender Equality, 2018). The aftermath of such events has given rise to the proliferation of LGBTQ candidates running for office, known as the "Rainbow Wave," with more than 400 LGBTQ candidates running for office in the November 2018 elec-

tions (Stack & Edmondson, 2018). Current LGBTQ candidates are appealing to larger audiences by representing diverse groups that treat variation in sexuality, race, and gender as assets and illustrating the ability to care about policy issues that are important to parents by being visible with their spouse and children. The "Rainbow Wave" is consistent with the findings of Dunn and Syzmanski's (2018) quantitative study of activism among 867 LGBTQ adults. Participants were more politically engaged when they were more aware of heterosexism, and when they linked their personal experiences of discrimination to a broader system of inequality (Dunn & Syzmanski, 2018). Political activism has been linked to higher global and psychological health (Lindsrom, 2004), and thus, civic engagement in LGBTQ rights may strengthen families.

## Religious Context

**Current Religious Climate** Local religious voices contribute to the overall climate for sexual minorities in itself, in part by interacting with legal and political systems (Oswald et al., 2010; see chapter "Religion in the Lives of LGBTQ-Parent Families"). In previous sections, we described the interaction of religion with law and politics; here we focus specifically on the climate within religious settings. Most religious denominations have an official position regarding the morality of same-sex desire and behavior, and the legitimacy of LGBTQ identities (Copeland & Rose, 2016; Siker, 2007). This stance, however, may not be shared by all congregations or adherents (e.g., the Baptist Peace Fellowship (2010) of North America is LGBTQ-affirming, but the larger Baptist denomination is not), but it does shape what is said and done within religious organizations as well as other community settings in which adherents are involved (Yip, 1997). Thus, variations in religious climate are integral parts of community climate.

Of the 236 denominations counted in the US Religion Census 2010 (Association of Statisticians of American Religion Bodies, 2018), very few are officially and unambiguously affirm-ing of LGBTQ people. For example, only nine major religious groups in the USA perform same-sex marriage: Episcopalian, Evangelical Lutheran Church in America, Presbyterian Church (U.S.A.), Metropolitan Community Church, Conservative and Reform Judaism, Unitarian-Universalist, Quaker, and United Church of Christ (Masci & Lipka, 2015). Nationwide, these affirming denominations account for just 10% of all congregations (35,601 of 344,894), and 31% of all religious adherents in the USA (5,755,258 of 141,364,420) [Association of Religion Data Archives (ARDA), 2010a, b].

Where an LGBTQ-parent family resides partly determines their access to religious affir-mation. For instance, LGBTQ-affirming denomi-nations are most prevalent in the northeast (ARDA, n.d.). LGBTQ parents and their children who live in other parts of the USA have fewer opportunities to access clerical or congregational support. In one study of 61 gay fathers living in Tennessee and California, those living in Tennessee—where Southern Baptists prevail—described more frequent stigma in religious set-tings than the fathers in California (Perrin, Pinderhughes, Mattern, Hurley, & Newman, 2016). Thus, LGBTQ parents and their children may be exposed to very different religious mes-sages across the USA.

**Religious Climate Outcomes** There is a grow-ing body of research showing that LGBTQ par-ents and their children are affected by religious messages regarding sexual and gender minori-ties, particularly with respect to their sexual and gender minority identities. LGBTQ parents and their children may experience tensions between their religious and sexual, gender, or family iden-tities due to the negative messages of some reli-gious groups in relation to sexual and gender minorities. For example, Tuthill (2016) inter-viewed 15 Hispanic lesbian mothers to learn how they navigate conflicts between being both Catholic and lesbian. Similar to studies of religi-osity among LGBTQ adults without children (e.g., Yip, 1997), Tuthill (2016) found that moth-ers reconciled their identities by taking a critical

stance toward the church as well as scripture and by identifying as spiritual rather than religious. Lytle, Foley, and Aster (2013) reported similar findings with a sample of 10 adult children with gay and lesbian parents: namely, most of these children, upon learning that their parents were LGBTQ, described changing their religious beliefs or practices to be more supportive of hav-ing LGBTQ parents.

In addition to effects on parent and child iden-tities, religious context shapes the socialization strategies of LGBTQ parents. In one online sur-vey, 75 LGBTQ parents were asked to describe how their religion or spirituality influenced their parenting (Rostosky, Abreu, Mahoney, & Riggle, 2017). Respondents reported that they used reli-gion and spirituality to teach morality and values, including the importance of critical thinking in the face of religious hostility. Indeed, they encouraged their children to question religious teachings while also being open to the views of others. Similarly, the lesbian mothers in Tuthill (2016) encouraged their children to participate in traditional religious services and activities and to develop religious identities, but also to question church teachings.

These parenting strategies connect to the sense of belonging that parents and their children feel within local religious contexts. Most of the par-ents in the Rostosky et al.'s (2017) study actively sought supportive religious congregations and activities to develop a sense of belonging within their children. The mothers in Tuthill's (2016) study felt somewhat supported within their ethnic communities because others saw them as uphold-ing cultural and religious norms. On the other hand, many of the fathers in the Perrin et al. (2016) study avoided, or felt shut out of, com-munity settings where there was religious hostil-ity. It seems then that religious climate is related to parenting practices—in that, the sense of sup-port or hostility within the local religious context influences how LGBTQ parents are socializing their children more broadly—as well as commu-nity attachment for LGBTQ-parent families.

Similar to the above discussion regarding political activism, religious hostility can also motivate LGBTQ people to organize within their denominations to promote LGBTQ-affirming change (Comstock, 1993). Lustenberger (2014) conducted an ethnography of how Jewish same-sex couples raising children in Israel invested energy into establishing Jewish-Israeli identities for their children. Israel is a religious state, and the Orthodox rabbinate that has majority control is decidedly anti-LGBTQ. To promote social change that would protect their families, the parents fought for, and obtained, piecemeal legal recognition of their families. Furthermore, they used conversion rituals to ensure that children born to non-Jewish mothers would have full citizenship, and childbirth celebrations to promote belonging within extended families. Therefore, it is important to remember that while current community climates are affecting the lives of LGBTQ parents and their families, this climate remains variable and may in fact be the impetus that drives community change.

## Workplace Context

**Current Workplace Climate** Federal, state, and local laws, as well as employer policies and practices, shape the economic structure of a given residential community, which influences community climate. There is no federal law protecting sexual minority employees in general, or parents specifically, from employment discrimination. Although Title VII, which, in part, prohibits discrimination in the workplace against employees based on sex, has been interpreted to include protections for employees' sexual orientation or gender identity, the Department of Justice has indicated this may not be true under future administrations in the USA (Ruggiero & Park, 2017). Furthermore, employment discrimination by sexual orientation remains legal in 26 US states, and gender identity discrimination is legal in 37 US states (MAP, 2018).

The lack of legal protections at the federal and state levels leaves decisions about organization-wide protective policies in the hands of individual employers (see chapter "LGBTQ Parents and the Workplace"). Fortunately, the majority of large companies have decided to offer such protections to employees. For instance, the majority (91%) of Fortune 500 companies have instated an employment nondiscrimination policy by sexual orientation; 83% have similar rules specifically for gender identity (Fidas & Cooper, 2018). These policies demonstrate significant improvement, given that 10 years ago, only 88% and 25% of Fortune 500 companies, respectively, employed such policies (Fidas & Cooper, 2018). These company policies have been found to have a more significant effect than state or municipal laws on employee perceptions of workplace climate (Ragins & Cornwell, 2001). Thus, even though US federal law or specific states may not provide employment protections, some sexual minority employees may access support and benefits through their workplace and may feel that their local employment context is affirming.

In addition to the policies within a specific workplace, the social climate of an organization can also affect employees' experiences. LGBTQ employees may perceive their work environment to be supportive, hostile, or tolerant toward sexual and gender minorities; some research shows that ambiguity in the work climate—experiences of simultaneous support and hostility—can also leave LGBTQ employees unsure of the level of support (Holman, Fish, Oswald, & Goldberg, 2018). However, it seems that the workplace social climate may be changing for the better, in some ways. For instance, in 2012, 43% of surveyed employees felt uncomfortable hearing an LGBTQ colleague talk about their personal life; in 2018, this number decreased to 36% (Fidas & Cooper, 2018). Therefore, the work climate for LGBTQ parents varies greatly depending on the state, local, and institutional climates.

**Workplace Climate Outcomes** Research on LGBTQ adult workers has found a link between workplace climate and well-being. For example, a survey of 379 gays and lesbians found that a company's written nondiscrimination policies was associated with less job discrimination and more accepting co-workers; this more supportive climate was in turn related to increased job satisfaction (Griffith & Hebl, 2002). Workplace nondiscrimination policies have also been associated with higher disclosure of sexual orientation at work (Rostosky & Riggle, 2002), more positive relationships with supervisors and increased organizational citizenship behaviors (Tejeda, 2006), and decreased levels of perceived discrimination (Ragins & Cornwell, 2001). In turn, greater support from supervisors has been associated with fewer reported depression and anxiety symptoms among sexual minority parents (Goldberg & Smith, 2013). In sum, workplace climates that affirm the existence of LGBTQ employees communicate messages of acceptance and belonging that lead to more optimal individual outcomes (Button, 2001).

Conversely, exposure to hostility and prejudice in the workplace correlates with higher rates of psychological distress (Velez, Moradi, & Brewster, 2013), more frequent absenteeism from work (Huebner & Davis, 2007), and lower levels of job satisfaction (Dispenza, 2015; Ragins, Singh, & Cornwell, 2007). Additionally, workplace heterosexism—indexed in some studies as the frequency of experiencing certain behaviors, such as being called a derogatory term about one's sexual orientation—has been correlated with depression among LGBTQ employees (Smith & Ingram, 2004). LGBTQ employees who perceive anything less than support in the work environment may choose not to disclose their identities in the workplace. For example, in the 2018 Human Rights Campaign Foundation's study of 804 LGBTQ employees, 46% reported being closeted at work, and 28% reported that they had lied about their personal life to colleagues (Fidas & Cooper, 2018). Invisibility can be painful for LGBTQ parents in particular, especially if work colleagues are discussing their families and they feel that they must stay silent.

The workplace climate for LGBTQ parents may have both direct and indirect effects for partners and children at home. In one case study of three sexual minority employees, Holman (2019) showed that discriminatory experiences in the workplace affected not only the psychological well-being of the employee but also their rela-

tionships with their romantic partners. Other scholars have also found that relationship quality and satisfaction inversely correlate with stress related to minority identity (Doyle & Molix, 2015; Rostosky & Riggle, 2002; Todosijevic, Rothblum, & Solomon, 2005). Although scholars have not yet extended this examination of the effects of workplace climate on children, these findings suggest that workplace climate may influence the family relationships of LGBTQ parents.

## School Context

**Current School Climate** Given the fact that school-aged children spend the majority of their waking hours in educational and extra-curricular settings, and that LGBTQ parents are involved in PTAs and other school affairs (Kosciw & Diaz, 2008), the supportiveness of a given classroom, school, or district most likely impacts the quality of life for LGBTQ parent families (see chapter "LGBTQ-Parent Families and Schools"). Indeed, a national survey of middle and high school-aged children with LGBTQ parents ($N = 154$) and LGBTQ parents with school-aged children ($N = 558$) found that many students reported mistreatment by peers and staff. For example, some students recalled reprimands after disclosing their family structure, as well as being excluded from school events or class projects because they have an LGBTQ parent (Kosciw & Diaz, 2008).

State education laws do not protect most children of LGBTQ parents from discrimination. Only six states (plus the District of Columbia) have laws prohibiting bullying in school by "association" with an LGBTQ person (e.g., a parent) (MAP, 2018). Only two of those six states legally prohibit discrimination in school by association with an LGBTQ person (MAP, 2018). Furthermore, seven states have laws that bar teachers from discussing gender or sexual minorities in a positive light (MAP, 2018); in those states, it is against the law to talk positively at school about LGBTQ-parent families.

The absence of explicit legal protections influences how administrators and teachers perform their jobs and thus contributes to the school climate. Consider the fact that North Carolina, Virginia, and New York do not have laws protecting or supporting LGBTQ-parent families in the schools. In North Carolina, a qualitative study of preschool administrators ($N = 203$) found that those with strong religious views were unlikely to attempt inclusive practices (Church, Hegde, Averett, & Ballard, 2018). Administrators with more positive attitudes toward LGBTQ populations described their inclusive practices as perfunctory rather than transformational (Church et al., 2018). Glass, Willox, Barrow, and Jones' (2016) qualitative study of 23 LG parents of preschoolers and 8 preschool teachers in Virginia found that both groups struggled with knowing when and how to be inclusive. Similarly, a survey of 116 school psychologists working in elementary schools throughout NY State reported that LGBTQ-parented families were acknowledged in their schools, but the climate and curriculum were not inclusive (Bishop & Atlas, 2015).

**School Climate Outcomes** School climate affects families through school selection, parental engagement, and parental satisfaction. Regarding school choice, lesbian and gay parents in Goldberg and Smith's (2014a) study sought out supportive preschools, often identifying the presence of other LGBTQ-parent families in the school as a good indicator of affirmation and support. The relationship between school climate and parental engagement is more complicated than the relationship between school climate and choice. The LG parents in Goldberg and Smith's (2014b) study were more engaged (e.g., more likely to volunteer and speak to teachers) when they perceived the school to be more hostile, but the other parents to be more welcoming and inclusive. It may be that this juxtaposition created an environment where LG parents felt supported in an advocacy role. These parents had problems with teachers when they were out but socially excluded (see Kosciw & Diaz, 2008, who found that an adverse school climate increased parent discomfort when attending parent-teacher

conferences). In a different paper from the same study, LG parents who were more social with, and felt more accepted by, other parents reported higher school involvement and better relationships with teachers (Goldberg & Smith, 2014c). LG parental school involvement and perceived acceptance by other parents predicted more positive psychological adjustment in children in a longitudinal analysis of this sample (Goldberg & Smith, 2017).

Children's own experiences in school may also relate to their well-being. For instance, Bos, Gartrell, Peyser, and van Balen (2008) found that children with lesbian mothers were more resilient in the face of stigma when they attended a school that included LGBTQ issues in the curriculum. Conversely, stigmatizing experiences at school hurt children's psychological health (Bos et al., 2008). These experiences may occur even in schools that parents describe as supportive. Farr, Oakley, and Ollen (2016) surveyed 96 LG parents of 50 elementary-aged children and 48 teachers who reported on the children. Ninety-five of the 96 parents rated their school as supportive, and yet 8% said that their child was bullied (the 4 children confirmed this). Furthermore, using a measure of psychological adjustment, the teachers scored the bullied children as having behavioral problems. In sum, schools are an integral part of residential communities, and the school climate for LGBTQ-parent families can help or hinder the well-being of children and families.

## Effects of Diversity in Residential Community Climate

As described above, residential communities are complex webs of subsystems, each of which can impact LGBTQ parents and their families in significant ways. Religious affirmation, supportive legislation, political activism, and recognition and support from schools and workplaces can all strengthen LGBTQ-parent families by promoting mental health and a sense of social inclusion. Oswald et al.' (2018) study of LGBQ parents residing in nonmetropolitan Illinois found that LGBQ parents who perceived their residential communities to be supportive ($n = 17$) were more likely to live in counties with legal support, participate in LGBTQ-focused social and political activities, have children with more exposure to other LGBTQ-parent families, and attend church less frequently when compared to LGB-parent families who perceived their communities as tolerant ($n = 38$). Conversely, a variety of studies that we have reviewed here demonstrate that LGBQ parents report increased depression, anxiety, stress, and defensiveness, a sense of vulnerability, and decreased support and disclosure in the face of exposure to negative contexts. A few studies that we reviewed also provided evidence that the community climate also affects the children and families of LGBTQ parents. As discussed below, these findings are limited by the paucity of research on trans and bisexual parents, as well as those living in non-US contexts.

## Implications for Practice

Although most of the above-discussed research examined the family-community interface at one time-point, it is essential to remember that communities change over time (Holman, 2016). Attitudes, beliefs, policies, and legislation are all variable, and changes in these aspects of community climate affect LGBTQ-parented families (Ogolsky et al., 2018). It is also important to remember that such shifts toward support for LGBTQ-parent families reflect the successful mobilization of citizens who, over time, created infrastructures that are LGBTQ-affirming. These movements stem from LGBTQ individuals and their allies who experience stigma and discrimination and decide to resist and advocate for change. Thus, a negative community climate can contribute to empowerment when those affected mobilize themselves to make a positive difference. Indeed, the family members of LGBTQ individuals in Horne, Rostosky, Riggle, and Martens' (2010) interview study were more likely to be political activists when they were more knowledgeable about, and affirming of,

LGBTQ personal and political struggles (see Arm et al., 2009).

Furthermore, LGBTQ people confronted by hostile religious beliefs have organized to promote LGBTQ-affirmation within their congregations and denominations (Comstock, 1993). LGBTQ adults who lived in states that voted to prohibit same-sex marriage constitutionally in 2006 were more involved in LGBTQ activism and more likely to vote in that election—despite concurrent reports of increased depression and stress (Riggle, Rostosky, & Horne, 2009). In the fight against Amendment 2 in Colorado (a 1992 state constitutional amendment that banned legal protections against sexual orientation discrimination; it was overturned in 1996 by *Romer v. Evans*), LGBTQ activists created new structures, such as a safe schools coalition, and heterosexual allies became more active and visible (Russell, Bohan, McCarroll, & Smith, 2010).

Relying on negative pressure to stimulate organizing for change can, however, result in the dissolution of the movement upon meeting movement goals. In Colorado, for example, LGBTQ community cohesion and mobilization fizzled after Amendment 2 was struck down, probably because there was no longer an imminent threat against which to organize (Russell et al., 2010). Some LGBTQ activists in Colorado considered it a success that the LGBTQ community was less visible and that local non-LGBTQ organizations began addressing LGBTQ concerns. However, the reduced LGBTQ community visibility and cohesion felt like a failure to people who valued having a cohesive LGBTQ community (Russell et al., 2010). The problem of disinvestment in the LGBTQ community was also observed by Ocobock (2018) among a sample of 116 married and unmarried same-sex partners in Massachusetts. Married participants with children were significantly more likely to report reduced participation in LGBTQ-specific activities after marrying, suggesting that access to marriage decreased LGBTQ community involvement, which suggests they are less involved in political activism. While some participants believed that LGBTQ community involvement was not necessary after achieving marriage equality, others felt that community support and political activism for others in the LGBTQ community broadly was still needed (Ocobock, 2018).

## Directions for Future Research

Researchers must also operationalize community climate as it changes over time, and investigate the social and economic impact that shifts in policies, practices, and beliefs have on the community. The literature shows that the community climate affects LGBTQ-parent families. Specifically, LGBTQ-affirming communities are positive for LGBTQ-parent families. However, this understanding is based primarily on studies of sexual minority parents in the USA. At this point, very little work has examined if this is also true for transgender parents in the USA, or LGBTQ parents worldwide.

Issues of gender expression and disclosure in community context may look very different compared to the experiences of sexual minority parents and their children. There is a growing body of literature examining the unique experiences for transgender parents and their children, specific to the issue of sexual orientation (see Stotzer, Herman, & Hasenbush, 2014). Despite the emerging research focus on this population, the current literature has not thoroughly examined the influence of contextual climate on these families. Dierckx, Motmans, Mortelmans, and T'sjoen (2015) reviewed 38 empirical research papers on transgender-parent families and found that only a few even considered the effects of social and community factors on family relationships and individual well-being (e.g., Freedman, Tasker, & di Ceglie, 2002; Haines, Ajayi, & Boyd, 2014). While it seems scholars are paying attention to resources and characteristics external to transgender parents, the connection between climate and family well-being is not yet empirically established.

Further, we cannot assume that a framework for assessing residential community climate based on US society adequately fits the widely varied sociocultural contexts around the world. The elements of climate discussed in this chapter may not be relevant in all locales, and additional features of climate may need to be considered (e.g., Kahlina, 2015). Indeed, LGBTQ people who immigrate share experiences of culture shock, a sense of uncertainty or anxiety as they adjust to new legal, social, political, and cultural climates (Gedro, Mizzi, Rocco, & van Loo, 2013). Thus, a more global perspective would help this line of research move forward. The take-home message of this chapter is that specific characteristics of residential communities matter considerably for LGBTQ-parent families. Scholars in multiple national contexts could explore these varied aspects of community climate for LGBTQ-parented families worldwide to provide a more complex and nuanced understanding of the relationship between place and well-being.

## References

Acosta, K. L. (2013). *Amigas y Amantes: Sexually nonconforming Latinas negotiate family*. New Brunswick, NJ: Rutgers University Press.

Albelda, R., Badgett, M. V. L., Gates, G., & Schneebaum, A. (2009). *Poverty in the lesbian, gay, and bisexual community*. UCLA: Williams Institute. Retrieved from http://www2.law.ucla.edu/williamsinstitute/pdf/LGBPovertyReport.pdf

Altman, I., & Low, S. (Eds.). (1992). *Place attachment*. New York, NY: Plenum.

Arm, J. R., Horne, S. G., & Leavitt, H. M. (2009). Negotiating connection to GLBT experience: Family members' experience of anti-GLBT movements and policies. *Journal of Counseling Psychology, 56*, 82–96. https://doi.org/10.1037/a0012813

Association of Religion Data Archives. (2010a). *U.S. membership report*. Retrieved from http://www.thearda.com/rcms2010/r/u/rcms2010_99_us_name_2010.asp

Association of Religion Data Archives. (2010b). *U.S. congregational membership: Maps*. Retrieved from http://www.thearda.com/mapsReports/maps/ardausmaps.asp

Baptist Peace Fellowship. (2010). *Statement on justice and sexual orientation*. Retrieved from http://www.bpfna.org/sxorient#Baptist_Peace_Fellowship_Statement_on_Justice_and_Sexual_Orientation

Baumle, A. K., Compton, D. R., & Poston, D. L., Jr. (2009). *Same-sex partners: The demography of sexual orientation*. Albany, NY: SUNY Press.

Berkowitz, D. (2008). *Schools, parks, and playgrounds: Gay fathers negotiate public and private spaces*. Paper presented at the National Council on Family Relations in Little Rock, AK.

Bishop, C. M., & Atlas, J. G. (2015). School curriculum, policies, and practices regarding lesbian, gay, bisexual, and transgender families. *Education & Urban Society, 47*, 766–784. https://doi.org/10.1177/0013124513508580

Bos, H. M. W., Gartrell, N. K., Peyser, H., & van Balen, F. (2008). The USA National Longitudinal Lesbian Family Study (NFFLS): Homophobia, psychological adjustment, and protective factors. *Journal of Lesbian Studies, 12*, 455–471. https://doi.org/10.1080/10894160802278630

Bos, H. M. W., van Balen, F., van den Boom, D. C., & Sandfort, T. G. M. (2004). Minority stress, the experience of parenthood and child adjustment in lesbian families. *Journal of Reproductive and Infant Psychology, 22*, 291–304. https://doi.org/10.1080/02646830412331298350

Button, S. B. (2001). Organizational efforts to affirm sexual diversity: A cross-level examination. *Journal of Applied Psychology, 86*, 17–28. https://doi.org/10.1037/0021-9010.86.1.17

Carroll, M. (2015). *Beyond legal equality for LGBT families.* Retrieved from: http://contexts.org/blog/beyond-legal-equality-for-lgbt-families/

Church, J., Hegde, A. V., Averett, P., & Ballard, S. M. (2018). Early childhood administrators' attitudes and experiences in working with gay- and lesbian-parented families. *Early Childhood Development & Care, 188*, 264–280. https://doi.org/10.1080/03004430.2016.1213725

Comstock, G. D. (1993). *Gay theology without apology.* Cleveland, OH: Pilgrim Press.

Copeland, M., & Rose, D. (2016). *Struggling in good faith: LGBTQI inclusion from 13 American religious perspectives.* Woodstock, VT: Skylight Paths Publishing.

Creative Family Connections. (2016). *Surrogacy law by state.* Retrieved from: https://www.creativefamilyconnections.com/us-surrogacy-law-map/

Dang, A., & Frazer, S. (2005). *Black same-sex households in the United States (2nd edition): A report from the 2000 Census.* Washington, DC: NGLTF Policy Institute and the National Black Justice Coalition. Retrieved from http://www.thetaskforce.org/downloads/reports/reports/2000BlackSameSexHouseholds.pdf

De Reus, L. A., Few, A. L., & Blume, L. B. (2005). Multicultural and critical race feminisms: Theorizing families in the third wave. In V. L. Bengtson, A. C. Acock, K. R. Allen, P. Dilworth-Anderson, & D. M. Klein (Eds.), *Sourcebook of family theory and research* (pp. 447–460). Thousand Oaks, CA: Sage.

Dierckx, M., Motmans, J., Mortelmans, D., & T'sjoen, G. (2015). Families in transition: A literature review. *International Review of Psychiatry, 28*, 36–43. https://doi.org/10.3109/09540261.2015.1102716

Dispenza, F. (2015). An exploratory model of proximal minority stress and the work-life interface for men in same-sex, dual-earner relationships. *Journal of Counseling & Development, 93*, 321–332. https://doi.org/10.1002/jcad.12030

Doyle, D. M., & Molix, L. (2015). Social stigma and sexual minorities' romantic relationship functioning: A meta-analytic review. *Personality & Social Psychology Bulletin, 41*, 1363–1381. https://doi.org/10.1177/0146167215594592

Dunn, T. L., & Syzmanski, D. M. (2018). Heterosexist discrimination and LGBQ activism: Examining a moderated mediation model. *Psychology of Sexual Orientation & Gender Diversity, 5*, 13–24. https://doi.org/10.1037/sgd0000250

Economic Research Service. (2019). *What is rural?* United States Department of Agriculture. Retrieved from https://www.ers.usda.gov/topics/rural-economy-population/rural-classifications/what-is-rural

Eggert, D. (2015). *LGBT adoption just got harder in Michigan.* U.S. News & World Report. Retrieved from http://www.usnews.com/news/us/articles/2015/06/11/new-michigan-law-lets-adoption-agencies-decline-referrals

Farr, R. H., Oakley, M. K., & Ollen, E. W. (2016). School experiences of young children and their lesbian and gay adoptive parents. *Psychology of Sexual Orientation & Gender Diversity, 3*, 442–447. https://doi.org/10.1037/sgd0000187

Fidas, D., & Cooper, L. (2018). *A workplace divided: Understanding the climate for LGBTQ workers nationwide.* Human Rights Campaign. Retrieved from https://assets2.hrc.org/files/assets/resources/AWorkplaceDivided-2018.pdf?_ga=2.166252860.325565919.1539091406-797221855.1534519897

Freedman, D., Tasker, F., & di Ceglie, D. (2002). Children and adolescents with transsexual parents referred to a specialist gender identity development service: A brief report of key developmental features. *Clinical Child Psychology & Psychiatry, 7*, 423–432. https://doi.org/10.1177/1359104502007003009

Gates, G. J. (2013). *LGBT parenting in the United States.* Los Angeles, CA: The Williams Institute, UCLA School of Law. Retrieved from http://williamsinstitute.law.ucla.edu/wp-content/uploads/LGBT-Parenting.pdf

Gates, G. J., & Ost, J. (2004). *The gay and lesbian atlas.* Washington, DC: The Urban Institute Press.

Gedro, J., Mizzi, R. C., Rocco, T. S., & van Loo, J. (2013). Going global: Professional mobility and concerns for LGBT workers. *Human Resource Development International, 16*, 282–297. https://doi.org/10.1080/13678868.2013.771869

Glass, V. Q., Willox, L., Barrow, K. M., & Jones, S. (2016). Struggling to move beyond acknowledgment: Celebrating gay and lesbian families in preschool environments. *Journal of GLBT Family Studies, 12*, 217–241. https://doi.org/10.1080/1550428X.2015.1039685

Goldberg, A. E. (2009). Lesbian and heterosexual pre-adoptive couples' openness to transracial adoption.

*American Journal of Orthopsychiatry, 79*, 103–117. https://doi.org/10.1037/a0015354

Goldberg, A. E., Gartrell, N. K., & Gates, G. (2014). *Research report on LGB-parent families*. Los Angeles, CA: The Williams Institute, UCLA School of Law. Retrieved from: https://williamsinstitute.law.ucla.edu/wp-content/uploads/lgb-parent-families-july-2014.pdf

Goldberg, A. E., & Smith, J. Z. (2011). Stigma, social context, and mental health: Lesbian and gay couples across the transition to adoptive parenthood. *Journal of Counseling Psychology, 58*, 139–150. https://doi.org/10.1037/a0021684

Goldberg, A. E., & Smith, J. Z. (2013). Work conditions and mental health in lesbian and gay dual-earner parents. *Family Relations, 62*, 727–740. https://doi.org/10.1111/fare.12042

Goldberg, A. E., & Smith, J. Z. (2014a). Preschool selection considerations and experiences of school mistreatment among lesbian, gay, and heterosexual adoptive parents. *Early Childhood Research Quarterly, 29*, 64–75. https://doi.org/10.1016/j.ecresq.2013.09.006

Goldberg, A. E., & Smith, J. Z. (2014b). Perceptions of stigma and self-reported school engagement in same-sex couples with young children. *Psychology of Sexual Orientation & Gender Diversity, 1*, 202–212. https://doi.org/10.1037/sgd0000052

Goldberg, A. E., & Smith, J. Z. (2014c). Predictors of school engagement among same-sex and heterosexual adoptive parents of kindergarteners. *Journal of School Psychology, 52*, 463–478. https://doi.org/10.1016/j.jsp.2014.08.001

Goldberg, A. E., & Smith, J. Z. (2017). Parent-school relationships and young adopted children's psychological adjustment in lesbian-, gay-, and heterosexual-parents families. *Early Childhood Research Quarterly, 40*, 174–187. https://doi.org/10.1016/j.ecresq.2017.04.001

Goldberg, A. E., Smith, J. Z., McCormick, N., & Overstreet, N. M. (2019). Health behaviors and outcomes of parents in same-sex couples: An exploratory study. *Psychology of Sexual Orientation & Gender Diversity., 6*, 318. https://doi.org/10.1037/sgd0000330

Griffith, K. H., & Hebl, M. R. (2002). The disclosure dilemma for gay men and lesbians: "Coming out" at work. *Journal of Applied Psychology, 87*, 1191–1199. https://doi.org/10.1037//0021-9010.87.6.1191

Haines, B. A., Ajayi, A. A., & Boyd, H. (2014). Making trans parents visible: Intersectionality of trans and parenting identities. *Feminism & Psychology, 24*, 238–247. https://doi.org/10.1177/0959353514526219

Haney-Caron, E., & Heilbrun, K. (2014). Lesbian and gay parents and determination of child custody: The changing legal landscape and implications for policy and practice. *Psychology of Sexual Orientation & Gender Diversity, 1*, 19–29. https://doi.org/10.1037/sgd0000020

Hanhardt, C. B. (2016). Safe space out of place. *QED: A Journal in GLBTQ Worldmaking, 3*, 121–125. https://doi.org/10.14321/qed.3.3.0121

Hatzenbuehler, M. L., McLaughlin, K. A., Keyes, K. M., & Hasin, D. S. (2010). The impact of institutional discrimination on psychiatric disorders in lesbian, gay, and bisexual populations: A prospective study. *American Journal of Public Health, 100*, 452–459. https://doi.org/10.2105/AJPH.2009.168815

Holman, E. G. (2016). Community climate. In A. E. Goldberg (Ed.), *The SAGE encyclopedia of LGBTQ studies* (pp. 252–255). Los Angeles, CA: Sage.

Holman, E. G. (2019). The effects of minority stressors in the workplace on same-sex relationships: A collective case study of female couples. *Journal of Lesbian Studies, 23*, 196–223. https://doi.org/10.1080/10894160.2019.1520541

Holman, E. G., Fish, J., Oswald, R. F., & Goldberg, A. (2018). Reconsidering the LGBT Climate Inventory: Understanding support and hostility for LGBQ employees in the workplace. *Journal of Career Assessment*. Advanced online publication, *27*, 544. https://doi.org/10.1177/1069072718788324

Holman, E. G., & Oswald, R. F. (2013). Nonmetropolitan GLBTQ parents: When and where does their sexuality matter? *Journal of GLBT Family Studies, 7*, 436–456. https://doi.org/10.1080/1550428X.2011.623937

Horne, S. G., Rostosky, S. S., Riggle, E. D. B., & Martens, M. P. (2010). What was Stonewall? The role of GLB knowledge in marriage amendment-related affect and activism among family members of GLB individuals. *Journal of GLBT Family Studies, 6*, 349–364. https://doi.org/10.1080/1550428X.2010.511066

Huebner, D. M., & Davis, M. C. (2007). Perceived antigay discrimination and physical health outcomes. *Health Psychology, 26*, 627–634. https://doi.org/10.1037/0278-6133.26.5.627

Kahlina, K. (2015). Local histories, European LGBT designs: Sexual citizenship, nationalism, and "Europeanisation" in post-Yugoslav Croatia and Serbia. *Women's Studies International Forum, 49*, 73–83. https://doi.org/10.1016/j.wsif.2014.07.006

Kastanis, A., & Wilson, B. (2014). *Race/ethnicity, gender, and socioeconomic wellbeing of individuals in same-sex couples*. Los Angeles, CA: The Williams Institute, UCLA School of Law. Retrieved from https://williamsinstitute.law.ucla.edu/wp-content/uploads/Census-Compare-Feb-2014.pdf

Kazyak, E., & Stange, M. (2018). Backlash or a positive response? Public opinion of LGB issues after Obergefell v. Hodges. *Journal of Homosexuality, 65*, 2028–2052. https://doi.org/10.1080/00918369.2017.1423216

Kazyak, E., & Woodell, B. (2016). Law and LGBQ-parent families. *Sexuality & Culture, 20*, 749–768. https://doi.org/10.1007/s12119-016-9335-4

Kosciw, J. C., & Diaz, E. M. (2008). *Involved, invisible, ignored: The experiences of lesbian, gay, bisexual, and transgender parents and their children in our nation's K–12 schools*. New York, NY: GLSEN in partnership with COLAGE and the Family Equality Council.

Lindsrom, M. (2004). Social capital, the miniaturization of community and self-reported global and psychological health. *Social Science & Medicine, 59*, 595–607. https://doi.org/10.1016/j.socscimed.2003.11.006

Lustenberger, S. (2014). Questions of belonging: Same-sex parenthood and Judaism in transformation. *Sexualities, 17*, 529–545. https://doi.org/10.1177/1363460714526117

Lytle, M. C., Foley, P. F., & Aster, A. (2013). Adult children of gay and lesbian parents: Religion and the parent-child relationship. *The Counseling Psychologist, 41*, 530–567. https://doi.org/10.1177/0011000012449658

Martin, B. (2007). Activism, social and political. In G. L. Anderson & K. G. Herr (Eds.), *Encyclopedia of activism and social justice* (pp. 20–27). Thousand Oaks, CA: Sage.

Masci, D., & Lipka, M. (2015, December 21). *Where Christian churches, other religions stand on gay marriage*. Pew Research Center. Retrieved from http://www.pewresearch.org/fact-tank/2015/12/21/where-christian-churches-stand-on-gay-marriage/

McLaren, S. (2009). Sense of belonging to the general and lesbian communities as predictors of depression among lesbians. *Journal of Homosexuality, 56*, 1–13. https://doi.org/10.1080/00918360802551365

McLaren, S., Jude, B., & McLachlan, A. J. (2008). Sense of belonging to the general and gay communities as predictors of depression among gay men. *International Journal of Men's Health, 7*, 90–99. https://doi.org/10.3149/jmh.0701.90

Mendez, S. (2014). *Race, place, and sexuality: A contextual understanding of LGB identity salience.* Unpublished master's thesis, University of Illinois at Urbana-Champaign. Retrieved from: https://www.ideals.illinois.edu/handle/2142/50424

Mendez, S. N. (2017). *Parenting processes in black and mixed-race LGQ parent families: Racial and queer socialization.* Unpublished doctoral dissertation, University of Illinois at Urbana-Champaign. Retrieved from: https://www.ideals.illinois.edu/handle/2142/98192

Mendez, S. N., Holman, E. G., Oswald, R. F., & Izenstark, D. (2016). Minority stress in the context of rural economic hardship: One lesbian mother's story. *Journal of GLBT Family Studies, 12*, 491–511. https://doi.org/10.1080/1550428X.2015.1099493

Meyer, I. H. (2003). Prejudice, social stress, and mental health in lesbian, gay, and bisexual populations: Conceptual issues and research evidence. *Psychological Bulletin, 129*, 674–697. https://doi.org/10.1037/0033-2909.129.5.674

Moore, M. (2011). *Invisible families: Gay identities, relationships, and motherhood among Black women.* Los Angeles, CA: University of California Press.

Movement Advancement Project (MAP) (2018). Retrieved from http://lgbtmap.org

National Center for Transgender Equality. (2018). *The discrimination administration: Anti-transgender and anti-LGBT actions.* Retrieved from https://transequality.org/the-discrimination-administration

O'Connell, M., & Lofquist, D. (2009, May). *Counting same-sex couples: Official estimates and unofficial guesses.* Paper presented at the Population Association of America, Detroit, MI. Retrieved from http://www.census.gov/population/www/socdemo/files/counting-paper.pdf

*Obergefell v. Hodges.* 135 S. Ct. 2584 (2015). Retrieved from: https://www.supremecourt.gov/opinions/14pdf/14-556_3204.pdf

Ocobock, A. (2018). Status or access? The impact of marriage on lesbian, gay, bisexual, and queer community change. *Journal of Marriage & Family, 80*, 367–382. https://doi.org/10.1111/jomf.12468

Ogolsky, B. G., Monk, J. K., Rice, T. M., & Oswald, R. F. (2018). As the states turned: Implications of the changing legal context of same-sex marriage on well-being. *Journal of Social & Personal Relationships.* Advanced online publication, *36*, 3219. https://doi.org/10.1177/0265407518816883

Ogolsky, B. G., Monk, J. K., Rice, T. M., & Oswald, R. F. (2019). Personal well-being across the transition to marriage equality: A longitudinal analysis. *Journal of Family Psychology.* Advance online publication, *33*, 422. https://doi.org/10.1037/fam0000504

Oswald, R. F., Cuthbertson, C., Lazarevic, V., & Goldberg, A. E. (2010). New developments in the field: Measuring community climate. *Journal of GLBT Family Studies, 6*, 214–228. https://doi.org/10.1080/15504281003709230

Oswald, R. F., & Kuvalanka, K. A. (2008). Same-sex couples: Legal complexities. *Journal of Family Issues, 29*, 1051–1066. https://doi.org/10.1177/0192513X08316274

Oswald, R. F., & Lazarevic, V. (2011). You live *where*? Lesbian mothers' attachment to nonmetropolitan communities. *Family Relations, 60*, 373–386. https://doi.org/10.1111/j.1741-3729.2011.00663.x

Oswald, R. F., Routon, J. M., McGuire, J. K., & Holman, E. G. (2018). Tolerance versus support: Perceptions of residential community climate among LGB parents. *Family Relations, 67*, 47–54. https://doi.org/10.1111/fare.12292

Pearson, K. H. (2018). Child custody in the context of LGBTQ relationship dissolution and divorce. In A. E. Goldberg & A. P. Romero (Eds.), *LGBTQ divorce and relationship dissolution* (pp. 195–220). New York, NY: Oxford University Press.

Perrin, E. C., Pinderhughes, E. E., Mattern, K., Hurley, S. M., & Newman, R. A. (2016). Experiences of children with gay fathers. *Clinical Pediatrics, 55*, 1305–1317. https://doi.org/10.1177/0009922816632346

Pew Research Center. (2017, June 26). *Support for same-sex marriage grows, even among groups that had been skeptical.* Retrieved from: http://www.people-press.org/2017/06/26/support-for-same-sex-marriage-grows-even-among-groups-that-had-been-skeptical/

Prokos, A. H., & Keene, J. R. (2010). Poverty among cohabiting gay and lesbian, and married and cohabiting heterosexual families. *Journal of Family Issues, 31*, 934–959. https://doi.org/10.1177/0192513X09360176

Ragins, B. R., & Cornwell, J. M. (2001). Pink triangles: Antecedents and consequences of perceived workplace discrimination against gay and lesbian employees. *Journal of Applied Psychology, 86*, 1244–1261. https://doi.org/10.1037/0021-9010.86.6.1244

Ragins, B. R., Singh, R., & Cornwell, J. M. (2007). Making the invisible visible: Fear and disclosure of sexual orientation at work. *Journal of Applied Psychology, 92*, 1103–1118. https://doi.org/10.1037/0021-9010.92.4.1103

Riggle, E. D. B., Rostosky, S. S., & Horne, S .G. (2009). Marriage amendments and lesbian, gay, and bisexual individuals in the 2006 election. *Sexuality Research & Social Policy, 6*, 80–89. doi:https://doi.org/10.1525/srsp.2009.6.1.80

Riggle, E. D. B., Rostosky, S. S., & Horne, S. G. (2010). Psychological distress, well-being, and legal recognition in same-sex couple relationships. *Journal of Family Psychology, 24*, 82–86. https://doi.org/10.1037/a0017942

Rodriguez, L., & Gaitlin, D. (2013). *Metro areas with the highest percentages of same-sex couples raising children are in states with constitutional bans on marriage.* Retrieved from: https://williamsinstitute.law.ucla.edu/press/press-releases/metro-areas-with-highest-percentages-of-same-sex-couples-raising-children-are-in-states-with-constitutional-bans-on-marriage/

*Romer v. Evans*, 517 U.S. 620 (1996). Retrieved from https://supreme.justia.com/cases/federal/us/517/620/

Rostosky, S. S., Abreu, R. L., Mahoney, A., & Riggle, E. D. B. (2017). A qualitative study of parenting and religiosity/spirituality in LGBTQ families. *Psychology of Religion & Spirituality, 9*, 437–445. https://doi.org/10.1037/rel0000077

Rostosky, S. S., & Riggle, E. D. B. (2002). 'Out' at work: The relation of actor and partner workplace policy and internalized homophobia to disclosure status. *Journal of Counseling Psychology, 49*, 411–419. https://doi.org/10.1037/0022-0167.49.4.411

Rostosky, S. S., Riggle, E. D. B., Horne, S. G., Denton, F. N., & Huellemeier, J. D. (2010). Lesbian, gay, and bisexual individuals' psychological reactions to amendments denying access to civil marriage. *American Journal of Orthopsychiatry, 80*, 302–310. https://doi.org/10.1111/j.1939-0025.2010.01033.x

Rostosky, S. S., Riggle, E. D. B., Horne, S. G., & Miller, A. D. (2009). Marriage amendments and psychological distress in lesbian, gay, and bisexual adults. *Journal of Counseling Psychology, 56*, 56–66. https://doi.org/10.1037/a0013609

Ruggiero, D., & Park, M. (2017). DOJ *files amicus brief that says title VII does not protect sexual orientation.* CNN. Retrieved from: https://www.cnn.com/2017/07/26/politics/doj-amicus-brief-title-vii-sexual-orientation/index.html

Russell, G. M., Bohan, J. S., McCarroll, M. C., & Smith, N. G. (2010). Trauma, recovery, and community: Perspectives on the long-term impact of anti-LGBT politics. *Traumatology, 17*, 14–23. https://doi.org/10.1177/1534765610362799

Russell, G. M., & Richards, J. A. (2003). Stressor and resilience factors for lesbians, gay men, and bisexuals confronting antigay politics. *American Journal of Community Psychology, 31*, 313–328. https://doi.org/10.1023/A:1023919022811

Shapiro, D. N., Peterson, C., & Stewart, A. J. (2009). Legal and social contexts and mental health among lesbian and heterosexual mothers. *Journal of Family Psychology, 23*, 255–262. https://doi.org/10.1037/a0017973

Shecter, E., Tracy, A. J., Page, K. V., & Luong, G. (2008). Shall we marry? Legal marriage as a commitment event in same-sex relationships. *Journal of Homosexuality, 54*, 400–422. https://doi.org/10.1080/00918360801991422

Short, L. (2007). Lesbian mothers living well in the context of heterosexism and discrimination: Resources, strategies, and legislative change. *Feminism & Psychology, 17*, 57–74. https://doi.org/10.1177/0959353507072912

Siker, J. S. (2007). *Homosexuality and religion: An encyclopedia.* Westport, CT: Greenwood Press.

Smith, N. G., & Ingram, K. M. (2004). Workplace heterosexism and adjustment among lesbian, gay, and bisexual individuals: The role of unsupportive social interactions. *Journal of Counseling Psychology, 51*, 57–67. https://doi.org/10.1037/0022-0167.51.1.57

Southern Poverty Law Center. (2017). *Anti-LGBT.* Retrieved from https://www.splcenter.org/fighting-hate/extremist-files/ideology/anti-lgbt

Spivack, C. (2010). The law of surrogate motherhood in the United States. *The American Journal of Comparative Law, 58*, 97–114.

Stack, L., & Edmondson, C. (2018, August 4). A 'rainbow wave'? 2018 has more LGBT candidates than ever. *The New York Times.* Retrieved from https://www.nytimes.com/2018/08/04/us/politics/gay-candidates-midterms.html

Stern, M. J. (2017). *Supreme court orders states to list same-sex parents on birth certificates; Gorsuch dissents.* Retrieved from https://slate.com/human-interest/2017/06/supreme-court-orders-states-to-list-same-sex-couples-on-birth-certificates.html

Stotzer, R. L., Herman, J. L., & Hasenbush, A. (2014). *Transgender parenting: A review of existing research.* The Williams Institute. Retrieved from: https://escholarship.org/uc/item/3rp0v7qv

Sullivan, M. (2004). *The family of woman: Lesbian mothers, their children, and the undoing of gender.* Berkeley, CA: University of California Press.

Tejeda, M. J. (2006). Nondiscrimination policies and sexual identity disclosure: Do they make a difference in employee outcomes? *Employee Responsibilities & Rights Journal, 18*, 45–59. https://doi.org/10.1007/s10672-005-9004-5

Todosijevic, J., Rothblum, E. D., & Solomon, S. E. (2005). Relationship satisfaction, affectivity, and gay-specific stressors in same-sex couples joined in civil unions. *Psychology of Women Quarterly, 29*, 158–166. https://doi.org/10.1111/j.1471-6402.2005.00178.x

Tuthill, Z. (2016). Negotiating religiosity and sexual identity among Hispanic lesbian mothers. *Journal of Homosexuality, 63*, 1194–1210. https://doi.org/10.1080/00918369.2016.1151691

Velez, B. L., Moradi, B., & Brewster, M. E. (2013). Testing the tenets of minority stress theory in workplace contexts. *Journal of Counseling Psychology, 60,* 532–542. https://doi.org/10.1037/a0033346

Wellman, B. (2002). Physical place and cyberplace: The rise of personalized networking. *International Journal* *of Urban & Regional Research, 25,* 227–252. https://doi.org/10.1111/1468-2427.00309

Yip, A. (1997). Dare to differ: Gay and lesbian Catholics assessment of official Catholic positions on sexuality. *Sociology of Religion, 58,* 165–180. https://doi.org/10.2307/3711875

# LGBTQ-Parent Families in Non-Western Contexts

Pedro Alexandre Costa and Geva Shenkman

This chapter examines the research on LGBTQ-parent families in non-Western contexts. Although some chapters in this book look into specific areas of inquiry (e.g., adoption) in order to pinpoint under-researched areas and help push the field forward, we propose to take a step back to reflect upon the knowledge produced in contexts other than Europe and the United States of America (USA), which is useful in bringing a more integrated perspective to the field. Thus, we review the research from non-Western contexts using culturally situated lenses while embracing the diversity of LGBTQ-parent families in these contexts. This position is in line with a cross-cultural theoretical perspective, which has dominated this field of study, and suggests exploring variations in human behavior, taking into account the specific cultural context alongside the symbolic systems of beliefs and norms surrounding sexuality in each environment (Herdt, 1997).

For the purpose of this chapter, we reviewed work from four main regions: (a) Asia, with an overall overview of the state of LGBTQ-parent families in the region; (b) the Middle East, with an in-depth look into LGBTQ-parent families in Israel; (c) Africa, with an in-depth look into LGBTQ-parent families in South Africa; and (d) Latin America, with a focus on the research on LGBTQ-parent families in Mexico and in Brazil. The decision to take an in-depth look into LGBTQ-parent families in the aforementioned countries was not decided a priori but rather it was informed by the number of studies conducted in these countries. Further, given the breadth of available research, it was also possible to examine the studies that focused on LGBTQ parents separately from the studies that examined children with LGBTQ parents in these four countries. In fact, the research on LGBTQ-parent families in these regions are not as scarce as we had expected. There has been a growing interest in the field along with important social transformations and legal advances regarding the human rights of LGBTQ people, especially in the last decade (Barrientos, 2016). However, one of the major difficulties in identifying the studies from these regions and integrating their findings into the broader knowledge base in the field is the language in which the studies were published. This was particularly evident in the case of the Latin America region, where the studies have been almost exclusively published in Spanish or in Portuguese.

Before we review the research from each of these regions, we provide some sociohistorical background to allow for a situated analysis that

P. A. Costa (✉)
William James Center for Research, ISPA – Instituto Universitário, Lisbon, Portugal
e-mail: pcosta@ispa.pt

G. Shenkman
Baruch Ivcher School of Psychology, Interdisciplinary Center (IDC) Herzliya, Herzliya, Israel
e-mail: geva.shenkman@idc.ac.il

© Springer Nature Switzerland AG 2020
A. E. Goldberg, K. R. Allen (eds.), *LGBTQ-Parent Families*,
https://doi.org/10.1007/978-3-030-35610-1_20

takes into account social, contextual, religious, and legal factors, and their impact not only on the situation of LGBTQ-parent families but also on the research and lines of inquiry into LGBTQ-parent families. While there is value in focusing on research from non-Western contexts, as opposed to Euro-American contexts, there is a great heterogeneity across the four regions in a number of ways. Social attitudes and legal frameworks vastly differ both across and within the regions. In Israel, LGBTQ people are given some opportunities to have children, and even encouraged to do so, which is in sharp contrast with the mostly negative attitudes, persecution, and even criminalization of LGBTQ people across the Middle East (Lavee & Katz, 2003; Muedini, 2018). According to the Latinobarómetro (2015), a survey research program involving 18 countries from Latin America, while in some countries (e.g., Uruguay) over 50% of the population is supportive of same-gender parented families, in others (e.g., Venezuela) about 90% are against recognizing these families under the law. Further, in most sub-Saharan African countries same-gender relationships are criminalized while in South Africa same-gender couples are given constitutional protection from discrimination (Lubbe, 2008a; Msibi, 2011). These differences and specificities are examined in detail in each region.

Some heterogeneity was also identified regarding the theoretical approaches to the study of LGBTQ-parent families across the four non-Western regions. Most studies included in this review were not clearly articulated within a theoretical approach, as most served as pioneering a field of inquiry in the region. For example, studies from across Latin America consisted of mostly exploratory qualitative studies focused on the experiences of LGBTQ-parent families in relation to their social contexts, but without a clear theoretical rationale. In contrast, studies from South Africa showed a greater engagement with theoretical underpinnings to the study of LGBTQ parents and their children, through the use of social constructionist approaches, and phenomenological and social identity theories to examine the experiences of these families. Furthermore, some of these South African studies

(e.g., Kruger, Lubbe-De Beer, & Du Plessis, 2016; Lubbe, 2008b) employed a strengths and resilience-based lens to discuss their findings especially regarding children of LGBTQ parents. Noteworthy, none of the studies from Africa, Latin America, or Asia used comparative designs between LGBTQ-parent and heterosexual-parent families. Comparative designs have nonetheless characterized most studies from Israel, with emphasis on the potential positive outcomes that may be fostered by LGBTQ parenthood (e.g., Shenkman, Ifrah, & Shmotkin, 2018; Shenkman & Shmotkin, 2019).

## Methodology

To locate the studies from the four non-Western regions, we conducted searches in several databases such as PsycNET, Proquest, Ebsco Discovery Service, Sociological Abstracts, Scielo, and Google Scholar, among others, using several combinations of keywords such as "same-sex," "same-gender," "gay," "lesbian," "queer," bisexual" with "families," "parents," "fathers," "mothers," "parenting," and in several languages: English, Hebrew, French, Portuguese, and Spanish. Further, we also consulted reference lists for published papers and contacted expert scholars in the field from the different regions. We sought a wide search of potential studies from each of the four regions and included studies with different methodologies and from different scientific fields (e.g., Anthropology, Psychology, Sociology). Although we followed the steps for a systematic review, we could not conduct a pure systematic review focusing only on LGBTQ-parent families for two main reasons. First, we decided to include studies on the sociocultural-legal context of each region and its relation to sexual minorities and parenting to allow a more compressive understanding of the experiences and difficulties of LGBTQ relations. Second, the overwhelming majority of studies from the four regions were qualitative, and thus results were not easily summarized. Further, given the diversity and number of regions, contexts, and studies included in this review, we could not include every study that we came across. Instead, we adopted a narrative approach that would summarize the main lines of inquiry in each of the four regions and by doing so implemented a cross-cultural theoretical perspective.

## LGBTQ-Parent Families in Asia

While studies concerning same-gender relationships and the pursuit of legalization of same-gender marriage has gained attention in some countries in Asia such as Taiwan and Japan (e.g., Jeffreys & Wang, 2018; Tamagawa, 2016), the number of studies on LGBTQ-parent families is quite limited in this region. One explanation for the scarcity of studies on LGBTQ-parent families in the case of China, for example, relates to the state controls over the media and social organizations, thus ensuring that LGBTQ issues, including controversial issues such LGBTQ parenting, will not become a major feature of public discussion or research (Jeffreys & Wang, 2018). The stigmatization of LGBTQ people is prevalent with over 70% of the general population endorsing that "same-sex sexual behavior is always wrong," and many Chinese gay men maintain secretive same-gender relationships while married to women (Xie & Peng, 2018). Religious beliefs, namely, Taoism, Confucianism, and Buddhism, are deeply embedded in Chinese culture and are partly responsible for the rejection of same-gender relationships, which are perceived as a violation to both egalitarian and family values (Hildebrandt, 2019; Liu et al., 2011). Further, China is still a largely traditional society, mainly influenced by Communism, in spite of rapid economic growth in the last two decades and the increasing influence of neo-capitalism and liberal values (Ji, Wu, Sun, & He, 2017).

In Taiwan, the legalization of same-gender marriage has gained recent support from the Taiwanese parliament (Lee, 2016). However, there is also vast public protest against marriage equality and LGBTQ-parent families on the grounds that it will undermine religious and traditional family values in the country. Similarly to China, Taiwan's religious traditions of Buddhism,

Confucianism, and Taoism exert their negative influence against same-gender relationships, such as restricting sexual morality and enforcing traditional gender roles (Lee, 2016). In contrast, Japan is considered a relatively "gay friendly" that does not have any real anti-homosexuality laws, and Japanese police do not typically raid gay spots (Tamagawa, 2016). Nevertheless, negative attitudes toward LGBTQ parents are still prevalent (Ipsos, 2013). In addition, with few reproductive technologies legally available to Japanese people in general, and the strong social resistance to child adoption by unmarried couples, same-gender couples have extremely few options for legally starting a family in Japan (Tamagawa, 2016). Thus, research on LGBTQ-parent families is quite scarce.

## LGBTQ-Parent Families in the Middle East

In the last decade, the social visibility of LGBTQ people in the Middle East has increased. However, LGBTQ people in most Middle Eastern countries are still marginalized, and homosexuality is even considered as illness (Başoğlu, 2015). In this section, we review research from diverse Middle Eastern nations, and then specifically from Israel.

### LGBTQ-Parent Families in the Middle Eastern Region

LGBTQ people in these environments, which are heavily influenced by Islam, tend to suffer from discrimination, harassment, stigma, and in extreme cases the death penalty (Needham, 2012). For most imams and Muslim populations, homosexuality is interpreted as being a prohibited act against God, the faith, and the family. The Quran, Islam's holy religious text, is commonly cited and interpreted to support these views (Muedini, 2018). In most of these countries, there is lack of legislation protecting LGBTQ rights in general and LGBTQ-parent families in particular, and in some cases, such as in Iran, Iraq, and Sudan, the regional laws and penal codes are reinforced to reduce homosexual visibility (Henrickson, 2018; Karimi & Bayatrizi, 2018). Countries such as Lebanon, Egypt, Turkey, Jordan, Iran, and Syria are often characterized by more conservative, homonegative, and heterosexist norms regarding homosexuality and same-gender parenting (Muedini, 2018). In Iran, for example, according to Islam and Iran's law, fertility treatment cannot be offered to single mothers or to gay men (Samani, Dizaj, Moalem, Merghati, & Alizadeh, 2007; Yadegarfard & Bahramabadian, 2014). This conservative and heterosexist environment is not a fertile ground for research on LGBTQ-parent families, and indeed we found almost no evidence in the academic databases for research on LGBTQ-parent families in Lebanon, Egypt, Turkey, Jordan, Iran, and Syria.

## LGBTQ-Parent Families in Israel

Israel is characterized with more enlightened and liberal norms regarding homosexuality, according to Western standards (Kama, 2011), though this societal context also contains some contradictions when considering parenthood and LGBTQ populations together (Shenkman, 2012). On the one hand, Israeli society highly esteems childbearing and parenting, such that being a parent is a main pathway to social acceptance by a society that sanctifies family values and continuity (Ben-Ari & Weinberg-Kurnik, 2007; Lavee & Katz, 2003; Tsfati & Ben-Ari, 2019). Similarly, there are higher birth rates in Israel in comparison to most countries in Europe and the USA, and child-oriented policies such as receiving birth allowances and tax deductions based on the number of children are well grounded in the state's dogma (Lavee & Katz, 2003). In addition, women in Israel are entitled to extensive Health Maintenance Organization (HMO) coverage for In Vitro Fertilization (IVF) procedures, regardless of their sexual orientation (Birenbaum-Carmeli & Dirnfeld, 2008). On the other hand, only in 1988 did the Israeli Knesset, i.e., the Israeli Parliament, repeal the British Mandate's rule that made homosexuality a crim-

inal offense (Shokeid, 2003). Also, Israel is largely characterized as a patriarchal society, which still adheres to masculine stereotypes that are further strengthened by continuous warfare conditions with Palestine, alongside the prominence of the army in most citizens' lives, as army service is mandatory and at the age of 18 Israeli men are drafted for 3 years and women for 2 years (Sion & Ben-Ari, 2009). In sum, it is challenging to become a LGBTQ parent in this societal context, amidst the context of militarism and traditional masculine roles, along with the reliance of the Jewish religion on the biblical law that firmly denigrates homosexuality, as explicitly stated in Leviticus, 20:13: "If there is a man who lies with a male as those who lie with a woman, both of them have committed a detestable act; they shall surely be put to death" (translation from the New American Standard Bible).

While Israeli law secured advanced legislation regarding the rights of LGBTQ people (Gross, 2014; Kama, 2011), same-gender marriage in Israel is not yet settled at this time. Similarly, though different-gender couples are allowed to pursue surrogacy within the boundaries of Israel, the law does not permit same-gender couples to use these services, and gay men who wish to become parents via surrogacy turn to highly expensive overseas surrogacy services in South East Asia and North America (Teman, 2010). In addition, adoption opportunities are extremely limited for LGBTQ people in Israel, as newborns are rarely available for adoption in Israel in general, and for international adoption opportunities are scarce for LGBTQ people as well (Gross, 2014; Inhorn, Birenbaum-Carmeli, Tremayne, & Gürtin, 2017).

**LGBTQ parents** Being a parent (of any kind) is an important path toward acceptance by a society that sanctifies family values and continuity (Tsfati & Ben-Ari, 2019). Additionally, gay fatherhood can be considered a huge triumph over the widespread message that gay men are not supposed to become parents (Armesto, 2002). Researchers in Israel suggested that successfully overcoming legal, social, and financial difficulties in the journey to parenthood might result in better subjective well-being (SWB). For example, Erez and Shenkman (2016) compared 90 Israeli gay fathers with 90 individually matched heterosexual counterparts and found that gay fathers reported significantly higher levels of SWB in comparison to heterosexual fathers. Additionally, Shenkman and Shmotkin (2014) compared 45 gay fathers with 45 individually matched gay men who were not fathers on indicators of SWB, depressive symptoms, and meaning in life. Results indicated that gay fathers reported higher levels of SWB and meaning in life alongside lower levels of depressive symptoms in comparison to single gay men. Whereas previous studies among heterosexual participants suggested that being a parent was related to decreased levels of SWB and increased levels of meaning in life, Shenkman and Shmotkin's (2014) study suggested that gay fathers had elevated levels of both SWB and meaning in life, thus deviating from the pattern found in heterosexual samples (e.g., Nomaguchi & Milkie, 2003).

Other research also suggests positive psychological outcomes in the meaning in life domain among Israeli gay fathers in comparison with heterosexual fathers. In Shenkman and Shmotkin's (2016) study, 82 Israeli gay fathers who became fathers mainly through surrogacy were individually matched with 82 heterosexual fathers and were compared on meaning in life and self-perceived parental role, defined as parents' subjective assessments of their self-efficacy, competence, and investment in parenthood. Results showed that higher self-perceived parental role was associated with higher meaning in life among gay fathers but not among heterosexual fathers. A similar pattern of results also emerged when higher self-perceived parental role was associated with less adverse mental health indicators (depressive symptoms, neuroticism, and negative emotions) among gay but not heterosexual fathers (Shenkman & Shmotkin, 2019). In another study, 76 middle-aged and older Israeli gay men who had become fathers in a heterosexual relationship were compared with 110 middle-aged and older gay men who were not fathers,

and with 114 middle-aged and older heterosexual fathers (Shenkman et al., 2018). Results showed that self-reported personal growth was higher among gay fathers than among heterosexual fathers. The authors suggested that gay fathers, who were conceived their children within a previous heterosexual relationship and presently identified as exclusively gay, have overcome multiple difficulties as part of the complex course of coming out to oneself, spouse, and children. Coping successfully with such hardships could result in a construction of new meaning in life, which might explain the higher levels of personal growth found among older gay, compared with heterosexual, fathers. In addition, both personal growth and purpose in life were higher among gay fathers compared to gay men who were not fathers. Taken together, these findings suggest that becoming a gay father in Israel, a familistic society that promotes childrearing though also poses difficulties for gay men who wish to become fathers, may relate to a stronger sense of meaning in life and SWB among those who succeed in becoming fathers.

Gay fatherhood in Israel has also been studied through qualitative methods. Erera and Segal-Engelchin (2014) conducted in-depth interviews with nine Israeli gay fathers who were co-parenting with a heterosexual woman. This route to parenthood is quite prevalent in Israel and reflects traditional cultural values of a family with different-gender parents (Segal-Engelchin, Erera, & Cwikel, 2005). Interviews revealed key motivations for establishing a hetero-gay family such as the belief in the essential mother, the belief in biological parenting, and the belief that the child's best interests dictate having two different-gender parents. Another qualitative study of 16 Israeli gay prospective fathers, most of whom expected a child through surrogacy in India, explored the emotional experience of pregnancy (Ziv & Freund-Eschar, 2015). Men often felt frustration and anxiety due to their distance from the physical pregnancy and, specifically, their inability to experience the physical presence of the fetus, thus posing difficulties with development of their parental identity during the pregnancy. In another qualitative study, 39 Israeli gay fathers, who became fathers through surrogacy, were interviewed (Tsfati & Ben-Ari, 2019). The authors suggested that gay parenthood subverts existing concepts of parenthood, in particular the notion of motherhood as a social construct derived from an essentialist framework, which commonly articulates heteronormative ideologies. Taken together, the findings mentioned above reflect the dialectics of gay fathers' parenting experiences, which are shaped by the heteronormative discourse on parenthood, yet resist its gendered attributes.

Compared to work on gay fathers, research on lesbian mothers has received somewhat less attention in Israel. Two comparative studies focused mainly on the lack of differences between lesbian and heterosexual mothers. In the first study, Shechner, Slone, Meir, and Kalish (2010) compared 30 two-mother lesbian families with 30 two-parent heterosexual mothers on levels of psychological distress, well-being, parental distress, and social support and found no differences between the two family types on any of these variables. In the second study, Shenkman (2018) studied 57 lesbian mothers who were individually matched with 57 heterosexual mothers and examined the association between basic need satisfaction in the couple relationship (the support the individual gets from the other person in the relationship for their sense of autonomy, competence, and relatedness) and personal growth as a function of sexual orientation. While results revealed no differences between the two groups on basic need satisfaction in the couple relationship, the positive association between basic need satisfaction in the couple relationship and personal growth was significant only among lesbian mothers. The authors interpreted this finding in terms of the particular characteristics of lesbian couples, such as high emotional support, equal division of labor, and the absence of traditional gender roles, which they theorized may have contributed to a sense of personal growth in the context of lesbian motherhood, which is planned, intentional, and often achieved after struggling with minority stress.

Other studies have focused more on the lived experiences of lesbian mothers in Israel. Ben-Ari

and Livni (2006), for example, explored the constructed meanings that both biological (using sperm donation) and nonbiological mothers related to their motherhood experience among eight lesbian couples who were parenting children together. The children's ages ranged between 2 months to 13 years. Although lesbian couples reported valuing a sense of equality in their relationships, the birth of a child was an event that created two different statuses of motherhood, a biological mother and a nonbiological mother, which had social and legal implications.

**Children of LGBTQ parents** Research on children's psychosocial adjustment as a function of parental sexual orientation is quite scarce in Israel. We identified only one study in our literature search. Shechner, Slone, Lobel, and Shechter (2013) compared 15 Israeli single lesbian mothers, 21 two-mother lesbian families, 16 single heterosexual mothers by choice, and 24 two-parent heterosexual mothers, on children's adjustment, children's perception of peer relations, and children's perceived self-competence. Results showed that children of lesbian mothers reported more prosocial behaviors and less loneliness than children from heterosexual parented families, and no differences emerged for perceived self-competence across family type. The authors concluded that mother's sexual orientation did not affect children's adjustment negatively, although single parenthood, regardless of sexual orientation, was associated with greater difficulties for children, manifested by more externalizing behavior problems and aggressiveness.

## LGBTQ-Parent Families in Africa

Same-gender relationships across the African continent are highly discouraged, outlawed, or criminalized. In 38 out of 53 African countries, same-gender behavior is illegal (Msibi, 2011). However, there has been a growing debate in the region, especially in sub-Saharan Africa, about the rights of LGBTQ people, and some legal advancements have been made (Jacques, 2013).

## LGBTQ-Parent Families in the African Region

In the Southern region of Africa, some instances of same-gender relationships and even same-gender marriages between women are both legally and socially acceptable, whereas same-gender relationships between mostly or exclusively non-heterosexuals may be tolerated if one of the members of the couple adopts cross-gender behaviors and identity (Bonthuys, 2008). Nevertheless, having a same-gender relationship does not necessarily translate into living openly as a couple or even identifying as gay or lesbian (Bonthuys, 2008). A study investigating same-gender intimate relationships between girls in Ghana reported that these relationships were characterized by an intimate bond between girl friends (*supi*) in which "they behave like a man and a woman" (Dankwa, 2009, pp. 195). These relationships are not socially accepted, but there is evidence that they are common among teenage girls or between a teenage girl and an older woman and occur within a context of ambiguity and secrecy.

Further, ethnographic studies have documented young LGBTQ people involved in secretive same-gender relationships and living a double life, that is, maintaining different-gender relationships openly while having same-gender partners hidden in Mozambique and in Cape Verde (Miguel, 2016; Souza, 2014). Few engage in open same-gender relationships for fear of social rejection and to avoid the perceived *subversiveness* of adopting an LGBTQ identity. Scholars suggest that non-heterosexuals may be involved in same-sex romantic and/or sexual behaviors yet are unwilling to adopt a LGBTQ identity in contexts where such identities are denied and/or persecuted (e.g., Msibi, 2011, 2013). Furthermore, some authors have argued that LGBTQ identities in African contexts may be seen as Western constructs and thus not necessarily embraced by individuals who engage in same-gender relationships (Msibi, 2013; see chapter "Race and Ethnicity in the Lives of LGBTQ Parents and Their Children: Perspectives from and Beyond North America"). Furthermore, the rejection of LGBTQ identities may serve as a self-protective strategy against discrimination and persecution or reflect internalized stigma associated with same-gender sexualities (Msibi, 2013).

## LGBTQ-Parent Families in South Africa

In contrast with other African countries and much like in most Western countries, South Africa has framed the rights of LGBTQ people within a human rights framework. The evolving recognition of same-gender relationships can be seen in South Africa, crystallized in one of the most important milestones which was the Constitutional protection against discrimination based on sexual orientation (Lubbe, 2008a). Slowly after that, specific rights such as marriage and parenting were legally extended to same-gender couples. However, that is not to say that the South African society is without prejudice or discrimination of LGBTQ people. On the contrary, social attitudes toward same-gender relationships are still prevalently negative (Breshears & Lubbe-De Beer, 2016). We found that research on LGBTQ-parent families in South Africa is limited yet flourishing in recent years. All of the studies we were able to locate employed a qualitative methodology, sampled through convenient and snowball procedures. Thematically, all of the studies with LGBTQ-parent families that we located focused on the social experiences of these families. The studies with parents and children in LGBTQ-parent families investigated how they navigated potentially discriminating contexts and how they managed family disclosure, particularly in the school context.

**LGBTQ parents** Breshears and Lubbe-De Beer's (2016) study focused on the perceptions and experiences of social oppression of 21 LGBTQ mothers and fathers (including five couples) and their 12 children. Only one child in the sample had been planned within a same-gender relationship, and adopted by a lesbian couple, while the others had been conceived in a previous heterosexual relationship. LGBTQ parents in this study reported feeling a growing acceptance of LGBTQ-parent families largely because of the existence of legal protection for same-gender relationships and families. Nevertheless, they also argued that there was still a notable gap between the country's progressive laws and social attitudes. Similarly, the 10 LG parent families in Kruger et al. (2016) study discussed social justice, and how they hoped that society would evolve to be more inclusive, which should extend beyond legal protections through educating society about LGBTQ-parent families and thus changing people's attitudes toward these families. In another study (Van Ewyk & Kruger, 2017), 10 lesbian couples with planned children through adoption and assisted reproduction described generally positive experiences of motherhood. Yet despite a positive adjustment to motherhood and overall positive experiences within the family, these mothers still felt as though they had to prove they were just as good at parenting as heterosexual people, which to some extent seems to stem from greater public scrutiny of LGBTQ parents.

Nevertheless, although Black sexual minorities are much more likely to be victimized because of their identities and relationships, and to feel disempowered (Breshears & Lubbe-De Beer, 2016), the samples in the cited studies were almost exclusively composed of White, middle-class urban LGBTQ parents (Breshears & Lubbe-De Beer, 2016; Kruger et al., 2016; Van Ewyk & Kruger, 2017). Considering how sexual minorities in same-gender relationships may not identify with LGBTQ identities across the region (Msibi, 2013), efforts to recruit more diverse samples of LGBTQ parents may prove challenging yet necessary for a more complete picture of LGBTQ-parent families in South Africa.

**Children of LGBTQ parents** In South Africa, not only have the experiences of LGBTQ parents been documented but also the experiences of their children/adolescents and adults. A qualitative study of 20 adults who had been raised by LG parents investigated the experiences of having a parent come out to them (Breshears &

Lubbe-De Beer, 2014). Participants were mostly young adults ($M_{age}$ = 29), and most learned about their parent's sexual identity during their late adolescent years ($M_{age}$ = 17). Participant interviews highlighted that a parent coming out to their children is an ongoing process and not a one-time conversation. Some participants stated that children may need time to adjust to the new information and to be assured of the possible ramifications of this disclosure, namely, parents' separation/divorce. Further, some participants suggested that notwithstanding the difficulties that LGBTQ parents may feel in coming out to their children, they should take the lead in the process and initiate the conversations instead of waiting for their children to ask them.

Other studies have looked into the disclosure of being part of an LGBTQ-parent family from the children's perspectives. Lubbe (2007, 2008c) followed eight children (aged 9–19 years), six of them White, from five mostly middle-class lesbian parented families, over a 3- to 4-month period to investigate the disclosure of having an LGBTQ-parent family in school. Although dependent on the specific school (e.g., private or public school), Lubbe (2007) found that children with LG parents tended to be silent about their families as a strategy to protect themselves from teasing and bullying by their peers. For example, Lubbe reported that conservative and religious schools offered a less supportive context for children to openly discuss their family. However, choosing to disclose or to stay silent is not always a one-time choice. Most children in Lubbe's (2008c) study based their decisions to hide or not to hide their family on the perceived safeness to disclose their family configuration in different contexts and with different people, acutely aware of the possibility of not being accepted. Further, a case study of a 14-year-old boy of a lesbian mother highlighted how children's characteristics also can inform their decisions regarding the disclosure of having an LGBTQ-parent family (Lubbe, 2008b). This case study illustrated how children adjust their disclosure strategy in a socially intelligent way by observing and anticipating their peers' reactions. Disclosure practices also depended upon their own feelings about their family in that children who were more confident on and proud of their family configuration were more likely to openly discuss it, especially with their peers (e.g., Lubbe, 2007).

## LGBTQ-Parent Families in Latin America

The general context of LGBTQ-parent families in Latin America varies widely. Despite geographical and cultural similarities, this region is composed of over 20 countries in 2 continents (North America and South America), ranging from Mexico in the North to Argentina and Chile in the South, each with its own historical and social background. Among Latin American countries, some of the shared values are grounded in the historical sociopolitical influence of the Catholic Church, where a heteronormative and patriarchal society is the norm. According to Barrientos and Nardi (2016), social prejudice against LGBTQ individuals may not be as openly expressed and violent as it once was across the region, yet opposition to same-gender marriage and parenting is still highly prevalent. Nevertheless, in spite of within-region differences, there is a growing number of countries that legally recognize same-gender relationships and families, namely, Argentina, Brazil, and Uruguay, where the level of support for LGBTQ-parent families also tends to be the highest in the region (Latinobarometro, 2015).

Outside of Brazil and Mexico, at which we will take closer look, there are a small number of studies on LGBTQ-parent families in this region. Qualitative studies from Chile (Díaz, González, & Garrido, 2018; Riquelme, 2017) recruited small yet diverse samples of LGBTQ parents and asked them about creating a family in spite of a lack of legal recognition of kinship. Notwithstanding the participants' different perspectives of *family*, the parents in Riquelme's (2017) study highlighted the importance of recognizing same-gender relationships—not only to provide legal protection to different family arrangements, but also as a means of symbolic

recognition of the affective bonds between same-gender partners. In the same vein, an Argentinian qualitative study (Libson, 2010) found that although some LG parents were critical of marriage as a heteronormative institution, they still acknowledged the importance of same-gender marriage because it implied a recognition of parent-child relationships, or the possibility of having children within a same-gender relationship. It is thus noteworthy that social and legal concerns regarding kinship in LGBTQ-parent families seems to be driving the research agenda in Latin America.

Furthermore, very little research has examined the experiences of children of LGBTQ parents. In fact, with the exception of one study from Mexico (Salinas-Quiroz et al., 2018) and two studies from Brazil (Hernández & Uziel, 2014; Palma & Strey, 2015), research has relied almost exclusively on parents' qualitative accounts to examine the experiences of LGBTQ-parent families, particularly in relation to their social adjustment and experiences of stigma. These studies have raised awareness to the effects of both social attitudes toward these families and legal recognition of parental roles on the well-being of both LGBTQ parents and their children and highlighted the diversity of experiences among these families based on parents' gender, race, education level, and socioeconomic level.

### LGBTQ-Parent Families in Brazil

In Brazil, same-gender marriages were legalized in 2015, thus effectively providing legal protection to same-gender relationships and families. Before 2015 and outside of the legal jurisdiction, many LGBTQ people have raised children through so-called *Brazilian adoption*, which consists of parents raising and legally registering a child as their own with the consent of the biological parents, and through *informal adoption*, which is a similar situation to Brazilian adoption but without any legal kinship recognition (Vitule, Couto, & Machin, 2015). According to the research produced in Brazil, both types of adoptions are quite common and have made it possible for LGBTQ people to become parents in face of legal obstacles to formally adopt a child or to access assisted reproductive technologies. However, the majority of documented LGBTQ-parent families in Brazil are headed by parents who have had children within heterosexual relationships, and few researches have studied trans or queer parented families (Palma, Strey, & Krugel, 2012).

**LGBTQ parents** Most of the published research with Brazilian LGBTQ-parent families that we were able to locate used qualitative designs and small samples, ranging from 2 to 14 families in each study. This literature, though groundbreaking, has exclusively relied on self-selected convenience samples. In contrast, one of the strengths of these studies has been the diversity of family configurations and family experiences that has been captured. Nevertheless, most of the reviewed studies have either recruited LGBTQ parents who have had children through Brazilian or informal adoptions, or who have had children in previous heterosexual relationships, and have tended to focus on social acceptance and experiences of stigma among LGBTQ-parent families. Further, an overarching finding across the different studies from Brazil is LGBTQ parents' pressure to adjust to a heteronormative pattern of family, by feeling the need to justify their parental practices and their family configuration, or even to just "be perfect" (Garcia et al., 2007; Sanches, Pelissoli, Lomando, & Levandowski, 2017).

Lira, Morais, and Boris (2016, 2017) interviewed four lesbian mothers: a lesbian couple with an adopted child and two lesbian women who had a child in a previous heterosexual relationship. The authors reported that these mothers not only faced prejudice from their own families of origin but also struggled with their own internalized stigma, and some even entered a different-gender relationship to pursue a heteronormative family and thus avoid social prejudice (Lira et al., 2017). Further, a study with three lesbian couples with children from a previous heterosexual relationship found that

mothers reported difficulties in their parent-child relationships because their children had not accepted their same-gender relationship (Sanches et al., 2017). Moreover, some mothers felt discriminated against in their children's school, and some opted to not disclose their family configuration in this context, anticipating and protecting themselves from negative reactions (Sanches et al., 2017). It is worth noting that the prejudicial experiences that these mothers have faced or the anticipation of prejudice may have shaped their pathway to parenthood. Many of these lesbian mothers chose not to disclose their sexual orientation and entered a different-gender relationship in order to have children and fulfill heteronormative family expectations.

Recent studies with planned LGBTQ-parent families have provided a different picture from that of families with children from previous heterosexual relationships. A study about the experiences of prejudice and discrimination of five same-gender couples with planned children through adoption and assisted reproduction found that none of the couples reported direct forms of prejudice as a family (Tombolato, Maia, Uziel, & Santos, 2018). However, institutional stigma persisted in denying these families all the same rights that different-gender couples have by default, and these families described adopting a confrontational stance to become visible and guarantee equal treatment in social spheres (Tombolato et al., 2018). Further, a study involving nine women (one single woman and four same-gender couples) who had children through assisted reproduction reported an asymmetry between biological and nonbiological mothers in their parental roles (Pontes, Féres-Carneiro, & Magalhães, 2017). The authors found that for these families, stigma manifested itself in the lack of recognition of the nonbiological mothers' role within the family, and some of them ensured the recognition of their parental role by legally adopting their partner's child.

Other Brazilian studies have focused on lesbian mothers' parenting aspiration and pathways to parenthood. Grossi (2003) reported that among lesbians who aspire to motherhood, assisted reproduction and in particular ROPA (Reception of Oocytes from Partner) was their elected pathway to parenthood, mostly because of the importance they placed upon a biogenetic connection with a child. Further, Vitule and her colleagues (2015) interviewed 2 single women and 12 same-gender couples about their pathways to parenthood, corroborating lesbian women's preference for biological kinship and the desire to experience pregnancy. For lesbian couples who could not access assisted reproduction due to financial or other constrains, the biological connection between the two mothers and the child could also be achieved through the insemination of one of the partners with the sperm of the other partner's brother (Grossi, 2003; Lira et al., 2017). However, beyond the importance of biological kinship, there are also other factors that motivate Brazilian lesbian women toward pursuing these pathways to parenthood. Even if just on a symbolic level, having a biological connection with the non-gestational child would make the mothers feel more secure about their role in the family as a "full mother figure" (Pontes et al., 2017). In contrast, among sexual minority men the preference for adoption was unanimous, although some reported having fantasized about having biological children through surrogacy arrangements, but abandoning the idea for fear of having a third person (the gestational mother) involved, or because of the financial difficulties associated with pursuing surrogacy overseas. In addition, men tended to be keener on raising older children, and not necessarily babies (Vitule et al., 2015).

**Children of LGBTQ parents** Only two papers about the well-being of children raised in same-gender households in Brazil were located, and these focused on the well-being of children in relation to the school context (Hernández & Uziel, 2014; Palma & Strey, 2015). Hernández and Uziel (2014) conducted an ethnographic study with 14 girls and women aged 5–50 years and their lesbian mothers. The authors found different perspectives in relation to the school setting: Whereas for some mothers it was difficult to disclose their family configuration at their children's schools, others reported a sense of responsibility for being visible as a family and for instigating discussions about family diversity to help change people's perceptions. However, some children reported facing unpleasant peer experiences related to having two mothers, and thus adopted protective strategies: namely, becoming selective about whom to disclose their family (Hernández & Uziel, 2014), similar to South African children (e.g., Lubbe, 2007). Palma and Strey (2015) interviewed 11 women in same-gender couples about their children's experiences at school, half of them in public schools and the other half in private schools. A few mothers discussed how some schools accepted different family configurations because they were already attentive to "children with special needs," drawing an unconscious parallel between children with disabilities and/or handicaps and children with same-gender parents (Palma & Strey, 2015). Further, according to these mothers, some children were consciously afraid of social prejudice and reported having hidden that one of their parents was in fact a parent, referring to them as an uncle/aunt, someone who just shared the house with them, or a parent's friend.

These two studies provided some evidence that schools are still not fully integrating LGBTQ-parent families and that is partially due to the influence of Christian and Evangelical faiths in public schools, which are more likely to reinforce heteronormative views of family and silencing discussions about diverse families. In contrast, private schools are described as being more inclusive and open to new family forms, and some parents mentioned how their children's private school had a "family day" instead of a "father's/mother's day" (Palma & Strey, 2015). It is thus noteworthy that the experiences of same-gender parented families in Brazil seem to be dependent to some extent on their race, social class, economic status, and place of living, as these affect LGBTQ parents' pathways to parenthood, but they also play an important role on how parents interact with different social contexts, on the possibility of choosing private vs. public schools, and on their child's social experiences.

## LGBTQ-Parent Families in Mexico

According to national statistics, there are about 250,000 nuclear LGBTQ-parent families in Mexico, from which nearly 70% have children and are mostly headed by lesbian/bisexual mothers (Aguirre, 2015). The legal framework of LGBTQ-parent families in Mexico is also diverse: In Mexico City same-gender marriage and adoption by same-gender couples were legalized in 2009, and in 2015 the Supreme Court of Justice ruled that denying marriage to same-gender couples was unconstitutional and mandated each state to legally correct this discrimination. However, only 20 out of a total of 32 Mexican states have so far recognized the right to marriage and to adopt a child regardless of gender or sexual orientation (Costa & Salinas-Quiroz, 2018). Further, attitudes toward same-gender families in Mexico are suggested to be halfway between the most negative (El Salvador, Paraguay, and Venezuela) and the most positive (Argentina, Brazil, and Uruguay) in the region (Latinobarómetro, 2015).

**LGBTQ parents** Most studies on LGBTQ-parent families in Mexico have examined the experiences of gay fathers (Aguirre, 2015; Laguna-Maqueda, 2016, 2017; Velasco, 2006), which is somewhat similar to the state of research on LGBTQ-parent families in Israel (e.g., Shenkman & Shmotkin, 2014). Laguna-Maqueda (2016, 2017) interviewed eight gay fathers who have had children through different paths. The parental experiences of these gay fathers were not only shaped by a prejudicial society, but especially by their own internalized stigma. "Among the fathers who have had children in different-gender relationships, some reported a concern with doing harm to their children because of their sexual identity, or policing their behavior in a gendered way so that their sons would be "masculine" and not grow up to be "homosexual" (Laguna-Maqueda, 2016). In contrast, a study with four gay fathers, three of whom had become parents through adoption provided a very different picture (Aguirre, 2015). These gay fathers had a mean age of 48 years, had high education

levels and a middle-to-high socioeconomic level, and possibly because of their high levels of resources they were all able to easily accommodate bringing a child into their family, and were able to take time off work to be with their children during their first months. The authors found that these couples did not explicitly fall into traditional gendered parental roles, as the division of parenting tasks relied more on the fathers' personality characteristics than on a set of pre-established rules (Aguirre, 2015). Similar results were found by Velasco (2006) in a qualitative study involving 11 gay fathers who have had children through different means. These fathers reported modeling their approach to parenthood after their own parents, but also underscored how they sought a greater emotional closeness with their children then they had with their own fathers.

Menassé (2017) and Menassé, Cosme, and Rodríguez (2014) investigated the attitudes of 10 mental health professionals toward LGBTQ families and the experiences of eight LGBTQ families with mental health professionals. The accounts of LGBTQ parents revealed a high level of prejudice toward these families. Namely, parents felt that therapists demonstrated a tendency to diagnose children a priori with some deficit because they were being raised by same-gender couples (Menassé et al., 2014). The deficits identified by the professionals were not necessarily based on parental sexual identity, but on the perceived impact of the lack of a traditional gendered parental figures. These findings can be understood in the context of a study by Menassé (2017) that found that prejudices regarding homosexuality were common among Mexican mental health professionals. Some of these professionals described their concerns about children being raised without the needed gendered role models, and one expressed the concern that the children would model their sexuality after their parents and grow up to be homosexual.

**Children of LGBTQ parents** Salinas-Quiroz and his colleagues (2018) provided an in-depth mixed-methods look into the *quality of care,* grounded in Ainsworth's attachment theoretical model (Ainsworth, Blehar, Waters, & Wall, 1978), in families headed by same-gender parents in Mexico. The study's sample consisted of three planned same-gender parented families, namely, two two-mother families with children conceived through donor insemination and one two-father family with an adopted child. Although the authors did not have a comparison group, they reported that same-gender parents showed similar levels of *parental sensitivity* to their children's needs and *security* offered to their children (Ainsworth et al., 1978) to that of different-gender parents from other studies in Latin America, adding that "their children remarkably used *both of their parents* [emphasis added] as a safety haven, as well as a base from which to explore their surroundings" (Salinas-Quiroz et al., 2018, p.8). This study represents an innovative approach to the development of children with LGBTQ parents since little attention overall has been given to child attachment security to their same-gender parents, despite the large number of studies about the psychosocial adjustment of children in LGBTQ-parent families from the USA and the UK.

## Directions for Future Research

One of the main paradigms that has dominated the field of LGBTQ-parent families relies on large-scale comparative studies with heterosexual-parent families, often described as the *no differences in outcomes* approach (Stacey & Biblarz, 2001). The research within this paradigm have helped to normalize LGBTQ-parent families by showing that a parent's sexual or gender identity does not negatively affect their children's development. These studies have also informed the debate regarding the recognition of same-gender marriage and parenting across the Western(ized) world and facilitated important legal advances and greater social acceptance of these families. While most of these studies have used generally large samples and quantitative research designs, this has not been

the case in non-Western regions. With the exception of studies from Israel (which mainly use quantitative study designs, reflecting their alignment with the still dominant Western paradigm of comparative studies using heterosexual-parent families as the norm; Johnson, 2012), the overwhelming majority of studies from Asia, Africa, the Middle East, and Latin America employed a qualitative approach to investigate the well-being of parents and children in diverse families. In some ways, these studies have pioneered new topic areas and given voice to both parents and children to help identify the unique challenges and difficulties faced by LGBTQ-parent families. We believe that the reliance on qualitative studies in the aforementioned regions may have been shaped by social and political climates that are not supportive of studies on LGBTQ identities, relationships, and families, thus hindering the researcher's ability to recruit large numbers of LGBT-parent families. However, we also acknowledge that some researchers may have intentionally conducted qualitative studies based on their theoretical grounding or research purpose. Further, small qualitative studies may not be seen as similarly helpful or effective in informing public debate as large-scale studies that focus on the well-being and the effects of social stigma on the psychosocial adjustment of these families.

The nature and design of the research in these regions largely depend on the social contexts; more conservative and religious contexts are not a fertile ground for large-scale quantitative studies on LGBTQ-parent families. Researchers may struggle with getting institutional support to conduct research involving LGBTQ people, as well as in engaging participants that are open about their sexual identity or behavior. Further, LGBTQ identities are not universal and throughout non-Western countries sexual and gender minorities may not necessarily identify with any of these categories despite maintaining same-gender romantic and/or sexual relationships. Studies using combined methodological approaches (qualitative and quantitative) are highly recommended in non-Western contexts as they may capture a more complete picture of the realities of LGBTQ-parent families in those rapidly changing regions. Lastly, we invite studies comparing LGBTQ-parent families from different countries and social contexts, namely Western and non-Western contexts, so that the similarities and differences in LGBTQ-parent families' lived experiences could be revealed.

In doing this review we also realized that in different social contexts, such as in the case of Israel and Mexico, studies on LGBTQ-parent families have almost exclusively examined the experiences of (cisgender) gay fathers, which highlights the need for research beyond the experiences of cisgender lesbian and gay parents, such as studies on plurisexual (e.g., bisexual, pansexual) parents, and trans or gender nonconforming parents in these non-Western contexts. Across the four regions included in this review, only very few bisexual parents were sampled and these were mostly merged with gay and lesbian parents, a research practice that has been underscored in a recent review on gay and bisexual fatherhood (Carneiro, Tasker, Salinas-Quiroz, Leal, & Costa, 2017). Regarding trans and gender nonconforming parent families, we were unable to locate any research from across the non-Western regions, which is aligned with the Western-based research trend mainly focused on cisgender gay and lesbian parents (see, e.g., van Eeden-Moorefield, Few-Demo, Benson, Bible, & Lummer, 2018). For plurisexual and gender nonconforming parents, the multiple challenges associated with being a minority in mostly heterosexist societies but also within the LGBTQ community makes them harder to recruit, and possibly to engage, in research on LGBTQ-parent families. Yet it is for this reason that it is so important that future research seek to give voice to these families in order to capture a more complete picture of the diversity of LGBTQ-parent families. Further, we suspect that the gender and sexual identities of researchers might also be linked to the accessibility and easiness to recruit such samples, and future studies should further explore this intriguing intersection between researchers' gender and sexual identities and LGBTQ-parent family type under study.

## Implications for Practice

In reviewing the studies from non-Western contexts, we found that intersecting with sociocultural aspects, other important factors shape the experiences of LGBTQ-parent families, namely parents' class and socioeconomic status, education level, and both parents and children's race/ethnic background. For example, studies from Brazil illustrated the different experiences of children in private or in public schools. While children in private schools were somewhat celebrated for having LGBTQ parents, children in public schools were not able to speak openly about their family configuration. Studies from South Africa further reported that some children with LGBTQ parents may feel oppressed by educators and school administrators' open religious views and opposition to homosexuality. Educators and practitioners need to become aware of their role in fostering acceptant and open environments within the school context that will allow children with LGBTQ parents to feel safe not to hide their family configuration, not to feel ashamed or embarrassed about having a diverse family, and not to be harassed by their peers.

These factors play an important role in determining how positive and empowered LGBTQ parents feel about themselves, but also how social contexts accept and integrate them. In some of the contexts reviewed here, it would be dangerous for people in same-gender relationships to live openly because their basic human rights are not recognized. In other contexts, LGBTQ people are *doing family* in ways that emulate or that are actual heterosexual relationships, because they are faced with a difficult choice: to live a same-gender relationship with the possibility of never having children or to establish a heterosexual relationship in order to have children. However, it is a testament to the strength of parenting desire among LGBTQ people how they find original ways of creating a family, and circumvent discriminatory laws and practices in face of prejudicial societies.

## Conclusion

Different social and cultural contexts construct different realities and experiences of LGBTQ-parent families and shape the research approaches in relation to these families. Westernized understandings of sexual and gender identities and relationships may not fully encompass or reflect the realities of LGBTQ-parent families from non-Western contexts without attention to their unique history and political climate (e.g., Breshears & Lubbe-De Beer, 2016). In light of this, this chapter focusing on non-Western contexts pushes Western understandings of LGBTQ-parent families by interpreting the research findings and the sometimes lack of research in the field within a cross-cultural perspective. One of the most important facets of these contexts is the impact of religion in shaping both the research in the field and the experiences of LGBTQ-parent families. Religion has been used in support of stigmatizing, discriminating, and often persecuting LGBTQ people (see chapter "Religion in the Lives of LGBTQ-Parent Families"), as still is the case across the non-Western regions reviewed in this chapter. Further, same-gender behavior is outlawed in several of these regions under the auspices of the dominant religion(s), regardless of specific denominations. Our review found evidence that in spite of differences between them, Islamism in the Middle East and parts of Africa, Christianity in other parts of Africa, Catholicism in Latin America, and Confucianism, Taoism, and Buddhism in Asia, all these denominations shared negative views of LGBTQ people. These negative views have an important impact on social understandings and acceptance of diverse sexual and gender identities, LGBTQ-parent families, and in particular, children with LGBTQ parents. Specifically, studies from South Africa and from Brazil reported how religious beliefs within school settings reinforced stigma against LGBTQ-parent families and thus constrained children's openness and confidence about their family.

There have been exciting new developments in the field of LGBTQ-parent families in non-Western contexts and most of the studies reviewed were published in the last decade. These developments have been facilitated by social transformations and legal advancements in the different societies. As these continue to evolve into more open and accepting societies of LGBTQ relationships and families, so will the research conducted in the four regions. More research is needed to continue to examine the impact of these changes for the well-being of LGBTQ parents and their children that may encourage both researchers and practitioners to further recognize and explore the resilience exercised by LGBTQ-parent families in non-Western contexts.

## References

Aguirre, S. G. (2015). Parenting practices of some gay men in Mexico City. Between taboos and new bets for their practice. *Sociedad y Economía, 29*, 39–62.

Ainsworth, M. D. S., Blehar, M. C., Waters, E., & Wall, S. (1978). *Patterns of attachment*. Hillsdale, NJ: Erlbaum.

Armesto, J. C. (2002). Developmental and contextual factors that influence gay fathers' parental competence: A review of the literature. *Psychology of Men & Masculinity, 3*, 67–78. https://doi.org/10.1037/1524-9220.3.2.67

Barrientos, J. (2016). The social and legal status of gay men, lesbians and transgender persons, and discrimination against the populations in Latin America. *Sexualidad, Salud y Sociedad – Revista Latinoamericana, 22*, 331–354. https://doi.org/10.1590/1984-6487. sess.2016.22.15.a

Barrientos, J., & Nardi, H. C. (2016). Introduction: Sexual minorities' discrimination in Iberian and Latin American countries. *Journal of Homosexuality, 63*, 1443–1445. https://doi.org/10.1080/00918639.2016.1 222823

Başoğlu, B. (2015). Legal status of same-sex couples within the framework of Turkish civil law. In M. Sáez (Ed.), *Same-sex couples: Comparative insights on marriage and cohabitation* (pp. 189–208). Dordrecht, the Netherlands: Springer.

Ben-Ari, A., & Livni, T. (2006). Motherhood is not a given thing: Experiences and constructed meanings of biological and nonbiological lesbian mothers. *Sex Roles, 54*, 521–531. https://doi.org/10.1007/ s11199-006-9016-0

Ben-Ari, A., & Weinberg-Kurnik, G. (2007). The dialectics between the personal and the interpersonal in the experiences of adoptive single mothers by choice. *Sex Roles, 56*, 823–833. https://doi.org/10.1007/ s11199-007-9241-1

Birenbaum-Carmeli, D., & Dirnfeld, M. (2008). The more the better? IVF policy in Israel and women's views. *Reproductive Health Matters, 16*, 1–10. https://doi.org/10.1016/S0968-8080(08)31352-4

Bonthuys, E. (2008). Possibilities foreclosed: The civil union act and lesbian and gay identity in southern Africa. *Sexualities, 11*, 726–739. https://doi.org/10.1177/1363460708096915

Breshears, D., & Lubbe-De Beer, C. (2014). A qualitative analysis of adult children's advice for parents coming out to their children. *Professional Psychology: Research and Practice, 45*, 231–238. https://doi.org/10.1037/a0035520

Breshears, D., & Lubbe-De Beer, C. (2016). Same-sex parented families' negotiation of minority social identity in South Africa. *Journal of GLBT Family Studies, 12*, 346–364. https://doi.org/10.1080/1550428X.2015.1080134

Carneiro, F. A., Tasker, F., Salinas-Quiroz, F., Leal, I., & Costa, P. A. (2017). Are the fathers alright? A systematic and critical review of studies on gay and bisexual fatherhood. *Frontiers in Psychology, 8*, 1636. https://doi.org/10.3389/fpsyg.2017.01636

Costa, P. A., & Salinas-Quiroz, F. (2018). A comparative study of attitudes toward same-gender parenting and gay and lesbian rights in Portugal and in Mexico. *Journal of Homosexuality.* Advance online publication. https://doi.org/10.1080/00918369.2018.1519303

Dankwa, S. O. (2009). "It's a silent trade": Female same-sex intimacies in post-colonial Ghana. *NORA – Nordic Journal of Feminist and Gender Research, 17*, 192–205. https://doi.org/10.1080/08038740903117208

Díaz, S. S., González, S. P., & Garrido, P. (2018). Being a mother outside heteronormativity: Vital trajectories and challenges of Chilean homoparental families. *Psicoperspectivas, 17*, 1–12. https://doi.org/10.5027/psicoperspectivas-vol17-issue1-fulltext-1202

Erera, P. I., & Segal-Engelchin, D. (2014). Gay men choosing to co-parent with heterosexual women. *Journal of GLBT Family Studies, 10*, 449–474. https://doi.org/10.1080/1550428X.2013.858611

Erez, C., & Shenkman, G. (2016). Gay dads are happier: Subjective well-being among gay and heterosexual fathers. *Journal of GLBT Family Studies, 12*, 451–467. https://doi.org/10.1080/1550428X.2015.1102668

Garcia, M. R. V., Wolf, A. G., Oliveira, E. V., Souza, J. T. F., Goncalves, L. O., & Oliveira, M. (2007). "Nao podemos falhar": A busca pela normalidade em familias homoparentais. In M. Grossi, A. P. Uziel, & L. Mello (Eds.), *Conjugalidades, parentalidades e identidades lésbicas, gays e travestis* (pp. 277–299). Rio de Janeiro, Brazil: Garamond.

Gross, A. (2014). The politics of LGBT rights in Israel and beyond: Nationality, normativity & queer politics. *Colombia Human Rights Law Review, 46*, 82–151. Retrieved from https://heinonlineorg.ezprimo1.idc.ac.il/HOL/Page?handle=hein.journals/colhr46&div=14&g_sent=1&casa_token=&collection=journals&t=1558332641

Grossi, M. P. (2003). Gênero e parentesco: Familias gays e lésbicas no Brasil. *Cadernos Pagu, 21*, 261–280. https://doi.org/10.1590/s0104-83332003000200011

Henrickson, M. (2018). Promoting the dignity and worth of all people: The privilege of social work. *International Social Work, 61*, 758–766. https://doi.org/10.1177/0020872816685616

Herdt, G. (1997). *Same sex, different cultures: Exploring gay and lesbian lives.* Boulder, CO: Westview Press.

Hernández, J. G., & Uziel, A. P. (2014). Famílias homoparentais e escola: Entre a vigilância e a transformação. *Momento, 23*, 9–24.

Hildebrandt, T. (2019). The one-child policy, eldercare, and LGB Chinese: A social policy explanation for family pressure. *Journal of Homosexuality, 66*, 590–608. https://doi.org/10.1080/00918369.2017.1422946

Inhorn, M. C., Birenbaum-Carmeli, D., Tremayne, S., & Gürtin, Z. B. (2017). Assisted reproduction and Middle East kinship: A regional and religious comparison. *Reproductive Biomedicine & Society Online, 4*, 41–51. https://doi.org/10.1016/j.rbms.2017.06.003

Ipsos. (2013, June). *Same-sex marriage: Citizens in 16 countries assess their views on same-sex marriage for a total global perspective.* Paris, France: Global @dvisor. Retrieved from https://www.ipsos.com/sites/default/files/news_and_polls/2013-06/6151-ppt.pdf

Jacques, G. (2013). Sexual minorities in Africa: A challenge for social work. *Journal of Gay and Lesbian Social Services, 25*, 158–177. https://doi.org/10.1080/10538720.2013.782835

Jeffreys, E., & Wang, P. (2018). Pathways to legalizing same-sex marriage in China and Taiwan: Globalization and "Chinese values". In B. Winters, M. Forest, & R. Sénac (Eds.), *Global perspectives on same-sex marriage* (pp. 197–219). Cham, Switzerland: Springer.

Ji, Y., Wu, X., Sun, S., & He, G. (2017). Unequal care, unequal work: Toward a more comprehensive understanding of gender inequality in post-reform urban China. *Sex Roles, 77*, 765–778. https://doi.org/10.1007/s11199-017-0751-1

Johnson, S. M. (2012). Lesbian mothers and their children: The third wave. *Journal of Lesbian Studies, 16*, 45–53. https://doi.org/10.1080/10894160.2011.557642

Kama, A. (2011). Parading pridefully into the mainstream: Gay and lesbian immersion in the civil core. In G. Ben-Porat & B. Turner (Eds.), *The contradictions of Israeli citizenship: Land, religion and state* (pp. 180–202). Abingdon, UK: Routledge.

Karimi, A., & Bayatrizi, Z. (2018). Dangerous positions: Male homosexuality in the new penal code of Iran. *Punishment & Society.* Advance online publication. https://doi.org/10.1177/1462474518787465

Kruger, L., Lubbe-De Beer, C., & Du Plessis, A.-B. (2016). Resilience in gay and lesbian parent families: Perspectives from the chrono-system. *Journal of Comparative Family Studies, 47*, 343–366. Retrieved from https://www.utpjournals.press/doi/abs/10.3138/jcfs.47.3.343

Laguna-Maqueda, O. E. (2016). Arreglos parentales de varones gay en la Ciudad de México: De la paternidad negada a la transformación inadvertida del cuidado. *MSC – Masculinities. Social Change, 5*, 182–204. https://doi.org/10.17583/MCS.2016.2033

Laguna-Maqueda, O. E. (2017). Un huésped no invitado: Homofobia en los arreglos parentales de padres gay en la Ciudad de México. *Cotidiano, 202*, 31–43.

Latinobarómetro. (2015). *Grado de acuerdo: Matrimónio entre personas del mismo sexo*. Retrieved from www.latinobarometro.org

Lavee, Y., & Katz, R. (2003). The family in Israel: Between tradition and modernity. *Marriage & Family Review, 35*, 193–217. https://doi.org/10.1300/J002v35n01_11

Lee, P. H. (2016). LGBT rights versus Asian values: De/re-constructing the universality of human rights. *The International Journal of Human Rights, 20*, 978–992. https://doi.org/10.1080/13642987.2016.1192537

Libson, M. (2010). Many ways of not being. Gay/lesbian right and the recognition of family contexts. *Sexualidad. Salud y Sociedad, 6*, 105–126. https://doi.org/10.1590/S1984-64872010000100006

Lira, A. N., Morais, N. A., & Boris, G. D. J. B. (2016). The (in)visibility of female homoparental experience: Between prejudice and overcomings. *Psicologia: Ciencia e Profissao, 36*, 20–33. https://doi.org/10.1590/1982-3703000152014

Lira, A. N., Morais, N. A., & Boris, G. D. J. B. (2017). Conceptions and ways of family living: The perspective of lesbian women who have children. *Psicologia: Teoria e Pesquisa, 32*, 1–10. https://doi.org/10.1590/0102.3772e324213

Liu, H., Feng, T., Ha, T., Liu, H., Cai, Y., … Li, J. (2011). Chinese culture, homosexuality stigma, social support and condom use: A path analytic model. *Stigma Research and Action, 1*, 27–35. https://doi.org/10.5463/sra.v1i1.16

Lubbe, C. (2007). To tell or not to tell: How children of same-gender parents negotiate their lives at school. *Education as Change, 11*, 45–65. https://doi.org/10.1080/16823200709487165

Lubbe, C. (2008a). Mothers, fathers or parents: Same-gendered families in South Africa. *Agenda, 76*, 43–55. https://doi.org/10.1080/10130950.2008.9674931

Lubbe, C. (2008b). The gift of growing up in a same-gendered family: A case study. *Journal of Psychology in Africa, 18*, 89–96. https://doi.org/10.1080/14330237.2008.10820175

Lubbe, C. (2008c). The experiences of children growing up in lesbian-headed families in South Africa. *Journal of GLBT Family Studies, 4*, 325–359. https://doi.org/10.1080/15504280802177540

Menassé, A. A. (2017). Mental health professionals and their relationship with homo-parental families in Mexico. *Debate Feminista, 54*, 17–33. https://doi.org/10.1016/j.df.2017.07.002

Menassé, A. A., Cosme, J. A. G., & Rodríguez, M- M. G. (2014). Experiências de famílias homoparentales com profesionales de la psicología en Mexico, Distrito Federal. Una aproximación cualitativa. *Cuicuilco, 59*, 211–236.

Miguel, F. (2016). (Homo)sexualidades masculinas em Cabo Verde: Um caso para pensar teorias antropológicas e movimento LGBT em África. *Enfoque, 15*, 87–110.

Msibi, T. (2011). The lies we have been told: On (homo)sexuality in Africa. *Africa Today, 58*, 5–77. https://doi.org/10.2979/africatoday.58.1.55

Msibi, T. (2013). Denied love: Same-sex desire, agency and social oppression among African men who engage in same-sex relationships. *Agenda, 27*, 105–116. https://doi.org/10.1080/10130950.2013.811014

Muedini, F. (2018). *LGBTI rights in Turkey: Sexuality and the state in the Middle East*. Cambridge, UK: Cambridge University Press.

Needham, J. (2012). After the Arab spring: A new opportunity for LGBT human rights advocacy. *Duke Journal of Gender Low & Policy, 20*, 287–323.

Nomaguchi, K. M., & Milkie, M. A. (2003). Costs and rewards of children: The effects of becoming a parent on adults' lives. *Journal of Marriage and Family, 65*, 356–374. https://doi.org/10.1111/j.1741-3737.2003.00356.x

Palma, Y. A., & Strey, M. N. (2015). The school and family relationship: Family diversity composing the school context. *Revista de Psicología, 24*, 1–17. https://doi.org/10.5354/0719-0581.2015.36918

Palma, Y. A., Strey, M. N., & Krugel, G. (2012). Mommy and mommy? The narratives of homomaternal families. *Revista Iberoamericana de Psicologia: Ciencia e Tecnologia, 5*, 81–90.

Pontes, M. F., Féres-Carneiro, T., & Magalhães, A. S. (2017). Homoparentalidade feminina: Laço biológico e laço afetivo na dinâmica familiar. *Psicologia USP, 28*, 276–286. https://doi.org/10.1590/0103-656420150175

Riquelme, M. F. (2017). Haciendo família en el Chile del siglo XXI: Desafíos y possibilidades para personas LGBT. In J. Zandoná, A. M. Veiga, & C. Nichnig (Eds.), *Proceedings of the XI Seminário Internacional Fazendo Gênero* (pp. 1–9). Florianópolis, Brazil: UFSC.

Salinas-Quiroz, F., Rodríguez-Sánchez, F., Costa, P. A., Rosales, M., Silva, P., & Cambón, V. (2018). Can children have ordinary expectable environments in unconventional contexts? Quality of care organization in three Mexican same-sex planned families. *Frontiers in Psychology, 9*, 2349. https://doi.org/10.3389/fpsyg.2018.02349

Samani, R. O., Dizaj, A. V. T., Moalem, M. R. R., Merghati, S. T., & Alizadeh, L. (2007). Access to fertility treatments for homosexual and unmarried persons, through Iranian law and Islamic perspective. *Iranian Journal of Fertility and Sterility, 1*, 127–130. Retrieved from http://ijfs.ir/journal/article/abstract/2311

Sanches, I. R., Pelissoli, M. S., Lomando, E. M., & Levandowski, D. C. (2017). The social support network of homoaffective families constituted by women. *Gerais: Revista Interinstitucional de Psicologia, 10*, 176–193.

Segal-Engelchin, D., Erera, P., & Cwikel, J. (2005). The hetero-gay family: An emergent family configuration. *Journal of GLBT Family Studies, 1*, 85–104. https://doi.org/10.1300/J461v01n03_04

Shechner, T., Slone, M., Lobel, T. E., & Shechter, R. (2013). Children's adjustment in non-traditional families in Israel: The effect of parental sexual orientation and the number of parents on children's development. *Child: Care, Health and Development, 39*, 178–184. https://doi.org/10.1111/j.1365-2214.2011.01337.x

Shechner, T., Slone, M., Meir, Y., & Kalish, Y. (2010). Relations between social support and psychological and parental distress for lesbian, single heterosexual by choice, and two-parent heterosexual mothers. *American Journal of Orthopsychiatry, 80*, 283–292. https://doi.org/10.1111/j.1939-0025.2010.01031.x

Shenkman, G. (2012). The gap between fatherhood and couplehood desires among Israeli gay men and estimations of their likelihood. *Journal of Family Psychology, 26*, 828–832. https://doi.org/10.1037/a0029471

Shenkman, G. (2018). The association between basic need satisfaction in relationship and personal growth among lesbian and heterosexual mothers. *Journal of Social and Personal Relationships, 35*, 246–262. https://doi.org/10.1177/0265407516681192

Shenkman, G., Ifrah, K., & Shmotkin, D. (2018). Meaning in life among middle-aged and older gay and heterosexual fathers. *Journal of Family Issues, 39*, 2155–2173. https://doi.org/10.1177/01925 13X17741922

Shenkman, G., & Shmotkin, D. (2014). "Kids are joy": Psychological welfare among Israeli gay fathers. *Journal of Family Issues, 35*, 1926–1939. https://doi.org/10.1177/0192513X13489300

Shenkman, G., & Shmotkin, D. (2016). The association between self-perceived parental role and meaning in life among gay and heterosexual fathers. *Journal of Family Psychology, 30*, 552–561. https://doi.org/10.1037/fam0000213

Shenkman, G., & Shmotkin, D. (2019). The association between self-perceived parental role and mental health concomitants among Israeli gay and heterosexual fathers. *Journal of Homosexuality*. Advance online publication. https://doi.org/10.1080/00918369.2018.1 555392

Shokeid, M. (2003). Closeted cosmopolitans: Israeli gays between center and periphery. *Global Networks, 3*, 387–399. https://doi.org/10.1111/14710374.00068

Sion, L., & Ben-Ari, E. (2009). Imagined masculinity: Body, sexuality, and family among Israeli military reserves. *Symbolic Interaction, 32*, 21–43. https://doi.org/10.1525/si.2009.32.1.21

Souza, F. M. (2014). Discretos e declarados: Relatos sobre a dinâmica da vida dos homossexuais em Maputo, Moçambique. *Revista Olhares Sociais, 3*, 76–101.

Stacey, J., & Biblarz, T. K. (2001). (How) does the sexual orientation of parents matter? *American Sociological Review, 66*, 159–183. https://doi.org/10.2307/2657413

Tamagawa, M. (2016). Same-sex marriage in Japan. *Journal of GLBT Family Studies, 12*, 160–187. https://doi.org/10.1080/1550428X.2015.1016252

Teman, E. (2010). The last outpost of the nuclear family: A cultural critique of Israeli surrogacy policy. In D. Birenbaum-Carmeli & Y. S. Carmeli (Eds.), *Kin, gen, community: Reproductive technologies among Jewish Israelis* (pp. 107–122). New York, NY: Berghahn Books.

Tombolato, M. A., Maia, A. C. B., Uziel, A. P., & Santos, M. A. (2018). Prejudice and discrimination in the everyday life of same-sex couples raising children. *Estudos de Psicologia Campinas, 35*, 111–122. https://doi.org/10.1590/1982-02752018000100011

Tsfati, M., & Ben-Ari, A. (2019). Between the social and the personal: Israeli male gay parents, surrogacy and socio-political concepts of parenthood and gender. *Journal of GLBT Family Studies, 15*, 42–57. https://doi.org/10.1080/1550428X.2017.1413475

van Eeden-Moorefield, B., Few-Demo, A. L., Benson, K., Bible, J., & Lummer, S. (2018). A content analysis of LGBT research in top family journals 2000-2015. *Journal of Family Issues, 39*, 1374–1395. https://doi.org/10.1177/0192513X17710284

Van Ewyk, J., & Kruger, L.-M. (2017). The emotional experience of motherhood in planned lesbian families in the South African context: "… Look how good a job I'm doing, look how amazing we are". *Journal of Homosexuality, 64*, 343–366. https://doi.org/10.1080/00918369.2016.1190216

Velasco, M. L. H. (2006). Significado y ejercicio de los roles parentales entre varones homosexuales. *Revista de Estudios de Género La Ventana, 23*, 127–165.

Vitule, C., Couto, M. T., & Machin, R. (2015). Same-sex couples and parenthood: A look at the use of reproductive technologies. *Interface – Comunicacao, Saude, Educacao, 19*, 1169–1180. https://doi.org/10.1590/1807-57622014.0401

Xie, Y., & Peng, M. (2018). Attitudes toward homosexuality in China: Exploring the effects of religion, modernizing factors, and traditional culture. *Journal of Homosexuality, 65*, 1758–1787. https://doi.org/10.10 80/00918369.2017.1386025

Yadegarfard, M., & Bahramabadian, F. (2014). Sexual orientation and human rights in the ethics code of the psychology and counseling organization of the Islamic Republic of Iran (PCOIRI). *Ethics & Behavior, 24*, 350–363. https://doi.org/10.1080/10508422.2013.84 5733

Ziv, I., & Freund-Eschar, Y. (2015). The pregnancy experience of gay couples expecting a child through overseas surrogacy. *The Family Journal, 23*, 158–166. https://doi.org/10.1177/1066480714565107

# Separation and Divorce Among LGBTQ-Parent Families

Rachel H. Farr, Kyle A. Simon, and Abbie E. Goldberg

Many studies have investigated the couple relationships of lesbian, gay, bisexual, transgender, and queer (LGBTQ) individuals, especially those of same-sex couples. Much less is known, however, about processes of separation and divorce among LGBTQ adults whose couple relationships come to an end. With a growing number of countries worldwide providing marriage equality for same-sex couples and increased legal recognition of LGBTQ identities broadly, it is timely to also consider the increasing prospect of legal same-sex divorce and its possible consequences for the health and well-being of LGBTQ-parent families. A growing number of studies have compared married other-sex couples with same-sex couples who are married, in civil unions, or have other forms of legal relationship recognition. As many LGBTQ people are parents and are opting for legal marriage (Gates, 2015; Goldberg & Conron, 2018), it is likely that a greater number of children with LGBTQ parents will experience their parents' legal divorce. It is not necessarily new that some children with LGBTQ parents have experienced their parents' relationship dissolution, yet historically speaking, these couple relationships have not received legal recognition. Lack of legal recognition has resulted in unique forms of stress as well as certain possible advantages for families, as we will discuss (Goldberg & Allen, 2013; Goldberg & Kuvalanka, 2012).

As divorce (or relationship dissolution) can be especially stressful and challenging to couples when children are involved, this chapter is devoted to knowledge regarding relationship dissolution among LGBTQ-parent families. A central question in considering this topic is: What happens for LGBTQ individuals in couples who are parents, and to their children, following separation or divorce? To address this, we draw on (a) available research on couple separation and divorce among LGBTQ adults, (b) the limited existing research about the experiences and outcomes for children and parents in LGBTQ-parent families who experience separation and divorce, and (c) relevant parallel literature about children who experience separation and divorce in the context of cisgender heterosexual parent families.

## Overview and Theory

Much of the research about dissolution and divorce among LGBTQ adults, consistent with broader literature on LGBTQ-parent families, has either lacked clear integrated theoretical

R. H. Farr (✉) · K. A. Simon
Department of Psychology, University of Kentucky, Lexington, KY, USA
e-mail: rachel.farr@uky.edu; kyle.simon@uky.edu

A. E. Goldberg
Department of Psychology, Clark University, Worcester, MA, USA
e-mail: agoldberg@clarku.edu

© Springer Nature Switzerland AG 2020
A. E. Goldberg, K. R. Allen (eds.), *LGBTQ-Parent Families*,
https://doi.org/10.1007/978-3-030-35610-1_21

frameworks or has drawn from a limited number of theories, namely, minority stress, ecological, feminist, family systems, and queer theory (Farr, Tasker, & Goldberg, 2017; van Eeden-Moorefield, Few-Demo, Benson, Bible, & Lummer, 2018). Much of the atheoretical work on LGBTQ-parent families has been motivated by issues of public debate and policy, such as questions surrounding same-sex marriage, rather than building from established theories in the social sciences or humanities. Regardless, we approach our literature review in this chapter from theoretical and conceptual frameworks that have been commonly applied to studies of LGBTQ-parent families, including those relevant to relationship dissolution (e.g., ambiguous loss theory; Allen, 2007). These broad frameworks also include developmental, ecological systems, family systems, and gender theories, as well as perspectives about economic, legal, and policy concerns and challenges to heteronormativity (Farr et al., 2017; Gartrell, Bos, Peyser, Deck, & Rodas, 2011; Kurdek, 2004; van Eeden-Moorefield, Martell, Williams, & Preston, 2011; Wiik, Seierstad, & Noack, 2014).

Throughout this chapter, we highlight specific issues that face families with LGBTQ parents who divorce, including unique family and relationship dynamics, lack of cultural models for LGBTQ people who divorce, and legal and practical concerns. We devote particular attention to unique family dynamics and concerns facing transgender individuals and their families as related to processes of couple separation and divorce. We emphasize what is known from the literature about couple dissolution and divorce among LGBTQ *parents*, yet the literature is complicated by studies that include samples of both parents and child-free couples, as well as studies that predated same-sex marriage. Thus, we clarify and contextualize wherever possible who is represented within research samples and whether legal relationship recognition was an option. Finally, we offer evidence-based recommendations and implications for families who may be vulnerable to or experiencing divorce or dissolution, including guidance particularly for LGBTQ parents and their children. It is important to note that available studies have generally focused attention on LG-parent families and more recently begun to include BTQ-parent families. Thus, much of our literature review focuses on studies of LG couples and parents, though we incorporate attention to diverse sexual and gender minority identities wherever possible.

## Risk for Couple Dissolution and the Role of Children Among LGBTQ Adults

### Dissolution Rates for Same-Sex Couples

Beginning in the 1980s and 1990s, researchers documented a higher dissolution rate for same-sex couples[1] as compared with heterosexual couples (Blumstein & Schwartz, 1983; Kurdek, 1998). This earlier work, largely inspired by the need for research in court custody cases (Farr et al., 2017), was limited, however, in comparing unmarried LG couples to married heterosexual couples (e.g., Kurdek, 2004; Oswald & Clausell, 2006). As social and legal climates have shifted, at least some studies indicate that same- and other-sex couples break-up at similar rates, and this similarity appears particularly true among same-sex couples who are married, in marriage-like relationships (e.g., civil unions, domestic partnerships, or other couple relationships with legal obligations differing from marriage), or who are parents (Goldberg & Garcia, 2015; Manning, Brown, & Stykes, 2016; Rosenfeld, 2014).

Research conducted internationally has revealed a variety of trends in rates of same-sex couple dissolution. In a study conducted in Taiwan, same-sex couple relationships were found to be characterized by greater instability than married couples overall (Shieh, Hsiao, & Tseng, 2009). In the United Kingdom (UK), Lau

---

[1] Although we use "same-sex," "female and male," and "lesbian and gay" interchangeably to refer to couples for consistency with terms used in original sources, we acknowledge that individual partners within couples may represent greater diversity (e.g., queer, bisexual, etc.).

(2012) employed two large population studies with data from 1974 to 2004 and found that cohabiting (nonmarried) same-sex couples were twice as likely to dissolve their relationships as were cohabiting (nonmarried) heterosexual couples and that male same-sex couples were more likely to break up than female same-sex couples. In countries such as Norway and Sweden, same-sex married couples have been found to be more likely to break up than married heterosexual couples, and in contrast to Lau's findings in the UK, female couples were twice as likely as male couples to break up (Andersson, Noack, Seierstad, & Weedon-Fekjaer, 2006).

## Dissolution Rates Among Same-Sex Couples with Children

Some studies regarding separation and divorce among same-sex couples with children have revealed contrasting findings related to the likelihood of breaking up based on parenting status. In Norway, Wiik et al. (2014) found that after 18 years, female same-sex couples were more likely to break up (45%) than male same-sex couples (40%). Having children, however, was protective for female same-sex couples but increased the risk for male same-sex couples (Wiik et al., 2014). In the United States of America (USA), among lesbian parents with children conceived through donor insemination, 40 of 73 couples (55%) had dissolved their relationships by the time children were 17 years old, as compared with a 36% divorce rate among heterosexual couples with 17-year-old children in the US National Survey of Family Growth (Gartrell, Bos, & Goldberg, 2011). Other studies in the USA comparing same-sex and other-sex couples who adopted children have revealed that lesbian couples were more likely to break up than gay or heterosexual parents over a 5-year timespan (Farr, 2017a; Goldberg & Garcia, 2015). Still other studies, such as those in Norway and Sweden, have not found differences in divorce rates among couples with children as a function of sexual orientation (i.e., lesbian, gay, heterosexual; Andersson et al., 2006).

## Predictors of Same-Sex Couple Dissolution

Even with possible differences in separation and divorce rates among same- and other-sex couples, correlates of dissolution—namely, relationship satisfaction, commitment, discrepant or low-income levels, lower educational attainment, younger ages, and partner age gaps—are similar for couples across studies (Andersson et al., 2006; Balsam, Rostosky, & Riggle, 2017; Balsam, Rothblum, & Wickham, 2017; Lau, 2012; Shieh, 2016; Shieh et al., 2009). Available data suggest that many factors that predict relationship dissatisfaction and disruption for cisgender heterosexual couples also do so among LG couples (Gottman et al., 2003; Kurdek, 2004). In comparing heterosexual parent couples with LG and heterosexual nonparent couples, Kurdek (2006) reported that predictors of relationship quality, stability, and commitment—namely, expressiveness, positive perception of one's partner, social support—were similar across couples, regardless of parenting status.

Although some same-sex couples may be more likely to get or stay married when they have children (Andersson et al., 2006; Balsam, Beauchaine, Rothblum, & Solomon, 2008; Goldberg & Conron, 2018; Wiik et al., 2014), some research has indicated that stresses related to parenting may contribute to experiences of separation and divorce among LGBTQ adults. Similar to heterosexual parenting couples (Amato, 2010; Lansford, 2009), many same-sex couples with children who dissolve their relationships cite parenting issues as a factor in their break-up. Studies among lesbian couples have indicated that differences in or disagreements about parenting are reported as common contributors to the relationship termination (Goldberg, Moyer, Black, & Henry, 2015; Turteltaub, 2002). Similarly, inequities in (and dissatisfaction with) the division of childcare responsibilities have been identified among lesbian adoptive mothers as reason for dissolution (Farr, 2017b; Goldberg et al., 2015). As research has demonstrated a tendency of LGBTQ adults to value egalitarianism and equity in their relationships, it may be particularly stressful when equity is lacking in coparenting responsibilities (e.g., Farr, 2017b; Goldberg et al., 2015).

Taken together, available research indicates that same-sex unions may be more at risk for dissolution than heterosexual unions, but it also appears that same- and other-sex couples end their relationships for similar reasons. Furthermore, the possible higher risk of dissolution for same-sex couples may be moderated by gender identity, the presence of children, and, as we discuss in the next section, marriage and other legal recognition.

## Legal Recognition of Couple Relationships and Parenting Among LGBTQ Adults

In general, legal recognition (e.g., marriage) is understood to have a "stabilizing" effect on intimate relationships, creating emotional, social, legal, and financial incentives to stay and financial barriers to leaving (Balsam et al., 2008; Rosenfeld, 2014). Most research indicating higher same-sex dissolution risk has resulted from comparisons of nonmarried cohabiting same-sex couples with married heterosexual couples. Yet new evidence is emerging that compares married other-sex couples to same-sex couples in marriages, civil unions, or other legal relationships. For example, in the UK, same-sex couples in civil partnerships were actually found to show fewer dissolutions than married heterosexual couples (Ross, Gask, & Berrington, 2011). Similarly, among couples in the USA, dissolution rates were lower across a 3-year period among same-sex couples with legal relationship recognition (i.e., civil unions) and married heterosexual couples as compared to same-sex couples not in civil unions (Balsam et al., 2008). Interestingly, more recently, this same research group observed that same-sex couples who had legalized their union over a 12-year period were no more likely to stay together than were those who had not (Balsam, Rothblum, et al., 2017). Rosenfeld (2014) also found that same-sex couples in marriages or marriage-like relationships in the USA were no more likely than heterosexual married couples to end their relationships.

There is some evidence that when same-sex couples have children together, they may be more likely to get married or stay married. In Balsam et al.'s (2008) study (in the USA), men in civil unions were found to be more likely to have children than male same-sex couples not in civil unions. In a study of same-sex couples in Vermont (civil unions), Massachusetts (marriages), and California (domestic partnerships), female couples were more likely to report having children than were male couples (Rothblum, Balsam, & Solomon, 2008). Recent research in the USA also reveals that married same-sex couples are more likely than unmarried same-sex couples to have children (Goldberg & Conron, 2018). In Rosenfeld's (2014) study, however, the presence of children in the household was not found to be associated with the dissolution of same-sex marriages or "marriage-like" relationships.

Now that marriage is available to same-sex parents, and thus to many LGBTQ persons in the USA, the implication is that divorce and custody battles will also become more common simply by nature of marriage. Among LGBTQ parenting couples, children may not be biologically related to either or both parents, yet marriage (as well as legal divorce from that marriage) may provide cohesive relationships between parents and children recognized as one family (Dodge, 2006). Historically, and particularly prior to same-sex marriage rights in the USA, only one partner might be the legal parent rights to the couple's children (if the partner had not adopted or could not legally adopt the children via co-parent or second-parent adoption; Gartrell, Bos, Peyser, et al., 2011; van Eeden-Moorefield et al., 2011).[2] The legal parent, who is commonly a biological parent, particularly among female same-sex couples who have children via donor insemination, often has much greater power than the other parent (Goldberg & Allen, 2013). Indeed, biological parents have traditionally been favored by judges over any other parental figures who have been involved in childrearing

---

[2]It is important to note that even with the availability of same-sex marriage, legal parenting rights for same-sex partners may still be called into question by some courts in the USA.

responsibilities (Goldberg & Allen, 2013). There is evidence that this bias continues to operate, even when same-sex couples who were legally married are divorcing and negotiating custody arrangements. Given that federal marriage equality granted through *Obergefell v. Hodges* (2015) did not confer full parenting recognition (legal parenthood) via same-sex marriage, nonbiological parents within married same-sex couples are particularly vulnerable in custody disputes (Farr & Goldberg, 2018). Without legal protections, the nonlegal parent might in turn be forced to sever relationships with children after same-sex relationship dissolution, which could be devastating to parents and children involved (Allen, 2007). Both the potential sudden and also ambiguous loss of a parent as a consequence of couple relationship dissolution has the potential to adversely affect children, and this loss is more likely that of the nonlegal, nonbiological parent (Allen, 2007).

## Outcomes for LGBTQ Parents and Their Children After Divorce

### Adjustment of LGBTQ Parents Post-Dissolution

Patterns of adjustment facing LGBTQ individuals in couples post-divorce are likely similar in many ways to those of cisgender heterosexual couples who split up. In addition, family processes following divorce among LGBTQ-parent families are presumably comparable in many ways to those among families headed by cisgender heterosexual parents. For example, LGBTQ-parent families who experience divorce may also be met with financial challenges (e.g., due to the financial hardship of going from one residence to two residences). Lesbian adoptive mothers who are separated have also been found to report financial insecurity and worries (Goldberg et al., 2015), and other research indicates that same-sex couples who divorce may be at increased risk for financial difficulties (van Eeden-Moorefield et al., 2011). Indeed, research with heterosexual parents also documents substantial changes in financial status after divorce, often with marked declines for women, who often have primary custody of (and caretaking responsibilities for) children (Greene, Anderson, Forgatch, DeGarmo, & Hetherington, 2012; Lansford, 2009).

## Child Adjustment After Their LGBTQ Parents' Couple Relationship Ends

Existing literature is scant about children's adjustment following the dissolution of their LGBTQ parents' couple relationship, so we first briefly review what we know from the ample knowledge base about children who experience the divorce of their cisgender heterosexual parents. We do this to draw parallels to the likely similarities with the experiences of children with LGBTQ parents, as well as to highlight where experiences may be unique for these children. There is clear consensus that although children who experience their cisgender heterosexual parents' divorce are at greater risk for adjustment problems than are children from nondivorced families, the great majority do not develop behavioral difficulties related to their parents' divorce (Greene et al., 2012; Lansford, 2009). Many children demonstrate responses that are considered normative reactions to parental divorce, such as anger, confusion, anxiety, and sadness upon experiencing their parents' divorce, but are often resilient in the face of this family transition with consistent parental support and involvement (Greene et al., 2012). Amato (2010) discusses the concept of psychological pain resulting from divorce as distinct from effects on psychological adjustment; although the adjustment of many children of divorce is not adversely affected in any enduring way, it is the case that psychological pain often persists.

Ample research from the past 30 years clearly indicates that children with LGBTQ parents develop on par with their peers with cisgender heterosexual parents (for reviews, see Biblarz & Stacey, 2010; Goldberg, Gartrell, & Gates, 2014; Moore & Stambolis-Ruhstorfer, 2013; Patterson, 2017). Thus, the adjustment of children who experience the dissolution of their LGBTQ parents' relationship is likely to be similar to children who experience their heterosexual parents' divorce. We expect that future research will reveal that some children who experience their LGBTQ parents' divorce will show persistent decreases in adjustment (at least in the short-term), but most will show typical adjustment over the long-term. Indeed, qualitative interview data from young adults with separated LGBTQ parents also suggest that they may experience ongoing sadness associated with their parents' relationship dissolution (Goldberg & Allen, 2013). Another similarity to cisgender heterosexual parent families is that children with LGBTQ parents describe financial challenges following couple relationship dissolution. For example, Turteltaub (2002) found that children with separated lesbian mothers mention financial hardships related to having two residences, having less space, and moving frequently. Similarly, just as parental conflict is related to children's lower well-being among divorced cisgender heterosexual parent families (Amato, 2010; Lansford, 2009), parenting disagreements post-separation are likely to be detrimental for children with LGBTQ parents. It is imperative, however, to mention that such conflict is often most intense around the time of the divorce and often dissipates over time. As such, any negative child outcomes tied to parental conflict during dissolution and divorce may not endure. Available evidence from studies of separated lesbian mothers support this notion: mothers who report amicable relationships with former partners describe their children as coping better than expected (Gartrell, Rodas, Deck, Peyser, & Banks, 2006).

In contrast, some post-separation issues that children face in the wake of their LGBTQ parents' relationship dissolution are unique (Gahan, 2018). Just as legal marriage might confer social and practical benefits to parents and children in LGBTQ-parent families, legal divorce might serve to disadvantage children by diminishing access to material resources, destabilizing (at least temporarily) family relationships, and potentially exposing children to stigma given their combined status of having divorced and sexual minority parents (Lansford, 2009; Oswald & Clausell, 2006). It should be noted, however, that relationship dissolution may have negative

effects regardless of whether the couple relationship had been legally recognized. In one study, young adults ($N = 20$) who had experienced their same-sex parents' relationship dissolution noted that the pain they felt about the break-up was accentuated by the lack of legal relationship recognition (Goldberg & Allen, 2013). They felt that the end of their parents' relationship was minimized—and as a result, they felt that outsiders often did not understand or empathize with their experience. Children of lesbian mothers have also noted difficulties in disclosing about their parents' separation, in part because of pervasive heteronormative assumptions about having a mother and father, yet they also felt positively about their families and were protective of their mothers (Turteltaub, 2002). In another study of 40 separated lesbian mother families (formed through donor insemination) with adolescent children, results showed that children generally showed positive life satisfaction and well-being in the years following the separation (Gartrell, Bos, Peyser, et al., 2011). Thus, although there may be unique challenges for children of LGBTQ parents, they also demonstrate resilience in their short- and long-term adjustment to their parents' relationship dissolution.

## Separation and Divorce Experienced by Transgender Persons and Their Children

Given the lack of research focusing on transgender persons more generally, it is unsurprising to find that there is little to no work on the experiences of transgender persons and divorce. The research that does exist indicates that transgender individuals face unique challenges related to couple relationship dynamics (Joslin-Roher & Wheeler, 2009; Meier, Sharp, Michonski, Babcock, & Fitzgerald, 2013; Simpson, 2017). The transitioning process for transgender people may lead to relationship dissolution or divorce if an individual is transitioning during the relationship (Meier et al., 2013), and particularly if it is it in the context of that long-term relationship that the individual first realizes, and comes to term with, their transgender identity (Simpson, 2017). One partner's gender transition may raise key questions related to both partners' individual sexual identities as well as their identity as a couple—which may or may not be a unique source of relationship strain. For example, if a transgender man is still in a relationship with a lesbian woman, what does that mean for them as a couple as related to their individual identities? One study that included 140 transgender men in relationships prior to transitioning reported that half of the relationships ($n = 70$) ended due to transition-related reasons (e.g., differing sexual identities, inability for relationship to adjust to changes; Meier et al., 2013). Possible discrepancies in identity are likely to increase stress between partners as they navigate new social dynamics, gender roles, and sexualities for which they do not have models (Joslin-Roher & Wheeler, 2009).

As existing work regarding divorce among transgender parents is primarily qualitative, we next review several studies to provide understanding of this newly emerging and important area of study among LGBTQ-parent families. It seems that divorce may be particularly common for transgender women who transition later in life, after having raised children in the roles of father and husband. Simpson's (2017) interviews with 10 transgender women who transitioned "late-in-life" (between 40 and 65 years) found evidence that all 10 women experienced divorce in part because of their transition. Many of these women referenced the pressure and harm that rigid gender roles associated with being fathers and husbands in families exerted on themselves and their relationships. Given the age of these transgender women, many had also internalized the belief that raising a child in a household without a father was detrimental to their children, which delayed their coming out and transitioning (Simpson, 2017).

Research has also addressed the experiences of spouses of transgender individuals across their partner's transition. Alegría's (2010) interviews about the reactions of cisgender women to their partner disclosing and transitioning as a male-to-female person revealed largely positive experiences. While all the cisgender wives in this study

($N = 17$) expressed shock and grief over the loss of their husband several years prior, all of them were still married, and many had already been married for over a decade. Almost all (16 of 17) described that they were able to communicate openly and have some say in the timeline of their partner's transition (e.g., needing additional time before their partner started chemical transitioning) while providing space for their partner to be their authentic selves. Finally, several reported that the realization that they *could* divorce and leave their partners led to an increased commitment to their marriage as an act of self-determination and empowered their relationship dynamics (Alegría, 2010).

Some transgender parents experience positive outcomes and dynamics following their divorce. For instance, von Doussa, Power, and Riggs (2017) found that some transgender parents divorced after coming out but were still amicable with spouses and their children. One transgender woman in their sample shared that her divorce from her cisgender, heterosexual wife allowed both members of the couple to develop new lives while maintaining a positive relationship. Another participant described how experiencing a family rupture after coming out removed the secrecy surrounding their identity, which allowed a space for positive identity exploration for all members of the family. Indeed, although some transgender parents do report child rejection and the denial of visitation rights following a divorce, often parent-child relationships are mutually positive (Church, O'Shea, & Lucey, 2014).

One way in which marriages and parent-child relationships are positively maintained is by extending the time between social and physical gender transitioning (Alegría, 2010). Slowing their path to transitioning, but not stopping it, is one way in which transgender parents successfully navigate their new family role. Additionally, encouraging dialectical thinking (i.e., both/and instead of either/or), a perspective from ambiguous loss theory (Boss, 2013), for all family members also seems to ease the family transition. For example, in Dierckx, Mortelmans, Motmans, and T'Sjoen's (2017), interviews with children of transgender parents who transitioned after becoming a parent revealed that what was helpful for the entire family was being able to simultaneously acknowledge, without fear of stigmatization, that their parent had previously been their father and that they now have two mothers. Thus, it is important to consider the complexity and nuances of dissolution and divorce experiences among transgender individuals and their families: family ruptures can be both painful and negative, but also create new spaces for family members to support one another and develop family resilience.

## Intersectionality Related to LGBTQ-Parent Couple Separation and Divorce

We know little about unique factors that may facilitate the endurance or dissolution of couple relationships among LGBTQ adults. Less attention has been paid to the roles of age, race, economic status, gender identity and expression, immigration status, geographic location, urbanicity/rurality, and pathways to parenthood in shaping same-sex relationship trajectories and outcomes. Related to gender, future research is needed to provide clarity regarding the mixed results about couple dissolution rates among LGBTQ adults. Numerous studies across cultural contexts have reported conflicting results regarding whether female or male same-sex couples are more likely to break up (e.g., Andersson et al., 2006; Farr, 2017a; Lau, 2012; Rosenfeld, 2014; Shieh, 2016; Wiik et al., 2014). Thus, the potentially unique contributions of gender identity to dissolution rates and processes among couples with LGBTQ-identified members are not yet well understood. In addition, few studies about relationship dissolution among LGBTQ adults have included large samples that are racially and socioeconomically diverse. Thus, research is needed that attends to how race and class intersect with sexual orientation and relational context to shape processes and outcomes related to marriage and relationship dissolution among couples who are parents.

Several studies have examined the role of geographic location, largely in terms of rates of couple relationship dissolution as related to access to legal relationship recognition in different countries worldwide. This research has revealed that geographic location translates to differential rates of couple relationship longevity across countries with variable same-sex marriage laws, as well as parent-child relationship dynamics, such that a lack of legal parenting recognition is linked with anxiety for children and parents involved (Balsam et al., 2008; Gartrell, Bos, Peyser, et al., 2011; Ross et al., 2011). Demographic research has also revealed variations in the numbers of same-sex parents across states, including higher numbers of racial minority than White same-sex parents, and a higher proportion of racial minority same-sex parents live in Southern states as compared to other parts of the USA (Gates, 2013). Thus, with marriage equality recognized in the USA, it would be ideal to examine how LGBTQ-parent families, in different regions and locales, experience parental relationship recognition (i.e., marriage) and divorce similarly and differently. For example, do parents and children in urban, more progressive areas experience different community responses to parental marriage and divorce? Where do they seek support during and after relationship dissolution? Current research suggests that LGBTQ individuals feel more isolated in rural contexts and have fewer community resources (e.g., local LGBTQ community centers), which may be associated with increased minority stressors or a lack of social recognition (Oswald & Culton, 2003; see chapter "LGBTQ-Parent Families in Community Context"), and in turn lead to relationship dissolution (Oswald, Goldberg, Kuvalanka, & Clausell, 2008). To the best of our knowledge, however, no research has focused on the differences (or similarities) in relationship dissolution among LGBTQ-parent families based on geographic location (Moore, 2015; Moore & Stambolis-Ruhstorfer, 2013).

Finally, LGBTQ adults' diverse pathways to parenthood (e.g., assisted reproduction, adoption, step-parenting, etc.) in relation to risk for and processes surrounding couple separation and divorce have not been studied systematically. Research, however, suggests that families formed through adoption, for example, may encounter unique issues that can create stress, such as their children's multiple prior placements, history of abuse or neglect, and consequent attachment and emotional/behavioral issues (Goldberg, 2010). Indeed, in Goldberg et al.'s (2015) study of lesbian adoptive mothers who were dissolving their relationships, women sometimes cited their children's special needs (i.e., attachment or behavioral difficulties) as contributing to stress and their ensuing relationship dissolution.

## Future Research Directions

Research regarding marriage and divorce among couples with LGBTQ members is in its infancy, yet available data have several important policy implications. Langbein and Yost (2009), using nationally representative data across US states from 1990 to 2004, evaluated the claim that same-sex marriage will have negative societal impacts, particularly on other-sex marriage, other-sex divorce, and abortion rates, as well as the number of children born to single mothers and who reside in female-headed households. They found no statistically significant "adverse" effects of same-sex marriage in terms of lower numbers of other-sex marriages, higher rates of divorce, abortion, or single mother households. In fact, states that permitted same-sex marriage showed fewer children in female-headed households and lower abortion rates.

Much of the current research involving transgender parents has largely occurred in the context of transgender parents who transitioned after having become a parent and many of whom are 40 years of age or older. Both qualitative and quantitative research with individuals who are transgender and have transitioned before becoming a parent is needed to further support existing findings. Finally, many studies in this area have included participants who were predominantly White and well-educated (e.g., bachelor's degree and above). Research with transgender people of color as well as those with lower income or education may be particularly informative. Additional research is needed to more rigorously and longitudinally investigate the impact of separation and divorce on children and parents in LGBTQ-parent families. Future work should also examine stepparent family formation among LGBTQ couples and dissolution of multiparent families. This research should incorporate mixed method designs, assessing the perspectives of children and parents, to provide a more comprehensive picture of couple relationship dissolution among LGBTQ people. Studies comparing effects related to separation and divorce for unmarried and married LGBTQ parents would be informative in addressing the role of legal relationship recognition. Cross-cultural studies could be used to compare contextual effects, including legal recognition and the roles of parent gender identity, socioeconomic status, race, culture, and immigration status in couple relationships and dissolution among LGBTQ adults.

## Implications for Practice: Recommendations for LGBTQ-Parent Families Experiencing Separation and Divorce

Research on heterosexual divorce reveals that custody mediation and the use of collaborative attorneys are promising alternatives to more adversarial court procedures between divorcing parents, and these methods are associated with positive outcomes for parents and children (Emery, Sbarra, & Grover, 2005; Kim & Stein, 2018). LGBTQ people in the process of divorce should also be encouraged to do so collaboratively, if at all possible, and to go through mediation, particularly if children are involved. Extant research on this topic, though scarce, indicates that unmarried lesbian mothers typically negotiate custody arrangements together after separating, without court involvement, and the majority report sharing custody (Gartrell et al., 2006; Goldberg et al., 2015; Goldberg & Allen, 2013).

The propensity for sharing parenting involvement and custody might represent unique strengths among divorcing couples with LGBTQ members, since some appear more likely to engage in such shared involvement as compared with heterosexual divorcing parents (Gartrell, Bos, Peyser, et al., 2011), although more research is certainly needed in this area. This is important, given that shared custody is associated with positive outcomes for children who have experienced the divorce of their heterosexual parents, especially if their parents' relationship remains amicable (Emery, 2011; Lansford, 2009). Shared custody has also been found to be more likely among former lesbian partners when both partners were the legal parents of the children (Gartrell, Bos, Peyser, et al., 2011; Goldberg et al., 2015), again highlighting the importance of legal relationship recognition (Balsam, Rostosky, et al., 2017; Goldberg & Allen, 2013; Riggle, Wickham, Rostosky, Rothblum, & Balsam, 2017).

Support services related to coparenting could be particularly useful, as studies have pointed to how undermining coparenting or discrepancies in parenting may contribute to same-sex relationship dissolution (Farr, 2017b; Goldberg et al., 2015). Associations between undermining coparenting and children's externalizing behaviors have been found among LG-parent families (Farr & Patterson, 2013), so interventions aimed at supportive coparenting among separated LGBTQ parents could benefit children. Interventions should be sensitively tailored to the needs and experiences of LGBTQ-parent families, such as incorporating recognition of how societal stigmas related to being LGBTQ impact couples as they partner up, end relationships, and possibly form new relationships (Balsam, Rostosky, & Riggle, 2017; Gahan, 2018).

## Conclusion

Although legal relationship recognition for LGBTQ partners in couple relationships has increased in many countries worldwide, this also signifies that the prevalence of LGBTQ adults, as well as their children, who experience separation and divorce may increase. Our review

of existing research indicates that many experiences of LGBTQ-parent families who live through divorce are similar to those of cisgender heterosexual parent families, yet some experiences are likely to be unique for LGBTQ-parent families headed with LGBTQ parents. Practice and policy designed to support LGBTQ-parent families in the wake of divorce should incorporate attention to issues specific to LGBTQ people, such as the role of societal stigma. Longitudinal research addressing the timing and predictors of dissolution for couples with LGBTQ members holds promise for better understanding rates of dissolution, as well as outcomes for children and parents in these families after separation and divorce.

## References

Alegría, A. (2010). Relationship challenges and relationship maintenance activities following disclosure of transsexualism. *Journal of Psychiatric and Mental Health Nursing, 17*, 909–916. https://doi.org/10.1111/j.1365-2850.2010.01624.x

Allen, K. R. (2007). Ambiguous loss after lesbian couples with children break up: A case for same-gender divorce. *Family Relations, 56*, 175–183. https://doi.org/10.1111/j.1741-3729.2007.00450.x

Amato, P. R. (2010). Research on divorce: Continuing trends and recent developments. *Journal of Marriage and Family, 72*, 650–666. https://doi.org/10.1111/j.1741-3737.2010.00723.x

Andersson, G., Noack, T., Seierstad, A., & Weedon-Fekjaer, H. (2006). The demographics of same-sex marriages in Norway and Sweden. *Demography, 43*, 79–98. https://doi.org/10.1353/dem.2006.0001

Balsam, K. F., Beauchaine, T. P., Rothblum, E. D., & Solomon, S. E. (2008). Three-year follow- up of same-sex couples who had civil unions in Vermont, same-sex couples not in civil unions, and heterosexual married couples. *Developmental Psychology, 44*, 102–116. https://doi.org/10.1037/00121649.44.1.102

Balsam, K. F., Rostosky, S. S., & Riggle, E. D. B. (2017). Breaking up is hard to do: Women's experience of dissolving their same-sex relationship. *Journal of Lesbian Studies, 21*, 30–46. https://doi.org/10.1080/10894160.2016.1165561

Balsam, K. F., Rothblum, E. D., & Wickham, R. E. (2017). Longitudinal predictors of relationship dissolution among same-sex and heterosexual couples. *Couple and Family Psychology, 6*, 247–257. https://doi.org/10.1037/cfp0000091

Biblarz, T. J., & Stacey, J. (2010). How does the gender of parents matter? *Journal of*

*Marriage and Family, 72*, 3–22. https://doi.org/10.1111/j.1741-3737.2009.00678.x

Blumstein, P., & Schwartz, P. (1983). *American couples: Money, work, sex.* New York, NY: William Morrow.

Boss, P. (2013). Resilience as tolerance for ambiguity. In D. Becvar (Ed.), *Handbook of family resilience* (pp. 285–297). New York, NY: Springer.

Church, H. A., O'Shea, D., & Lucey, J. V. (2014). Parent-child relationships in gender identity disorder. *Irish Journal of Medical Science, 183*, 277–281. https://doi.org/10.1007/s11845-013-1003-1

Dierckx, M., Mortelmans, D., Motmans, J., & T'Sjoen, G. (2017). Resilience in families in transition: What happens when a parent is transgender? *Family Relations, 66*, 399–411. https://doi.org/10.1111/fare.12282

Dodge, J. A. (2006). Same-sex marriage and divorce: A proposal for child custody mediation. *Family Court Review, 44*, 87–103. https://doi.org/10.1111/j.1744-1617.2006.00069.x

Emery, R. E. (2011). *Renegotiating family relationships: Divorce, child custody, and mediation* (2nd ed.). New York, NY: Guilford.

Emery, R. E., Sbarra, D. A., & Grover, T. (2005). Divorce mediation: Research and reflections. *Family and Conciliation Courts Review, 43*, 22–37. https://doi.org/10.1111/j.1744-1617.2005.00005.x

Farr, R. H. (2017a). Does parental sexual orientation matter? A longitudinal follow-up of adoptive families with school-age children. *Developmental Psychology, 53*, 252–264. https://doi.org/10.1037/dev0000228

Farr, R. H. (2017b). Factors associated with relationship dissolution and post-dissolution adjustment among lesbian adoptive couples. *Journal of Lesbian Studies, 21*, 88–105. https://doi.org/10.1080/10894160.2016.1142354

Farr, R. H., & Goldberg, A. E. (2018). Sexual orientation, gender identity, and adoption law. *Family Court Review, 56*, 374–383. https://doi.org/10.1111/fcre.12354

Farr, R. H., & Patterson, C. J. (2013). Coparenting among lesbian, gay, and heterosexual couples: Associations with adopted children's outcomes. *Child Development, 84*, 1226–1240. https://doi.org/10.1111/cdev.12046

Farr, R. H., Tasker, F., & Goldberg, A. E. (2017). Theory in highly cited studies of sexual minority parent families: Variations and implications. *Journal of Homosexuality, 64*, 1143–1179. https://doi.org/10.1080/00918369.2016.1242336

Gahan, L. (2018). Separated same-sex parents: Troubling the same-sex parented family. *Sociological Research Online, 23*, 245–261. https://doi.org/10.1177/1360780418754699

Gartrell, N., Bos, H., Peyser, H., Deck, A., & Rodas, C. (2011). Family characteristics, custody arrangements, and adolescent psychological well-being after lesbian mothers break up. *Family Relations, 60*, 572–585. https://doi.org/10.1111/j.1741-3729.2011.00667.x

Gartrell, N., Bos, H. M. W., & Goldberg, N. G. (2011). Adolescents of the U.S. National Longitudinal Lesbian Family Study: Sexual orientation, sexual behavior, and sexual risk exposure. *Archives of Sexual Behavior, 40*, 1199–1209. https://doi.org/10.1007/s10508-010-9692-2

Gartrell, N., Rodas, C., Deck, A., Peyser, H., & Banks, A. (2006). The National Lesbian Family Study: Interviews with mothers of 10-year-olds. *Feminism and Psychology, 16*, 175–192. https://doi.org/10.1177/0959-353506062972

Gates, G. J. (2013). *LGBT parenting in the United States.* The Williams Institute. Retrieved from https://williamsinstitute.law.ucla.edu/wp-content/uploads/LGBT-Parenting.pdf

Gates, G. J. (2015). Marriage and family: LGBT individuals and same-sex couples. *Future of Children, 25*, 67–87.

Goldberg, A. E. (2010). The transition to adoptive parenthood. In T. W. Miller (Ed.), *Handbook of stressful transitions across the life span* (pp. 165–184). New York, NY: Springer.

Goldberg, A. E., & Allen, K. R. (2013). Same-sex relationship dissolution and LGB stepfamily formation: Perspectives of young adults with LGB parents. *Family Relations, 62*, 529–544. https://doi.org/10.1111/fare.12024

Goldberg, A. E., & Garcia, R. (2015). Predictors of relationship dissolution in lesbian, gay, and heterosexual adoptive parents. *Journal of Family Psychology, 29*, 394–404. https://doi.org/10.1037/fam0000095

Goldberg, A. E., Gartrell, N., & Gates, G. (2014). *Research report on LGB-parent families.* The Williams Institute. Retrieved from https://escholarship.org/uc/item/7gr4970w

Goldberg, A. E., & Kuvalanka, K. A. (2012). Marriage (in)equality: The perspectives of adolescents and emerging adults with lesbian, gay, and bisexual parents. *Journal of Marriage and Family, 74*, 34–52. https://doi.org/10.1111/j.1741-3737.2011.00876.x

Goldberg, A. E., Moyer, A. M., Black, K., & Henry, A. (2015). Lesbian and heterosexual adoptive mothers' experiences of relationship dissolution. *Sex Roles, 73*, 141–156. https://doi.org/10.1007/s11199-014-0432-2

Goldberg, S. K., & Conron, K. J. (2018). *How many same-sex couples in the U.S. are raising children?* The Williams Institute. Retrieved from https://williamsinstitute.law.ucla.edu/research/parenting/how-many-same-sex-parents-in-us/

Gottman, J. M., Levenson, R. W., Gross, J., Frederickson, B. L., McCoy, K., Rosenthal, L., . . . Yoshimoto, D. (2003). Correlates of gay and lesbian couples' relationship satisfaction and relationship dissolution. *Journal of Homosexuality, 45*, 23–43. doi:https://doi.org/10.1300/J082v45n01_02

Greene, S. M., Anderson, E. R., Forgatch, M. S., DeGarmo, D. S., & Hetherington, E. M. (2012). Risk and resilience after divorce. In F. Walsh (Ed.), *Normal family processes: Growing diversity and complexity* (4th ed., pp. 102–127). New York, NY: Guilford Press.

Joslin-Roher, E., & Wheeler, D. P. (2009). Partners in transition: The transition experience of lesbian, bisexual, and queer identified partners of transgender men.

*Journal of Gay & Lesbian Social Services, 21*, 30–48. https://doi.org/10.1080/10538720802494743

Kim, S. A., & Stein, E. (2018). Gender in the context of same-sex divorce and relationship dissolution. *Family Court Review, 56*, 384–398. https://doi.org/10.1111/fcre.12355

Kurdek, L. A. (1998). Relationship outcomes and their predictors: Longitudinal evidence from heterosexual married, gay cohabiting, and lesbian cohabiting couples. *Journal of Marriage and Family, 60*, 553–568. https://doi.org/10.2307/353528

Kurdek, L. A. (2004). Are gay and lesbian cohabitating couples really different from heterosexual married couples? *Journal of Marriage and Family, 66*, 880–900. https://doi.org/10.1111/j.0022-2445.2004.00060.x

Kurdek, L. A. (2006). Differences between partners from heterosexual, gay, and lesbian cohabiting couples. *Journal of Marriage and Family, 68*, 509–528. https://doi.org/10.1111/j.1741-3737.2006.00268.x

Langbein, L., & Yost, M. J. (2009). Same-sex marriage and negative externalities. *Social Science. Quarterly, 90*, 292–308. https://doi.org/10.1111/j.1540-6237.2009.00618.x

Lansford, J. E. (2009). Parental divorce and children's adjustment. *Perspectives on Psychological Science, 4*, 140–152. https://doi.org/10.1111/j.1745-6924.2009.01114.x

Lau, C. Q. (2012). The stability of same-sex cohabitation, different-sex cohabitation, and marriage. *Journal of Marriage and Family, 74*, 973–988. https://doi.org/10.1111/j.1741-3737.2012.01000.x

Manning, W., Brown, S., & Stykes, B. (2016). Same-sex and different-sex cohabiting couple relationship stability. *Demography, 53*, 937–953. https://doi.org/10.1007/s13524-016-0490-x

Meier, S. C., Sharp, C., Michonski, J., Babcock, J. C., & Fitzgerald, K. (2013). Romantic relationships of female-to-male trans men: A descriptive study. *International Journal of Transgenderism, 14*, 75–85. https://doi.org/10.1080/15532739.2013.791651

Moore, M. R. (2015). LGBT populations in studies of urban neighborhoods: Making the invisible visible. *City & Community, 14*, 245–248. https://doi.org/10.1111/cico.12127

Moore, M. R., & Stambolis-Ruhstorfer, M. (2013). LGBT sexuality and families at the start of the twenty-first century. *Annual Review of Sociology, 39*, 491–507. https://doi.org/10.1146/annurev-soc-071312-145,643

Oswald, R. F., & Clausell, E. (2006). Same-sex relationships and their dissolution. In M. A. Fine & J. H. Harvey (Eds.), *Handbook of divorce and relationship dissolution* (pp. 499–513). Mahwah, NJ: Erlbaum.

Oswald, R. F., & Culton, L. S. (2003). Under the rainbow: Rural gay life and its relevance for family providers. *Family Relations, 52*, 72–81. https://doi.org/10.1111/j.1741-3729.2003.00072.x

Oswald, R. F., Goldberg, A., Kuvalanka, K., & Clausell, E. (2008). Structural and moral commitment among same-sex couples: Relationship duration, religiosity, and parental status. *Journal of Family Psychology, 22*, 411–419. https://doi.org/10.1037/0893-3200.22.3.411

Patterson, C. J. (2017). Parents' sexual orientation and children's development. *Child Development Perspectives, 11*, 45–49. https://doi.org/10.1111/cdep.12207

Riggle, E. D. B., Wickham, R. E., Rostosky, S. S., Rothblum, E. D., & Balsam, K. F. (2017). Impact of civil marriage recognition for long-term same-sex couples. *Sexuality Research & Social Policy, 14*, 223–232. https://doi.org/10.1007/s13178-016-0243-z

Rosenfeld, M. J. (2014). Couple longevity in the era of same-sex marriage in the United States. *Journal of Marriage and Family, 76*, 905–918. https://doi.org/10.1111/jomf.12141

Ross, H., Gask, K., & Berrington, A. (2011). Civil partnerships five years on. *Population Trends, 145*, 172–202. https://doi.org/10.1057/pt.2011.23

Rothblum, E. D., Balsam, K. F., & Solomon, S. E. (2008). Comparison of same-sex couples who were married in Massachusetts, had domestic partnerships in California, or had civil unions in Vermont. *Journal of Family Issues, 29*, 48–78. https://doi.org/10.1177/0192513X07306087

Shieh, W. (2016). Why same-sex couples break up: A follow-up study in Taiwan. *Journal of GLBT Family Studies, 12*, 257–276. https://doi.org/10.1080/1550428X.2015.1057887

Shieh, W., Hsiao, Y., & Tseng, H. (2009). A comparative study of relationship quality of same- sex couples and married couples in Taiwan. *Archive of Guidance and Counseling, 31*(2), 1–21.

Simpson, E. K. (2017). Influence of gender-based family roles on gender transition for transgender women. *Journal of GLBT Family Studies, 14*, 356–380. https://doi.org/10.1080/1550428X.2017.1359722

Turteltaub, G. L. (2002). *The effects of long-term primary relationship dissolution on the children of lesbian parents* (Doctoral dissertation). Retrieved from Dissertation Abstracts International (AAI3053022).

van Eeden-Moorefield, B., Few-Demo, A. L., Benson, K., Bible, J., & Lummer, S. (2018). A content analysis of LGBT research in top family journals 2000–2015. *Journal of Family Issues, 39*, 1374–1395. https://doi.org/10.1177/0192513X17710284

van Eeden-Moorefield, B., Martell, C. R., Williams, M., & Preston, M. (2011). Same-sex relationships and dissolution: The connection between heteronormativity and homonormativity. *Family Relations, 60*, 562–571. https://doi.org/10.1111/j.1741-3729.2011.00669.x

von Doussa, H., Power, J., & Riggs, D. W. (2017). Family matters: Transgender and gender diverse peoples' experience with family when they transition. *Journal of Family Studies*. Advance online publication. doi:https://doi.org/10.1080/13229400.2017.1375965

Wiik, K. A., Seierstad, A., & Noack, T. (2014). Divorce in Norwegian same-sex marriages and registered partnerships: The role of children. *Journal of Marriage and Family, 76*, 919–929. https://doi.org/10.1111/jomf.12132

# Losing a Child: Death and Hidden Losses in LGBTQ-Parent Families

Katherine R. Allen and Christa C. Craven

The death of a child is a devastating loss. Nothing in the experience or discourse of parenthood prepares a parent for the untimely or traumatic death of their child (Albuquerque, Ferreira, Narciso, & Pereira, 2017; Craven & Peel, 2014; Feigelman, Jordan, McIntosh, & Feigelman, 2012; Hill, Cacciatore, Shreffler, & Pritchard, 2017; Peel, 2010; Rosenblatt, 2000). In this chapter, we address the invisible topic of losing a child and explore the experiences and implications of child loss on LGBTQ-parent families. As a family scholar who experienced the loss of an adult child by suicide, and an anthropologist who suffered a second-trimester miscarriage, we approach this subject both as researchers and bereaved queer parents. We address the limited sources of knowledge on this issue, piecing together theoretical perspectives, autoethnography and personal narrative, and empirical research in order to chart this understudied area. We build upon common experiences of loss, death, bereavement, grief, and healing for families experiencing the death of a child. From that foundation, we explore unique features of LGBTQ-parent families that reflect their challenges in heteronormative society that lead to stigma, prejudice, and other forms of sexual minority stress that compound their hidden losses over the life course (Allen, 2019; American Psychological Association, 2009; Craven, 2019; Craven & Peel, 2017; Dahl, 2018; Goldman & Livoti, 2011; Nadal, Whitman, Davis, Erazo, & Davidoff, 2016; Scherrer & Fedor, 2015).

In this chapter, we focus on two types of child loss that result in the loss of a child's life: (a) loss of an adolescent or adult child by suicide and (b) reproductive loss through miscarriage or stillbirth. We acknowledge that there are many other traumatic ways of losing a child that are relevant to LGBTQ-parent families—such as the loss of custody or visitation with a child through parental divorce or relational dissolution (Allen, 2007; see chapter "Separation and Divorce Among LGBTQ-Parent Families"), through a failed adoption (Craven, 2019; Craven & Peel, 2014), through chronic illnesses such as cancer or drug overdose and issues related to mental illness (Bostwick et al., 2014; Feigelman et al., 2012), and through sudden or unexpected accidents and disasters (Murray, 2017)—that are also understudied (or have never been studied before) and deserve further scholarly attention. With this in mind, we propose directions for future research and implications for practice and support for LGBTQ-parent families experiencing child loss.

K. R. Allen (✉)
Department of Human Development and Family Science, Virginia Tech, Blacksburg, VA, USA
e-mail: kallen@vt.edu

C. C. Craven
Anthropology and Women's, Gender & Sexuality Studies, The College of Wooster, Wooster, OH, USA
e-mail: ccraven@wooster.edu

© Springer Nature Switzerland AG 2020
A. E. Goldberg, K. R. Allen (eds.), *LGBTQ-Parent Families*,
https://doi.org/10.1007/978-3-030-35610-1_22

## The Loss of a Child's Life: Compounded Stigma for LGBTQ Parents

The loss of a child is accompanied by a tremendous amount of intensely personal emotions, including grief, fear, anger, sorrow, and despair. At the same time, the loss of a child is associated with stigma—both internalized, through self-blame, and externalized, through blaming others (Sheehan et al., 2018). At the personal level, stigma can be manifested as self-blame, by personally indicting oneself for not being able to bear a child that lives (Cacciatore, Froen, & Killian, 2013) or to keep one's adolescent or adult child safe from a suicide attempt (Frey, Hans, & Cerel, 2017) or a violent, tragic death (Bolton, 2009; Rosenblatt, 2000; Song, Floyd, Seltzer, & Greenberg, 2010). At the interpersonal level, stigma can be felt from concern that others hold the grieving parent responsible, triggering an inability to communicate with family and friends about the loss (Feigelman et al., 2012; Hooghe, Rosenblatt, & Rober, 2018). At the institutional level, stigma is embedded in social institutions that hold parents responsible for their children "turning out well" (Ryff, Schmutte, & Lee, 1996), and thus, there are few established cultural rituals surrounding the loss of a child (Cacciatore & Raffo, 2011; Craven & Peel, 2017; Layne, 2003), and few institutional resources for parents and family members to consult to help with their grieving process (Frey, Hans, & Sanford, 2016; Jaques, 2000; Jordan, Price, & Prior, 2015; Peel & Cain, 2012). The loss of a child is a uniquely painful, disorienting, and isolating experience at every level (Murphy, 2008).

Adding to the interacting complexities of intense emotion and pervasive stigma are the unique experiences facing parents who also happen to be members of sexual and gender minority groups—that is, lesbian, gay, bisexual, transgender, and queer parents. In addition to personal, interpersonal, and institutional levels of stigma noted above for all of those who face the loss of a child, LGBTQ bereaved parents frequently experience homophobia and heterosexism that intensify the cultural silences surrounding child death, such as discriminatory laws and institutional policies about who is considered "next of kin" and thus able to make decisions about autopsies and funeral arrangements (Craven, 2019; Wojnar, 2007, 2009; Wojnar & Swanson, 2006). In addition, few support resources exist for LGBTQ parents to turn to when they have lost a child, which can lead to feelings of isolation (Craven & Peel, 2014, 2017; Peel, 2010; Peel & Cain, 2012). LGBTQ parents may also experience overt discriminatory sentiments from family or others, or internalized concerns (Craven, 2019), exemplified in comments such as "lesbians shouldn't be parents in the first place," or "perhaps a miscarriage was God's way of telling them they shouldn't have children as a gay person." Even seemingly empathetic responses, such as suggestions for partners to "just swap" if one has had difficulty conceiving or had a miscarriage (Walks, 2007) or that LGBTQ parents can just "try again" (particularly those who have invested substantially in reproductive technologies or adoption proceedings) can intensify the grief of LGBTQ parents (Craven, 2019; Walks, 2007).

## Theoretical Perspectives for Studying Child Loss in LGBTQ-Parent Families

Given the understudied nature of child loss in LGBTQ-parent families, we propose two theoretical perspectives that are relevant to define and understand how parents experience the loss of a child, grieve, and move forward. Although a great deal of the loss and bereavement literature in general builds upon attachment theory (e.g., Murray, 2017; Scott, Diamond, & Levy, 2016), among the most neglected areas of research in studies of loss and death are more critical perspectives that address the survivors of traumatic loss (such as the loss of a child to suicide or homicide; Feigelman et al., 2012) or the loss of a child through stillbirth or miscarriage (which has often been characterized as a non-event; Cacciatore et al., 2013). Thus, we address critical theories that are ripe for the integration of sexual minority experience, stress, and stigma within the context of traumatic loss and grief. First, we address the disenfranchised grief framework that already appears in the LGBTQ literature on a related topic, which is of spousal bereavement. Second, we address intersectional and feminist framings that can be extended to examine child loss and grief.

## Perspectives on Disenfranchised Grief

Building on work by Doka (2008), bereavement scholars typically characterize family or relational loss in the LGBTQ community as a form of disenfranchised grief (Green & Grant, 2008; Patlamazoglou, Simmonds, & Snell, 2018). Integrating biological, psychological, and sociological perspectives on grief, disenfranchised grief "results when a person experiences a significant loss and the resultant grief is not openly acknowledged, socially validated, or publicly mourned" (Doka, p. 224).

Disenfranchised grief has been used to explain the bereavement reactions to the loss of a same-sex partner, particularly in later life (Scherrer & Fedor, 2015). In the context of normative events across the life course, the death of one's spouse is one that most individuals anticipate, but for older cohorts of LGBTQ adults, the lack of legal marriage (until the US Supreme Court ruling legalized same-sex marriage in 2015), inheritance rights, legal recognition of family ties, and even being out to family and friends have placed them at increased risk for experiencing a partner's death as an unacknowledged loss (de Vries, 2009; McNutt & Yakushko, 2013; Patlamazoglou et al., 2018). Although scholarship is now accumulating on the topic of same-sex partner bereavement, as noted above, as well as the topic of end of life care for LGBTQ individuals (Acquaviva, 2017; de Vries & Gutman, 2016), we suggest that disenfranchised grief is also an important way to frame the understudied topic of bereaved LGBTQ parents. Social workers have also described this grief as a "double disenfranchisement" for LGBTQ bereaved parents, who experience stigma both because of experiencing a miscarriage and homophobic or transphobic responses to LGBTQ reproduction and parenting more generally (Cacciatore & Raffo, 2011).

There are a variety of ways that critical perspectives about grief and loss, including disenfranchised grief, ambiguous loss, and complex trauma can be applied to LGBTQ-parent families in the area of child loss. For example, Boss's (2006) ambiguous loss framework, where a person may be psychologically absent but physically present, or physically absent but psychologically present, has been applied in the LGBTQ-family literature to the break-up of a lesbian-parent family and the loss of a nonbiological child (Allen, 2007). McGuire, Catalpa, Lacey, and Kuvalanka (2016) applied ambiguous loss to family members of trans people, who, for example, experience the loss of a daughter or sister when their child or sibling undergoes gender transition. Ambiguous loss theory could have application to failed adoptions as well, where losing a child is grieved by an adoptive family, though the child has not died (Craven, 2019). Regarding complex trauma, researchers cannot assume that people have only experienced one type of loss; many of the participants in Christa's research, for example, had experienced multiple traumas/losses, such as stillbirth followed by adoption loss or miscarriage followed by the unexpected death of a known donor (Craven, 2019).

## Intersectional and Feminist Perspectives

Intersectional and feminist perspectives are essential for studying child loss among LGBTQ-parent families with attention to the diversity of experiences with homophobia and heterosexism as they intertwine with racism, cultural biases, and other forms of adversity (Allen & Henderson, 2017; Collins & Bilge, 2016; Craven, 2019; Davis & Craven, 2016; McLaughlin, Casey, & Richardson, 2006). These approaches are especially relevant because the experiences of White, middle-class lesbians and gay men have been the most widely documented in the LGBTQ-family literature (Badgett, 2018; Browne & Nash, 2010; Compton, Meadow, & Schilt, 2018; Craven, 2019; Gates, 2015). This focus excludes many LGBTQ families, which the US census shows are twice as likely to include African-American and Latinx parents as White ones, and who have lower median incomes than heterosexual married couples (Gates & Romero, 2009, p. 232); furthermore, the census is only inclusive of families headed by same-sex couples. Intersectional perspectives that investigate the matrix of domination, including multiple oppressions and resilience in creating and sustaining families as experienced by queer people of color are especially important to examine (Acosta, 2013; see chapter "Race and Ethnicity in the Lives of LGBTQ Parents and Their Children: Perspectives from and Beyond North America"; cárdenas, 2016; Moore, 2011). In the pregnancy loss and infertility bereavement literature, women with less educational and financial resources frequently lack social support (Cacciatore, Killian, & Harper, 2016; Paisley-Cleveland, 2013), as well as the help they may need to conceive again, if that is their goal (Almendrala, 2018; Bell, 2014).

The intersectional approach of reproductive justice theorists has been particularly useful in moving beyond the individualized focus on *choice* among many reproductive rights groups to one of *access* to resources such as high-quality healthcare, education, and support not only for legal abortion and contraception, but also the right to have and parent children in safe and healthy environments (Ross, Roberts, Derkas, Peoples, & Toure, 2017; Ross & Solinger, 2017). Promoting access to safe and supportive healthcare and mental health resources following a tragic loss is an important extension of this work. By centering an intersectional feminist analysis, a reproductive justice approach also serves as an important corrective to previous research that has assumed the whiteness and affluence of LGBTQ people seeking to form families (Ross, 2017).

## Situating Personal Experience and Research on Child Loss in LGBTQ-Parent Families

Our perspectives on the topic of child loss are inevitably shaped by our own experiences as queer parents who have lost children. Qualitative researchers have argued that autoethnography, in which the researcher narrates her own personal experience through a critical, theorized lens, is particularly useful in pioneering new areas of research on highly stigmatized topics (Adams & Manning, 2015; Allen & Piercy, 2005; Davis & Craven, 2016; see chapter "Qualitative Research on LGBTQ-Parent Families"; Sachs, 2019). In this tradition, we both share our personal experiences here—and elsewhere (Allen, 2007, 2019; Craven, 2019)—to speak past the stigma, pain, grief, invisibility, and lack of understanding associated with LGBTQ bereavement. In doing so, we aim to move beyond merely a reflexive engagement centered around our own experiences, but rather use autoethnography as an empirical tool to consider how our particular social locations and experiences intersect with institutional, geographical, political, and material aspects of our positionality, as well as others who have experienced similar losses (see Nagar, 2014; Narayan, 2012).

In this spirit, we are intent on decentering narratives of LGBTQ experience that rely upon a linear progression from marriage to achieving pregnancy to having children. In a political moment when LGBTQ lives are often presented as ones of moral inferiority or, more progressively, as a seamless narrative of progress towards enhanced marital and familial rights, there is more pressure than ever for queer people to marry (legally), have children, and create public narratives of LGBTQ progress (Craven, 2019). In this context, losses, challenges, and disruptions to stories of "successful" LGBTQ family-making, such as divorce, are often silenced, both personally and politically (Romero & Goldberg, 2019). Writing about child loss and death offers an important counterpoint to heteronormative and homonormative political narratives.

The first type of loss we explicitly address in this chapter is the death of an adult child through suicide; this experience has never been investigated in the scholarly literature from the perspective of LGBTQ-parent families. We introduce this topic through Katherine's autoethnographic account of her own son's death by suicide as a way to open the conversation in the empirical literature and to spur further work. The second type of loss we explore, that of reproductive loss, is a topic that Christa has not only personally experienced but has also examined in her research and writing (Craven, 2019; Craven & Peel, 2014, 2017). Thus, we use a combination of autoethnography, theory, and empirical research to orient the study of child loss in LGBTQ-parent families.

## A Child's Death by Suicide: Katherine's Reflections

In January 2011, at the age of 23, my son, Matthew, took his own life. I received the highly disorienting phone call at 4:00 a.m. from a police officer telling me to come to the hospital in a city about an hour away because my son had been involved in an accident. Crawling on the floor searching for my glasses that I had knocked off the night stand in my flailing, semi-conscious effort to answer the telephone, I could not comprehend what the officer was saying. I kept asking, "is he okay, is he okay," and the officer would only say, "he went over a bridge." I finally heard myself saying, "Is my son alive?" and the officer would not answer my question. Recalling this moment years later, I can still feel the sensation of having my head and my heart disconnect as I sprawled on the floor and tried to write down what the officer was telling me to do: come to the hospital, have someone drive you, the doctors will talk to you there.

As the days after Matt's death by suicide unfolded, I read the note my son left to his lover (Matt's word for his partner), a young man with whom my son had been very close for 3 years. The romantic portion of their relationship had recently cooled, and his friend had told Matt that he loved him but he "wasn't *in* love with him." Losing this relationship that he had nurtured and pursued for 3 years was devastating, as his note revealed. At the time of Matt's death, I did not know that their relationship had ended, only that it had "cooled." Just 2 days before he died, Matt had spent a typical Sunday evening with me, having dinner, doing his laundry, and sharing an educational computer game he had created for his work. Although he did not tell me he and his lover had broken up, he did tell me that he had a

lot of things going on that he couldn't discuss with me or his friends and that he was now ready to see a counselor. I wrote down the name and contact information for a respected therapist in our town, and he said he would call her on Monday. He left that evening and I felt a sense of relief about how he was doing—my "primal instincts" as a mother to nurture my son were momentarily satisfied: he had eaten a good meal at my home, we had laughed and talked about personal issues, and I felt that although he seemed in somewhat low spirits, he was on the right track because he was ready to establish a therapeutic relationship. I have worked with a therapist my entire adult life, and I had been open with my son about the mental health challenges in our family among his biological kin and the need to be vigilant and proactive in getting support and professional help, and thus I felt my son was realistic and knowledgeable about the challenges he could face as he grew into adulthood. As I was soon to discover from the narratives of other bereaved parents that I eventually read, I did not see the events of the next day coming.

Matt's note that he sent to his partner moments before he fell from the bridge that took his life was not recriminating toward anyone but himself. He began his note with, "So, I'm taking the coward's way out," and yet before I read his note (provided to me by Matt's partner—to whom his note was addressed, and also given to me by the police detective who investigated his case in order to rule out bullying and "foul play"), my first reaction was, "Where did he find the courage to jump from that bridge?" This interplay between cowardice and courage was my first glimpse into the complicated thoughts and emotions and the lack of a congruent story line to explain the events or make sense of them that led to my son's decision to take his own life. I learned from his note that he felt hopeless about his own sadness and loss over the relationship not working out, despite his many efforts to establish and maintain a partnership with the young man he loved. Since his death, I have learned how relationship conflict and loss can be a common component of completed suicides (Rivers, Gonzalez, Nodin, Peel, & Tyler, 2018; Skerrett, Kolves, & De Leo, 2017).

Yet, Matt also wrote about how he "never really liked living anyway," a phrase that breaks my heart into a million pieces whenever I recall it. As his mother, I could not save him. I could not save my son.

Not being able to save one's child is only one of the many heartbreaking things about losing a child before their time. As feminist philosopher Sara Ruddick (1989) proposed in her theory of maternal thinking, a mother has three aims: to preserve the life of the child, to foster the child's growth, and to render the child acceptable to the mother's own society. These are often contradictory mandates, as when a mother raises a child who is eventually expected to go to war, and yet it is stitched into the discourse and experience of motherhood in our society that a mother is responsible for the life of her child. I have resonated with this framing of maternal thinking, especially with its analysis of the inherent contradictions of motherhood, as I raised my children and conducted my professional life. To not be able to save my son, despite my deepest love for him, has been a devastating loss, like no other. The bereavement literature, and the wisdom of friends and professionals who have walked this path before me, tell me that it is a loss from which no one can completely return, yet life can and does improve and move forward. What has helped me to restructure my emotions and cognitions about this loss is to actively engage the grief process through psychotherapy, meditation, massage, walking, gardening, writing, and other contemplative practices as well as the conscientious and compassionate support of family, friends, and professionals in the communities to which I belong (Frey, Fulginiti, Lezine, & Cerel, 2018; Hunt & Hertlein, 2015; Kasahara-Kiritani, Ikeda, Yamamoto-Mitani, & Kamibeppu, 2017; Meris, 2016; Sugrue, McGiloway, & Keegan, 2014; Vachon & Harris, 2016). Now that 8 years have passed, I am reaching out to other bereaved parents and have started a bereavement support group for parents, grandparents, and siblings who have experienced the death of an adolescent or adult child, as there are no such support groups for this experience in my community.

The death of my son by suicide is a loss that compounds another major loss our family experienced two decades ago, when our lesbian-mother family dissolved. After 12 years together, my former partner moved out and we lost contact with her and her biological son (born into our relationship, and whose father is my brother's husband), particularly after she partnered with another woman and merged their families. Our relationship dissolution occurred before the advent of legal marriage, divorce, or custody rights for the second parent, as I have chronicled in two other autoethnographic accounts (Allen, 2007, 2019). Thus, my son, Matt, born to me and my former husband (my first marriage) was raised primarily in a lesbian-parent family (my second marriage, albeit not a legal one) for 12 years, until he was age 13, when my former partner left our family. Then Matt and I lived as a single-parent family for several years, until I eventually partnered with my current husband (Matt's stepfather), with whom I have lived for the past 15 years (my third marriage).

Thus, as my biological child, Matt had lived in several family configurations, and one of my ongoing challenges has been to constantly wonder, agonize over, and assess the degree to which my own queer intimate relationship history of three sequential long-term partnerships (i.e., one legal marriage and divorce from a man; one intentional lesbian partnership that dissolved with a woman; a second legal marriage with a man) had on his subsequent traumatic reaction to his own experience of relational loss. The therapeutic practice that has worked well for me has been to disentangle my son's death from my own relationship choices and history, but given the social prescriptions about a parent's responsibility for the life and death of their child, it is something I constantly wrestle with and engage. Worry about my fault and responsibility in my son's death is a traumatic by-product of this devastating loss, and it requires daily vigilance, examination, and emotion work to keep it at bay. This emotion work also involves the deliberate cognitive dismantling of the narrow heteronormative lens that is embedded in the broader society, that condemns me for my son's death, when in fact, I know that there are a million reasons I cannot understand or piece together for why he made the decision he did to end his life.

Another piece of the puzzle is that my son, as a young man who identified as "more gay than straight" was also dealing with his own sexual minority experience, in the context of a society in which LGBTQ youth are at heightened risk for suicide (Haas et al., 2011). Males are far more likely than females to complete a suicide; the worldwide aggregate ratio is 3.5 male suicides to 1 female suicide, particularly in industrialized countries (Canetto & Cleary, 2012). Adolescent sexual minorities are at a heightened risk as well (Bostwick et al., 2014; Caputi, Smith, & Ayers, 2017), though Russell and Toomey (2012) found that suicide as a risk factor for LGBTQ youth levels off in adulthood. The complexities of LGBTQ suicide risk and being a member of the second generation of sexual minority individuals in his family are just two pieces of a larger frame that cannot be encapsulated into a simple equation and answered by the search for causes. I take heart in the work of Kuvalanka and Goldberg (2009) and see chapter "The "Second Generation:" LGBTQ Youth with LGBTQ Parents" about the second generation of LGBTQ youth and parents, as I know that the story about our lives is far more complex and resilient than the limited heteronormative interpretation suggests. Where I am now, 8 years out, is in embracing and loving my son, helping to keep his memory alive, and trying to study, understand, and document through my writing and research the meanings this loss has for LGBTQ-parent families and their children.

## Reproductive Losses: Christa's Reflection

A more extensive account of my personal experience with miscarriage appears in the first chapter of my book *Reproductive Losses: Challenges to LGBTQ Family-Making* (Craven, 2019). While I do not reiterate that reflection in its entirety here, there

are a few experiences that are important to highlight, many of which were echoed in my subsequent interviews with 54 LGBTQ people who had experienced reproductive loss. After suffering a miscarriage during my second trimester of pregnancy in 2009, the isolation my partner and I initially experienced was, for lack of a better term, shattering. The resources we found focused exclusively on heterosexual couples—typically also White, middle-class, and Christian. And ironically, despite our career paths as a Labor and Delivery Nurse and a researcher who has studied reproductive health and childbirth, neither of us knew any other queer families who had experienced reproductive loss when we were confronted with our own.

What I did learn quite quickly via Internet searches was that miscarriages were far more common than I had thought—25% of all "recognized" pregnancies (McNair & Altman, 2012)—which likely meant an even higher percentage for those of us who were actively trying to conceive and using home pregnancy tests early on. In fact, miscarriage is a part of "normal" pregnancy for a great number of us. Yet this reality is often hidden in pregnancy advice books and rarely mentioned by well-intended healthcare practitioners, friends, or family (Craven, 2019; Layne, 2003; Peel & Cain, 2012). In fact, a 2015 survey of over 1000 adults in the USA showed that 55% thought miscarriage was rare, occurring in 5% or less of pregnancies (Bardos, Hercz, Friedenthal, Missmer, & Williams, 2015). In part, this is because of the pervasive cultural silencing of experiences with pregnancy loss (Layne, 2003). For bereaved LGBTQ parents, however, there are multiple layers of invisibility as we combat the general cultural silence surrounding pregnancy loss, as well as struggling with homophobia and heteronormative assumptions about who should (and should not) have children. Further, political efforts to downplay queer "failure" (i.e., divorce) often create a silence around queer family-making efforts that do not produce a "success story" and uphold a universalizing (and damaging) narrative of "queer progress."

This cultural silencing is particularly damaging for parents who have not physically carried children, often termed in the empirical literature as nongestational or nonbiological parents (sometimes inaccurately in the case of in vitro fertilization with a partner's egg), and more colloquially as social mothers or co-mothers—though all of these designations place emphasis on their parenting role as somehow secondary (Craven, 2019). In our case, although many friends and family offered me emotional support following our loss, the emotional needs of my partner, B, often seemed like an afterthought (B is my partner's nickname, which is how most everyone knows her). Although I had clearly had *different* experiences (like the physical trauma of surgery and the physical and emotional pain of my breastmilk coming in several days afterwards), the emotional scars of losing the dream of raising our daughter Lily together was a jointly shared trauma.

Yet bereavement material sent from the hospital was addressed solely to me and all of the information provided assumed a heterosexual married couple. Although sending "follow-up materials" under a patient's name is standard practice at most hospitals, it was also a glaring reminder that B was not only prohibited legally from being recognized as our child's parent, but also invisible in her grief. Both of us chafed at the fact that I was coded as a "single mother" in the medical records, despite the fact that B had been with me throughout the entire ordeal. We felt broken and alone, and having our grief assessed by others based on whether we had a biological connection and/or legal relationship to our child intensified our pain and belied our intention to parent together and be recognized as a family.

An exchange with gay male friends shortly after our loss was particularly poignant in breaking the initial isolation we felt. We learned that they had also lost a child. After the couple had bonded with an infant in their home for 10 days as part of an open adoption, his birth mother chose to reclaim him. They were eventually able to adopt other children, but nearly a decade later, the birth mother used social media to find them. Although she recognized that they might not want to speak with her, she reached out to let them know that the child was doing well and that

she appreciated the time they had spent with him. The complexities and ambiguities of reproductive losses that do not involve the death of a child remain understudied both among LGBTQ and heterosexual adoptive parents.

Although this chapter focuses primarily on parents experiencing the death of a child, my broader study of reproductive loss addresses LGBTQ experiences with adoption loss, infertility, and sterility as a result of taking hormones for gender transition or other medical procedures (Craven, 2019). As an anthropologist, after unwittingly becoming a participant-observer—bearing witness not only to my own experience, but also B's pain—I wanted to understand what was at stake for other queer people who face reproductive loss.

Thus, a central aim of my project has been to contribute to a broader picture of LGBTQ experiences with reproductive loss and grief, especially among groups that have previously received little attention in studies of queer reproduction and parenting, such as nongestational or "social" parents (including adoptive parents), queer people of color, and trans and nonbinary people. B and my experiences were unmistakably marked and privileged by our social location as White, professional, cisgender women. Yet even those privileges did not protect us from homophobic laws and policies, and heteronormative assumptions about what makes one a "real" parent. Importantly, the stories among those I interviewed further challenge the assumed affluence and whiteness of LGBTQ families (particularly those formed with assisted reproductive technology and via adoption or surrogacy). For many LGBTQ people and families—and, really, all individuals and families who encounter challenges as they try to form families—reproductive loss encompasses far more than the loss of the child. It includes the loss of imagined futures and often sometimes hidden losses, like financial strains and relationship tensions, which are difficult to talk about in relation to emotional (and sometimes physical) trauma of reproductive loss. For LGBTQ intended parents, these are frequently amplified by discriminatory laws and homophobic/transphobic responses.

I argue in my book *Reproductive Losses* (Craven, 2019) that pregnancy and adoption loss, as well as infertility and sterility, are part of many LGBTQ people's reproductive journeys and, as such, they are worthy of acknowledgment and commemoration. Because reproductive loss is often experienced in isolation, reconceptualizing queer reproductive losses as communal losses can create an important link to the creative, generative, and often politicized responses to historical queer losses, such as The NAMES Project (AIDS memorial quilt) in response to the HIV/AIDS pandemic, Transgender Day of Remembrance for those who have been killed through transphobic violence, and the art and fiction memorializing the Stonewall riots. Thus, from its beginnings, my study has had a public focus. I wrote *Reproductive Losses* for a broad audience—including healthcare and adoption professionals, counselors and therapists, scholars of reproduction, and bereaved intended parents—and launched an open-access companion website that includes an archive of commemorative strategies and advice from participants, among other resources at http://www.lgbtqreproductiveloss.org. The website also includes an interactive tool which allows for ongoing contributions to this digital resource with the hope of continuing this conversation long into the future.

## Implications for LGBTQ Parents and Practitioners

Reaching out to LGBTQ parents and their broader communities is a primary way to bring the scholarship of child loss to parents, clinicians, educators, and others who are working with bereaved parents. Internet resources and parent support groups on social media often provide the first resource for grieving parents (Perluxo & Francisco, 2018). For example, Walker (2017) described how she created Alliance of Hope, which is now the largest online community of suicide loss survivors in the world. Other resources include Bereaved Parents of the USA (https://www.bereavedparentsusa.org/), Baby in Heaven: An Infohub for Grieving Parents (https://

babyinheaven.com/), International Stillbirth Alliance (www.stillbirthalliance.org), and Compassionate Friends (https://www.compassionatefriends.org/). These organizations include tabs on their respective websites "For the Newly Bereaved" among other resources for coping with loss. Just reading through lists of the "wide and often frightening variety of emotions" after the loss of one's child, and that "these feelings and experiences are natural and normal" can be reassuring to parents, who are likely experiencing "profound sadness; crying all the time or at unexpected times; difficulty sleeping; anxiety; denial; inability to concentrate; a deep longing and emptiness; intense questioning; needing to tell and retell the story of your loved one's death" (For the newly bereaved, n.d.). These types of resources can also be helpful to family members experiencing the loss, as well as a place to start for practitioners, therapists, educators, and others working with families.

Most self-help resources that are available about child loss, however, are geared toward heterosexually-identified families. Topics directly related to LGBTQ parent family loss might be included (though often not), but are not often readily apparent. Yet a few online groups do exist. On the Compassionate Friends website, LGBTQ issues can be found under the topic "diversity and grief" (www.compassionatefriends.org). The creator of Baby in Heaven asked Christa to write a section specifically for grieving LGBTQ parents addressing the unique aspects of loss of a child during pregnancy, birth, or adoption (Craven, 2017). Because having access to inclusive resources is crucial to supporting bereaved LGBTQ parents and families (Craven, 2019; Craven & Peel, 2014, 2017; Peel, 2010; Peel & Cain, 2012), Ari Lev created an online support group for LGBTQ bereaved parents (https://www.facebook.com/groups/tcflgbtqlossofachild/).

Education and training for medical, healthcare, social work, nursing, counseling, religious, and educational professionals is also needed to help them understand their own attitudes about LGBTQ individuals and communities (Allen, 2013; Craven & Peel, 2017; Murray, 2017), in much the same way that Acquaviva (2017) argues for helping to transform professional practice in hospice and palliative care. Therapists need to address the intersecting adversities that many LGBTQ intended parents face, such as the layered effects of homophobia, transphobia, racism, and assumptions of affluence (Craven, 2019), as well as the internalized stigma associated with grieving the loss of a child (Sheehan et al., 2018). In a study of mothers grieving the loss of a young child, Gear (2014) described aspects of informal social support networks that are helpful to bereaved mothers, including authenticity and being "in tune" with the needs of the bereaved parent and also offering practical assistance in ways that respect the bereaved parents' choice to accept or reject it. With this advice in mind, Katherine began a support group for parents who have experienced the loss of older children in her community.

Support groups, whether online or in person, can also be useful locations to debunk negative reactions parents who have experienced the traumatic loss of a child may have received, such as the seven categories outlined by Feigelman et al. (2012), each with an example:

(a) Avoidance: "People who I thought would be at the funeral or send a sympathy card didn't show any acknowledgment of the death."
(b) Unhelpful advice: "Haven't you grieved enough already?"
(c) Absence of a caring interest: "If I started talking about my lost child, they quickly changed the subject."
(d) Unempathic spiritual explanations: "He's in a better place now."
(e) Blaming the child: "He was so reckless in how he lived."
(f) Blaming the parent: "Didn't you see it coming?"
(g) Other negative responses: "At least you have other children." (pp. 50–51)

As noted above, these comments are often intensified by homophobic assumptions, as well as heterosexist platitudes that downplay the intentionality and financial investment many LGBTQ people put into family-making, such as "You can always try again" (Craven, 2019).

The use of a social justice framework for trauma survivors is highly applicable for practitioners working with bereaved LGBTQ parents and their families (Meris, 2016). One of the major antidotes to the devastating impact of traumatic loss and disenfranchised grief is the use of compassion as a therapeutic model for both individual counseling and community social justice work. Vachon and Harris (2016) proposed the GRACE model developed to promote compassion for clinician-patient interactions: "G—Gather your attention. R—Recall your intention. A—Attune by checking in with yourself, then the patient. C—Consider what will really serve by being truly present in the moment. E—Engage, enact ethically, and then end the interaction" (p. 276). The GRACE model helps to prevent burnout in caregivers and health care practitioners while still maintaining the capacity to be present and respond with compassion.

Finally, family resilience (Power et al., 2016) is defined "as a capacity to overcome adversity, or to thrive despite challenges or trauma" (p. 67). It is more complex than individual resilience, because it involves a systemic view of relationship processes that enable individuals in families to support one another through major life challenges. Family resilience allows us to see how individuals make meaning out of adversity (p. 69). Queer resiliency can offer important possibilities for acknowledging and valuing LGBTQ experiences of reproductive loss—both as a valid part of queer family-making and as a communal loss—particularly in the face of homophobic responses to LGBTQ families, as well as politicized narratives of queer progress that rely upon the public image of successful, stable LGBTQ families (Craven, 2019).

## Future Research Directions

There are many possible research directions that are evident from our examination of child loss in LGBTQ-parent families. As noted, we have covered through autoethnography and review of the literature, only two kinds of child loss—reproductive child loss and the loss of an adult child to suicide. There is also little research on child loss as a result of relationship dissolution, failed adoption (among queer or heterosexual families), infertility and sterility among LGBTQ people, and the loss experiences of nongestational parents, queer people of color, or trans/nonbinary people. More work is needed on LGBTQ family-making in general that moves beyond previous research centered on White, middle-class and affluent, cisgender lesbian and gay (and some bisexual; see Bergstrom-Lynch, 2015; Luce, 2010; Peel, 2010) people and families (notable exceptions include Acosta, 2013; cárdenas, 2016; Moore, 2011). This research (and application of its findings) is especially important for those individuals are less likely to seek—or have less access to—social or professional support for child loss (see Almendrala, 2018; Bell, 2014; Cacciatore et al., 2016; Craven, 2019; Mullings, 2005; Paisley-Cleveland, 2013).

There are also many other family relationships that need to be examined, particularly the reactions and recovery of siblings who survive the death of their own sibling, live through a parent's miscarriage, or must give up a new sibling when they return to their birth family. A literature is starting to amass regarding sibling responses to loss and yet much more work can be done in order to specifically address the loss of a child on siblings in LGBTQ-parent families. Furthermore, other intra- and intergenerational family relationships, including those of cousins, grandparents, and close friends of a child who dies should be considered in research throughout the life course. In sum, expanding research in these areas, among others, is necessary to create more inclusive and affirming support resources for LGBTQ people who have experienced child loss, as well as the professionals, family, and friends who support them.

# References

Acosta, K. L. (2013). *Amigas y amantes: Sexually nonconforming Latinas negotiate family*. New Brunswick, NJ: Rutgers University Press.

Acquaviva, K. D. (2017). *LGBTQ-inclusive hospice and palliative care: A practical guide to transforming professional practice*. New York, NY: Harrington Park Press.

Adams, T. E., & Manning, J. (2015). Autoethnography and family research. *Journal of Family Theory & Review, 7*, 350–366. https://doi.org/10.1111/jftr.12116

Albuquerque, S., Ferreira, L. C., Narciso, I., & Pereira, M. (2017). Parents' positive interpersonal coping after a child's death. *Journal of Child and Family Studies, 26*, 1817–1830. https://doi.org/10.1007/s10826-017-0697-5

Allen, K. R. (2007). Ambiguous loss after lesbian couples with children break up: A case for same-gender divorce. *Family Relations, 56*, 175–183. https://doi.org/10.1111/j.1741-3729.2007.00444.x

Allen, K. R. (2013, January). Teaching about loss and resilience in families with LGBT members. *The Forum: The Quarterly Publication of the Association for Death Education and Counseling, 39*(1), 19–20.

Allen, K. R. (2019). Family, loss, and change: Navigating family breakup before the advent of legal marriage and divorce. In A. E. Goldberg & A. P. Romero (Eds.), *LGBTQ divorce and relationship dissolution: Psychological and legal perspectives and implications for practice* (pp. 221–232). New York, NY: Oxford University Press.

Allen, K. R., & Henderson, A. C. (2017). *Family theories: Foundations and applications*. Malden, MA: Wiley.

Allen, K. R., & Piercy, F. P. (2005). Feminist autoethnography. In D. Sprenkle & F. P. Piercy (Eds.), *Research methods in family therapy* (2nd ed., pp. 155–169). New York, NY: Guilford.

Almendrala, A. (2018, October 17). Most Americans who can't get pregnant have no way to access treatment. Huffington Post. Retrieved from https://www.huffingtonpost.com/entry/fertility-treatment-access_us_5bc51497e4b0d38b58706b15

American Psychological Association. (2009). *Report of the American Psychological Association Task Force on Appropriate Therapeutic Responses to Sexual Orientation*. Retrieved from https://www.apa.org/pi/lgbt/resources/therapeutic-response.pdf

Badgett, M. V. L. (2018). Left out? Lesbian, gay, and bisexual poverty in the U.S. *Population Research and Policy Review, 37*, 667–702. https://doi.org/10.1007/s11113-018-9457-5

Bardos, J., Hercz, D., Friedenthal, J., Missmer, S. A., & Williams, Z. (2015). A national survey on public perceptions of miscarriage. *Obstetrics and Gynecology, 125*, 1313–1320. https://doi.org/10.1097/AOG.0000000000000859

Bell, A. V. (2014). *Misconception: Social class and infertility in America*. New Brunswick, NJ: Rutgers University Press.

Bergstrom-Lynch, C. (2015). *Lesbians, gays, and bisexuals becoming parents or remaining child-free: Confronting social inequalities*. Lanham, MD: Lexington Books.

Bolton, I. (with Mitchell, C.). (2009). *My son...my son...a guide to healing after death, loss or suicide*. Roswell, GA: Bolton Press Atlanta.

Boss, P. (2006). *Loss, trauma, and resilience: Therapeutic work with ambiguous loss*. New York, NY: W. W. Norton.

Bostwick, W. B., Meyer, I., Aranda, F., Russell, S., Hughes, T., Birkett, M., & Mustanski, B. (2014). Mental health and suicidality among racially/ethnically diverse sexual minority youths. *American Journal of Public Health, 104*, 1129–1136. https://doi.org/10.2105/AJPH.2013.301749

Browne, K., & Nash, C. J. (Eds.). (2010). *Queer methods and methodologies: Intersecting queer theories and social science research*. London, UK: Routledge.

Cacciatore, J., Froen, J. F., & Killian, M. (2013). Condemning self, condemning other: Blame and mental health in women suffering stillbirth. *Journal of Mental Health Counseling, 35*, 342–359. https://doi.org/10.17744/mehc.35.4.15427g822442h11m

Cacciatore, J., Killian, M., & Harper, M. (2016). Adverse outcomes in bereaved mothers: The importance of household income and education. *SSM-Population Health, 2*, 117–122. https://doi.org/10.1016/j.ssmph.2016.02.009

Cacciatore, J., & Raffo, Z. (2011). An exploration of lesbian maternal bereavement. *Social Work, 56*, 169–177. https://doi.org/10.1093/sw/56.2.169

Canetto, S. S., & Cleary, A. (2012). Men, masculinities and suicidal behavior. *Social Science & Medicine, 74*, 461–465. https://doi.org/10.1016/j.socscimed.2011.11.001

Caputi, T. L., Smith, D., & Ayers, J. W. (2017). Suicide risk behaviors among sexual minority adolescents in the United States, 2015. *Research Letter. JAMA, 318*(23), 2349–2351. https://doi.org/10.1001/jama.2017.16908

cárdenas, m. (2016). Pregnancy: Reproductive futures in trans of color feminism. *TSQ: Transgender Studies Quarterly, 3*(1–2), 48–57. https://doi.org/10.1215/23289252-3334187

Collins, P. H., & Bilge, S. (2016). *Intersectionality*. Cambridge, UK: Polity Press.

Compton, D. R., Meadow, T., & Schilt, K. (Eds.). (2018). *Other, please specify: Queer methods in sociology*. Oakland, CA: University of California Press.

Craven, C. (2017, July 26). Resources & support for LGBTQ parents. Retrieved from https://babyinheaven.com/support-grieving-lgbtq-parents/

Craven, C. (2019). *Reproductive losses: Challenges to LGBTQ family-making*. New York, NY: Routledge.

Craven, C., & Peel, E. (2014). Stories of grief and hope: Queer experiences of reproductive loss. In M. F. Gibson (Ed.), *Queering motherhood: Narrative and theoretical perspectives* (pp. 97–110). Bradford, ON: Demeter Press.

Craven, C., & Peel, E. (2017). Queering reproductive loss: Exploring grief and memorialization. In E. R. M. Lind & A. Deveau (Eds.), *Interrogating pregnancy loss: Feminist writings on abortion, miscarriage and stillbirth* (pp. 225–245). Bradford, ON: Demeter Press.

Dahl, U. (2018). Becoming fertile in the land of organic milk: Lesbian and queer reproductions of femininity and motherhood in Sweden. *Sexualities, 21*, 1021–1038. https://doi.org/10.1177/1363460717718509

Davis, D.-A., & Craven, C. (2016). *Feminist ethnography: Thinking through methodologies, challenges & possibilities*. Lanham, MD: Rowman & Littlefield Press.

de Vries, B. (2009). Aspects of death, grief, and loss in lesbian, gay, bisexual, and transgender communities. In K. Doka & A. Tucci (Eds.), *Living with grief: Diversity and end-of-life care* (pp. 243–257). Washington, DC: Hospice Foundation of America.

de Vries, B., & Gutman, G. (2016). End-of-life preparations among LGBT older adults. *Generations, 40*(2), 46–48.

Doka, K. J. (2008). Disenfranchised grief in historical and cultural perspective. In M. S. Stroebe, R. O. Hansson, H. Schut, & W. Stroebe (Eds.), *Handbook of bereavement research and practice: Advances in theory and intervention* (pp. 223–240). Washington, DC: American Psychological Association.

Feigelman, W., Jordan, J. R., McIntosh, J. L., & Feigelman, B. (2012). *Devastating losses: How parents cope with the death of a child to suicide or drugs*. New York, NY: Springer.

Frey, L. M., Fulginiti, A., Lezine, D., & Cerel, J. (2018). The decision-making process for disclosing suicidal ideation and behavior to family and friends. *Family Relations, 67*, 414–427. https://doi.org/10.1111/fare.12315

Frey, L. M., Hans, J. D., & Cerel, J. (2017). An interpretive phenomenological inquiry of family and friend reactions to suicide disclosure. *Journal of Marital and Family Therapy, 43*, 159–172. https://doi.org/10.1111/jmft.12180

Frey, L. M., Hans, J. D., & Sanford, R. L. (2016). Where is family science in suicide prevention and intervention? Theoretical applications for a systemic perspective. *Journal of Family Theory & Review, 8*, 446–462. https://doi.org/10.1111/jftr.12168

Gates, G. J. (2015). Marriage and family: LGBT individuals and same-sex couples. *The Future of Children, 25*(2), 67–87. https://doi.org/10.1353/foc.2015.0013

Gates, G. J., & Romero, A. P. (2009). Parenting by gay men and lesbians: Beyond the current research. In H. E. Peters & C. M. K. Dush (Eds.), *Marriage and family: Perspectives and complexities* (pp. 227–243). New York, NY: Columbia University Press.

Gear, R. (2014). Bereaved parents' perspectives on informal social support: "What worked for you?". *Journal of Loss and Trauma, 19*, 173–188. https://doi.org/10.1080/15325024.2013.763548

Goldman, L., & Livoti, V. M. (2011). Grief in GLBT populations: Focus on gay and lesbian youth. In R. A. Neimeyer, D. L. Harris, H. R. Winokuer, & G. F. Thornton (Eds.), *Grief and bereavement in contemporary society: Bridging research and practice* (pp. 249–260). New York, NY: Routledge.

Green, L., & Grant, V. (2008). 'Gagged grief and beleaguered bereavements?' An analysis of multidisciplinary theory and research relating to same sex partnership bereavement. *Sexualities, 11*, 275–300. https://doi.org/10.1177/1363460708089421

Haas, A. P., Eliason, M., Mays, V. M., Mathy, R. M., Cochran, S. D., D'Augelli, A. R., . . . Clayton, P. J. (2011). Suicide and suicide risk in lesbian, gay, bisexual, and transgender populations: Review and recommendations. *Journal of Homosexuality, 58,* 10–51. doi:https://doi.org/10.1080/00918369.2011.534038

Hill, P. W., Cacciatore, J., Shreffler, K. M., & Pritchard, K. M. (2017). The loss of self: The effect of miscarriage, stillbirth, and child death on maternal self-esteem. *Death Studies, 41,* 226–235. https://doi.org/10.1080/07481187.2016.1261204

Hooghe, A., Rosenblatt, P. C., & Rober, P. (2018). "We hardly ever talk about it": Emotional responsive attunement in couples after a child's death. *Family Process, 57,* 226–240. https://doi.org/10.1111/famp.12274

Hunt, Q. A., & Hertlein, K. M. (2015). Conceptualizing suicide bereavement from an attachment lens. *American Journal of Family Therapy, 43,* 16–27. https://doi.org/10.1080/01926187.2014.975651

Jaques, J. D. (2000). Surviving suicide: The impact on the family. *The Family Journal: Counseling and Therapy for Couples and Families, 8,* 376–379. https://doi.org/10.1177/1066480700084007

Jordan, J., Price, J., & Prior, L. (2015). Disorder and disconnection: Parent experiences of liminality when caring for their dying child. *Sociology of Health & Illness, 37,* 839–855. https://doi.org/10.1111/1467-9566.12235

Kasahara-Kiritani, M., Ikeda, M., Yamamoto-Mitani, N., & Kamibeppu, K. (2017). Regaining my new life: Daily lives of suicide-bereaved individuals. *Death Studies, 41,* 447–454. https://doi.org/10.1080/07481187.2017.1297873

Kuvalanka, K., & Goldberg, A. (2009). "Second generation" voices: Queer youth with lesbian/bisexual mothers. *Journal of Youth and Adolescence, 38,* 904–919. https://doi.org/10.1007/s10964-008-9327-2

Layne, L. L. (2003). *Motherhood lost: A feminist account of pregnancy loss in America.* New York, NY: Routledge.

Luce, J. (2010). *Beyond expectation: Lesbian/bi/queer women and assisted conception.* Toronto, ON: University of Toronto Press.

McGuire, J. K., Catalpa, J. M., Lacey, V., & Kuvalanka, K. A. (2016). Ambiguous loss as a framework for interpreting gender transitions in families. *Journal of Family Theory & Review, 8,* 373–385. https://doi.org/10.1111/jftr.12159

McLaughlin, J., Casey, M. E., & Richardson. (2006). Introduction: At the intersections of feminist and queer debates. In D. Richardson, J. McLaughlin, & M. E. Casey (Eds.), *Intersections between feminist and queer theory* (pp. 1–18). Basingstoke, UK: Palgrave.

McNair, T., & Altman, K. (2012). Miscarriage and recurrent pregnancy loss. In K. J. Hurt, M. W. Guile, J. L. Bienstock, H. E. Fox, & E. E. Wallach (Eds.), *The Johns Hopkins manual of gynecology and obstetrics* (4th ed., pp. 438–447). Philadelphia, PA: Lippincott Williams & Wilkins.

McNutt, B., & Yakushko, O. (2013). Disenfranchised grief among lesbian and gay bereaved individuals. *Journal of LGBT Issues in Counseling, 7,* 87–116. https://doi.org/10.1080/15538605.2013.758345

Meris, D. (2016). Transformation through socially sensitive experiences. In D. L. Harris & T. C. Bordere (Eds.), *Handbook of social justice in loss and grief: Exploring diversity, equity, and inclusion* (pp. 179–190). New York, NY: Routledge.

Moore, M. R. (2011). *Invisible families: Gay identities, relationships, and motherhood among Black women.* Berkeley, CA: University of California Press.

Mullings, L. (2005). Resistance and resilience: The Sojourner Syndrome and the social context of reproduction in Central Harlem. *Transforming Anthropology, 13,* 79–91. https://doi.org/10.1525/tran.2005.13.2.79

Murphy, S. A. (2008). The loss of a child: Sudden death and extended illness perspectives. In M. S. Stroebe, R. O. Hansson, H. Schut, & W. Stroebe (Eds.), *Handbook of bereavement research and practice: Advances in theory and intervention* (pp. 375–395). Washington, DC: American Psychological Association.

Murray, C. I. (2017). Death, dying, and grief in families. In C. A. Price, K. R. Bush, & S. J. Price (Eds.), *Families and change: Coping with stressful events and transitions* (5th ed., pp. 359–380). Los Angeles, CA: Sage.

Nadal, K. L., Whitman, C. N., Davis, L. S., Erazo, T., & Davidoff, K. C. (2016). Microaggressions toward lesbian, gay, bisexual, transgender, queer, and genderqueer people: A review of the literature. *Journal of Sex Research, 53,* 488–508. https://doi.org/10.1080/00224499.2016.1142495

Nagar, R. (2014). *Muddying the waters: Coauthoring feminisms across scholarship and activism.* Urbana, IL: University of Illinois Press.

Narayan, K. (2012). *Alive in the writing: Crafting ethnography in the company of Chekhov.* Chicago, IL: University of Chicago Press.

Paisley-Cleveland, L. (2013). *Black middle-class women and pregnancy loss: A qualitative inquiry.* Lanham, MD: Lexington Books.

Patlamazoglou, L., Simmonds, J. G., & Snell, T. L. (2018). Same-sex partner bereavement: Non-HIV-related loss and new research directions. *Omega—Journal of Death and Dying, 78,* 178–196. https://doi.org/10.1177/0030222817690160

Peel, E. (2010). Pregnancy loss in lesbian and bisexual women: An online survey of experiences. *Human Reproduction, 25,* 721–727. https://doi.org/10.1093/humrep/dep441

Peel, E., & Cain, R. (2012). Silent' miscarriage and deafening heteronormativity: A British experiential and critical feminist account. In S. Earle, C. Komaromy, & L. L. Layne (Eds.), *Understanding reproductive loss: Perspectives on life, death and fertility* (pp. 79–92). New York, NY: Routledge.

Perluxo, D., & Francisco, R. (2018). Use of Facebook in the maternal grief process: An exploratory qualitative study. *Death Studies, 42,* 79–88. https://doi.org/10.1080/07481187.2017.1334011

Power, J., Goodyear, M., Maybery, D., Reupert, A., O'Hanlon, B., Cuff, R., & Perlesz, A. (2016). Family resilience in families where a parent has a mental illness. *Journal of Social Work, 16,* 66–82. https://doi.org/10.1177/1468017314568081

Rivers, I., Gonzalez, C., Nodin, N., Peel, E., & Tyler, A. (2018). LGBT people and suicidality in youth: A qualitative study of perceptions of risk and protective circumstances. *Social Science & Medicine, 212*, 1–8. https://doi.org/10.1016/j.soscimed.2018.06.040

Romero, A. P., & Goldberg, A. E. (2019). Introduction. In A. E. Goldberg & A. P. Romero (Eds.), *LGBTQ divorce and relationship dissolution: Psychological and legal perspectives and implications for practice* (pp. 1–6). New York, NY: Oxford University Press.

Rosenblatt, P. C. (2000). *Parent grief: Narratives of loss and relationship.* New York, NY: Taylor & Francis.

Ross, L. (2017). Reproductive justice as intersectional feminist activism. *Souls: A Critical Journal of Black Politics, Culture, and Society, 19*, 286–314. https://doi.org/10.1080/10999949.2017.1389634

Ross, L., Roberts, L., Derkas, E., Peoples, W., & Toure, P. B. (Eds.). (2017). *Radical reproductive justice: Foundation, theory, practice, critique.* New York, NY: The Feminist Press.

Ross, L., & Solinger, R. (2017). *Reproductive justice: An introduction.* Oakland, CA: University of California Press.

Ruddick, S. (1989). *Maternal thinking: Toward a politics of peace.* Boston, MA: Beacon Press.

Russell, S. T., & Toomey, R. B. (2012). Men's sexual orientation and suicide: Evidence for U.S. adolescent-specific risk. *Social Science & Medicine, 74*, 523–529. https://doi.org/10.1016/j.socscimed.2010.07.038

Ryff, C. D., Schmutte, P. S., & Lee, Y. H. (1996). How children turn out: Implications for parental self-evaluation. In C. D. Ryff & M. M. Seltzer (Eds.), *The parental experience in midlife* (pp. 383–422). Chicago, IL: University of Chicago Press.

Sachs, A. D. (2019). Tying tight or splitting up: An adult's perspective of his parents' same-sex relationship dissolution. In A. E. Goldberg & A. P. Romero (Eds.), *LGBTQ divorce and relationship dissolution: Psychological and legal perspectives and implications for practice* (pp. 245–262). New York, NY: Oxford University Press.

Scherrer, K. S., & Fedor, J. P. (2015). Family issues for LGBT older adults. In N. A. Orel & C. A. Fruhauf (Eds.), *The lives of LGBT older adults: Understanding challenges and resilience* (pp. 171–192). Washington, DC: American Psychological Association.

Scott, S., Diamond, G. S., & Levy, S. A. (2016). Attachment-based family therapy for suicidal adolescents: A case study. *Australian and New Zealand Journal of Family Therapy, 37*, 154–176. https://doi.org/10.1002/anzf.1149

Sheehan, L., Corrigan, P. W., Al-Khouja, M. A., Lewy, S. A., Major, D. R., Mead, J., … Weber, S. (2018). Behind closed doors: The stigma of suicide loss survivors. *Omega—Journal of Death and Dying, 77*, 330–349. https://doi.org/10.1177/0030222816674215

Skerrett, D. M., Kolves, K., & De Leo, D. (2017). Pathways to suicide in lesbian and gay populations in Australia: A life chart analysis. *Archives of Sexual Behavior, 46*, 1481–1489. https://doi.org/10.1007/s10508-016-0827-y

Song, J., Floyd, F. J., Seltzer, M. M., & Greenberg, J. S. (2010). Long-term effects of child death on parents' health-related quality of life: A dyadic analysis. *Family Relations, 59*, 269–282. https://doi.org/10.1111/j.1741-3729.2010.00601.x

Sugrue, J. L., McGiloway, S., & Keegan, O. (2014). The experiences of mothers bereaved by suicide: An exploratory study. *Death Studies, 38*, 118–124. https://doi.org/10.1080/07481187.2012.738765

Vachon, M. L. S., & Harris, D. L. (2016). The liberating capacity of compassion. In D. L. Harris & T. C. Bordere (Eds.), *Handbook of social justice in loss and grief: Exploring diversity, equity, and inclusion* (pp. 265–281). New York, NY: Routledge.

Walker, R. S. (2017). After suicide: Coming together in kindness and support. *Death Studies, 41*, 635–638. https://doi.org/10.1080/07481187.2017.1335549

Walks, M. (2007). Breaking the silence: Infertility, motherhood, and queer culture. *Journal of the Association for Research on Mothering. Special Issue: Mothering, Race, Ethnicity, Culture, and Class, 9*, 130–143.

Wojnar, D. (2007). Miscarriage experiences of lesbian couples. *Journal of Midwifery & Women's Health, 52*, 479–485. https://doi.org/10.1016/j.jmwh.2007.03.015

Wojnar, D. (2009). *The experience of lesbian miscarriage: Phenomenological inquiry.* Köln, Germany: Lambert Academic Publishing.

Wojnar, D., & Swanson, K. M. (2006). Why shouldn't lesbian women who miscarry receive special consideration? *Journal of GLBT Family Studies, 2*(1), 1–12. https://doi.org/10.1300/J461v02n01_01

# Part III

# Applied Topics

# The Law Governing LGBTQ-Parent Families in the United States

## Julie Shapiro

Many LGBTQ people, alone or in couples, want to add children to their families. There are a variety of ways this can be done, and individuals or couples may explore several paths before settling on a plan (Goldberg, Gartrell, & Gates, 2014). One initial choice is often whether to pursue adoption or some form of assisted reproduction. Either of these choices will lead to more choices. For example, if one chooses adoption, does one pursue domestic or foreign adoption? Can a couple adopt a child together? Choosing assisted reproduction[1] leads to other questions, and generally different ones for women (who typically have access to ova and need sperm) and men (who generally have access to sperm but need both ova and a woman to gestate the child). LGBTQ couples becoming parents will face yet more questions: For example, whatever the method by which one person attains legal parentage, will the other person's parental rights also be secure? If not, can steps be taken to secure them?

As complicated and layered as these choices are, it is essential to understand that each choice brings with it its own set of legal considerations. Failure to consider the legal ramifications of the various courses of action being considered can result in future difficulties for the individuals and families involved. Understanding the basic outlines of the law of parentage as it pertains to LGBTQ people can assist individuals in understanding their options and in assessing their legal positions and, perhaps more importantly, it can also help them understand why attention to legal status issues is so critical.

Even as the laws regarding recognition of lesbian and gay family relationships have changed dramatically in the last few years, the basic truth remains the same: There are significant legal questions that every LGBTQ person and/or LGBTQ couple must consider as they form their families (Joslin, Minter, & Sakimura, 2018).

The very fact of LGBTQ people becoming parents remains controversial. This results in

---

[1] Assisted reproduction generally uses some form of ART (assisted reproductive technology). These include insemination with sperm from a donor (who may be known or unknown), in vitro fertilization, and surrogacy. Assisted reproduction stands in contrast to non-assisted reproduction, which is conception via heterosexual intercourse. If a child is conceived via heterosexual intercourse, it is virtually certain that both the male and the female participants will be legal parents. This is rarely the outcome queer women contemplating parenthood want and so should only be considered in rare cases.

J. Shapiro (✉)
Seattle University School of Law, Faculty Fellow
Fred T Korematsu Center for Law and Equality,
Seattle, WA, USA
e-mail: shapiro@seattleu.edu

© Springer Nature Switzerland AG 2020
A. E. Goldberg, K. R. Allen (eds.), *LGBTQ-Parent Families*,
https://doi.org/10.1007/978-3-030-35610-1_23

365

both state-by-state variation in the law and near-constant change in law. It is practically impossible to accurately summarize the current state of the law at any given moment. Even if it were possible to do so at any given moment, the summary would quickly become unreliable and outdated. Unreliable or incomplete legal information may create serious hazards for LGBTQ people planning for parenthood. The goal of this chapter is, therefore, not to provide a specific account of the law as it stands today. Instead, this chapter provides a brief introduction to the major legal principles that shape the law. For more specific and concrete analysis of individual situations, one would be well advised to consult a lawyer familiar with the relevant law in the relevant jurisdiction.[2]

In order to be legally secure in their relationship to a child, a person needs to be recognized as a legal parent. The process by which LGBTQ adults become parents (adoption, assisted reproduction, or nonassisted reproduction) is critical to analysis of legal parentage. As LGBTQ people planning to become parents consider whether to pursue adoption or ART, the law governing legal status should inform their decision-making. For those using ART, one or more adults (if there is more than one adult) may gain recognition as a legal parent without taking any legal action. For other individuals, including all adoptive parents, legal action will be needed to secure recognition as a legal parent. In later sections, this chapter considers each path to parenthood in greater detail.

Once recognition as a legal parent is attained, subsequent legal issues become significantly less complicated. The rights of legal parents are well understood and do not vary based on the sexual or gender identity of the parents. For instance, resolution of a custody dispute for an LGBTQ couple where both parties are legal parents is legally indistinguishable from a heterosexual child custody case. Similarly, resolution of a custody dispute between an LGBTQ legal parent and a cisgender heterosexual legal parent should not depend on the sexual or gender identity of the LGBTQ parent. The individual facts of the case will be critical, but the two adults stand on equal legal footing[3] (Joslin et al., 2018, §6.1). The deciding factor will be the best interests of the particular child or children involved[4] (Pearson, 2019). By contrast, if a person is not a legal parent, they will be at a nearly insurmountable legal disadvantage in litigation against a legal parent or parents.

Thus, the most critical legal question encountered by LGBTQ people contemplating parenthood, and particularly LGBTQ couples,[5] is who will have recognition as a legal parent. This chapter uses the initial question of recognition as a legal parent as the organizing structure for a larger discussion of the legal issues facing LGBTQ parents and prospective parents.

---

[2]National legal organizations that focus on lesbian, gay, and transgender rights may be helpful in locating a knowledgeable local attorney. The websites of both Lambda Legal Defense and Education Fund (http://www.lambda-legal.org/) and The National Center for Lesbian Rights (http://www.nclrights.org/) offer legal help desks.

*Protecting Families: Standards for LGBT Families* is jointly produced by GLAD (Gay and Lesbian Advocates and Defenders) and NCLR. This publication provides critical guidance for queer couples who are engaged in co-parenting disputes. The standards can be reviewed at http://www.glad.org/protecting-families

[3]This is not to say that an LGBTQ parent will be treated fairly when litigating against a non-LGBTQ parent. Discrimination undoubtedly exists in fact even if it is not legally permissible.

[4]The best interest of the child is an indeterminate test which, by design, allows each judge to consider each case on its own particular facts. What is seen to be best for one child may be different from what is seen to be best for another. Judges are given broad discretion to consider a very wide range of factors in making their decision. Because of the wide latitude that judges are given, it can be very difficult to predict the outcome of the test and it can be very expensive to litigate a case.

[5]A small number of states recognize the possibility of more than two legal parents. Recognition may be possible where three or more people are involved in the initial decision to create a family or where a family with two legal parents separates and a new partner of one of the original parents gains recognition. California and Washington have explicit statutory language that permits this. In other states, such as Massachusetts, individual courts have allowed it. This recognition is NOT commonly available. Knowledgeable local lawyers must be consulted. For the purpose of this chapter, the focus will be on sole or dual parentage.

## Overview: The General Structure of Family Law in the United States

Most family law in the United States (US) is state (as opposed to federal) law. This means that as a general rule, family law is made by state legislatures or state courts rather than by the US Congress or federal courts. However, the US Constitution establishes some essential rights in this area, and all states must recognize and/or protect those basic rights. This is the basis for the US Supreme Court decision directing all states to grant access to marriage to same-sex couple.

Once those basic rights are established, the details, and to some degree the scope, of those rights are up to the individual states. While it is easy to point to broad commonalities (e.g., every jurisdiction has marriage, all have recognized legal parent/child relationships, all legally recognized parents have strong rights and obligations vis-à-vis their children), the specifics of the law (e.g., how one enters into marriage, who is eligible to marry, when is a person recognized as a legal parent) can and do vary significantly state-to-state. Each of the 50 states as well as the District of Columbia and the US territories has its own body of law (Joslin et al., 2018).

For married heterosexual-parent families, the most important aspects of family law—namely, marriage and the recognition of parent/child relationships—are well established and essentially uniform across all states. While there are state-to-state differences in the finer points of marriage eligibility (minimum age for marriage varies, for instance), unrelated adult heterosexuals who are not already married are generally eligible to marry in all states. Equally important, all states readily accord respect to virtually all different-sex marriages performed out-of-state, so if a heterosexual couple marries in New York, they can travel freely around the United States, knowing that all other states will recognize their marriage. Further, all states will grant heterosexual married couples a similar set of rights arising from marriage. There is essentially no state-to-state variation in this regard. Thus, the state-law nature of family law is rarely a source of difficulty or even comment for heterosexual married couples. If a heterosexual couple marries and has children in one state, both members of the couple will typically be recognized as legal parents in every other state.

Same-sex couples, including same-sex married couples, cannot be confident that they will be afforded similar recognition. The law regarding marriage for same-sex couples has, of course, changed dramatically in recent years, and many significant protections have been obtained. After the Supreme Court's decision in *Obergefell v. Hodges* (2015), same-sex couples are permitted to marry throughout the United States. In addition, each state must recognize valid same-sex marriages from other states. Thus, Alabama must recognize a California marriage between two women or two men. Further, the LGBTQ married couple must be accorded all of the core rights of marriage just as heterosexual couples are. But crucially, it is not yet firmly established that rights to *parentage* that arise from marriage must also be recognized. States that have historically been generally resistant to equal rights for LGBTQ people continue to be resistant to recognition of parental rights for LGBTQ people (Knauer, 2019).

To be clear, *Obergefell* did much to equalize the legal status of same-sex and different-sex married couples. It alleviated many important problems faced by LGBTQ couples. So, for instance, in the past, the law of marriage for transgender people varied from state to state. A transman and cisgender woman might be deemed to be married in some states (because they were recognized as being a male/female couple), but their marriage might not be recognized in other states (because that state saw only a female/female couple because of the state's refusal to allow legal gender change).[6] This problem has been eliminated as the validity of a marriage no longer depends on the genders of those getting married.

At the same time, where legal status as a parent is claimed based on marriage, the degree

---

[6]This was the situation in both Kansas and Texas. Survivors of these marriages, whether transgender or cisgender, faced harsh results as their marriages were deemed invalid.

to which recognition of marriage requires recognition of status as a parent may still be contested in some jurisdictions. While the Supreme Court has taken some positive steps toward extending broad recognition, *Pavan v. Smith* (2017), it has not issued definitive guidance. As is discussed further below, some individual judges have been unwilling to extend the same presumptions of legal parentage to LGTBQ married couples as are available to different-sex married couples. Thus, it is still the case that the parental rights of married LGBTQ couples vary more widely and are more contested than those of married different-sex couples even in the postmarriage recognition period (NeJaime, 2016).

Given that interstate travel is common, this variation can be problematic even for couples who live in states where the law is clear. A married lesbian couple with children living in Massachusetts may be quite confident in their legal status while in Massachusetts, but should their travels take them to Alabama, and should circumstances—perhaps unanticipated emergencies—arise there, an Alabama court's determination of their parental status may not match the status they would have had in Massachusetts. Thus, LGBTQ couples must still take care to ensure recognition of parental rights across all states. Recognition of marriage equality has not led to uniform recognition of LGBTQ parent/child relationships.

For example, there is a common legal presumption, used in virtually all states, that the husband of a woman who gives birth to a child is a legal parent of the child.[7] The presumption dates back to feudal England when, of course, the only legally recognized marriages were those between men and women. The presumption is still available to different-sex married couples, but states have reached differing conclusions on whether it should be extended to lesbian couples. Thus, where a married woman gives birth to a child,

some states will automatically recognize her spouse, whether male or female, as a legal parent. Other states will not extend automatic recognition to a female spouse.[8]

This inconsistency can have important ramifications. Suppose P (who is female) and C (child) live in state A and that the law in state A recognizes a legal parent–child relationship between P and C because P is married to the woman who gave birth to C. Now suppose that there is a neighboring state, B. State B is required to recognize P's marriage, whether the spouse is of the same sex or not. But state B may contend that it does not have to recognize P's status as a legal parent. As to this obligation, the law is unsettled.

This question of legal parental status is of immense practical importance. Will state B allow P to authorize medical care for C, as a legal parent is undoubtedly able to do? Can P visit C in a hospital? Can P enroll C in school? If P died, would C inherit as a child of P? If P and the other legal parent separate, does P stand on an equal footing in terms of the rights to care, custody, and control of the child? These questions cannot always be answered generally. Even as many things have changed in recent years, LGBTQ parents still inhabit a world rife with legal uncertainty.

As was noted above, there is little direct federal family law. Constitutional cases like *Obergefell* are the exception rather than the rule. Instead, generally speaking, the federal government will recognize family relationships that are recognized under the relevant state's law.[9] Thus,

---

[7]In fact, this presumption is the basis on which the vast majority of heterosexual married men are recognized as legal parents. Nothing beyond the marriage of the man and woman is required in order to secure the husband's parental status.

[8]The situation for gay male couples is even more complicated. Historically, the presumption only applied to a *man* whose wife gave birth to a child. It did not apply to a *woman* whose husband fathered a child. But with the advent of surrogacy one might argue that where a married man provides the sperm used in creating an embryo carried to term by a surrogate, his spouse—whether husband or wife—should automatically be recognized as a legal parent of a child. Courts, however, have not embraced this argument.

[9]Often, it is clear which state's law will be used, as when a family has lived for an extended period of time in a single state. But this is not always so. As families travel and/or relocate, questions about which state's law the federal government will use may arise.

if the parent–child relationship between P and C is recognized by state A, it will generally be recognized by the federal government (Joslin et al., 2018, §6.7). This recognition provides the child with access to federal programs based on the parent/child relationship, such as social security survivor benefits or veteran's benefits.

The next section of this chapter examines general family law principles that apply in all states. It also considers constitutional law—which is to say those family law principles found to be rooted in the United States Constitution. Because the Constitution is binding in all states, principles of constitutional law necessarily apply to all states. It is only because the principles introduced here are stated relatively abstractly that generalizations can be offered. The specifics of family law vary significantly state to state. Thus, the outcomes of particular cases may vary state to state.

## The Importance of Legal Parenthood

"Parent" is a word with many meanings. In common speech, it is often coupled with different modifiers. There can be stepparents and social parents, natural parents and adoptive parents, and so on. The critical category for law is, unsurprisingly, that of *legal parent*. A legal parent is a person who the law recognizes as a parent of the child in question. People who function as social parents may or may not be legal parents, just as legal parents may or may not be social parents.

It is difficult to overstate the importance of being a legal parent. Legal parents are assigned an array of rights and obligations with regard to a child. Legal parents make critical decisions about education, religious upbringing and medical care, as well as countless lesser decisions in day-to-day life. As long as the actions of a legal parent do not endanger the child, neither the state nor other individuals who are not themselves legal parents can interfere with the legal parent's decisions. At the same time, legal parents have obligations to care for, protect, and support their children and can be subject to prosecution where they fail to fulfill their obligations. Legal parents

have great latitude within their families and can invoke powerful protections to prevent outside interference (Polikoff, 1990, 2009).

Importantly, throughout the United States, as in most countries throughout the world, the legal rights of those recognized in law as parents are far superior to the legal rights of individuals who are not legal parents. Legal parents can decide whom their children see and spend time with. This means that legal parents can effectively exclude nonparents from their children's lives.

The US Supreme Court has recognized that the rights of a legal parent are constitutionally protected (*Troxel v. Granville*, 2000). In *Troxel*, a trial judge ordered visitation between two children and their paternal grandparents over the objections of the children's mother. (The children's father was deceased.) The trial judge did so because he found that visiting the grandparents would be beneficial to the children. The US Supreme Court concluded that the trial judge's action violated the constitutionally protected parental rights of the mother. (The mother's status as a legal parent was never in doubt.) The Supreme Court did so even though it might well have been beneficial to the children to visit with the grandparents. The choice of who the children were to see properly lay with their mother, and the state (here acting through the trial judge) could not interfere with her choice absent specific circumstances. The Court did not define what those circumstances might be. The fact that the judge thought seeing the grandparents was a better decision was not enough.

While those precise circumstances where a legal parent's decision might remain ill-defined, the general import of *Troxel* is clear: All states are required to recognize and enforce strong parental rights. Absent extraordinary circumstances, a legal parent's decisions about who the child spends time with will stand.

The circumstances under which a legal parent's judgment will be overridden are narrow but have historically been of some concern to LGBTQ-parent families. A legal parent loses the protections described above where the parent is found to be unfit. In the past, there have been cases where unfitness has been premised on a parent's identification as lesbian or gay. For some courts, proof that a parent was a lesbian or a gay man constituted proof that the parent was unfit (*N.K.M. v. L.E.M.*, 1980). This was known as the "per se" rule. These cases arose where a heterosexual relationship that had produced children dissolved and one of the parties subsequently identified himself or herself as gay or lesbian. The heterosexual parent would invoke the sexuality of the parent newly identified as LGBTQ as a basis for disqualifying that parent from receiving custody (Joslin et al., 2018, §1).

In more recent years, the idea that the parental sexual *identity* could disqualify one from custody has been rejected in favor of a test focused on actual parental *conduct* (sexual or otherwise) and an inquiry into whether that conduct has caused harm to the child (Joslin et al., 2018; Shapiro, 1996). This is often called a "nexus" test. Courts are instructed to focus on parental conduct rather than parental identity. Further, courts must determine whether there is a connection (or nexus) between parental conduct and actual harm to the child. Only if there is such a connection is parental conduct relevant.

Use of the nexus test is now nearly universal. Only conduct which is shown to cause harm to the child may be a basis for a finding of unfitness (Joslin et al., 2018). This test requires an individualized analysis based on the specific facts of each case. In the hands of a fair judge, it places LGBTQ parents on an equal footing with all other parents with regard to unfitness inquiries.[10] Findings of parental unfitness are relatively rare and the overwhelming majority of LGBTQ people who have obtained legal recognition as parents will be fit parents.

The shift to a nexus test has not, however, eliminated the possibility of discrimination against LGBTQ parents. This can be of particular concern in custody cases that arise after the dissolution of a heterosexual union. If one partner identifies as LGBTQ that person may be subject to judicial bias—conscious or implicit—in determination of child custody. Judges can rule against

LGBTQ parents without direct reference to the parent's status as LGBTQ (Pearson, 2019). Instead, they might discuss stability, or the nature of the choices the LGBTQ parent has made and their potential impact on the child. In one recent case, the Washington State Supreme Court recognized this form of bias and sought to create protections against it (*In re Marriage of Black*, 2017).

In sum, the only person who can directly challenge a fit legal parent's decisions in court is another fit legal parent. Where two fit legal parents disagree over the custody/control of a child or children, a court will determine the outcome in a conventional custody case. In such a case, the best interests of the child become the court's guiding principle. But if a fit legal parent has a disagreement with a person who is *not* a legal parent, the fit legal parent has an immense and typically an insurmountable advantage. It is the fit legal parent's right to determine the outcome and courts will be loath to interfere. Where they do interfere, they will grant the fit legal parent's decision great deference, typically affirming whatever actions the fit parent proposes.

Historically, the majority of family cases involving LGBTQ parents arose upon dissolution of heterosexual relationships where one party subsequently identified as LGBTQ. As is noted above, these cases do still exist and present concerns about possible judicial bias. A more typical custody case today arises when two (or occasionally more than two) people who identify as LGBTQ form a family and raise a child together. If the adults separate and disagree over the continuing care and custody of the child, litigation may result. If both of the adults have status as a legal parent, then these cases present as ordinary custody cases where two legal parents compete. But in the most troubling cases, the dynamic is quite different. One person claims that they are the sole legal parent. They assert that the former partner or spouse, who may have functioned as a parent for any number of years, is not a legal parent. If this argument succeeds, the end is virtually certain—the nonlegal parent's relationship with the child (and the child's relationship with that person) has no pro-

---

[10] Sexual conduct by a heterosexual parent that is shown to cause harm to the child will also be considered.

tection. An early example of this which remains good law almost 30 years later is *Alison D. v. Virginia M.* (1991). The legal parent alone is entitled to decide with whom the child spends time. If they prefer that the child not see the former partner, the child will not see that person.

These cases illustrate the power of the legal parent and the necessity of attention to legal status in family formation. These problematic outcomes are best avoided if LGBTQ people forming families take steps to ensure recognition of legal parentage in both parties.[11] The following section examines the law governing the methods by which LGBTQ people bring children into their relationships.

## Bringing Children into a Family

Broadly speaking, there are two alternative paths to legal parenthood: One can become a parent to an already existing child via adoption or one can participate in the creation of a new child via the process of conception/birth. Each path has its own complications and potentials, particularly for LGBTQ prospective parents. In the first two of the following sections, these options are examined in more detail. Because the original formation of a family sometimes only involves recognition of one legal parent, legal devices for securing rights for additional legal parents are then considered.

## Adoption

Adoption is a process by which a child acquires a new parent or set of parents who take the

place of an earlier parent or set of parents[12] (Farr & Goldberg, 2018). While adoptions can be (and often are) arranged in advance of the birth of a child, there is always some period of time after the birth of the child during which the birth parent(s) can revoke their consent to the adoption. This period varies from place to place and may be quite short, but it is important to recognize that it exists.

There is no general right to adopt. Thus, prospective parents must apply to the state for approval in order to adopt. The process for assessing prospective parents is typically delegated to either a state or private agency, but the legal process for the adoption and the requirements for adoptive parents are essentially similar in the public and private systems in any given state. The approval process may be quite time consuming, intensive, intrusive, and expensive (Goldberg, 2010). It typically includes a home study as well as criminal background checks. Home studies are generally an evaluation of the fitness of the prospective parent(s) to raise a child or children and may or may not include an actual visit to the home.

Prospective LGBTQ adoptive parents may face some special concerns. Some private agencies will not provide services for LGBTQ prospective parents. While this obviously discriminatory practice is controversial, the current federal administration has approved of

---

[11] Litigation of these cases can be destructive for the lesbian and gay communities as well as for the individuals involved. This is the motivation for the pamphlet "Protecting Families"—a co-production of GLAD and NCLR. http://www.glad.org/uploads/docs/publications/protecting-families-standards-for-lgbt-families.pdf

[12] The important exception to this generalization is second-parent or stepparent adoption, which are discussed in more detail below. (Absent adoption, a stepparent is typically not a legal parent. Step-parent adoptions are generally available in all states. The availability of second-parent adoptions is more limited.) A second-parent adoption or a step-parent adoption allows the court to add an adoptive parent to a family without terminating the rights of the existing parent or parents. This is unusually in that typically completion of an adoption terminates the parental rights of the preadoption parents. (That outcome is consistent with the general intent of most individuals adopting.) A second-parent adoption or a step-parent adoption recognizes that sometimes the intent of the prospective adoptive parent is to co-parent with the existing legal parent. Thus, the second parent or step-parent is granted parental rights and the original parent's rights are not terminated.

discriminatory foster care rules as an exercise of religious freedom (Cha, 2019). As a result, these restrictions on provision of services may actually be more common now than they were in the recent past (Joslin et al., 2018, §2.8.). If LGBTQ prospective parents are using a private agency, it should be selected with care (see chapter "LGBTQ Adoptive Parents and Their Children").

Beyond agency discrimination, adoption law should apply to all people, whether LGBTQ or not, similarly. All states permit married couples, including LGBTQ married couples, to adopt assuming they meet general qualifications. Discrimination against married LGBTQ couples in this setting has been found to be unconstitutional (Pavan v. Smith, 2017).

Additionally, all states permit adoption by unmarried individuals who are generally qualified. No state prohibits adoption based on an individual's status as LGBTQ. In other words, single and married LGBTQ people are generally eligible to adopt in all states.

The prospect for unmarried LGBTQ couples seeking to adopt jointly is more complicated, but this is because they are unmarried rather than because they are LGBTQ. Some states limit joint adoptions to married couples only. Unmarried couples, whether LGBTQ or not, cannot adopt jointly. In those states, couples who wish to adopt jointly must marry.

In most states where joint adoption by unmarried couples is not possible, one member of the same-sex couple would still be eligible to adopt, as nonmarital cohabitation is not a bar to adoption.[13] While this may be an important avenue to parenthood for a same-sex couple, it is at best an imperfect solution. The end result is a family where one member of the couple has status as a legal parent and the other does not. As is discussed earlier, this can have very serious consequences. The nonlegal parent will be at a severe disadvantage in the event

that the relationship between the adults dissolves or the legal parent dies. Further, benefits and obligations that ordinarily run between parent and child may not be recognized or imposed. Thus, it is possible that a child will not receive social security if the nonlegal parent dies or is injured. The nonlegal parent may not be able to make medical decisions for the child in the event of an emergency or to visit the child in a hospital. Further, a child may have difficulty establishing an entitlement to financial support from a nonlegal parent (Polikoff, 2009).

Lawyers may be able to prepare documents which will ameliorate some of the legal disadvantages experienced by the nonlegal parent and should be consulted, but these documents may not be honored in all states, and the powers granted by them may be revoked in the event the legal parent wishes to do so. Other possible avenues by which a nonlegal parent may gain legal protection are discussed below.

Unmarried couples seeking to remain unmarried and to complete a joint adoption may wish to consider relocating to a more hospitable state. Most states require residence for a period of time (the precise time varies but is often around 6 months) before a couple can invoke that state's adoption laws.

Once an adoption is properly completed, adoptive parents are full legal parents. Thus, they have the full range of parental rights regarding custody and control of their children as well as the full set of parental obligations. A dispute over custody of a child between two adoptive parents or between an adoptive parent and a natural legal parent should be handled as any dispute between two recognized legal parents of the child would be. In most instances, this means that a court will attempt to determine the best interests of the child and that the two parents stand on an equal footing at the beginning of this inquiry (Pearson, 2019).

Adoption is generally said to be irrevocable, though all parental rights can be terminated due to unfitness. It is extremely difficult to challenge

---

[13] A small number of states still bar a person cohabiting outside of marriage from adopting.

a completed adoption.[14] It is important, however, for prospective parents to be forthright and honest with adoption evaluators during the evaluative process involved in adoption. Fraud (which is deliberately misstating facts) and/or concealment of significant facts about past conduct or about one's qualifications as an adoptive parent may undermine the validity of an adoption. While candid disclosure of some matters (a criminal record or a history of mental illness, for instance) may make the path to adoption more difficult, it ensures that once completed the adoption will stand. In some instances, as when adoptive parents are traveling with their child, LGBTQ parents who have completed an adoption may find themselves in a hostile legal environment and allegations of fraud could provide a basis for a hostile court to invalidate an adoption. Consultation with experienced legal counsel before or during the adoption is strongly advised so that any potential issues can be properly addressed.

Transgender people may face unique challenges during adoption (Farr & Goldberg, 2018; Joslin et al., 2018, §9.6–9.9). While no state specifically addresses the eligibility of transgender people as adoptive parent, doubtless individual agencies and judges would consider this a significant factor (Joslin et al., 2018). Similarly, many judges and agencies would view the failure to disclose transgender status as a meaningful omission. Thus, careful consultation with a lawyer is essential.

Many LGBTQ people consider international adoptions (Joslin et al., 2018). As is true with the states, different countries have different rules about who is permitted to adopt. Some permit single people but not unmarried couples. Some do not permit LGBTQ people to adopt. Issues about the extent to which full disclosure is required or advisable are not uncommon. Individualized legal advice is strongly recommended as international adoption adds additional layers of complexity to the adoption process. Lack of candor during the adoption process may be a basis on which the adoption itself can be undermined.

**The portability of adoption** Given the confusing array of state laws governing adoption, it is valuable to note that once an adoption is properly concluded in one state, all other states must recognize the adoption. Thus, if a second-parent adoption is completed in state A, state B must recognize the adoption even if state B would not have permitted it. This is true not only of traditional adoptions but also of second-parent adoptions and step-parent adoptions, discussed further below (Joslin et al., 2018).

This result is required by the Full Faith and Credit Clause of the US Constitution. That Clause obliges the states to give full effect to a valid court judgment from another state (USCA CONST Art. IV §1). Consistent with this doctrine, in 2016, the US Supreme Court unanimously reversed an Alabama Supreme Court decision refusing to recognize an adoption completed in Georgia by a lesbian partner (*V.L. v. E.L.*, 2016). Alabama was required to recognize the adoption even though it might not have permitted it had the couple begun a new proceeding in Alabama. The state was required to treat the adoption just as it would one of its own adoptions. This means that adoptions are portable and can be effective as one travels from state-to-state. It is prudent to carry some proof of adoption as one travels state-to-state.

**Birth certificates** When an adoption is completed, it is common for a court to order that a new birth certificate be prepared for the child. The new birth certificate will list the legally recognized parents of the child, post-adoption. Thus, in the case of a second-parent

---

[14]A North Carolina Supreme Court opinion, *Boseman v. Jarrell*, is a disturbing exception to this rule (*Boseman v. Jarrell*, 2010). In this case, the North Carolina Supreme Court voided a second-parent adoption years after it was completed. In addition, the court appears to have voided all other second-parent adoptions completed in North Carolina. While the case is an extreme outlier, it is also a sobering reminder that on rare occasions, adoptions can be challenged long after the fact. The court based its decision on the absence of statutory authority supporting second-parent adoptions. This is potentially problematic because many states allow second-parent adoptions without statutory support. However, no court has followed the North Carolina Supreme Court.

adoption, the name of the second parent will be added. The original birth certificate is then typically sealed.

A certified copy of the postadoption birth certificate can be produced by adoptive parents in order to demonstrate their status as legal parents.[15] The birth certificate allows parents to register a child for school or enroll a child for health insurance. It is also required in order to obtain a passport.

Some states continue to resist placing the names of two parents of the same sex on a birth certificate even where they have adopted jointly in another state or a second-parent adoption is completed in the couple's home state.[16] For example, Louisiana declined to issue a new birth certificate to two gay men who had adopted a child born in Louisiana. The men had completed an adoption in New York State and thus were both legal parents. The men sued in federal court. Louisiana lost the early rounds of this litigation but prevailed in the United States Court of Appeal for the Fifth Circuit (*Adar v. Smith*, 2011). The United States Supreme Court declined to review the decision which means that it is a final decision. Louisiana does not have to issue a birth certificate with the two men's names on it. This decision does not have any impact on the validity of the adoption but does create practical difficulties for the family. In order to enroll the child in school or take other actions where a birth certificate would ordinarily suffice, copies of legal papers documenting the adoption might be required.

A more recent decision appears to resolve this issue for *married* LGBTQ couples. In *Pavan v.*

*Smith* (2017), the US Supreme Court required Arkansas to list the names of both members of a married lesbian couple on a birth certificate because both names of a heterosexual couple would be listed. To refuse to both names for the married lesbian couple was deemed to be inconsistent with the Court's earlier holding on marriage equality in *Obergefell v. Hodges* (2015). Given that the Supreme Court made no reference to the *Adar* case, this may be another area in which the rights of married vs. unmarried LGBTQ couples diverge.

It may be fair to say that there is less discrimination based on LGBTQ status in the post-*Obergefell* world. Instead, there is discrimination based on marital status. Couples who do not wish to marry may find themselves at a disadvantage with regard to legal parentage (Polikoff, 2008).

## Assisted Reproduction

The alternative to adoption for LGBTQ-parent families is some form of assisted reproduction (ART). ART offers an array of options. The law has been slow to respond to rapidly developing technology, and legal responses vary widely state-to-state and country-to-country (Joslin et al., 2018 §3.). It is, therefore, difficult to make any general statements about ART and parentage. Further, as the ART industry has developed, ART transactions often touch on multiple states if not multiple countries (see chapter "Gay Men and Surrogacy"). Since the different entities often have different laws, this further complicates the legal picture.

Though prices vary widely, one can generally say that ART can be expensive and may strain the budgets of many LGTBQ people. Legal counsel is typically an additional expense. Efforts to cut costs have led some people to use social media to find the needed participants for ART and to prepare their own legal or quasi-legal documents. While it is undoubtedly a way to reduce expenses up front, in the longer term this is a high-risk strategy because documents that fail to comply with legal standards may be deemed invalid. In the absence of a valid agreement, in many states,

---

[15] That said, the mere fact that a person's name is placed on a birth certificate does not give them the rights of a legal parent. The key point is that the birth certificate with the parent's name on it evidences the parent's status as a recognized legal parent. It does not transform the person into a legal parent.

[16] Birth certificates are issued by the state in which the child was born which may not be the state in which the adoption was completed. Ordinarily issuance of a new birth certificate with the adoptive parents' names on it is routine.

a sperm donor or a surrogate may be deemed to be a legal parent even where this is not the intention of the people involved in the arrangement. Only skilled legal advice can effectively protect all of the parties' expectations.

Given the nature of human reproduction, the needs of women seeking to become parents are different from the needs of men. Single women, whether lesbian, bisexual, or queer, and lesbian couples need a source of sperm, while single men and gay male couples need an egg and also a woman to gestate and give birth to the child.[17] Thus, lesbians and gay men generally use different ART techniques and so encounter different legal issues. The following section considers these distinct issues.

**ART for lesbians** Lesbians have used assisted insemination (AI) to become pregnant for many years. As a general matter, when a woman gives birth to a child, she is automatically recognized as a legal parent of that child (Jacobs, 2006).[18] Whether she is a lesbian, bisexual, or identifies as queer has no bearing on this question. The two main legal questions presented by assisted insemination are the potential parental rights of the man who provides the sperm and the legal status of a nonpregnant lesbian partner or spouse. These are considered in turn.

First, regarding legal issues around the rights of the sperm provider, women using third-party sperm have several options. They can use sperm from a man they know, they can use sperm from a man who can be identified in the future, usually at the election of the child, or they can use sperm from a man who is expected to remain anonymous and unidentified.

The last option is less common than it once was. While some sperm banks may still offer sperm from an anonymous provider, truly anonymous donors are increasingly rare. This is true for both practical and policy-related reasons. Practically speaking, the availability and common use of DNA testing often makes the identity of a man providing sperm readily discoverable. At the same time, just as openness and honesty has become the dominant practice in adoption, so it has become the norm for ART (Joslin et al., 2018, §3.12–3.15). Concerns about the health and well-being of donor-conceived children has led many to advocate for a system where at least basic information will be made available to a child at the child's request when the child reaches a designated age (Londra, Wallach, & Zhao, 2014). While this is the practice of many sperm banks in the United States, it is also required by law in some states. Thus, it is probably more accurate to characterize the choice presented to lesbian prospective parents as between a sperm provider who will be known to the child during childhood and one whose identity may become known later in life.

The decision as to the source of sperm is one that involves both legal and nonlegal factors. Thus, one may choose a known provider so that one's child can have a relationship with that person during childhood. Alternatively, one might choose a donor who can be identified when the child reaches adulthood so that the child can locate the person at that time if the child desires to do so. There is a great deal of current discussion about the potential social or psychological value of these options, but there are important legal ramifications that should be considered as well (Golombok, 2015).

This is an area where the law varies significantly state-to-state. In many states, a man who provides sperm for the insemination of a woman not his wife will not be recognized as a legal parent of any resulting child. In some states, his status will depend on whether there is an agreement regarding parental status in place or on whether or not the insemination was conducted by a medical professional. The first task should be to determine the relevant law. Establishing relevant law typically requires consultation with a lawyer or a local LGBTQ rights organization. It is crucial

---

[17]Transmen may retain the capacity to provide egg and womb and transwomen may have frozen sperm. To date, courts have apparently treated a transman who has given birth as they would treat a woman who gave birth.

[18]There are limited exceptions in some states for women who are acting as surrogates (*Johnson v. Calvert*, 1993). These are not of considered here. Surrogacy is discussed below.

that the information obtained be both current and reliable. It is not enough to rely on an agreement between the donor and the recipient.

If the law states that a sperm provider is not a legal parent, then a woman may freely choose a known or an identifiable provider without concern that he will acquire parental rights. But if a provider is deemed to be a legal father, then use of a known provider means that the provider will be a legal parent of the child. This may or may not be consistent with the woman's lesbian parental plan. It will almost always make it more difficult for a woman's lesbian partner to establish parental rights.

Use of an anonymous provider ensures that no man will step forward to claim the legal rights of a parent and the rights of the unknown man can generally be terminated by proper legal proceedings if termination is required. The same is generally true if the provider's identity is only to be revealed to the child later in life.

While a known provider can give up his legal rights after the birth of a child, it is also possible that the provider may change his mind and elect not to give up his rights. Further, some judges may refuse to allow him to give up his rights if it creates a single-parent family. Thus, using a known provider in those jurisdictions where a sperm provider is deemed to be a legal parent requires extremely careful consideration, preferably including input from a legal professional. In those states where the legal status of the provider depends on an agreement between the parties, care must be taken to ensure that the agreement is properly crafted and expresses the clear understanding of all those involved. In most states, however, while agreements between the parties may be useful in order to clarify the intent of the parties, they will not have legal effect.

Second, regarding legal issues around the legal status of the nonpregnant female partner, the woman who gives birth automatically gains recognition as a legal parent. If that woman is married, in many states her wife will also automatically gain recognition as a legal parent. But this may not be true for an unmarried partner. Again, the law here varies state to state. As is noted above, even where a married partner gains recognition as a legal parent in the home state, it is not yet clear that all states must recognize her status.

In some states, a second-parent adoption may secure the rights of the partner. Over time, she may also qualify as a de facto parent.[19] In addition, some states permit a woman in a same-sex relationship to execute a Voluntary Acknowledgment of Parentage (VAP) when her partner gives birth to a child. Each of these possibilities is discussed in section "Adding Parents".

**ART for gay men** Gay men who are considering ART generally use some form of surrogacy. In surrogacy, a woman agrees to become pregnant and give birth without intending to be a parent to the child. Instead, she acts for another individual or individuals who are planning to be the parent or parents of the child. Those individuals are often called the "intended parents." The surrogate may be the source of the ovum (in which case the practice is called "traditional surrogacy") or the ovum may be obtained from a third party (Joslin et al., 2018). If the pregnant woman is genetically unrelated to the fetus she carries, this is called gestational surrogacy.

There are additional divisions among types of surrogates. Some women (such as close relatives or friends of the men intending to be parents) serve as surrogates without compensation. Often, surrogates are compensated and are women previously unknown to the intended parents.

As with most other aspects of family law, the law governing surrogacy varies a great deal state-to-state. In some states (California is one), surrogacy is relatively well accepted and the legal course of action is well understood, but in other states, surrogacy is either illegal or of questionable status.

---

[19] A de facto parent is a person who is a parent, in fact, but is not recognized as a legal parent. So, for example, a woman who has participated in the process of conceiving and raising a child born to her lesbian partner might be a parent, in fact, but not in law. Should the women separate, the parent, in fact, has no legal protection for her relationship with the child. De facto parentage, when available, recognizes her parental rights and ensures she can remain in contact with the child. This is discussed in more detail below.

Because of the complexity of the legal issues involved, surrogacy should never be pursued without consultation with a lawyer who has some expertise in the matter (see Joslin et al., 2018).

Surrogacy is also frequently transnational (see chapter "Gay Men and Surrogacy"). Because some US states provide a clear path to parenthood through surrogacy, they may be destinations for gay couples or single men whose home countries are not similarly accommodating. But that the same time, surrogacy in the United States is quite expensive, and other countries may offer surrogacy at far lower prices.[20] Thus, gay men and couples from the United States may consider surrogacy abroad. Caution in engaging in international surrogacy is necessary as complex transnational legal problems can arise.

In the absence of specific law authorizing surrogacy, a judge in some states may conclude that any woman who gives birth to a child is a legal parent, whether the woman is genetically related to the child or not.[21] While this does not necessarily mean that surrogacy is barred in those states, it does mean that the surrogate has to confirm her intention to relinquish parental rights *after* the birth of the child. If, after the birth of the child, the surrogate changes her mind and wishes to maintain her status as a legal parent, she can do so.[22] For many intended parents, the prospect that the surrogate might reconsider creates difficult uncertainty, though in reality the instances in which a surrogate changes her mind appear to be quite rare.

In any surrogacy arrangement, an extensive written agreement is common (Joslin et al.,

2018). A written agreement is an expression of the understandings of the surrogate and the intended parents as to the expectations of all the parties. Even though the agreement may not be legally enforceable, it may be useful to draft an agreement in order to clarify the expectations. In general, the surrogate must retain the right to control her own medical care and the option to terminate or not terminate her pregnancy. In addition, in most states where surrogacy is permitted, all parties are required to undergo a psychological assessment and counseling. Further, separate legal counsel for the intended parent(s) and the surrogate is a common requirement. These features, as well as the actual ART involved, explain why surrogacy can be quite expensive.

## Adding Parents

LGBTQ couples who form families may find that the initial steps of family formation leave them with only one legal parent. It might be the woman who gives birth or a man who provides the sperm in surrogacy. It may be that only one member of the couple could complete a foreign adoption. However, it occurs, the situation in which there is only one legal parent should be addressed since, as is discussed above, it creates a serious power imbalance within the couple.

One way to secure rights in the second parent is through a second-parent adoption. They may not be available to all couples in all locations. Some couples will find it easier to use Voluntary Acknowledgments of Parenthood. In the absence of either of these, a second-parent adoption, a person may qualify as a de facto parent. Each of these options is discussed below.

It is worth noting that while parties may enter into various forms of parenting agreements, these agreements are often revocable at the will of the legal parent and so do not provide a great deal of protection for the nonlegal parent (Allen, 2019; Kauffman, 2019). To supplement an agreement, legal documentation may be pre-

---

[20]Typically, the prices are lower because surrogates are paid less. There may be moral or ethical concerns arising from the treatment of foreign surrogates.

[21]This is essentially an application of the near-universal presumption that a woman who gives birth to a child is a legal mother. Statutes authorizing surrogacy create exceptions to the presumption, identifying circumstances under which it will not be applied. In states where there are no statutes relating to surrogacy, the presumption typically retains its force.

[22]This is what happened in the well-known *In re Baby M* (1988) case. Ultimately, William Stern, the intended father, and Mary Beth Whitehead, the surrogate, shared legal custody of the child.

pared, but this may not increase the security of the nonlegal parent.

## Second-Parent Adoptions

Second-parent adoptions have been a critical legal tool in the formation of LGBTQ-parent families. They are to be distinguished from traditional adoptions (Polikoff, 2009). As is noted above, in adoption the general case is that a new parent or parents take the place of the original parent or parents. On many occasions, however, LGBTQ couples wish to add an additional parent while maintaining the status of the original parent. Second-parent adoptions make this possible. Second-parent adoptions are modeled on stepparent adoptions, which are widely available in proper cases.[23] In the absence of an adoption, stepparents are not legal parents. Second-parent adoptions (as opposed to step-parent adoptions) are not available in all states.[24] This may present a challenge for unmarried couples.[25]

Second-parent adoptions allow the creation of LGBTQ-parent families with two recognized legal parents. For example, if one member of a lesbian couple gives birth to a child, she will be recognized as a parent by the operation of law.[26] Often, the woman who gives birth will be referred to as a "natural parent." She becomes a legal parent without having to take any legal action. But it is critical to note that this is not the operation of nature but rather the operation of law which is arranged to recognize her rights without the necessity of legal action. In the same way, where a woman who is married to a man gives birth, he automatically becomes a parent and he also will often be referred to as a natural parent for the same reason—the law is arranged so that no legal action is required to secure his parental rights. She and her partner may wish to secure recognition for the partner as a second legal parent of the child. While the partner may be able to adopt the child, an ordinary adoption would require the termination of the first woman's parental rights. Thus, at the end of the day, the child would still only have one legal parent, albeit a different legal parent. A second-parent adoption allows the addition of the second woman as a parent without the first woman losing legal status. Once the adoption is completed, the parental status of both women is fully secured.

While the situation just described may be the most common instance where a second-parent adoption is concluded, there are other circumstances where they are useful. If only one member of an LGBTQ couple completes an overseas adoption (in order to comply with the laws of the other country), the second person may complete a second-parent adoption upon return to their home state. Similarly, one member of an LGBTQ couple may complete an adoption in a state where joint adoptions by unmarried couples is not permitted. Here, too, the other member of the couple may be able to complete a second-parent adoption in the couple's home state. Or one member of a male same-sex couple may claim legal parentage by virtue of his genetic connection to a child born to a surrogate. As with adoption gener-

---

[23] With the advent of marriage equality, step-parent adoptions may also be useful to LGBTQ people. However, where an LGBTQ couple plans to form a family, the non-child-bearing parent is not truly analogous to a step-parent. (Traditionally step-parents join families at some time after the birth of a child.) Thus, second-parent adoptions, where available, may be more suitable.

[24] It is difficult to compile a definitive list of the states where second-parent adoptions are permitted, but the websites noted in footnote 1 are generally kept up-to-date. In some jurisdictions, there are no authoritative precedents or statutes, so the matter may be left to the discretion of individual judges. This means that some judges are sympathetic and supportive and will approve second-parent adoptions while others will not. Overall, second-parent adoptions can be concluded in most major cities even where there is no authoritative legal ruling allowing them, provided one can find a supportive judge. Typically, local lawyers are knowledgeable about judicial selection.

It is clear that some states do not permit second-parent adoptions. (See the discussion of the North Carolina case above.)

[25] Married LGBTQ parents should be able to use the procedures for step-parent adoptions.

[26] Often, she is referred to as a natural parent, but the critical thing here is the operation of law, not nature. The law generally recognizes a woman who gives birth as the mother of a child. The important exception here is surrogacy which is discussed above.

ally, once a second-parent adoption is properly completed, all other states must recognize and respect it.

When a second-parent adoption is completed, the rights of the original parent are necessarily diminished. Before the adoption, the original parent is the sole legal parent. As such, she or he stands largely unrivaled when it comes to decision-making for the child. In agreeing to a second-parent adoption, the original parent agrees to the recognition of a second-parent who is co-equal. No longer is the first parent's position unrivaled. While there are many substantial reasons why a second-parent adoption is desirable, it is nevertheless important to note that the original parent, in granting consent to the second-parent adoption, is agreeing to share control of and responsibility for the child. While a second-parent adoption can only be completed with the consent of the original parent, once it is given the consent is irrevocable.

In this regard, second-parent adoptions are quite different from less formal arrangements where a legal parent allows another person to coparent a child. While in some states the other person may acquire some legal status (see the discussion of de facto parentage, below), in general the relationship between the child and a person who has not completed an adoption is vulnerable to interference from the legal parent. The legal parent is generally entitled to change her or his mind and terminate the relationship between the coparent and the child even when it can be shown to cause some harm to the child. Drafting a coparenting agreement may be a helpful tool in delineating the expectations and understandings of the parties, but it will typically not be given legal force.

While many children are raised by single parents or in two-parent families, some children have more than two social parents. One situation where this may arise is where two parents separate and continue to share custody of the child although they live apart. If one or both of those parents repartner, the child may have three or four social parents. Additionally, some children may be part of intact family groups with more than two social parents. In some circum-

stances, some states will recognize three (and possibly more) legal parents. While this remains a minority view, the number of places permitted recognition of more than two parents has been steadily increasing (Joslin et al., 2018, §7.14).

## Voluntary Acknowledgments of Parentage

For many years, when an unmarried woman gave birth, men were permitted to execute Voluntary Acknowledgments of Paternity (VAPs). When properly executed, these documents had the effect of making the men legal parents to the children concerned. Further, federal law required that all other states recognize the parental status of the men who executed VAPs. VAPs are not generally available to same-sex couples.

This has begun to change. The newest iteration of the Uniform Parentage Act (a model law that may be influential in many states) now allows any intended parent to execute a Voluntary Acknowledgment of *Parentage*. Apart from keeping the initials (VAP), the new legal provisions follow the old rules for the VAPs—in particular, the requirement that all states recognize a person who has properly executed a VAP as a legal parent. Some states have already enacted these provisions, and thus, VAPs are now available in a few places. Where they are available, they provide a simple and inexpensive method for gaining secure legal status for a second parent. While only a small number of states permit the procedure at present, more states will adopt it in the future (Joslin et al., 2018). For any unmarried LGBTQ couple considering parenthood, it is worth checking with a lawyer to see if the option is available.

## De facto Parenthood

By now it should be clear that, absent legal action, it is quite possible for an LGBTQ family to consist of one legal parent, one nonlegal parent, and a child or children. This might be the case where only one member of an LGBTQ couple is permitted to adopt a child or where a woman establishes parental rights by giving birth while no provisions of state law confer similar legal rights on her partner. As has been explained, the nonlegal parent right to continue a relationship with the child is vulnerable in this situation. There are a regrettably large number of instances where the adult members of couples in this situation have separated and the legal mother has attempted to gain advantage by virtue of being the sole legal parent of the child (Pearson, 2019). Unfortunately, this has often been a successful tactic.

In response to these cases, a doctrine of de facto parentage was developed (Polikoff, 1990). De facto parentage, in its strongest form, grants legal recognition as a parent to a person who has acted like a parent for a substantial period of time. This doctrine exists in a variety of forms in a minority of states. There are no fixed definitions for what it means to act like a parent or for the required period of time, but the test is generally fairly stringent (Joslin, 2017; Joslin et al., 2018).

De facto parentage is only established after the fact. In all of the cases litigated, it was determined after a couple separates. While it provides a potential avenue for a person to continue his/her relationship with a child and may provide full parental rights, it does not give the person parental status *during* the relationship. It is also not clear whether this status is in any way portable, although if a person is determined by litigation to have been a de facto parent in the past, that judgment is very likely binding on other states (Joslin et al., 2018).

Establishing status as a de facto parent can be long, contested, and expensive. The court will examine the nature and duration of the relationship between the adult and the child, the extent to which the relationship was encouraged by the legal parent, and a variety of other factors. LGBTQ legal advocacy groups have worked long and hard to establish and fortify the de facto parent doctrine and where it is well established, claiming de facto status may be somewhat more routinized (Joslin et al., 2018). But even in the best of the jurisdictions entering the dispute with status as a legal parent is preferable.

## Separating with Children

Law is most important at two points in the life of most LGBTQ-parent families. First, law matters at the time the family is formed. Second, law matters when the family dissolves, particularly if the adults in the family separate[27] (Farr & Goldberg, 2018; Pearson, 2019).

It is often difficult for separating couples who have been raising children to reach agreement about the children, yet it is frequently better for all involved to reach agreement rather than choose the path of litigation. This advice is particularly true for LGBTQ-parent families. Courts are not always hospitable forums for these families (Pearson, 2019). While judges may be receptive to some arguments offered by individual LGBTQ litigants, some judges are most likely to be receptive to those that will, in the long run, injure LGBTQ communities. If litigation is necessary, then care should be taken that the arguments raised do not undermine the status of LGBTQ-parent families generally.[28]

At the time of separation, the most critical question for families with children will be whether the people separating are legal parents (Hertz, 2019). If they are, then the case will be handled as a conventional custody dispute. The court will in the end approve a plan for the division of decision-making authority with regard to the child as well as a plan for the child's residence. The plan will be drawn up based on an analysis of the best interests of the child.

If one of the parties is not a legal parent, that person could be at a substantial disadvantage if their former partner chooses to argue that they should not have any legal rights. Leading LGBTQ legal organizations have prepared a statement of principles outlining approaches to custody matters that allow the parties to vigorously air their

---

[27]If the adults do not separate, the relationship will eventually end with the death of one or both of the adults/parents. This, too, raises legal questions, but they are beyond the scope of this chapter.

[28]Those considering litigation should carefully consider the points raised in *Protecting Families*, a joint production of GLAD and NCLR that can be obtained at http://www.glad.org/protecting-families

disagreement without harming the communities to which they belong. Consideration of the broader effects of specific arguments that may be offered is warranted.[29]

For example, in 1991, the New York State Court of Appeals decided a case involving lesbian coparents who were separating (*Alison D v. Virginia M*, 1991). Though Alison D had acted as a social parent to the child, Virginia M argued that she was not entitled to recognition as a legal parent. The Court of Appeals agreed with Virginia M, and Alison D was found to have no right to maintain contact with the child. Beyond the effect on the parties in this case, the precedent has stood for nearly 30 years, and to this day, New York State does not recognize de facto parents. This lack of recognition has undermined the ability of LGBTQ people to create stable families.

If both the separating parties are legal parents, then there is a strong presumption that the child will continue to have contact with both parents and that both parents will continue to be involved with the children, both as decision makers and as sources of financial support. Thus, discussion will focus on allocation of decision-making authority (sometimes called legal custody) and on residential provisions (sometimes called physical custody).

In general, day-to-day decision-making authority is assumed to reside with whomever the child is living with at the time. This allocation of authority is premised on the assumption that day-to-day decisions are small ones. Typically, there is an expectation that major decisions (about elective medical procedures, religion, and education, for example) are expected to be made jointly between the parents even if the parents do not spend equal amounts of time with the child (Pearson, 2019).

Different states may have different starting presumptions for the allocation of residential time with the child. Factors such as the age of the children and the physical proximity of the parents' residences will be important.

As with litigation generally, most custody cases do not go to trial. The vast majority of

them settle as a result of negotiations between the parties. While the outlines of settlements are no doubt influenced by the governing law, they also reflect the parties' ability to work with each other and reach agreement about what is best for the children involved. Even where the parties separate, they will need to continue to work together as coparents for the life of the children.

## Conclusion

LGBTQ people have been creating families with children for decades, but legal protection of those families is still imperfect and uneven. While all states now recognize marriage between adults regardless of sex or gender, recognition of parental status remains uneven. Further, while many legal protections may travel with a family as it travels or moves state to state, not all will do so, at least with regard to some other states. Thus, in addition to the challenges any family with children confronts, LGBTQ families confront complex legal questions in many different contexts.

The trends over the last several years are encouraging, especially for those who choose to marry. But not all states have progressed at the same pace. LGBTQ families residing in or even traveling to hostile states may find their parental status under attack. The patchwork of laws will remain, and thus, for the foreseeable future, LGBTQ families will need to be aware of potential legal problems that may arise so that these problems can be addressed.

## References

Adar v. Smith, 639 F.3d 146 (5th Cir. 2011).

Alison D. v. Virginia M., 572 N.E.2d 27 (Court of Appeals of New York 1991).

Allen, K. R. (2019). Family, loss, and change: Navigating family breakup before the advent of legal marriage and divorce. In A. E. Goldberg & A. P. Romero (Eds.), *LGBTQ divorce and relationship dissolution: Psychological and legal perspectives and implications for practice* (pp. 221–232). Oxford, UK: Oxford University Press.

Boseman v. Jarrell, 704 S.E.2d 494 (Supreme Court of North Carolina 2010).

---

[29] See footnote 12.

Cha, A. E. (2019, February 8). Administration seeks to fund foster care groups that reject LGBTQ parents. *The Washington Post*. Retrieved from http://www.washingtonpost.com

Farr, R. H., & Goldberg, A. E. (2018). Sexual orientation, gender identity and adoption law. *Family Court Review, 56*, 374–383. https://doi.org/10.1111/fcre.12345

Full Faith and Credit Act, USCA CONST Art. IV §1.

Goldberg, A. E. (2010). The transition to adoptive parenthood. In T. W. Miller (Ed.), *Handbook of stressful transitions across the life span* (pp. 165–184). New York, NY: Springer.

Goldberg, A. E., Gartrell, N. K, & Gates, G. (2014). *Research report on LGB-parent families*. Retrieved from http://williamsinstitute.law.ucla.edu/wp-content/uploads/lgb-parent-families-july-2014.pdf

Golombok, S. (2015). *Modern families: Parents and children in new family forms*. Cambridge, UK: Cambridge University Press.

Hertz, F. (2019). Emerging legal issues in same-sex divorces: A lawyer's view of the unanticipated effects of heteronormative marital law. In A. E. Goldberg & A. P. Romero (Eds.), *LGBTQ divorce and relationship dissolution* (pp. 383–401). Oxford, UK: Oxford University Press.

In re Baby M., 109 N.J. 396 (New Jersey Supreme Court 1988).

In re Marriage of Black, 188 Wash.2d 144 (Washington Supreme Court 2017).

Jacobs, M. (2006). Procreation through ART: Why the adoption process should not apply. *Capital University Law Review, 35*, 399–411.

Johnson v. Calvert, 851 P.2d 776 (Supreme Court of California 1993).

Joslin, C. (2017). Nurturing parenthood through the UPA. *Yale Law Journal Forum, 127*, 589–613. https://doi.org/10.2139/ssrn.3097793

Joslin, C., Minter, S., & Sakimura, C. (2018). *Lesbian, gay, bisexual and transgender family law*. St Paul, MN: Thomson/West.

Kauffman, J. (2019). A lesbian parent's perspective on LGBTQ families of choice: Sharing custody when there is no legal requirement to do so. In A. E. Goldberg & A. P. Romero (Eds.), *LGBTQ divorce and relationship dissolution: Psychological and legal perspectives and implications for practice* (pp. 233–244). Oxford, UK: Oxford University Press.

Knauer, N. J. (2019). Implications of Obergefell for same-sex marriage, divorce, and paternal rights. In A. E. Goldberg & A. P. Romero (Eds.), *LGBTQ divorce and relationship dissolution* (pp. 7–30). Oxford, UK: Oxford University Press.

Londra, L., Wallach, E., & Zhao, Y. (2014). Assisted reproduction: Ethical and legal issues. *Seminars in Fetal and Neonatal Medicine, 19*, 264–271. https://doi.org/10.1016/j.siny.2014.07.003

N.K.M. v. L.E.M., 606 S.W.2d 169 (Missouri Court of Appeals, Western District, 1980).

NeJaime, D. (2016). Marriage equality and the new parenthood. *Harvard Law Review, 129*, 1185–1266.

Obergefell v. Hodges, 135 S.Ct. 2584 (Supreme Court of the United States 2015).

Pavan v. Smith, 137 S.Ct. 2075 (Supreme Court of the United States 2017).

Pearson, K. H. (2019). Child custody in the context of LGBTQ relationship dissolution and divorce. In A. E. Goldberg & A. P. Romero (Eds.), *LGBTQ divorce and relationship dissolution* (pp. 195–220). Oxford, UK: Oxford University Press.

Polikoff, N. (1990). This child does have two mothers: Redefining parenthood to meet the needs of children in lesbian-mother and other nontraditional families. *Georgetown Law Journal, 78*, 459–575.

Polikoff, N. (2008). *Beyond straight and gay marriage*. Boston, MA: Beacon Press.

Polikoff, N. (2009). A mother should not have to adopt her own child: Parentage law for children of lesbian couples in the twenty-first century. *Stanford Journal of Civil Rights & Civil Liberties, 5*, 201–270.

Protecting Families: Standards for LGBT Families. Retrieved from http://www.glad.org/protecting-families

Shapiro, J. (1996). How the law fails lesbian and gay parents and their children. *Indiana Lalli Journal, 721*, 623–671.

Troxel v. Granville, 530 U.S. 57 (Supreme Court of the United States 2000).

V.L. v. E.L., 136 S.Ct. 1017 (Supreme Court of the United States 2016).

# Clinical Work with LGBTQ Parents and Prospective Parents

Arlene Istar Lev and Shannon L. Sennott

In the past few decades, same-sex marriage and LGBTQ parenting have become embedded in the fabric of the social discourse within both the LGBTQ community and mainstream society. Child-rearing opportunities for queer and same-sex couples continue to expand despite contentious debates about the legal status for same-sex parented families and shifting social opinions about transgender, nonbinary, and gender nonconforming identities. Although still vilified in many parts of the world, in most Western countries, LGBTQ people, with or without legal rights, are building families and raising children. Although civil rights have increased in the past decades, political backlash has also increased, leaving LGBTQ-parent families both more visible and more vulnerable. Historically, LGBTQ parents were closeted and rearing children primarily from previous marriages. Increasingly, LGBTQ-identified people are planning families and raising children "out and proud," and presenting with more complex, matrixed, and intersectional clinical issues.

Becoming parents for most LGBTQ people requires conscious preparation and complex decision-making, and the needs and concerns presented by individuals vary across sexual and gender identity status. To conflate the issues and needs of those under the LGBTQ umbrella seeking to become parents muddies these multifaceted issues. Lesbian, gay, bisexual, queer, trans, and nonbinary people face different biological possibilities, social imperatives, and public bias in making choices to become parents. Nonbinary identities are gender identities that fall outside of the female–male or woman–man gender binary (Constantinides, Sennott, & Chandler, 2019). The acronym LGBTQ can conflate the important distinctions among individuals, especially regarding those who are nonbinary, bisexual, and pansexual, because people in heterosexual relationships are often assumed to be straight, and those in same-sex relationships are presumed to be gay or lesbian. There is a dearth of empirical research on bisexual parents (who are often conflated with lesbian and gay individuals) and for those who are single, polyamorous or consensually nonmonogamous, and pansexual.

## Clinical Competency in the Therapeutic Setting with LGBTQ Parents

Clinical approaches to working with LGBTQ parents ought to be informed by an integration of narrative, relational, and transfeminist

A. I. Lev (✉)
University at Albany, School of Social Welfare, and Choices Counseling and Consulting,
Albany, NY, USA

S. L. Sennott (✉)
Smith School for Social Work, Translate Gender, Inc., The Center for Psychotherapy and Social Justice,
Northampton, MA, USA

© Springer Nature Switzerland AG 2020
A. E. Goldberg, K. R. Allen (eds.), *LGBTQ-Parent Families*,
https://doi.org/10.1007/978-3-030-35610-1_24

perspectives. A narrative approach (White, 2007) separates people from their problems and allows for the emergence of unique stories. A relational approach includes both feminist and cultural lenses that offer clinical transparency between provider and client (Constantinides et al., 2019). A transfeminist perspective acknowledges that most trans and gender nonconforming individuals have had lived experiences, in the past or present, as a girl or woman and have suffered the direct repercussions of socially condoned misogyny and gender-based oppression. The utilization of a transfeminist therapeutic approach in working with LGBTQ individuals incorporates an awareness that there does not exist a hierarchy of authentic lived experience for women and to privilege one type of womanhood over another is inherently antifeminist (Constantinides et al., 2019; Sennott, 2011).

The therapeutic utilization of an eclectic and contextual clinical framework allows for a focus on the client's strengths through the exploration and emergence of the client's intersecting identities (i.e., race/ethnicity, class, ability, religion, education, size, citizenship, and age) (Sennott & Smith, 2011; Walsh, 2011, 2016). Therapists who work with LGBTQ clients need training in basic family systems theory and should have knowledge of the multiple options for family building in LGBTQ communities (Goldberg, 2010; Lev, 2004a). Clinicians also need to understand the coming out process and how this can affect the developmental life cycle of families, including families of origin, as well as the role of internalized homophobia or biphobia in development of believing one has the "right" to become parents (Ashton, 2011). Parenting places LGBTQ people under a social microscope as they come into contact with the medical profession, adoption specialists, daycare providers, and educational institutions (Lev, 2004b; Sennott, 2011). Clinicians must be prepared to examine the in-depth discourse these parents are bringing to therapy regarding values, legalities, gender, and unique family-building strategies.

## Queering the LGBTQ Family Life Cycle

Working with LGBTQ people requires an understanding of both the "normative" life cycle issues all couples and families face and the unique life cycle issues experienced by those with diverse sexual and gender identities. Life cycle models, in general, have come under great scrutiny for ignoring women's unique developmental processes (Gilligan, 1993; Jordan, Kaplan, Miller, Stiver, & Surrey, 1991). Additionally, the complex multidimensionality of class, race, ethnicity, and religion has routinely been minimized and ignored within standard family life cycle models (McGoldrick & Hardy, 2008). Psychological theories of LGBTQ people have focused on individual coming out processes. From a larger sociocultural perspective, there have been massive cultural shifts in the development of diverse and multicultural family forms, which LGBTQ is just one of many manifestations (Walsh, 2011). Increasingly, models of family life have moved from deficit perspectives to strengths based models, examining family resilience in the face of challenges (Unger, 2012; Walsh, 2016).

Numerous models have been developed to examine the specific coming out processes for lesbian and gay people (Cass, 1979; Troiden, 1993), and with various adaptations, those of bisexual people as well (Brown, 2002). Transgender coming out stages have also been examined developmentally, identifying the specific processes of identity development (Devor, 1997; Lev, 2004b; see chapter "Transgender-Parent Families"). There has been much criticism that these models are embedded within White, Western perspectives (Adams & Phillips, 2009; Cass, 1998; Morales, 1996), and minimize the complex issues for people of color who are also LGBTQ (Ashton, 2011; Bowleg, Burkholder, Teti, & Craig, 2008). Additionally, these models generally emphasize the coming out and identity integration processes itself, but not the larger issues of couple and family building, or how sexual orientation issues and gender identity are integrated into general life cycle development (McDowell, 2005). Lastly, they do not emphasize the profound strengths that can develop from facing the stressors and challenges inherent in the coming-out process (Vaughan & Waehler, 2010), and the unique ways that resilience can manifest (Harvey, 2012). Slater (1999) developed a lesbian life cycle model, focused specifically on couple development, and recognized that for many lesbians having children is not the primary focus of their relationship. Slater emphasized the ways that lesbian and gay people have built extended families within the queer community outside of their family of origin *and* without rearing a younger generation. Looking at LGBTQ-parent families through a traditional family life cycle lens ignores the alternative family structures that LGBTQ-parent families have built to nurture themselves, and specific queer intimacies that have emerged (Hammock, Frost, & Huges, 2018).

One of the central features in the early days of the gay and lesbian-feminist liberation movements was moving away from heterosexist notions of family and the rigid proscription of gender role expectations and parenting mandates. Although it was liberating to step outside of mainstream values, queer people who wanted children were left having to "choose" between being queer or being a parent, for queer parenting was still an oxymoron in the beginning of queer liberation (Lev, 2004a). Kelly McCormick was the founder of one of the first national organizations for lesbian mothers: "[Her] legacy in creating *Momazons* is that now this generation is able to decide whether they want to parent, whereas before, we were simply grieving that we couldn't" (Kelly's partner, Phyllis Gorman, personal communication, 2011).

Starting from the premise that some LGBTQ people *will* desire to have children, and that LGBTQ people build unique family structures and community affiliations, then it can also be assumed that LGBTQ people also have unique life cycle experiences that "queer" the study of the family life cycle. De-centering heterosexuality allows us to look at some of the ways that LGBTQ parents "do family" (Hudak & Giammattei, 2010), and "become parent" (Riggs, 2007), that recognizes the evolution of new family forms, and honors emerging values and norms that differ from the heteronormative expectations (Lev, 2010). Ashton (2011) utilizes McGoldrick, Carter, and Garcia-Preto (2010) work to examine the ways LGBTQ people are challenged moving through the typical stages of development due to the nature of cissexism, heterosexism, homophobia, and transphobia.

The first stage of development for young adults, leaving home, is affected by the challenging coming out processes for LGBTQ youth. Historically, this has meant that LGBTQ youth sometimes experience a lag developmentally (Rosario, Schrimshaw, & Hunter, 2004), where they do not experience life cycle socialization and dating patterns at the same age as their heterosexual, gender conforming peers. Youth are now coming out younger and able to explore dating and intimacy at developmentally appropriate ages, although this is impacted by geographic location, and the values of one's family of origin (LaSala, 2010). For youth who are gender nonconforming—transgender, nonbinary, or genderqueer—puberty can be a confusing and challenging time (Ehrensaft, 2016; Nealy, 2017; Sennott & Chandler, 2019). Often sexuality and exploration take a back-burner to the pressing issues of body incongruence, and the search for gender affirming medical treatments. It is hard to imagine in the current climate a healthy normative adolescence for a gender nonconforming child, even in the most supportive families and communities (Lev & Alie, 2012; Lev & Gottlieb, 2019; Meadow, 2018). Every aspect of dating and intimacy is affected by living in a body that is betraying one's authentic gender expression.

LGBTQ young adulthood may start painfully early, because youth have had to prematurely become independent due to the effects of homophobia within their families (Ryan, Huebner, Diaz, & Sanchez, 2009), and this may also delay the process of family building. Once relationships have been initiated, queer couples must negotiate the same developmental tasks as heterosexual couples, but do so within the frame of a larger homophobic and transphobic culture.

## Family-Building Strategies in LGBTQ Communities

In addition to the diversity across identities, LGBTQ family-building strategies vary greatly across race/ethnicity, class, religion, disability, and age. Research on lesbian parenthood has historically tended to examine middle-class White women and men, who become parents through donor insemination and adoption (Goldberg & Gianino, 2012; Patterson, 1995). Families of color may think about family building utilizing different lenses than White families, focusing on additional contexts, including how they will integrate their family of choice with their families of origin (Acosta, 2014). Research has shown that many working-class people and same-sex couples of color often become parents via previous heterosexual sexual encounters, and often view donor insemination, private adoption, and surrogacy as financially prohibitive (Moore, 2008, 2011; see chapter "Race and Ethnicity in the Lives of LGBTQ Parents and Their Children: Perspectives from and Beyond North America"). Additionally, some queer women of color seek out known donors, and eschew the use of sperm banks, because they are specifically seeking donors who mirror their own racial/ethnic/cultural identities (Karpman, Ruppel, & Torres, 2018). Social class often impacts prospective parents' relationships with the foster care system (see chapter "LGBTQ Foster Parents"). For some working-class prospective parents, adoption through foster care may be their only viable option to become parents, and they may fear discrimination and bias in this system. Despite the positive advances in foster care policies regarding lesbian and gay parents, some couples may assume they will be rejected or highly scrutinized for being queer (Downs & James, 2006; Lev, 2004b). Bisexual people in heterosexual relationships tend to hide these aspects of their identities from medical professionals and adoption agencies, and although both LGBTQ and heterosexual couples may be in open relationships, the more mainstream LGBTQ people *appear to be*, the

less resistance they will experience in their attempts to build their families (Manley, Legge, Flanders, Goldberg, & Ross, 2018). LGBTQ prospective parents with alternative family structures or who identify as gender queer, polyamorous, or pansexual are often erased by the in vitro fertilization (IVF) medical industrial complex and both public and private adoption programs (Acosta, 2014; Boyd, 2017; Epstein, 2014; Tye, 2013).

For those LGBTQ people who desire to become parents, there is a parallel to that of heterosexual people, in terms of the psychospiritual longing for parenthood, the financial strain associated with parenthood, and the need to reorganize one's life, work, and priorities to properly parent children. LGBTQ people may face infertility challenges and require the assistance of medical experts or adoption specialists (Goldberg, 2010; Goldberg, Downing, & Richardson, 2009). Like heterosexual couples, some LGBTQ people are older when beginning their parenting journey, in part because of increased options due to reproductive technologies. For LGBTQ people raised in more repressive times, they could never seriously entertain the possibility of becoming parents until they were older. Some LGBTQ people also become stepparents after becoming involved with someone who already has children (Lynch, 2004); sometimes, this is warmly welcomed and other times it is "the price" for falling in love. LGBTQ people who are stepparents must address all the same concerns as other stepparents, except they often do so without social or legal sanction for these relationships.

Sometimes, LGBTQ parents try to minimize the differences in their family structure in an effort to normalize their families. In one of our clinical practices, there was a 10-year-old boy in family therapy who said to his biological mother, "Everyone keeps asking me who Tammy is when she picks me up after school"; his mother responded, "Tell them it's none of their business." Although this answer may be technically accurate, it is not particularly helpful for a young child seeking language to explain his family to his friends at school. It actually further reinforces silence and increases the social discomfort for the child, who is not only isolated in school but does not have parents as allies in helping him negotiate the differences. Helping children speak openly about LGBTQ issues, in age-appropriate ways, is a parental duty specific to LGBTQ parents, but not all parents have the skills to initiate or structure the conversation.

Finally, it is important to note that LGBTQ parents are dealing with the same basic issues and concerns that all parents must address: exhaustion, managing a home and family, adult relationship struggles as co-parents as well as intimate partners, struggles with discipline strategies, and concerns for their children's well-being (real or imagined). As parents address issues such as a child's learning disability, mental health concerns, drug use, or academic problems, they may not be focused at all on LGBTQ-related concerns, but are simply seeking a supportive environment where their own families are respected.

## Clinical Considerations for Parenting with Lesbian and Bisexual Women

Lesbians seeking to retain custody of their children following a heterosexual divorce were the first group of sexual minorities to challenge the legal system's bias against queer parenting (Goldberg, 2010). The societal bias against lesbian motherhood centered on the assumption that children needed both a mother and father to develop traditional sex role behavior, including an eventual heterosexual orientation (Tasker & Golombok, 1997). It took the results of a decade of psychological research (Patterson, 2006) to prove to the courts that children reared by lesbian mothers exhibited psychological stability and heteronormative identities. This research and the subsequent legal decisions allowing lesbian mothers to retain custody of their children paved the way for other erotically marginalized people who are pathologized and oppressed for their gender identities or their

sexual identities, orientations, or practices (Constantinides et al., 2019).

Lesbians and bisexual women arguably have the easiest path to becoming parents, because they are biologically capable of conceiving and carrying a child. Donor insemination utilizing a sperm bank is readily available and accessible to most people with middle-class salaries, and donor insemination performed at home, or through known donor assistance, is a possibility for many LGBTQ people. Many can also choose to adopt domestically, either privately or through the child welfare system (Goldberg, 2010). As cultural mores shift, lesbian motherhood is less frequently challenged in the courts. However, lesbian (and gay male) couples cannot adopt internationally as a couple, but must have one partner move through the legal process as a single parent—a process that can be emotionally challenging to partnerships that already lack legal sanction and societal support (Goldberg, 2010, 2012).

Although there has been a plethora of research on lesbian parenting, much of it has focused on White, middle-class women, living in urban centers with access to affirmative communities (Goldberg, 2010; Lev, 2010). With few exceptions, there is a lack of research on the familial dynamics within lesbian families who are working-class, racial/ethnic minorities, living with disabilities, or who are butch/femme identified, especially regarding their pathways to parenting. Clinical experience suggests that although the literature reveals that lesbian couples tend toward egalitarian relationships, dividing chores, and responsibilities evenly (Goldberg, 2010), these may be class-based privileges not available to working-class women or disabled women. Housework is a classically gendered activity, yet some evidence suggests that in butch/femme couples and African-American lesbian couples, housekeeping duties were not divided along expected gender roles (Levitt, Gerrish, & Hiestand, 2003; Moore, 2008). Research has not yet explored the dynamics of butch/femme couples and how they negotiate decisions about pregnancy, breastfeeding, or the division of labor, raising questions about how gender actually functions within these couples (Lev, 2008). Therapists should explore issues of class, culture, racial identity, and gender with LGBTQ couples and not assume that research on White LGBTQ individuals reflects the dynamics of those who are minorities within minorities.

Lesbians and bisexual women seek therapy for numerous reasons. Sometimes, they are seeking information on family planning strategies or struggling with the complexities of infertility. Lesbian couples may have differing views on donor insemination, use of known versus unknown donors, and the importance of biological fathers in their children's lives. Questions about adoptions choices (domestic, international, foster care) are often salient. Most commonly, differences in parenting strategies, conflict, and exhaustion caused by the demands of children, and struggles in parenting children with special needs are reasons that lesbian couples seek out therapeutic guidance. Lesbian couples and individuals also seek out assistance when they are considering or going through the process of separation and divorce or coping with the fallout from infidelity. Increasingly, couples seek therapy who are contemplating opening up the relationship to having other sexual relationships. Lesbian couples, like all families, also seek therapy due to domestic violence, substance use or abuse, chronic and life-threatening health issues, and following the death of a family member.

The following vignette explores a monogamous lesbian relationship highlighting some of the complex issues that arise when two women of different racial backgrounds partner, each having children from previous relationships. The multiple intersecting identities of age, race, religion, and previous parental and marital status all affect this couple's ability to communicate and support one another, as both of these women are parenting in mid-life and have children spanning more than two decades. The therapist in this vignette is modeling a curious and nonjudgmental stance, which is critical to working with LGBTQ parents.

### Case of Jeanette and Gladys

Jeanette and Gladys sought out therapy because their 5-year relationship was "in trouble." Jeanette, a White woman in her mid-40s, was the mother of four children. The oldest three were from a previous marriage to a White man, who had left when the children were small. Gladys, who was African-American and in her mid-50s, identified as "seriously Christian." She had two grown children, conceived in a heterosexual relationship. Her husband had died of a heart attack 20 years earlier, and she raised her children as a single mother before coming out as a lesbian when her children were teenagers. The youngest child in their family was African-American, 4 years old. He was originally fostered by Jeannette, who did emergency foster care work for the State, and was later adopted by both women. They were both assertive and verbal about their issues and needs, and often spoke animatedly over one another.

Jeanette and Gladys owned their own home and struggled to pay the bills. Gladys worked as a nurse and was very proud of her work at the hospital where she had been for over 30 years. Jeanette worked as a teacher's aide in a public school, which made it easy to pick the kids up after school, including the little one who was in a day care center across the street. They both agreed the house was a "disaster" though they had different opinions as to whose fault that was.

Gladys was very critical of Jeanette's parenting. She felt Jeannette was "weak" and that the children ran wild. She stated she would "never tolerate that behavior from her (now grown) boys." Jeanette felt that Gladys was "too hard" on the kids, who were, after all "just kids." Gladys felt that Jeanette didn't support her when she disciplined the kids; Jeanette said, "I don't like when you talk to my kids that way."

There were numerous issues affecting the relationship between Jeanette and Gladys. Each had very different parenting styles and had experience raising children before they were a couple. Their entire relationship revolved around their children, and they had never had time together as a couple without children. Both women had extensive histories living as heterosexuals, and when the topic of lesbianism was introduced, both agreed that they did not like "that word" and both felt that "being gay was not really an issue." They had rarely discussed their relationship with their children, who referred to Jeannette as "Mommy" and Gladys as "Auntie," including their youngest who they had adopted together. The social worker who assisted them with adopting their foster child had never really explored their relationship dynamics. It was not clear whether Gladys really felt she was a full-fledged parent to this child, and her relationship with the older children was even more ambivalent, creating unclear roles within the family.

Utilizing a genogram (McGoldrick, Gerson, & Petry, 2008), the therapist was able to help map the family dynamics and history, allowing the couple to examine both of their previous marriages, as well as their relationships to their older children as single parents. This experience introduced a deeper conversation about what it meant for each of them to join together as a stepfamily. With therapeutic guidance, they also explored both of their cultural, racial, and religious backgrounds, and how that informed their parenting philosophies and beliefs about their role as parents. The therapist employed a narrative approach (White, 2007), allowing the women to reveal their unique stories, grounded in an understanding of the complex intersectionalities in these women's lives.

Additionally, the couple began to explore what it meant to be in a relationship with another woman, how that was different than their previous relationships with men, and how that might impact their children, including whether they were comfortable being seen as a lesbian-parent family. Utilizing a feminist therapeutic understanding (Sennott, 2011) that was affirming of diverse orientations and experiences allowed Gladys to say that she thought she could "love either a man or a woman," and Jeanette revealed that perhaps she had been "gay her whole life but didn't know it until she fell in love with Gladys." Both women were visibly softened by this statement.

It is easy for therapists to assume that because a couple is "out" that they are comfortable with their relationship and have accepted and adapted to being LGBTQ. However, there are many ways that people cope with their sexual orientation, and there are various steps in the process of integrating one's identity. As social mores regarding gay identity have shifted, people can come out with greater ease and are, therefore, less likely to feel confined by established social rules about their identity development or how they *should* experience it. It was important therapeutically that the therapist was able to support both Gladys and Jeanette in their unique experiences of their sexuality, historically and currently, and not assume that their sexual identities (i.e., labels and experiences) within their lesbian relationship were the same.

As Gladys began discussing her Christian beliefs in therapy, she became increasingly agitated. She revealed her fears that her grandmother, who had raised her, would feel strong disapproval knowing Gladys was "like that." For Gladys, being Christian and lesbian was a conflict that she had coped with through avoidance, or denial, rather than attempts at resolution. For Gladys to acknowledge the pain she felt in going to church and listening to her preacher criticize homosexuality was a powerful breakthrough. By creating a holding environment for Gladys's pain, therapy became a safe place to explore her relationship with God, Jesus, and religious tolerance. It was therapeutically important to honor the importance of Jesus and the role of the church in Gladys' life, not avoid these contentious and often tender topics with comments that were dismissive about religiosity, or revealed a politically charged call-to-arms regarding homophobia within the church. Gladys had to come into her sexuality knowing that her god approved of and loved her, a journey that a therapist can guide without necessarily sharing those values.

Within the context of therapy, the couple was able to explore what it meant to share parenting together and raise *their* child, an African-American child who was adopted, as well as the children who were stepchildren to Gladys. This created difficult conversations about race, with Gladys confronting Jeanette, "What do you know about raising a Black girl-child?" Previous to this discussion in therapy, Gladys and Jeanette had never discussed race, their interracial relationship, the adoption of an African-American child, or the blended racial configuration of their children. Additionally, they had never talked with their children—including Gladys' older children—about their relationship, their love, the nature of their families, or how the children should view their commitment to one another and to each of their six children. Forming a stepfamily is particularly challenging for gay and lesbian couples who are not only integrating a socially stigmatized identity (i.e., being gay), but also an identity that has historically been culturally invisible (i.e., stepparenting) (Bermea, van Eeden-Moorefield, Bible, & Petren, 2018; Lynch, 2004).

Having all of these topics out in the open did not make them vanish, but the couple no longer felt their relationship was "in trouble," rather, that they could begin to address their "troubles." Most significantly, they began to attend a welcoming Christian congregation, which served to provide a spiritual home for their family. Gladys and Jeanette are building a family that is coping with multiple, intersecting identities including being in a lesbian couple, having an interracial relationship, being adoptive parents, and forming a stepfamily. This process created numerous conflicts regarding household authority, especially the conflicting roles of having two mothers, with different parenting styles and histories, competing for the role of "the" mother, roles familiar to both of them in previous heterosexual marriages and as single parents.

## Clinical Considerations with Gay and Bisexual Men and Parenthood

Although societal prejudice about men raising children is fierce and the financial costs of becoming parents can be steep, gay fatherhood is increasingly common (Brown, Smalling, Groza, & Ryan, 2009; Downing, Richardson, Kinkler, & Goldberg, 2009; Gates, Badgett, Macomber, & Chambers, 2007) and research on their family-building process is increasing (Biblarz & Savci, 2010; see chapter "Gay Men and Surrogacy"). Gay and bisexual men are building families through domestic adoption, surrogacy, and partnerships with women.

Historically, when gay men were coming out and leaving heterosexual marriages, there was little chance of gaining custody of their children. The reasons for this were two-fold: first because of the prejudice toward fathers, in general, and the second was the specific prejudice toward gay males (Bigner & Bozett, 1990). The courts have historically favored mothers in custody battles in general; gay men were levied the additional prejudice of being "homosexual" within a cultural milieu that assumed gay men were sexual predators of children. Therefore, gay men often lost all rights to their children, sometimes even including visitation. In the past two decades, gay men are increasingly choosing to become parents after coming out (Berkowitz, 2007; Biblarz & Savci, 2010). As prejudice has lessened, gay men have increasing opportunities to become parents (Carneiro, Tasker, Salinas-Quiroz, Leal, & Costa, 2017; Goldberg, 2012). Compared to lesbians who are often able to conceive and carry children with or without societal support, gay men are at an obvious disadvantage. However, as more adoption agencies become welcoming toward gay men, they are taking advantage of these new potentialities. Additionally, gay men who are financially able are seeking out opportunities to build families through surrogacy (Bergman, Rubio, Green, & Padron, 2010; Lev, 2006a). Of course, gay men can also become parents from a previous marriage or through stepparenting.

Gay men are often sperm donors, and depending on the legal and social relationships, they can be chosen family relationships with these children (Lev, 2004a). It is common for clinical concerns about the use of known donors versus anonymous donors to arise for LGBTQ couples.

Gay men can seek clinical consultation for a number of reasons. Perhaps, they are seeking reassurance that being gay will not negatively affect their children; perhaps, they want support in becoming a single dad. Sometimes, the members of a couple have different opinions about how to become parents (adoption versus surrogacy). Additionally, gay men who want to adopt will need a home study evaluation, as do all prospective adoptive parents (Lev, 2006b; Mallon, 2007). The case below outlines Duncan and Mario's process of becoming parents and how they navigated multiple concerns regarding parenthood.

### Case of Duncan and Mario

Duncan and Mario had been partnered for a decade when they sought out counseling because they were hoping to become parents. Duncan, a 37-year-old gay man of European descent, entered therapy excited about becoming a parent; he came from a large family and was an uncle to numerous nieces and nephews. Mario, a 43-year-old gay man, came from an immigrant family with strong Christian values. Although he, too, had a large family, they were rejecting of his partnership with Duncan, and he feared that he would not have family support in choosing to become a parent. Mario experienced confusion and shame about his "homosexuality" (as he referred to it), and where his children would "fit" into his family. It was important to Mario that he pass his culture on to his children, yet he could not imagine having his children exposed to his family of origin's homophobia. Although both men were solidly employed, Duncan came from a

middle-class family, whereas Mario was raised in poverty. Duncan was open to various routes to parenting, including adoption and surrogacy, and did not see the finances as a major concern: "What else should we be spending money on that is more important than this?" Mario was concerned about the financial costs of having children, as well as rearing them. However, he also disclosed another concern, which was that "adopting children through foster care will mean we will have troubled children—I don't think I could do that."

Through the course of therapy, Mario was able to tell his parents that he was planning to have a child. To his surprise, although they had serious reservations, they also expressed (an odd kind of) support saying, "This will make your lifestyle more normal." After going through a foster-to-adopt program, they both felt that the children needing homes who were currently in the foster care system had needs beyond what they were able to provide. This decision was difficult for both men. Duncan expressed that he felt "guilty" that he was uncomfortable fostering children. He felt that he was "the kind of person" who "should" want to do this, yet he really didn't want to: "It just didn't feel right."

They then began to investigate possibilities for surrogacy which was difficult because of the extensive financial costs and legal challenges. They eventually decided to use a donor egg, and a separate gestational surrogate. It was important for Mario that their child was of Latino descent, so they chose to use his sperm. To their surprise, they ended up developing a warm relationship with their surrogate, who was present for their child's birth, and ended up maintaining an ongoing familial relationship with her.

Duncan and Mario came from very different families of origin and their core beliefs and values differed greatly. The first therapeutic task was to assist them in exploring their own dreams of parenting. It was important that the therapist validate each of the options available to them. It was especially salient in working with Duncan and Mario to acknowledge their reservations about adopting a child through foster care, without judgment or guilt. Gently, the couple was informed about the potentiality of any child to have "high needs," and that choosing another option would not eliminate that possibility, as all children can have or develop physical or mental challenges during their lifetimes. However, it was equally important that they not feel "guilty," and that the therapist honor their right to make choices that were the best fit for the family. Although Duncan was comfortable having the child be biologically Mario's, it was obvious that he had not thought much about the racial and cultural considerations that come with rearing a Latino child, which also became an important focus of therapy. Duncan's lack of conscious awareness of the racial identity of their future child highlighted the differences in their backgrounds, and the assumptions embedded in Duncan's white privilege. It also initiated a conversation about the home in which their child would be reared, including the cultural environment, religious, and ritualistic or moral aspects of family life.

Through the use of therapy, Duncan and Mario began to formulate what their family would look like structurally, particularly how they would create a nurturing environment. This process included an exploration of both partners' ideas of masculinity and gender roles. They soon realized that they had differing feelings about who would be the primary earner in the family and who would provide the primary caregiving to their children. Through discussion of this in therapy, they were able to plan ahead for a more equitable parenting relationship.

## Clinical Considerations with Transgender and Nonbinary Parents

Increasing numbers of people are coming out and seeking services for gender dysphoria, including referrals for medical and surgical treatments (Chang, Singh, & dickey, 2018; Ettner, Monstrey, & Eyler, 2007). Gender dysphoria is defined as "the psychological discomfort some individuals experience between their biological (or natal) sex and their experience of their core gender identity" (Lev, 2016, p. 987); however, it is important to note that many people seek transition-related services who do not experience "dysphoria," but rather seek increased comfort in their gender expression. Research indicates that 25–49% of the transgender population have children (Dierckx, Motmans, Mortelmans, & T'sjoen, 2016). When a trans person discloses their identity, the family can be thrown into a state of chaos and spouses often experience predictable stages of intense betrayal, anger, and grief (Lev, 2004b), even if the children do not know the cause of the marital distress they are affected by the ongoing discord in the home.

Disclosure of gender diversity has often foreshadowed separation and divorce (Dierckx et al., 2016). Historically, the pressure has come from laws and policies that would not allow legal marriages to continue following a gender transition or from LGBTQ communities insisting that separation from a heterosexual marriage was essential in order to live "authentically." Often transition has meant losing legal custody of children, although options for trans parents are increasing as society and families beginning to understand that relationships, families, and healthy parenting can continue following a change in gender identity or expression. One common presenting therapeutic concern is when an individual in a heterosexual couple comes out to their partner as transgender, often after many years of marriage and parenting together.

## Gender Transition after Parenthood

Working with trans people coming out later in life and with established families is a delicate process. Couples' work with trans partners is still in its infancy, though some clinical models have been developed (Constantinides et al., in press; Lev, 2004b; Malpas, 2006); work with trans parents and their children remains an underexplored area clinically. As seen in the case of Louis, the therapist's role is to aid in the negotiation of different opinions and levels of acceptance of the news.

### Case of Louis/Louisa

When Louis, a White heterosexual man, sought out therapy, the first thing he said was, "I've never spoken to anyone about this in my life." Louis was 35 years old, married to his high school sweetheart, with whom he had three children. He described his home life as generally happy, and he loved being a father. His work was stressful, but he was satisfied that he could support his family.

Over the course of 2 years of therapy, Louis came to the understanding that he desired to medically transition and live full-time as a woman. He had hidden his cross-dressing from his wife for decades, and he thought she would "freak out" when he told her. His sense of shame and isolation was extreme, but in his fantasy of transitioning, his reality testing was weak. On one hand, he could not imagine a life without moving forward to affirm his gender as a woman, and on the other hand, he lacked insight into how transitioning might affect his job, his wife, or his children. He saw himself having to make a choice to continue to live "as a man" (which meant continuing to be married to his wife and parenting his children) or to live "as a woman" (which meant leaving his wife and children); he saw no possibility for a middle ground—to live as a woman, and continue to be a parent to "his" children.

The first step in working with Louis was to create a safe place to explore his gender, including his current knowledge about the transition process, and his goals for the future. Another important focus was examining his relationship with his wife, the kind of marriage they had, what their intimacy was like, and why he had not shared this important part of himself with her before. Louis spent nearly a year in therapy exploring his gender dysphoria and various options on how to resolve it. As he became more secure and comfortable in his identity as a trans woman, he became clear that he wanted to live full-time and maintain his relationship with his wife if that was possible. As he moved into the second stage of emergence (Lev, 2004b), he began the process of self-disclosure with his wife. Part of that process including beginning to use female pronouns and the name Louisa.

As Louisa feared, her wife did "freak out," and they spent many months processing the issues of betrayal and grief that her wife struggled with, before Louisa's identity as a trans woman was discussed with their children. Often the greatest concern for the heterosexual wives of trans women is how the revelation of their partner's gender identity, or the parent's transition, will affect the children's own gender development and sexuality (Dierckx et al., 2016; White & Ettner, 2007), although there is no evidence that having a trans parent will negatively affect a child's developing sexual orientation or gender identity (Stotzer, Herman, & Hasenbush, 2014). The issues facing children are more about social acceptance and embarrassment within their own peer groups. The emerging literature reveals that the younger children are told of their parents' gender identification the easier it is to accept (White & Ettner, 2004). The therapist must create a supportive environment for the family through this difficult and challenging time; the more the therapist can normalize this life cycle transition, the easier it will be for the parents to support their children through the familial changes. Therapists need to validate the children's pain, betrayal, confusion, and fear and assist the transitioning adult to hear these fears without perceiving this as a rejection of their identity. The therapist is challenged to take a both/and view, supporting the person in authenticity, while also validating their parental role and ability to maintain close and loving relationships with their children (and hopefully their spouse as well). Therapists should take a strong stance against any attempts to alienate the trans parent from their children.

When a mother comes out as transgender and decides to transition, it is often difficult because the socially constructed identities and roles of motherhood are some of the most prescribed in Western culture. Given the position of privilege and power that most husbands have over their female partners, great care must be taken. In the case of Jared and Robert, it is clear how vulnerable Jared became after his transition from female to male as he is forced to create a new identity as a parent as well as manage extreme prejudice and discrimination from his ex-husband Robert.

### Case of Jared and Robert

Jared and Robert met when Jared was female identified at age 18. Jared, who was called JoLynn, saw Robert as a safe and protective escape from an abusive family of origin and married Robert only months after meeting him. Jared recounted the story of his first years with Robert, clear that he told Robert about how he felt "like a man on the inside" and that Robert said that he "didn't mind." Jared speculated that Robert was himself interested in men and thought that perhaps this was part of his attraction to Jared. They both wanted to be parents and so Jared agreed to live as a woman until they had their two children, Samantha and Lily. After giving birth to their second child, Jared became increasingly more depressed and anxious due to concerns related to gender identity and expression. Jared told Robert that he needed to transition as soon as possible in order to be the most stable and effective parent to their two daughters.

Robert was not able to accept this, and he became cruel, stating that he was not a "fag" and would not be married to a "fake man." Robert filed for divorce and demanded that Jared give up all parental rights to their children. Jared fought and won joint custody of their two children but the verbal abuse continued, as Robert berated Jared in front of the children. Jared's depression and isolation increased as Robert further ostracized him from the family, continuing to call him "JoLynn" and using female pronouns. He also insisted that their daughters keep calling Jared "Mommy" even though they had decided to call Jared "Maddy" in a family therapy session months earlier.

Legal advocacy and therapeutic work with Jared began with recognizing the complex matrix of both present and past traumas that inform Jared's self-esteem and trans identity development. Most importantly, Jared's ability to parent his two daughters was an empowering and connective force in his life, critical to his mental health and emotional stability. For Jared, neither his gender identity nor his transition was directly affecting his children's well-being; rather, it was the rupture in the family system caused by Robert's extremely rejecting reaction. When Jared's parenting was called into question due to Robert's transphobia and misogyny, it was critical that Jared's identity as Maddy be explored and cultivated within the therapeutic relationship as this was an unquestionable achievement for Jared and needed to be acknowledged and nurtured. Often parents who are transitioning have difficulty envisioning themselves as parents in their newly gendered bodies. They have internalized the transphobia that makes trans parenting an impossibility. Assisting newly transitioned clients in the exploration of their trans parenthood is critical to their new identity development and how they understand themselves as trans parents.

## Gender Transition Before Parenthood

Trans, genderqueer, and nonbinary people have been consciously becoming parents throughout the course of LGBTQ history (More, 1998), although it has only recently become public knowledge. When trans, genderqueer, and nonbinary people choose to begin families, they can face complex psychosocial and medical challenges, as well as discrimination from service providers. Although they are able to become parents more openly now, they are still vulnerable to scrutiny by social service providers when they seek assistance with adoption, surrogacy, and fertility issues. The Ethics Committee of the American Society for Reproductive Medicine (2015) specifically states, "Patients who deviate from the heteronormative family have historically been denied access to assisted reproductive technology (ART)" (p. 1111). This impacts those who transition in adulthood and then begin families, as well as those who transition as children or youth, and later in life seek to become parents.

When trans people seek out medical treatment for their gender dysphoria, discussions of fertility options should always be part of a routine assessment by both the psychotherapist and the medical doctors, according to The World Professional Association of Transgender Health (WPATH) and the Endocrine Society (Coleman et al., 2012; Hembree et al., 2009). Before beginning medical treatments, providers should obtain a signed informed consent and make sure clients are understand any known medical risks and the limited medical data on outcomes. Additionally, discussions about family creation should broadly include diverse representation of the gender spectrum, as well as all options including reproductive technologies, surrogacy, and foster/adoption (dickey, Ducheny, & Ehbar, 2016).

Those assigned male at birth (AMAB) who have sperm and testes may want to utilize sperm cryopreservation or testicular sperm extraction (TESE) before beginning hormonal treatment so that they can have biological children later in life with a female partner (De Sutter, 2001; Wallace,

Blough, & Kondapalli, 2014). Those assigned female at birth who have a uterus, eggs, and ovaries may want to utilize oocyte cryopreservation (De Roo, Tilleman, T'sjoen, & De Sutter, 2016; Maxwell, Noyes, Keefe, Berkeley, & Goldman, 2017). Transmasculine people are capable of getting pregnant if they still have their female anatomy, but they must stop taking testosterone first, which can be psychologically disorienting. Some get pregnant accidentally, after having stopped taking male hormones (Light, Obedin-Maliver, Sevelius, & Kerns, 2014). Fertility treatments may include taking high doses of feminizing hormone with fertility medication in order to conceive. When trans men become pregnant, they both challenge "patriarchal fatherhood" (Ryan, 2009, p. 147) and also transform the notions of parenthood and "motherhood." Transmasculine parents often identify as the father to the children that they have birthed (Epstein, 2009). Embryo cryopreservation (Wallace et al., 2014), surrogacy, and adoption are all routes to parenthood.

Within an affirmative care model (Edwards, Leeper, Leibowitz, & Sangganjanavanich, 2016; Janssen & Leibowitz, 2018; Keo-Meier & Ehrensaft, 2018), increasing numbers of young people are transitioning in childhood, and then medically—and sometimes surgically (Milrod, 2014)—in adolescence, raising a plethora of questions about fertility and nursing options (Estes, 2015; MacDonald et al., 2016). The ability to reproduce is impacted by medical and surgical interventions to treat adolescent gender dysphoria; fortuitously, medical knowledge on fertility preservation had been developed in oncofertility research treating childhood cancer treatment and has been adapted to work with transgender youth (Wallace et al., 2014).

Pubertal suppression (commonly referred to as "hormone blockers") are often prescribed to young trans adolescents to pause their puberty, but this also prevents maturation of the primary sex organs; cross-sex hormones started in later adolescence may also affect fertility, but has not been fully studied (Finlayson et al., 2016). The ability to reproduce into adulthood requires the preservation of sperm or eggs, or the cryopreservation of testicular or ovarian tissues (which remains experimental). Rates of fertility preservation by trans youth appear at this time to be low (Chen, Simons, Johnson, Lockart, & Finlayson, 2017), with many adolescents stating that they would prefer to adopt (Lev & Wolf-Gould, 2018). Fertility preservation for those with female anatomy is surgical invasive, requiring the introduction of increased female hormones; and for those with male anatomy requires masturbation which may cause dysphoria and be embarrassing, especially for young adolescents (Lev & Wolf-Gould, 2018). Treatments require additional waiting time before starting cross-sex hormones and often increase symptoms of gender dysphoria (Chen et al., 2017). These medical treatments are often prohibitively expensive; parents and youth do not always see eye-to-eye on their value (Lev & Wolf-Gould, 2018). There are, of course, other youth that care deeply about their ability to biologically produce their own children, and these adolescents are most likely to take advantage of fertility preservation, in some cases wait until their gonads fully mature to commence medical treatments. Lev and Wolf-Gould (2018) state, "The therapeutic team can offer a safe space to express and process this grief, or assist a child in living in a discordant gender until gametes are harvested for preservation of fertility" (p. 201).

Nonbinary people often experience their identities being erased when they decide to become gestational parents due to the social construction of motherhood. Many nonbinary people live on the fringes of even their own queer communities as they request their support systems to identify them as gestational parents and not mothers, or even a pregnant "person" instead of a pregnant "woman." Often trans and nonbinary pregnant people call nursing chestfeeding because they do not identify as having breasts (MacDonald et al., 2016). In the vignette that follows, a polyamorous couple, with one partner who identifies as trans masculine and the other as nonbinary, are raising two children under the pressures of larger social systems of oppression.

## Case of Len and Nico

Len (they/them pronouns), age 32, and Nico (he/him pronouns), age 30, a polyamorous White nonbinary/trans couple, came into therapy because they were contemplating a separation. They had been together for over a decade and had a commitment ceremony 8 years previously, but were not legally married. They shared the parenting of two children, Noa, 6 years old, and Lucinda, 3 years old, both gestated by Len, and conceived with known donor sperm (Nico's best friend from high school). Len was a "stay-at-home parent," who was homeschooling their children, and Nico worked as a contractor with a construction company. Nico and Len were loving parents to their children, but their relationship had felt hollow for the past few years, while they struggled with typical issues that families with young children face. They had little time for their relationship due to their parental philosophy of extreme hands-on parenting: they were reluctant to hire babysitters, and they practiced attachment parenting, including extended chestfeeding and co-sleeping. Although both parents believed strongly in these values, the lion's share of the work fell on Len, who was with the children every day, while Nico worked long hours to single-handedly support the family.

Separating presented unique challenges for Len and Nico. They had been unable to afford the legal paperwork to secure their family with a second parent adoption for Nico, though they did have their donor release his rights to the children directly after each of their births. Still, Nico had no legal ties or rights to his children. Nico was terrified that if the couple separated Len would not let him see the children if he moved out, and Len admitted, sheepishly, to using the power of their legal status to forestall Nico from leaving. Len had few employable skills and was extremely resistant to working out of their house while their children were small. They were completely financially dependent on Nico. The couple felt trapped in a relationship where they were no longer "in love" and unable to maintain a lifestyle they had carefully created unless they remained together. They were both deeply committed to the needs of their children, yet couldn't see spending another decade together until the children matured. Because they also both identified as polyamorous when they began their relationship, they were hopeful that with the support of therapy they could find a way to create an alternative family structure that would include each of them having emotional and romantic needs met by other partners; however, in the entire 10 years that they had been together, they had never officially opened their relationship up to the possibility of other connections.

Len and Nico's decade-long relationship and shared commitment to their children were strengths for them as parents; however, separation required a massive shift in the foundation of their lives together. The stability and security of their home life was not only threatened by the separation, but suddenly they were confronted with legal ambiguities, forcing them to face complex ethical dilemmas. Nico feared the loss of being a parent to his two children. He had no legal standing as a nongestational parent and depended on Len's good will to maintain his parenting role. Len was in a situation familiar to many people in heterosexual relationships, especially those who are stay-at-home parents. They feared the loss of the parenting lifestyle that they were accustomed to, including full financial support from Nico. The fact that Len was aware of the power they held as the legal and biological parent of the two children, and that they wielded this power in an attempt to keep Nico from leaving the relationship, was the crux of the relational

mistrust between the two—an idea they both accepted, when the therapist presented it. Their awareness of their unequal parental power can be viewed as an important strength, as there are many couples who do not want to admit that there are certain axes of privilege as a birth parent in a queer partnership. The therapist must provide a container for the couple and family that disallows using the homophobic legal system to minimize Nico's role as a parent. Although queer couples often form their families outside of the legal system, they sometimes resort to that very system during separations. The judicial system, embedded in homophobic constructs about families, will rarely respect the structure of queer families. When LGBTQ couples are separating, judges will often only honor the biological or legal partner; sadly, some LGBTQ people purposely seek out legal measures in order to wield power over their (ex) partners (Shuster, 2002).

Len felt powerless because Nico wanted to leave and understood that they would not be able to continue parenting, their primary job, in the way they had been. Len was losing not only their dream of their family, and the relationship they shared with Nico, but their entire way of life was threatened. Nico felt powerless to maintain an equal parenting relationship with Len, and feared he had no recourse; he was legally a stranger to his children. It took time to help Len understand the threat that Nico faced, especially because he had complete passing privilege and no one that he worked with knew that he was trans. This made him safer in his workplace in some ways but much less protected in emotional and legal ways within their relationship.

The values and ethical stance of the therapist in a case like Len and Nico's can significantly impact the outcome for this family. The therapist must hold the fears of each partner, especially in light of these power differentials, yet take a firm stance that, despite the lack of legal protections, both partners are parents to their children and must remain so in the eyes of their children as well as one another. The therapist must examine their own experiences and how that affects their values and opinions about this family.

For Len and Nico, their commitment to the kind of life they wanted for their children was able to supersede their disappointment, anger, and fear of ending their romantic relationship. The therapist was able to use the Alternative Family Structures Approach (AFSA) (Constantinides et al., in press) to begin the process of supporting Len and Nico in opening up their relationship to other partnerships and connections. Through the use of AFSA, both Len and Nico were able to grieve the loss of their 10-year commitment to one another as sexual partners, and it was important for the therapist to acknowledge and name their relationship as deeply binding and life altering commitment regardless of the lack of legal recognition.

Over time Len was able to tell Nico that they would not use their biological status to impede Nico's right to his children or his contact with them. They were able to write a contract stating this, but more importantly, they were able to create a separation ritual outlining the contract that served as a way to psychologically concretize their separation even more than a legally binding document (Imber-Black, 1988). Nico was able to commit to not abandoning the children financially, although he was clear with Len that he could not support Len indefinitely. They began to engage in conversations about how Len could return to school so they could become more employable, while still remaining home with the children while they were young. They eventually found a small apartment, and they began to develop an equitable parenting arrangement, where they would nest with the children separately and be with other new romantic interests at the apartment when they were not with the children. They continued to grieve, but their focus became helping their children cope with the changes in their family, rather than wielding domestic and judicial power over one another through the course of their separation. With the right amount of therapeutic support and the AFSA structure, Len and Nico were able to reorganize their family and assist the children in adjusting to the structural and relational changes. The entire family was eventually able to feel a sense of pride about their identities as a queer polyamorous family system.

# The Next Generation of LGBTQ Parents

Younger LGBTQ people no longer wonder if parenting is a possibility; now it is often an assumed reality and birthright. Therapeutic work with these clients is often more about naming goals and negotiating differences within a partnership. Parenting possibilities are wide open if therapists allow themselves to think outside of the box with LGBTQ prospective parents.

Even with this burgeoning fleet of new queer-identified parents, there are many clinical considerations for therapists to be mindful of, most poignantly the collective trauma of stigma, gender oppression, and the history of children being ripped away from LGBTQ parents in the past when they have come out to partners and family members. Therapists aid in building and empowering the clients' identities as parents while making space to explore possible fears and resentments that clients may have about how their families of origin and society may react to their parenthood. One thing that therapists can usually count on with the new generation of LGBTQ parents is that they are freer to make parenting decisions than LGBTQ people a decade ago, and this increasing freedom makes the therapeutic work rewarding and challenging. The following vignette depicts a case in which the clinician utilizes the relational aspects of their orientation to both create connection with the couple and to slow down the family-building process.

### Case of Grace and Karin
Loud, angry voices emanated from the waiting room, interrupting the session. Awkwardly excusing herself, the therapist walked to the waiting room, where two people in their early 20s sat, engaged in a fierce argument. The therapist introduced herself and asked the couple to please lower their voices and wait for their session to begin in about 15 minutes. One of them seemed embarrassed, but the other seemed

annoyed to be distracted from their argument. They immediately reengaged, albeit in lower voices, when the therapist walked back to her office.

When Grace and Karin came into the office, they immediately resumed their battle, barely acknowledging the therapist's presence. With pitched voices, Karin and Grace yelled over one another, making the therapist wish she had a referee whistle in her clinical bag of tricks. The therapist had to stand up and loudly insist that they stop arguing. After setting up basic communication rules (one person talks at a time), the therapist asked them to introduce themselves. Karin self-identified as using she/her pronouns, Latinx, queer femme, and disabled. She had long wavy hair, black lipstick, and multiple piercings, and reported that she was a college student in political science. Grace self-identified as using they/them pronouns, nonbinary, White, and fat, with a short crew cut and visible tattoo sleeves, said they had recently graduated from college and was working as a medical assistant in a local hospital.

Quieter now, but no less intense, Karin explained why she was seeking help from a therapist. "We want to have a child," Karin explained, adding, in a sarcastic tone, "at least I do." Grace quickly jumped in, "We both want the same thing. The issue is how to make it happen. You see, Karin wants to get pregnant, which I'm okay with, but it is *how* she wants to do it that worries me." For the first time, there was silence in the room.

Karin said, "I don't see what the big deal is." She turned to the therapist with a look that was both pleading and challenging. "I want to have a child the natural way, you know? I don't want to use a sperm bank," she said, her voice acerbic. "I want my children, *our* children, to know their biological father...I mean it's only right. What's the big deal about having sex with a guy anyway?" she asked pointedly.

Grace looked at the therapist with raised eyebrows, clearly expecting the therapist to take their side on this issue. "Tell me that's not gross," Grace said. "I mean, I don't care if someone likes sex with men, but to have sex with one just to make a baby, *my* baby, ugh!" The therapist paused thoughtfully. "How long have you two been together," she asked. Without pause, they simultaneously answered, "Three weeks."

Karin and Grace represent an emerging generation of young LGBTQ prospective parents. Born 20 years after Stonewall, reaching adulthood in a world where marriage equality is discussed on the evening news, and having received college credits for discussing the relationship between queer theory and postcolonial racism, Grace and Karin came to their queer relationship secure in the knowledge that they could become parents. Unlike an older cohort of LGBTQ parents, Grace and Karin do not verbalize concerns about how being queer might affect their children's development, or if queer parenthood might be a detriment in rearing a male child. They appear to have no concerns about the social world—their families of origin, their LGBTQ community, their jobs; they are solid in their inalienable right to become queer parents.

That they are also young in both age and relational status, and have not engaged in any detailed conversations about finances, child-rearing philosophies, or relationship stability, mirrors the same immaturity and naiveté of their non-LGBTQ peer group; that is, they are experiencing these developmental milestones at the appropriate time in the life cycle (Sassler, 2010). The idea that a young queer couple would fantasize and plan for their family as part of their courtship, that they imagine children as part of their human birthright, and that they are (somewhat) educated about how to create a family reflects a new era in LGBTQ family building. This new generation is not asking permission of the world and could care less what the research says about their families; they simply believe that having children is what couples in love can *do*. Perhaps, the reader is oddly relieved to discover that unlike heterosexual couples, conception will take a bit of planning—maybe even another 3 or 4 weeks!

Although on the surface, Karin and Grace's issues are similar to other young couples considering parenting, their presenting problem illustrates the unique interpersonal and emotional struggles that queer and same-sex couples face when choosing to become parents. Specifically, an additional concern is whether their relationship is legally sanctioned—although legal in all U.S. states, marriage and/or second-parent adoption is not necessarily practiced by all partners—and how that might affect their child's legal status, particularly if Karin were to become pregnant in what she viewed as the "natural way." Legal issues, including health insurance and paternity rights, financial responsibilities, extended family and community support, and the complex issues of parenting "style" and values, are all potential fodder for the clinical conversation.

## Conclusion

Clinical work with LGBTQ parents and prospective parents can be a rich and illuminating experience when therapists have properly educated themselves regarding the multitude of parenting possibilities for LGBTQ people. It is helpful to utilize an eclectic therapeutic approach that is informed by systemic, narrative, transfeminist, and relational perspectives. There is a new generation of LGBTQ prospective parents who are looking for clinicians able to work competently with the matrix of intersecting identities that parents may have. The challenge for clinicians is no longer to help LGBTQ parents fit into a heteronormative construct of parenting and child rearing. The new charge for therapists is to nurture and foster the endless possibilities and choices that are becoming a reality for LGBTQ parents and prospective parents.

## References

Acosta, K. L. (2014). We are family. *Contexts, 13*(1), 44–49. https://doi.org/10.1177/1536504214522008

Adams, H. L., & Phillips, L. (2009). Ethnic related variations from the cass model of homosexual identity formation: The experiences of two-spirit, lesbian and gay Native Americans. *Journal of Homosexuality, 56*, 959–976. https://doi.org/10.1080/00918360903318789

Ashton, D. (2011). Lesbian, gay, bisexual, and transgender individuals and the family life cycle. In M. McGoldrick, B. Carter, & N. Garcia-Preto (Eds.), *The expanded family lifecycle* (pp. 115–132). Boston, MA: Allyn and Bacon.

Bergman, K., Rubio, R. J., Green, R. J., & Padron, E. (2010). Gay men who become fathers via surrogacy: The transition to parenthood. *Journal of GLBT Family Studies, 6*, 111–141. https://doi.org/10.1080/15504281003704942

Berkowitz, D. (2007). A sociohistorical analysis of gay men's procreative consciousness. *Journal of GLBT Family Studies, 3*, 157–190. https://doi.org/10.1300/J461v03n02_07

Bermea, A., van Eeden-Moorefield, B., Bible, J., & Petren, R. (2018). Undoing normativities and creating family: A queer stepfamily's experience. *Journal of GLBT Family Studies, 15*, 357–372. https://doi.org/10.1080/1550428X.2018.1521760

Biblarz, T. J., & Savci, E. (2010). Lesbian, gay, bisexual, and transgender families. *Journal of Marriage and Family, 72*, 480–497. https://doi.org/10.1111/j.1741-3737.2010.00714.x

Bigner, J. J., & Bozett, F. W. (1990). Parenting by gay fathers. In F. W. Bozett & M. B. Sussman (Eds.), *Homosexuality and family relations* (pp. 155–175). New York, NY: Harrington Park Press.

Bowleg, L., Burkholder, G., Teti, M., & Craig, M. L. (2008). The complexities of outness: Psychosocial predictors of coming out to others among black lesbian and bisexual women. *Journal of LGBT Health Research, 4*, 153–166. https://doi.org/10.1080/15574090903167422

Boyd, J. P. (2017). *Polyamory in Canada: Research on an emerging family structure.* The Vanier Institute of the Family. Retrieved from: https://prism.ucalgary.ca/bitstream/handle/1880/107495/Boyd%20Polyamorous%20Families%201.pdf?sequence=1

Brown, S., Smalling, S., Groza, V. & Ryan, S. (2009). The experiences of gay men and lesbians in becoming and being adoptive parents. *Adoption Quarterly 12*(3–4), 229–246.

Brown, T. (2002). A proposed model of bisexual identity development that elaborates on experiential differences of women and men. *Journal of Bisexuality, 2*(4), 67–91

Carneiro, F. A., Tasker, F., Salinas-Quiroz, F., Leal, I., & Costa, P. A. (2017). Are the fathers alright? A systematic and critical review of studies on gay and bisexual fatherhood. *Frontiers in Psychology, 8*, 1636. https://doi.org/10.3389/fpsyg.2017.01636

Cass, V. C. (1979). Homosexuality identity formation: A theoretical model. *Journal of Homosexuality, 4*, 291–235. https://doi.org/10.1300/J082v04n03_01

Cass, V. C. (1998). Sexual orientation identity formation, a western phenomenon. In R. J. Cabaj & T. S. Stein (Eds.), *Textbook of homosexuality and mental health* (pp. 227–251). Washington, DC: American Psychiatric Association.

Chang, S. C., Singh, A. A., & Dickey, L. M. (2018). *A clinician's guide to gender-affirming care: Working with transgender and gender nonconforming clients*. Oakland, CA: Context Press.

Chen, D., Simons, L., Johnson, E. K., Lockart, B. A., & Finlayson, C. (2017). Fertility preservation for transgender adolescents. *Journal of Adolescent Health, 61*, 120–123. https://doi.org/10.1016/j.jadohealth.2017.01.022

Coleman, E., Bockting, W., Botzer, M., Cohen-Kettenis, P., DeCuypere, G., Feldman, J., ... Zucker, K. (2012). Standards of care for the health of transsexual, transgender, and gender nonconforming people, 7th version. *International Journal of Transgenderism, 13*, 165–232. https://doi.org/10.1080/15532739.2011.700873

Constantinides, D. M., Sennott, S. L., & Chandler, D. (2019). *Sex therapy with erotically marginalized clients: Nine principles of clinical support*. New York, NY: Routledge.

De Roo, C., Tilleman, K., T'sjoen, G., & De Sutter, P. (2016). Fertility options in transgender people. *International Review of Psychiatry, 28*, 112–119. https://doi.org/10.3109/09540261.2015.1084275

De Sutter, P. (2001). Gender reassignment and assisted reproduction: Present and future reproductive options for transsexual people. *Human Reproduction, 16*, 612–614. https://doi.org/10.1093/humrep/16.4.612

Devor, H. (1997). *FTM: Female-to-male transsexuals in society*. Bloomington, IN: Indiana University Press.

dickey, L. M., Duchen, K. M., & Ehbar, R. D. (2016). Family creation options for transgender and gender nonconforming people. *Psychology of Sexual Orientation and Gender Diversity, 3*, 173–179. https://doi.org/10.1037/sgd0000178

Dierckx, M., Motmans, J., Mortelmans, D., & T'sjoen, G. (2016). Families in transition: A literature review. *International Review of Psychiatry, 28*, 36–43. https://doi.org/10.3109/09540261.2015.1102716

Downing, J. B., Richardson, H. B., Kinkler, L. A., & Goldberg, A. E. (2009). Making the decision: Factors influencing gay men's choice of an adoption path. *Adoption Quarterly, 12*, 247–271. https://doi.org/10.1080/10926750903313310

Downs, A. C., & James, S. E. (2006). Gay, lesbian, and bisexual foster parents: Strengths and challenges for the child welfare system. *Child Welfare, 85*, 281–298. https://doi.org/0009-4021/2006/030281-18

Edwards-Leeper, L., Leibowitz, S., & Sangganjanavanich, V. F. (2016). Affirmative practice with transgender and gender nonconforming youth: Expanding the model. *Psychology of Sexual Orientation and Gender Diversity, 3*, 165–172. https://doi.org/10.1037/sgd0000167

Ehrensaft, D. (2016). *The Gender Creative Child*. NY: The Experiment.

Epstein, R. (2009). *Who's your daddy? And other writings on queer parenting*. Toronto, ON: Sumach Press.

Epstein, R. (2014). *Married, single or gay? Queerying and transforming the practices of assisted human reproduction* (Unpublished PhD dissertation). Toronto, ON: York University.

Estes, S. J. (2015). Fertility preservation in children and adolescents. *Endocrinology and Metabolism Clinics of North America, 44*, 799–820. https://doi.org/10.1016/j.ecl.2015.07.005

Ethics Committee of the American Society for Reproductive Medicine. (2015). Access to fertility services by transgender persons: An Ethics Committee opinion. *American Society for Reproductive Medicine Fertility & Sterility, 104*, 1111–1115.

Ettner, R., Monstrey, S., & Eyler, A. E. (Eds.). (2007). *Principles of transgender medicine and surgery*. New York, NY: The Haworth Press.

Gates, G., Badgett, M. V. L., Macomber, J. E., & Chambers, K. (2007). *Adoption and foster care by gay and lesbian parents in the United States*. Washington, DC: The Urban Institute.

Gilligan, C. (1993). *In a different voice: Psychological theory and women's development*. New York, NY: Harvard University Press.

Goldberg, A. E. (2010). *Lesbian and gay parents and their children: Research on the family life cycle*. Washington, DC: American Psychological Association.

Goldberg, A. E. (2012). *Gay dads: Transitions to adoptive fatherhood*. New York, NY: NYU Press.

Goldberg, A. E., Downing, J. B., & Richardson, H. B. (2009). The transition from infertility to adoption: Perceptions of lesbian and heterosexual preadoptive couples. *Journal of Social & Personal Relationships, 26*, 938–963. https://doi.org/10.1177/0265407509345652

Goldberg, A. E., & Gianino, M. (2012). Lesbian and gay adoptive parents: Assessment, clinical issues, and intervention. In D. Brodzinsky & A. Pertman (Eds.), *Lesbian and gay adoption: A new American reality* (pp. 204–232). New York, NY: Oxford University Press.

Hammock, P. L., Frost, D. M., & Huges, S. D. (2018). Queer intimacies: A new paradigm for the study of relationship diversity. *The Journal of Sex Research, 56*, 1–37. https://doi.org/10.1080/00224499.2018.1531281

Harvey, R. (2012). Young people, sexual orientation, and resilience. In M. Unger (Ed.), *The social ecology of resilience: A handbook of theory and practice* (pp. 3–25). New York, NY: Springer.

Hembree, W. C., Cohen-Kettenis, P., Delemarre-van de Waal, H. A., Gooren, L. J., Meyer, W. J., 3rd, Spack, N. P., ... Montori, V. M. (2009). Endocrine treatment of transsexual persons: An Endocrine Society clinical practice guideline. *Journal of Clinical*

*Endocrinology & Metabolism, 94,* 3132–3154. https://doi.org/10.1210/jc.2017-01658

Hudak, J. M., & Giammattei, S. V. (2010). Doing family: Decentering heteronormativity in "marriage" and "family" therapy. *AFTA Monograph Series: Expanding our Social Justice Practices: Advances in Theory and Training, 6,* 49–58. https://doi.org/10.1016/j.wsif.2012.03.003

Imber-Black, E. (1988). *Families and larger systems.* New York, NY: Guilford Press.

Janssen, A., & Leibowitz, S. (2018). *Affirmative mental health care for transgender and gender diverse youth: A clinical guide.* New York, NY: Springer.

Jordan, J. V., Kaplan, A. G., Miller, J. B., Stiver, I. P., & Surrey, J. L. (Eds.). (1991). *Women's growth in connection: Writings from the Stone Center.* New York, NY: Guilford Press.

Karpman, H. E., Ruppel, E. H., & Torres, M. (2018). "It wasn't feasible for us": Queer women of color navigating family formation. *Family Relations, 67,* 118–131. https://doi.org/10.1111/fare.12303

Keo-Meier, C., & Ehrensaft, D. (2018). *The gender affirmative model: An interdisciplinary approach to supporting transgender and gender expansive children.* Washington, DC: American Psychological Association.

LaSala, M. C. (2010). *Coming out, coming home: Helping families adjust to a gay or lesbian child.* New York, NY: Columbia University Press.

Lev, A. I. (2004a). *The complete lesbian and gay parenting guide.* New York, NY: Berkley.

Lev, A. I. (2004b). *Transgender emergence: Therapeutic guidelines for working with gender variant people and their families.* New York, NY: Routledge.

Lev, A. I. (2006a). Gay dads: Choosing surrogacy. *The British Psychological Society Lesbian and Gay Psychology Review, 7,* 72–76.

Lev, A. I. (2006b, March 31). Scrutinizing would-be parents (Gay): Gays looking to adopt will have to endure rigorous home studies. *Washington Blade,* pp. 6b, 7b.

Lev, A. I. (2008). More than surface tension: Femmes in families. *Journal of Lesbian Studies, 12,* 127–144. https://doi.org/10.1080/10894160802161299

Lev, A. I. (2010). How queer!—The development of gender identity and sexual orientation in LGBTQ-headed families. *Family Process, 49,* 268–290. https://doi.org/10.1111/j.1545-5300.2010.01323.x

Lev, A. I. (2016). Gender dysphoria. In N. A. Naples (Ed.), *Wiley-Blackwell encyclopedia of gender and sexuality studies* (pp. 987–990). Oxford, UK: Wiley-Blackwell.

Lev, A. I., & Alie, L. (2012). Addressing the needs of youth who are LGBT and their families: A system of care approach. In S. Fisher, G. Blau, & J. M. Poirier (Eds.), *Addressing the needs of youth who are LGBT and their families: A system of care approach* (pp. 43–66). Baltimore, MD: Brookes.

Lev, A. I. & Gottlieb, A. R. (2019). Families in Transition: Parent Perspectives on Raising Gender- Diverse Children, Adolescents, and Young Adult. NY: Harrington Park Press.

Lev, A. I., & Wolf-Gould, C. (2018). Collaborative treatment across disciplines: Physician and mental health counselor coordinating competent care. In C. Keo-Meier & D. Ehrensaft (Eds.), *The gender affirmative model: An interdisciplinary approach to supporting transgender and gender expansive children* (pp. 189–207). Washington, DC: American Psychological Association.

Levitt, H. M., Gerrish, E. A., & Hiestand, K. R. (2003). The misunderstood gender: A model of modern femme identity. *Sex Roles, 48,* 99–113. https://doi.org/10.1023/A:1022453304384

Light, A. D., Obedin-Maliver, J., Sevelius, J. M., & Kerns, J. L. (2014). Transgender men who experienced pregnancy after female-to-male gender transitioning. *Obstetrics and Gynecology, 124,* 1120–1127. https://doi.org/10.1097/AOG.0000000000000540

Lynch, J. M. (2004). Identity transformation: Stepparents in lesbian/gay stepfamilies. *Journal of Homosexuality, 48,* 45–60. https://doi.org/10.1300/J082v47n02_06

MacDonald, T., Noel-Weiss, J., West, D., Walks, M., Biener, M., Kibbe, A., & Myler, E. (2016). Transmasculine individuals' experiences with lactation, chestfeeding, and gender identity: A qualitative study. *BMC Pregnancy and Childbirth, 16,* 106. https://doi.org/10.1186/s12884-016-0907-y

Mallon, G. P. (2007). Assessing lesbian and gay prospective foster and adoptive families: A focus on the home study process. *Child Welfare, 86,* 67–86. https://doi.org/0009-4021/2007/020767-86

Malpas, J. (2006). From "otherness" to alliance: Transgender couples in therapy. *Journal of GLBT Family Studies, 2,* 183–206. https://doi.org/10.1300/J461v02n03_10

Manley, M. H., Legge, M. M., Flanders, C. E., Goldberg, A. E., & Ross, L. E. (2018). Consensual nonmonogamy in pregnancy and parenthood: Experiences of bisexual and plurisexual women with different-gender partners. *Journal of Sex & Marital Therapy, 44,* 721–736. https://doi.org/10.1080/0092623X.2018.1462277

Maxwell, S., Noyes, N., Keefe, D., Berkeley, A. S., & Goldman, K. N. (2017). Pregnancy outcomes after fertility preservation in transgender men. *Obstetrics & Gynecology, 29,* 1031–1034. https://doi.org/10.1097/AOG.0000000000002036

McDowell, T. (2005). Practicing a relational therapy with a critical multicultural lens. Introduction to a special section. *Journal of Systemic Therapies, 24,* 1–4. https://doi.org/10.1521/jsyt.2005.24.1.1

McGoldrick, M., Carter, B., & Garcia-Preto, N. (Eds.). (2010). *The expanded family lifecycle.* Boston, MA: Allyn and Bacon.

McGoldrick, M., Gerson, R., & Petry, S. (2008). *Genograms: Assessment and intervention* (3rd ed.). New York, NY: W. W. Norton.

McGoldrick, M., & Hardy, K. V. (Eds.). (2008). *Re-visioning family therapy: Race, culture, and gender in clinical practice.* New York, NY: Guilford Press.

Meadow, T. (2018). *Trans kids: Being gendered in the twenty-first century*. Oakland, CA: University of California Press.

Milrod, C. (2014). How young is too young: Ethical concerns in genital surgery of the transgender MTF adolescent. *Journal of Sexual Medicine, 11*, 338–346.

Moore, M. R. (2008). Gendered power relations among women: A study of household decision making in black lesbian stepfamilies. *American Sociological Review, 73*, 335–356. https://doi.org/10.1177/000312240807300208

Moore, M. R. (2011). *Invisible families: Gay identities, relationships, and motherhood among Black women*. Berkeley, CA: University of California Press.

Morales, E. (1996). Gender roles among Latino gay and bisexual men: Implications for family and couple relationships. In J. Laird & R. J. Green (Eds.), *Lesbians and gays in couples and families: A handbook for therapists* (pp. 272–297). San Francisco, CA: Jossey-Bass.

More, S. D. (1998). The pregnant man—An oxymoron? *Journal of Gender Studies, 7*, 319–325. https://doi.org/10.1080/09589236.1998.9960725

Nealy, E. C. (2017). *Transgender children and youth: Cultivating pride and joy with families in transition*. New York, NY: Norton.

Patterson, C. J. (1995). Lesbian mothers, gay fathers, and their children. In A. R. D'Augelli & C. J. Patterson (Eds.), *Lesbian, gay, bisexual identities over the lifespan: Psychological perspectives* (pp. 262–290). New York, NY: Oxford University Press.

Patterson, C. J. (2006). Children of lesbian and gay parents. *Current Directions in Psychological Science, 15*, 241–244. https://doi.org/10.1111/j.1467-8721.2006.00444.x

Riggs, D. (2007). *Becoming parent: Lesbians, gay men, and family*. Teneriffe, QLD: Post Pressed.

Rosario, M., Schrimshaw, E. W., & Hunter, J. (2004). Ethnic/racial differences in the coming-out process of lesbian, gay, and bisexual youths: A comparison of sexual identity development over time. *Cultural Diversity and Ethnic Minority Psychology, 10*, 215–228. https://doi.org/10.1037/1099-9809.10.3.215

Ryan, C. (2009). *Supportive families, healthy children: Helping families with lesbian, gay, bisexual, and transgender children*. Retrieved from: http://familyproject.sfsu.edu/publications

Ryan, C., Huebner, D., Diaz, R. M., & Sanchez, J. (2009). Family rejection as a predictor or negative health outcomes in white and Latino lesbian, gay, and bisexual young adults. *Pediatrics, 123*, 346–352. https://doi.org/10.1542/peds.2007-3524

Sassler, S. (2010). Partnering across the life course: Sex, relationships, and mate selection. *Journal of Marriage and Family, 72*, 557–571. https://doi.org/10.1111/j.1741-3737.2010.00718.x

Sennott, S., & Smith, T. (2011). Translating the sex and gender continuums in mental health: A transfeminist approach to client and clinician fears. *Journal of Gay and Lesbian Mental Health, 15*, 218–234. https://doi.org/10.1080/19359705.2011.553779

Sennott, S. L. (2011). Gender disorder as gender oppression: A transfeminist approach to rethinking the pathologization of gender non-conformity. *Women & Therapy, 34*, 93–113. https://doi.org/10.1080/02703149.2010.532683

Sennott, S. L., & Chandler, D. (2019). Supporting siblings through transition: A child-centered transfeminist therapeutic approach. In A. I. Lev & A. R. Gottlieb (Eds.), *Families in transition: Parenting gender diverse children adolescents and young adults* (pp. 290–307). New York, NY: Harrington Park Press.

Shuster, S. (2002). An ounce of prevention: Keeping couples out of court. *In the Family, 7*(3), 7–11.

Slater, C. (1999). *The lesbian family life cycle*. Chicago, IL: University of Illinois Press.

Stotzer, R., Herman, J. L., & Hasenbush, A. (2014). *Transgender parenting: A review of research*. Los Angeles, CA: The Williams Institute, UCLA School of Law. Retrieved from: http://williamsinstitute.law.ucla.edu/research/parenting/transgender-parenting-oct-2014/

Tasker, F., & Golombok, S. (1997). *Growing up in a lesbian family*. New York, NY: Guilford Press.

Troiden, R. R. (1993). The formation of homosexual identities. In L. D. Garnets & D. C. Kimmel (Eds.), *Psychological perspectives on lesbian and gay male experiences* (pp. 191–217). New York, NY: Columbia University Press.

Unger, M. (Ed.). (2012). *The social ecology of resilience: A handbook of theory and practice*. New York, NY: Springer.

Vaughan, M. D., & Waehler, C. A. (2010). Coming out growth: Conceptualizing and measuring stress-related growth associated with coming out to others as a sexual minority adult. *Journal of Adult Development, 17*, 94–109. https://doi.org/10.1007/s10804-009-9084-9

Wallace, S. A., Blough, K. L., & Kondapalli, L. A. (2014). Fertility preservation in the transgender patient: Expanding oncofertility care beyond cancer. *Gynecology Endocrinology, 30*(12), 868–871.

Walsh, F. (Ed.). (2011). *Normal family processes: Growing diversity and complexity* (4th ed.). New York, NY: Guilford Press.

Walsh, F. (2016). *Strengthening family resilience* (3rd ed.). New York, NY: Guilford Press.

White, M. (2007). *Maps of narrative practice*. New York, NY: W. W. Norton.

White, T., & Ettner, R. (2004). Disclosure, risks and protective factors for children whose parents are undergoing a gender transition. *Journal of Gay & Lesbian Psychotherapy, 8*, 129–145. https://doi.org/10.1080/19359705.2004.9962371

White, T., & Ettner, R. (2007). Adaptation and adjustment in children of transsexual parents. *European Child & Adolescent Psychiatry, 16*(4), 215–221.

# Clinical Work with Children and Adolescents Growing Up with LGBTQ Parents

Cynthia J. Telingator, Peter T. Daniolos, and Eric N. Boyum

Lesbian, gay, bisexual, transgender, and queer (LGBTQ) people desire to parent for many of the same reasons as cisgender, heterosexually oriented men and women, but the process of becoming parents may be more complex for these sexual and gender minorities which includes "coming out" for a second time, but now as an LGBTQ parent. This often means integrating one's own needs with familial and societal expectations and prohibitions. LGBTQ parents attempt to anticipate the unique issues their children may confront at different developmental stages but cannot alter the sociocultural and political impact of societal bias on their families. Although LGBTQ families are more visible and accepted today, all sexual and gender minority families continue to be affected by societal bias. The potential impact of this bias may differ for each member of the family. Gender diverse parents (i.e., trans and nonbinary parents) face challenges that are likely distinct from sexual minority parents, including types of stigma they may face, the coming-out processes, and transitions they must negotiate in their own lives (Biblarz & Savci,

2010; Haines, Ajayi, & Boyd, 2014; Pyne, Bauer, & Bradley, 2015; Tabor, 2019). A therapist working with LGBTQ-parent families should consider the struggles that each parent may have faced for being a sexual/gender minority across their life span. Clinical attention to the intersectionality in each individual's experience based on socioeconomic status (SES), religious, ethnic, and racial identity is essential. Early positive and negative experiences of the parent(s) both within their families and communities can influence their own social and developmental processes, and subsequently their parenting.

## Theoretical Considerations: Life Course and Minority Stress Theories Applied to LGBTQ-Parent Families

A life course perspective emphasizes that development is lifelong and continuous. The transition to parenthood is a significant life transition and is informed by continuities and discontinuities from all previous stages of development (Engel, 1977; Halfon & Hochstein, 2002). According to a life course perspective, the interaction between one's life stages and experiences cannot be understood in isolation, but is influenced at each developmental stage by one's previous development, as well as the responses of the environment in which one is raised (Johnson, Crosnoe, & Elder, 2011). A life course approach is used in this chapter to

C. J. Telingator (✉)
Harvard Medical School, Cambridge Health Alliance,
Cambridge, MA, USA
e-mail: cindy_telingator@hms.harvard.edu

P. T. Daniolos · E. N. Boyum
Child and Adolescent Psychiatry University of Iowa
Hospitals & Clinics, Iowa City, IA, USA
e-mail: peter-daniolos@uiowa.edu

© Springer Nature Switzerland AG 2020
A. E. Goldberg, K. R. Allen (eds.), *LGBTQ-Parent Families*,
https://doi.org/10.1007/978-3-030-35610-1_25

illuminate the importance of one's "coming out" process and how it may impact relationships within one's own generation, and across generations. Growing up as a sexual and/or gender minority person can influence the strengths and vulnerabilities one brings to parenting (Fredriksen-Goldsen et al., 2014).

For example, based on their own experiences of discrimination and stigma, LGBTQ parents may have a heightened level of anxiety around the safety and well-being of their children. This anxiety may impact their understanding of the needs and feelings of their children. A therapist may be in a unique position to help the parent to understand where there may be misattunement between the feelings and needs of the parent(s) and the child(ren) and help the family find a way to traverse those differences. The dynamics between parents and children in LGBTQ-parent families can be understood by developing an appreciation of how their lives and life courses are interwoven, and how the narrative of their experiences may converge and diverge (Settersten, 2015). A therapist can help parents to distinguish which issues are normative developmental struggles for parents and for children and what if any struggles may be particular to having parents who are sexual and/or gender minorities.

Considering the stress process framework along with the life course perspective can help the clinician to formulate each family member's vulnerabilities and the strengths, and those of the family as a whole. The stress process framework considers not only the stress that one experiences, but also the resources and support that are available to help mitigate stress. The sources and moderators of stress can influence the emotional, physical, and behavioral sequelae across the life course (Pearlin & Skaff, 1996). Although research has shown that stressful life events and repeated or chronic environmental challenges can impact individual vulnerability to illness, it has also revealed that having a sense of psychological well-being and living within a supportive environment can be protective (Fava & Sonino, 2007; Flier, Underhill, & McEwen, 1998; Ryff & Singer, 1996). LGBTQ people may face stressors including stigma, prejudice, and discrimination

due to both identity concealment and disclosure. Decisions about where, when, and with whom to share this aspect of one's identity can be possible sources of stress and distress at multiple points in one's life. The associated consequences of this process on mental health can differ based on gender, class, race, ethnicity, and religion (Meyer, 2003; Pachankis, Cochran, & Mays, 2015; Pearlin, Schieman, Fazio, & Meersman, 2005). Conditions in the sociocultural context in which one lives can compound personal experiences and can have long-term implications for the well-being of the individual (Meyer, 2003).

The stress that LGBTQ individuals experience due to being a member of a stigmatized minority group has been understood as a type of "minority stress." Minority stress theory posits that people from stigmatized social categories experience negative life events and additional stress due to their minority status (Meyer, 1995, 2003). Meyer (2003) further described four different minority stress processes applicable to LGBTQ adults: (a) experiences of prejudice; (b) expectations of rejection or discrimination; (c) hiding and concealing one's identity; and (d) internalized homophobia.

A secondary process that may be especially relevant to the experiences of LGBTQ-parent families is one of "microaggressions." Microaggressions are social or environmental, verbal and nonverbal, intentional and unintentional brief assaults on minority individuals (Balsam, Molina, Beadnell, Simoni, & Walters, 2011; Sue et al., 2007). These microaggressions can take the form of microassaults, microinsults, and microinvalidation (Balsam et al., 2011). Whether or not they are intended as an aggression, children may witness or experience these types of transgressions toward LGBTQ people as an assault on their parents, and secondarily on them. Experiences of microaggressions may occur in a variety of settings and be very confusing for children and adolescents. They may experience anxiety for the safety and well-being of their parents, and subsequently for themselves. Parents in turn may have their own anxiety concerning the safety and well-being of their children. This anxiety may be expressed by maintaining a kind of hypervigilance around the child's interactions with adults and peers at school and in the community, with the hope of protecting them. It may be difficult for family members to consciously identify these microaggressions and therefore impede the ability of the family to discuss the overt and covert stress it creates for the family system.

Linked lives is a perspective that connects both the theory of life course and the stress process. It recognizes the interaction and impact of an individual's life within one's family and across generations (Gilligan, Karraker, & Jasper, 2018). Thinking about becoming a parent may provoke anxiety as the individual faces the possibility that his or her children may experience rejection and discrimination solely based on the sexual orientation or gender identity of their parent(s). A study by Bos and van Balen (2008) revealed that one of the primary concerns of lesbians considering parenthood is the possibility of their child having negative experiences as a consequence of being raised in a nontraditional family, within a heterosexist and homophobic society. The children of LGBTQ parents have "membership by association" of a stigmatized minority group (Goldberg, 2007, p. 557).

Children who are born into a "different" family constellation may not feel "different," even though their parents are "different" from other parents. The children of LGBTQ parents do not necessarily experience the same minority group identity as their parents. Although children and adolescents may feel protective of the LGBTQ community and feel a part of this community by virtue of being a child with an LGBTQ parent, this aspect of their lives may or may not be pivotal to their identity (Goldberg, Kinkler, Richardson, & Downing, 2012). Parents may unwittingly overemphasize this aspect of their own identity to communicate their concerns about the discrimination their child may face. The constant reference to a parent's sexual orientation or gender identity may be confusing for the child, due to not understanding why it is an ongoing topic of conversation.

An ongoing dialogue between parents and children that is developmentally attuned is important to scaffold the child's experience of being raised in a "different" family structure, and to mitigate the homophobia and transphobia that may be misdirected toward them by peers based on their parents' sexual orientation or gender identity. Research on sexual minorities found that grade school and middle school years may be the hardest for children of LGBTQ parents (Goldberg, 2010; Ray & Gregory, 2001). Thus, therapists need to be aware of how children with LGBTQ parents may experience varying types of bias and harassment at different ages and developmental stages.

## Managing Stigma and Shame: As Children of LGBTQ Parents Grow Up

Children of LGBTQ parents often lack a peer group at school who share a similar family structure and with whom they can identify, and for that reason, they may feel different themselves. During grade school, it is not unusual for children to be exposed to the stigma directed toward people who are identified as LGBTQ. Children with parents who are sexual or gender minorities may be bullied due to the sexual orientation or gender identity of their parents, and they may experience comments and jokes as a personal affront, even when they are not directed specifically toward them or their families. Children of sexual and gender minority parents may not necessarily share these negative comments or experiences with their parents in order to protect their parents.

Goldberg (2007) found that children often develop an early awareness of homophobia and are aware of the impact of stigmatization and discrimination on individuals, families, and communities. In some cases, children are taught overtly or covertly either by their families, or from their experiences in school and with friends, or both, that it is not safe to talk openly to others about their family. Parents may conceal their sexual or gender identity in the community in which they are raising their children, or avoid certain social interactions altogether, in order to manage bias and stigma (Hines, 2006; Stein, Perrin, & Potter, 2004; Webster & Telingator, 2016). Bisexual adults are less likely to "come out" to family or their community compared to lesbian and gay identified adults due to unique social pressures and stigma (e.g., stereotypes and assumption about bisexuality; Pistella, Salvati, Ioverno, Laghi, & Baiocco, 2016). Depending on the community in which they are raised, children may need to closely monitor what they say to friends and other adults about their lives. They learn that their safety may be dependent on the need to "hide" aspects of their family. This need to maintain secrecy can impact children's capacity to form trusting relationships with peers and adults outside of the family where they can openly explore different parts of themselves and use these relationships to begin to separate from their parents. Living in secrecy also can fuel a stigmatized identity.

Both family and friends can be important sources of support to buffer the children's experience of heterosexism and gender discrimination. Based on her review of the literature, Goldberg (2010) concluded that both living in a community that was supportive, as well as having relationships with other children of LGBTQ parents, can help children of LGBTQ parents feel "less vulnerable and alone" (p. 161). Goldberg also concluded that open communication between parents and their children helps children of LGBTQ parents to cope effectively with heterosexism while they grow up.

The developmental tasks of adolescence may bring new challenges for the children of LGBTQ parents. Adolescents are often duly aware that their parents have been stigmatized for being a sexual and/or gender minority, and that their own sexuality and/or gender expression, or gender identity may reflect back on their parents. Based on societal prejudices, adolescent children of LGBQ parents may fear coming out as nonheterosexual themselves (Goldberg, 2010; Kuvalanka & Goldberg, 2009). Perlesz et al. (2006) found that due to societal, peer, and developmental pressures and their desire to appear "normal," adolescents with LGBTQ parents may remain more secretive with their peers about the nature of their family constellation. This secretiveness may cause them to isolate their parents from their social worlds. While some adolescents might try to "blend in," others cope by opening up about their family experience, choosing instead to confront and educate those around them, and at times even engaging in social activism. Yet another subset of children of LGBTQ parents show more detachment and less consciousness of such stigma and pressures (Kuvalanka, Leslie, & Radina, 2014).

LGBQ parents' own experiences of coming out may make them more sensitive to openly discussing issues around gender and sexuality with their children and more supportive of their children's questions about sexuality and gender (Kuvalanka & Goldberg, 2009). Gartrell and Bos (2010), in a longitudinal study of the children of lesbian parents, found that although parents may be open and accepting of their children exploring their sexuality, parents' anxiety and desire to protect their children from the stigmatization they had faced may complicate the messages they give their children about sexual orientation. Previous experiences of their own rejection, discrimination, and verbal/physical assaults due to their sexual and/or gender identity, as well as the intersection with other aspects of their identity and/or their child's identity, may heighten their fear for their child's safety and well-being if their children identify as LGBTQ.

As adults, children of LGBTQ parents show no differences from normative samples on a measure of adaptive, behavioral, and emotional functioning (Gartrell, Bos, & Koh, 2018). They describe themselves as being more tolerant and open minded as a direct consequence of being raised by parents who were sexual minorities, and who socialized their children to appreciate differences (Goldberg, 2007). Additionally, they often feel that a consequence of being in a home where the parent's sexual orientation was openly discussed allowed them to think more deeply about their own sexuality, and understand it more complexly (Goldberg, 2010). Further, as adolescents and adults, they often view themselves as more comfortable than children who were raised in heterosexual-parent homes to resist heteronormative expectations around gender and sexuality (Goldberg, 2007).

LGBTQ parents' desire to foresee struggles and protect their children from the stigma of having LGBTQ parents can be consuming at both conscious and unconscious levels. An awareness of the factors that have contributed to the resilience and vulnerability in the lives of both the parents and their children will help the therapist to contextualize the issues they face and consider how to approach the children and parents in a manner that takes into consideration their life course separately and together.

## Clinical Relevance of the Intersection of Parents' and Their Children's Life Course

To better understand LGBTQ-parent families, it is helpful to first understand the parents' history developmentally both in the context of their family of origin and throughout their life course. When taking a history, the clinician should include biological, social, and psychological vulnerabilities and strengths of each member of the family. The clinician should pay particular attention to the stress process over the life course both for the parents and the children. Stress endured by one individual may be unconsciously and subconsciously transmitted across and between generations (Leblanc, Frost, & Wight, 2015). This concept, which can be understood as stress proliferation, considers not only sociocultural and economic factors which may cause stress, but also the layers of stress one endures as being an ethnic, racial, sexual, and/or gender minority (Pearlin et al., 2005). Cultural differences and intersectionality of identity across, race, ethnicity, social class, religion, and community should be explored as they may impact stigma, stress, and resilience (Mink, Lindley, & Weinstein, 2014; Rosario, Scrimshaw, & Hunter, 2004). Vulnerabilities and supports that parents had at different developmental stages as well as supports that are currently available to the family impact not only the individual, but the family as a whole. Eliciting this information can help the

clinician to better understand family dynamics as well as symptoms that have brought the identified patient and their family to therapy. The clinician's understanding of the issues may be reformulated as one works with the family over time.

To better understand the children's experience, it is helpful to understand the developmental history of the parents, including the parents' experience of coming out, as well as their decision-making process around having children. Understanding the parent's life course in terms of the historical, social, and cultural context of each parent's path to self-identifying as an LGBTQ individual will help the therapist to appreciate the parent's own developmental experiences, and how these experiences may influence how they parent their children.

Therapists often work with parents who, starting at a young age, experienced emotional distancing from parents, peers, and their community due to being "different." Some LGBTQ individuals were raised in families and communities who were accepting of their sexual and gender identity. It is important to understand how ethnicity, race, religion, and/or class may also have informed the coming-out experiences of acceptance and rejection. Experiences of trauma, homophobia, and transphobia can occur across the life span. It is important to establish whether the parents currently are living in circumstances in which they feel safe. Individuals may have experienced rejection and discrimination in a multitude of ways, at each stage of their lives, starting in childhood. This may have included verbal and nonverbal communications of anger and disappointment and verbal and physical harassment from parents, peers, or other members of the community. Some may have internalized this stigma as a rejection of their core self, attempting to "cover" to keep stigmatized aspects of their identity from "looming large" (Goffman, 1963). This process of rejection may lead to a shame-based identity and result in the individual living with internalized homophobia and/or transphobia. Individuals will vary in how well they cope with this stress load, predisposing to psychological distress in some cases (Goldbach & Gibbs, 2017; Hatzenbuehler, 2009). This internalized sense of fear and shame also can have a long-term impact on individual self-esteem and may consciously or unconsciously influence one's parenting (Katz-Wise et al., 2017; Kaufman & Raphael, 1996). The following clinical vignettes highlight how the influence of the parents' life course and experiences of stress, specifically as a sexual and/or gender minority, can impact the lives of their children. The narrative of the parent(s) and child(ren) may include issues particular to LGBTQ families. These vignettes capture how the life course and stress process framework intersect across generations, influencing the resiliency and vulnerabilities of the children and their developmental trajectories.

## LGBTQ-Parent Families

### Clinical Vignette of a Child with Lesbian Parents: Melissa

Melissa is a 16-year-old Caucasian girl growing up in a city in Massachusetts. She is a little over five feet four inches, wearing her brown hair down to her shoulders. She takes pride in her appearance and her ability to connect with others. She loves sports and music and is a particularly gifted cross-country runner. She has many male and female friends and enjoys social activities as well as time spent alone. Her family is upper middle class and identifies as Caucasian. She volunteers for an organization that helps children who are living in poverty around the world, and she works for a community food bank once a month. She was referred to therapy due to concern about her sadness and a change in her behavior.

During the therapists' initial meeting with Melissa's parents, the following information was elicited. Melissa has two mothers, Denise and Jill. Her mothers are currently in their 40s. They first became a couple in their 20s and discussed their wish to have children early on. Their dream of having a child was complicated by Jill's diagnosis at age 23 of Lupus. She was aware that her medications would complicate a pregnancy. Because of this, Jill felt she would not feel safe

trying to conceive a child or carry a pregnancy. Denise wanted to carry a pregnancy and was medically healthy. When they were in their early 30s, they began to discuss having children more seriously and explored their options. They felt most comfortable with using a donor who would agree to be known when the child was 18, or to try to find a friend who would agree to donate sperm and be a known donor. Their desire to have their child know the person who donated sperm led them to consider the option of identifying a friend who would agree to be the donor.

Denise and Robert were in the field of technology and had become friends while working together. As Denise and Robert grew closer, she began to speak to him about her wish to have children. She told him of her ambivalence about using a sperm bank, and her wish to have her children know the identity of the sperm donor. Robert later spoke with Denise and told her that he and his partner Zack had discussed donating sperm to Jill and Denise to pursue this dream. Denise arranged a meeting for the four of them to discuss in greater detail this possible way of conceiving a child. One early discussion Jill and Denise had with Robert and Zack was to clarify who would be identified as parents. They all agreed that Denise and Jill would be the parents and that Robert and Zack would be involved in the child's life. Initially, the four of them did not deepen this discussion to include defined roles for Robert and Zack, exploring how the men's roles might be constructed by the child, or how they would be designated with regard to their name or role with the child. None of the adults knew exactly how this arrangement would take shape but agreed that they would work it out over time and that the child would know that Robert was the sperm donor and that all of them would spend time with the child, but the details of this arrangement were not considered at this early stage.

At the time of conception – early in 2001 – they all lived in a state that allowed for second parent adoption. Legally, in order for this to occur a known donor would need to agree to give up his parental rights to their child. Robert agreed to this stipulation. As a result, Jill would be allowed to be the second parent on the birth certificate, permitting her to have the legal rights of a second parent, ensuring that Jill and Denise would have full legal and physical custody. They agreed that Jill and Denise would make all financial, physical, and school-related decisions regarding the child. A lawyer was consulted and wrote a contract for the couples about this arrangement. No specifics were written into the contract about how much time the child would spend with Robert and Zack, but all agreed that the decision to conceive with a "known" donor was intended to give the child an opportunity to know Robert and to have a relationship with him and Zack.

The couple's daughter, Melissa, was born without complications. Although Robert had given up parental rights after Melissa's birth, both Denise and Jill became increasingly anxious that he would change his mind. If he did, it would mean that Jill would not be allowed to adopt Melissa and become her legal parent. While Denise and Jill had tried to anticipate issues their child might face in her life due to having lesbian parents, they had never considered that they would become fearful of their child being "taken away" by the men who helped to conceive her. They did not feel comfortable discussing this fear with Robert and Zack and began to pull away from them as the due date approached. When Melissa was born, all four of them were at the hospital, although only Jill was present during the delivery. Immediately after her birth, Robert and Zack spent some time with Melissa, but Jill asked them to leave so she and Denise could have time alone to "bond" with Melissa. Denise and Jill's fears had begun to create a barrier between Robert, Zack, and Melissa, which Melissa would experience as a small child, but not understand until much later.

Throughout grade school and middle school, Melissa's parents listened for any difficulties she might be having with peers or with teachers as a result of having two mothers. They tried to not overemphasize this difference, but they also wanted to allow Melissa to talk about struggles she might encounter for any reason, including having lesbian parents. Melissa did not share any experiences of rejection or discrimination that they could directly relate to having two mothers. Melissa had never experienced any bullying directed toward her or her family, but she was acutely aware of, and hurt by, the comments her peers made with regard to "gay" people.

Prior to entering high school, Melissa began to share less of her day-to-day experiences with her parents. Denise and Jill continued to be concerned, but they wanted to give her the space that she needed at this time in her life, while trusting that she would bring up any issues to them when they arose. Melissa did well socially and academically and was considered by her teachers as a leader. Her sensitivity and awareness of how other children were treated based on race, class, and disabilities were beyond what her teachers normally encountered in her age group.

Unbeknownst to her parents, going to high school was a difficult transition for Melissa. She began to allow herself to think about her own experience of her gender and sexuality. She identified as cisgendered. She recognized that she was attracted to both men and women and identified as bisexual, but she was not prepared to deal with her own conflicted feelings as she began to have intensified feelings toward a female friend. The conflict she felt centered around an unspoken pressure she felt to be a "normal" child of lesbian parents. Her loyalty to her parents and to the LGBTQ community fueled a desire to prove that children who were raised with gay or lesbian parents were just as healthy as children raised in heterosexual homes. Although she rejected the notion that there was any one healthy way to express herself in terms of gender or sexuality, she knew that society would define "healthy" as being heterosexual and gender conforming. Having been raised in a marginalized family, she had come to appreciate the spectrum of gender and sexuality that exists across and within individuals, and she felt that she did not yet know what all of this meant to her. As her freshman year progressed, Melissa had increasing difficulty focusing on her schoolwork, and her grades began to drop. She stopped bringing friends to her house and participating in afterschool activities. When her school counselor approached her to talk about her deteriorating grades, she began to open up about her struggles. Melissa agreed with the counselor that she should let her parents know as well, and the counselor helped them to identify a therapist.

The therapist initially met with Melissa, and then met separately with her mothers to get a family history. Melissa told the therapist that she had two mothers, and when the therapist asked what she knew about her conception, the family's story unfolded including Robert and Zack. She asked to meet with Melissa's mothers as well as with Zack and Robert separately as couples, and then all together over several sessions to get a history. The therapist wanted to hear both the individual and collective narratives about the process of the decision to have Melissa, and about the roles and relationships that each of them had had with Melissa since she was born.

Melissa liked this therapist because she asked about her family and made her comfortable speaking about Zack and Robert. She did not normally talk about them with her mothers, or with her friends. During the initial phase of therapy, Melissa primarily focused on her feelings toward her friend, and the difficulty she was having transitioning to high school. Feelings about her family were not addressed during this phase, since Melissa did not present them as being consciously related to her current struggle. Her therapist felt that it was important nevertheless to learn from Melissa about how she perceived her relationships with her mothers and Robert and Zack before presuming the significance each had in her life, or her relationship with each of them. The therapist believed that Melissa's symptoms would likely resolve with both individual and family therapy.

The therapist referred the family to a family therapist to work with Melissa's parents as well as Zack and Robert. Melissa's ongoing work in her individual psychotherapy helped her to understand that some of the disappointment she felt toward friends and family was related to her own difficulty expressing her own needs, for fear of not having them fulfilled. She also recognized her tendency to take care of others' needs while neglecting her own. She realized that the resulting feelings of isolation and loneliness had been

making her feel sad. She had been unable to allow herself to be intimate with others in a way that fulfilled her. As she explored these issues in therapy, she began to feel less sad and anxious and reengaged with her peers and school. As these immediate challenges were resolving, she tentatively began to express her disappointment in her family to her therapist. In the context of her therapy, she referred to her mothers as well as Robert and Zack as her family. To her, while her mothers were her parents, all four of them were a part of her family. She felt disappointed and angry when she thought about how her mothers, Zack, and Robert had not assisted her in figuring out these relationships earlier in life.

She was angry with her mothers at times but was primarily angry with Zack and Robert. She was not able to articulate what prompted this anger, but she was able to say that it was something that she wanted help to figure out. Thus, Melissa began a therapeutic process which lasted almost a year, during which she began to open up more about her feelings about growing up in her family. She felt very close to both of her mothers. She had always referred to Denise as "mommy," and Jill as "mama." Denise and Jill had chosen those names before Melissa was born, and since she was an infant, they had referred to each other as "mommy" and "mama." When friends or other adults asked her who her "real mother" was, Melissa felt intense anger and sadness. Both Denise and Jill were her "real mothers," and she felt this deeply. She could not understand the ignorance of others who felt that a biological connection made one of her mothers more real than the other.

Since she was young, Melissa had a sense that she needed to protect her mothers as she felt they were scrutinized for being lesbian, and thus was frustrated that her parents' concerns were often focused on her experience of having "gay" parents, as she often felt this was irrelevant in her day-to-day life. She sometimes felt annoyed by people who were overly curious and intrusive with regard to her family, as her peers with heterosexual parents were not asked such questions. For Melissa, her relationship with her parents was her main concern, not their sexual orientation. Her peers with the exception of her closest friends were not aware of Zack and Robert and the role in her life.

Melissa was eventually able to share her anger and sadness that the relationships between the significant adults in her life were constructed prior to her birth and there had not been any conversation within her family since that time to include her preferences in how these relationships would be managed going forward. She had spent much of her life confused about the expectations of how she related to each of her mothers, Robert and Zack, and continually feared stepping over some unspoken boundary. Her hopes that these family relationships would be spoken about were never realized. Therefore, she felt left alone to interpret what she was supposed to do and was so caught up in this that she never thought to explore what she *wanted* to do. She did not feel that her parents understood or asked what she wanted or needed from each of them, and that they had made assumptions about how much time she wanted to spend with whom. She had become frustrated with herself for letting her parents take the lead in defining her relationships. Through her work in therapy, Melissa began to recognize that she could allow herself to think about and articulate her wishes for her relationships with Denise, Jill, Robert, and Zack.

As a child, Melissa would spend several hours a couple of times a month with Robert and Zack. From an early age, she understood that they were important people to her family, but they were referred to not as her dads but as "Robert" and "Zack." The anxiety that Jill and Denise had felt leading up to her birth had never been articulated by anyone. As a child, Melissa could sense tension when all four of them were together but could not name it. As she got older and learned that Robert was her biological father, she began to understand Robert's and Zack's desire to spend time with her, but she still did not understand why her mothers seemed different when they were around. She loved her mothers, and also yearned to have more time with Robert and Zack. When she was around 7 or 8 years old she would fantasize that Robert and Denise would get married, and Zack and Jill would get married, and

they would all live together. As she got older this marriage fantasy waned, but her longing to be closer to Zack and Robert continued.

Melissa was angry that Zack and Robert were not more involved in her life, and they addressed her as "Melissa" instead of "my daughter." She referred to Robert and Zack by their proper names but this felt to her an uncomfortably distant and formal way to refer to them. She assumed that it must have been agreed that calling them anything other than Robert and Zack was not acceptable and was upset that she had never been asked what she wanted to call them. She often tried to imagine ways in which she could eliminate the awkwardness between her mothers and them, but she did not know how to accomplish this. When she was younger she made up reasons why they were not closer, and most of the fantasies included something that she had done to create this tension.

Now that she was older, Melissa understood that she was not fully responsible for the tension, but she still felt in part that it was her fault. She did not have any friends who had a family that closely approximated the complexity of her family and felt as a result that none of her friends could help her with this issue; in fact, she never talked about it with them. Over the course of therapy, Melissa began to express her sadness and anger about Robert and Zack's limited involvement in her life. Concurrent to Melissa's individual therapy, a family therapist was working with her and her family. Her mothers had agreed to work side by side with Robert and Zack to revisit their early history together. With Melissa's permission, her individual therapist worked closely with the family therapist to help guide family treatment.

In family therapy, Jill, Denise, Robert, and Zack expressed appreciation for the insight Melissa had given them into how the communication – or lack thereof – among the four of them had led to Melissa's misunderstandings and pain. Denise and Jill were able to tell Robert and Zack that although their wish was to use a known donor, they had not anticipated their fear that Robert and Zack would take Melissa away from them. They had realized that for each this dated to a time when they were young and believed that they would have to forsake having children if they were to live a life which was consistent with their sexual identity. As teens and in their 20s, most lesbian identified women were not having children outside the context of a heterosexual relationship. They realized that they harbored internalized homophobia from their youth, and this led them to fear that their child would be taken away from them. They had come to understand their own internalized homophobia and shame. They shared that these feelings had dissipated over the years as they became more comfortable with raising a child within the context of a lesbian-headed family and more secure in their relationship with Melissa. They realized that some of the anxiety that they felt about Robert and Zack was a projection of their early experiences, and their anxiety of not knowing who might cause them or their child harm. The therapist recognized that for Melissa, the very people who could have been helpful were the same ones whose fears may have led them to be hurtful.

Zack and Robert were able to speak to the family therapist about their deep sense of rejection and experience of anger and disappointment when her mothers sent them away after Melissa's birth. They felt an immediate familial connection to Melissa that they did not anticipate when they agreed to donate sperm. They had not anticipated how much they wanted to be parents. At the time, Melissa was conceived there were very few gay men who became parents outside the context of a heterosexual relationship. It was not something they had imagined as a possibility when they "came out." They did not realize that this was a role that they would cherish and want to expand, but felt constrained by what they had contractually agreed to and the early sense of rejection and distancing that they experienced with Jill and Denise. As Melissa got older and interacted with them, they wanted to spend more time with her alone to build their own relationships with her, but they were also afraid of being cut off from having any contact with Melissa if they requested to have more time with her. The therapist

interpreted that Melissa's feeling of rejection by them was a result of this unaddressed tension which became a barrier to a close relationship between them and Melissa.

A meeting was held with Melissa's therapist, Melissa, the family therapist, her mothers, and Robert and Zack. In this meeting, Melissa was able to tell Robert and Zack that she wanted them to spend more time with her. She also expressed her wish that she could use familial terms for them like "dad" and "daddy." Denise, Jill, Robert, and Zack were all responsive to this request. In a series of family meetings, the family therapist was able to help both couples and Melissa to understand the origin of some of the tensions that existed between the couples and help them to work together to renegotiate their relationships. Both couples were able to speak to their fears and wishes regarding Melissa, and this increased ability to openly communicate allowed them in a unified way to facilitate Melissa building relationships with Zack and Robert in a way that met her needs.

The work that Melissa, Denise, Jill, Robert, and Zack were able to do in individual and family therapy helped Melissa to articulate how her experience of her relationships in her family led to her sadness and anger that brought her to treatment, with her work in individual and family therapy helping her better understand this complex underlying dynamic. The family therapy allowed her to engage and reengage with her family in ways that felt more satisfying for her. Following this work, they terminated family therapy, but Melissa continued with individual therapy for a while. She was able to focus her individual therapy on working to separate from her parents, gain a better understanding of her own identity, and reengage with her peer group. Her mood further improved as did her grades. Over time, she terminated with her therapist with the understanding that she could return to do individual and family work at other points in her life when it might be useful to her and her family. Melissa's family had many of the qualities that are associated with better mental health outcomes in families regardless of the sexual orientation of the parent(s).

## Research Addressing Vulnerabilities and Resilience in LGBTQ Parents and Their Children

Golombok (2000) found that better mental health outcomes for children are associated with parents who have a close, positive, and meaningful connection with their children. Bos and Gartrell (2010) found that although homophobic stigmatization can have a negative impact on the psychological well-being of lesbian-mother families, being raised by "loving, nurturing, supportive parents can counteract these detrimental effects" (p. 569). This finding is consistent with earlier data that showed that warm and supportive relationships between parents and their children, as well as between children and their peers, may be protective for children, and may buffer them from the negative psychological consequences of real or perceived stigmatization (Bos & Van Balen, 2008; Frosch & Mangelsdorf, 2001; Golombok, 2000). A close and loving relationship with one's parents through adolescence continues to have a positive influence on children's well-being and psychosocial development (Udell, Sandfort, Reitz, Bos, & Dekovic, 2010). This is true for all families, regardless of the sexual orientation of the parent(s) (Lamb, 2012).

Bos and van Balen (2008) found that children with lesbian mothers who perceived higher levels of stigmatization for having lesbian parents had a lower sense of well-being. Girls who perceived high levels of stigma reported low self-esteem, and boys who perceived high levels of stigma were rated by their parents as being more hyperactive, which may have been a reflection of increased levels of anxiety. In both gay and lesbian parent families, parents' experience of stigma has been shown to result in higher levels of externalizing behaviors in their children, regardless of gender (Golombok et al., 2018). The negative effects of homophobic stigmatization on children's self-esteem and behavior have been shown to be counteracted by frequent contact with other offspring of same-sex parents, being in a school that teaches tolerance, and having mothers who perceive themselves as active members of the lesbian community (Bos & van

Balen, 2008). Yet it is also important to appreciate that undergoing stress can sometimes be a positive learning experience and lead to personal growth (Cox, Dewaele, van Houtte, & Vincke, 2010; Savin-Williams, 2008).

An ongoing dialogue between parents and children that is developmentally attuned is important both to scaffold the child's experience of being raised in a "different" family structure than many of their peers and to mitigate the homophobia that may be misdirected toward them.

based on their parents' sexual orientation. As with Melissa, this dialogue includes a narrative of their birth as well as an ongoing relevant narrative about their family constellation.

While most early research has focused on the psychosocial well-being of the children of lesbian mothers, some recent research has been dedicated to the relationships of gay fathers with their children. Gay men become fathers in a multitude of ways (Tornello & Patterson, 2015). Some gay men have children through previous heterosexual relationships. More recently, assistive reproductive technology, such as in vitro fertilization and/or surrogacy, has been options for gay men to become parents (Norton, Hudson, & Culley, 2013; see chapter "Gay Men and Surrogacy"). Some gay men have become fathers through adoption or fostering children, while others have chosen a family constellation in which they co-parent children with another person or couple. In some cases, they have a biological connection and shared parenting with a single woman or couple (Erera & Segal-Engelchin, 2014).

The path to parenthood for some gay men has included confronting internalized and external stigmatized representations of gay men as childless, pedophiles, or wanting to bring up children who themselves will become a sexual minority. This may result in a reluctance to have children due to internalized shame and stigma. (Goldberg, Downing, & Moyer, 2012). There are also legal and financial barriers for gay men to conceive children (Biblarz & Savci, 2010). It is not known whether such barriers to fatherhood might unconsciously affect parenting by gay men. However, various aspects of gay male fathers' parenting have been studied and suggest that gay male parent households tend toward egalitarian division of labor between the parents, and positive styles of parenting, in a similar manner to lesbian parent-headed households (Biblarz & Savci, 2010; Golombok et al., 2014).

Currently, there is little research on the experience of children who grow up with gay male fathers. The current literature primarily focuses on research involving children of gay adoptive fathers. Golombok et al. (2014) showed that children of gay male adoptive fathers are generally well adjusted, similar to those of lesbian adoptive mothers, and better adjusted than children of heterosexual families. Prospective, longitudinal data confirm that the adopted children of gay fathers have similar psychosocial outcomes as of the adopted children of lesbian and heterosexual parents (Farr, 2017). One recent study by Tornello and Patterson (2018) reported that of adult children of gay fathers, most (93.8%) conceived in this context showed normative rates of depression in adulthood. Predictors of better functioning in the adult children of gay fathers included disclosure by the father of his sexuality when the child was younger as well as ongoing feelings of closeness with their father into adulthood (Tornello & Patterson, 2018).

Research on children who were born to gay fathers through surrogacy is beginning to emerge. Surrogacy is very expensive and therefore the men who have access to surrogacy are often limited to those who are of high SES (see chapter "Gay Men and Surrogacy"). The surrogacy process involves not only high cost, but also, due to the complexity of the process, a strong desire and intent. Bergman, Rubio, Green, and Padrón (2010) found a strong increase in self-esteem in these men compared to gay men who were not parents, which appeared to be due to their sense of pride in being parents, and an increased sense of meaning and validation due to having had children. While preliminary research suggests that most children born to gay fathers through assistive reproductive technology will be told about their surrogate and possibly have some kind of relationship with her in childhood or adolescence, the psychological space for surrogates

within these family systems remains poorly understood (Blake et al., 2016; Carone et al., 2018).

## Transgender and Gender Queer Parent Families

### Clinical Vignette of a Child with a Transgender Parent: Isaiah

Isaiah is a 13-year-old African-American boy growing up in the St. Louis metropolitan area, living with his mother, father, and maternal grandmother. The family resides in a home in an area of town with a high proportion of African-American families. The family considers themselves middle class, though SES technically would fall in the lower-middle class spectrum. Isaiah is the only child in the family. He is very active in sports, including baseball, soccer, and cross-country running. He is also described as a "sensitive" boy very attuned to the needs of others, and in his maternal grandmother's words as having "a very big heart." His maternal grandmother, Cynthia, is a very significant and supportive member of his family. He is typically an average student, with regard to grades. Isaiah's homeroom teacher asked to meet with his parents due to her concern that he was being disrespectful with some of his teachers, withdrawing from other students and friends, and that his grades were deteriorating. Before meeting with his teacher, his parents had begun to wonder why he did not want to sign up for sports and why he was becoming more isolated, spending more time at home. After they met with his teacher, they felt that they needed help to understand what was going on with him. They asked their pediatrician for her input, and feeling that Isaiah was sad and anxious, she referred them to a therapist.

Isaiah's parents, Tina and Byron, met with the therapist before he met with Isaiah in order to share their concerns. The parents shared their narrative that they met in their 20s and had married several years before Isaiah was born. About a year into their relationship, Tina moved from her rural hometown to St. Louis to live with Byron. In both locales, the couple dealt with what they considered racially based harassment and decided that they wanted to move to a predominantly Black neighborhood in the city. In spite of this, they found that their family and neighbors felt ongoing pressure related to racial tensions in the city. They predominantly associated themselves with other Black families, and attended a traditional and predominantly Black church in which Byron was raised. Though they described trying to "lie low," they also developed an underlying sense of mistrust of the majority White population of the city, a sentiment that was shared among most of their peers. After marrying they briefly considered having children and, both knowing that they wanted to do so, had no difficulty conceiving Isaiah. Tina's pregnancy was complicated by depression, which she had dealt with intermittently during her life. She was treated for her depression and received mental health support from her obstetrician throughout the pregnancy. During Isaiah's early life, Tina stayed home to care for him and Byron continued to work, which often took him out of the home for days at a time. Despite this, Byron was very involved in Isaiah's life and fostered his early love of sports. Through sports the family became well connected with other families with young children in the area. When Isaiah turned eight, Tina's father died of cardiovascular disease, and Tina's mother Cynthia moved in with them. She became very involved in Isaiah's day-to-day activities and they developed a very close bond. Cynthia helped with parenting responsibilities, which allowed Tina to go back to work and help with the family finances.

At the initial visit, Byron and Tina shared with the therapist that Tina had recently disclosed a long-standing transgender identity with both Byron and Cynthia. Tina has held a consistent male gender identity since a very early age. Tina recalled that she had hoped that her relationship with Byron would "fix" her, describing how at the time she had internalized negative stereotypes in society at large which led her to believe that her experience of gender was unnatural and pathological. Tina clarified that she prefers romantic

and sexual relationships with males and felt at the time that developing this committed relationship with a male would make her feel "more like a woman." Nevertheless, the painful discrepancy between her internal gender identity and her identity in her relationship persisted. Her distress was heightened about her gender incongruence during her pregnancy. After the pregnancy, she knew that "at some point" she would come out as transgender, but worried about the timing of this and the impact it would have on her partner and their then-baby boy.

Byron recalled that Tina seemed down during the pregnancy, and when he asked Tina if she was sad Tina was dismissive of his concerns. This moroseness seemed to lift once Isaiah was born, though in retrospect Byron felt that he could sense some distraction or preoccupation in his partner. Tina recalled acting like a typical "mom" during Isaiah's infancy and early childhood. She and Isaiah were very visible in the community together, as mother and son.

Byron and Tina described parenting well together and feeling that parenting decisions were made equally and without significant disagreements. She had referred to herself as mom, but as he began to talk and refer to her as "mama" or "mommy," she recalled feeling disappointed. As she spoke about it with the therapist, she realized that she had held the fantasy that Isaiah would see who "she" was and naturally think and speak of her in masculine terms. Tina did not identify any one factor having led her to disclose her identity when she did, or how long it took her to get to the point of disclosure. She described it as a nonlinear process. She described the lingering psychological cost of hiding her identity, including the angst she felt with body changes that happened during her pregnancy, the hidden disappointment of having her son growing up not knowing who she really is, and feeling that she was keeping a secret from her partner. Counterbalancing this was a deep fear of abandonment by Byron, her family of origin, their community, and their church, becoming an "outcast," and losing her son.

As she had in other times of major life transitions, Tina at this time sought the counsel of their church's minister privately. While the pastor made it clear that their congregation would continue to accept all members of the family, he also discussed Tina's desire for gender transition as "a temptation" and suggested to Tina that the appropriate response would be to resist the desire to transition. Over the ensuing years, Tina described striving to become less visible, though not consciously. She began to develop a sense of "not being comfortable" with a vague sense of agoraphobia in certain settings, primarily at their church or around other families that she knew were more conservative with respect to LGBTQ issues.

Given her close relationship with Isaiah, Tina worried that he would pick up on her struggles and difficulty presenting as a female, so she took on more work outside the home and shifted more parenting responsibilities and caregiving of Isaiah to her mother. This, she felt, distanced her from Isaiah to some degree, as Cynthia came more and more to be regarded as Isaiah's caregiver. Cynthia attended more of his sporting events, school conferences, medical appointments, and church events. As she had started working more outside the home, Tina identified which of her coworkers seemed more accepting of LGBTQ people and eventually confided in one of them, Jason, about her situation. This experience was positive, and Jason remains one of Tina's best friends. Over time, Tina shared with Jason the internal conflict with which she was struggling, how to come out to her family and start a more public social transition. Jason continually encouraged her to live in a more authentic way. Tina considered this support essential to her eventual decision to come out to her family. Tina was experiencing the loneliness of not being authentic in relationships, and with the loss of the intimacy that she once shared with Isaiah. She began to wonder if some of the recent changes in his demeanor had to do with her withdrawal and distancing from the family. Given his sensitivity, Tina also thought he was aware that she was distressed but did not know the reason for this. She had noticed Isaiah making comments intermittently that he felt that Tina seemed to be working a lot and not seeking out family time in a way that

she once did, and he had mentioned once that when they were together she always seemed to be preoccupied.

The struggles that Tina had been enduring were shared with distress and anxiety in her narrative during this initial interview. Tina had recently disclosed her identity to her mother and husband, but had not told anyone else other than Jason, and had not yet started the process of publicly transitioning from female to male. The therapist realized he had not initially inquired about pronouns for either Tina or Byron, but as Tina began to speak, he apologized to both and inquired how he should address them in terms of name and pronouns. Tina stated that currently she wanted to use feminine pronouns and Tina. Byron stated that he wanted to use male pronouns and his given name. Tina and Byron had had several conversations since her initial disclosure to him about her gender identity, and Byron's experienced sense of disbelief about the situation. He stated that he was overwhelmed, and that he was "still trying to get his head around it." Through further discussion, the therapist found that Byron came from a very conservative, African-American family, in which he had been brought up with very rigid constructs of masculinity and femininity and developed a very low tolerance to gender nonconformity. Part of his disbelief stemmed from his not having been able to identify Tina's gender nonconformity prior to the disclosure, which he recognized stemmed largely from her efforts to hide this from everyone, including him. He was unsure whether he would have married Tina had he known about her transgender identity. He also admitted to a significant sense of betrayal that Tina had kept this significant aspect of her identity secret from him throughout their life together.

The therapist stated that since this was an evolving family issue, he wondered if it would be helpful to include Tina's mother in the evaluation prior to meeting with Isaiah, having been made aware of Cynthia's importance in the family system. With consent from both Tina and Byron, Cynthia joined the discussion at this point. Cynthia discussed the difficulty she was experiencing changing her perception of Tina's gender as being different than her natal sex. She repeated emphatically that she loved Tina and wanted her to be happy, so that she would support whatever changes she needed to make to be who she is. Cynthia and Byron both asked Tina when she thought that she would want to share her identity with others within the family. Tina felt she could not move forward in her life, or share anything with anyone else, until she felt that Isaiah was told and felt supported.

The therapist met with Isaiah prior to this family disclosure. At the initial visit, he used the time to establish a relationship with Isaiah and hear about his concerns. Over the next few weeks of therapy, Isaiah felt safe enough with his new therapist to describe his experience of feeling alone in the family. He felt that over the past 6 months that all the adults had been more preoccupied and were not attentive to him. He did not feel like his friends liked him, and he did not have much energy. He said that he did not want to do sports because it was not fun for him anymore. As he spoke about his own experience over the past 6 months, it appeared that he was aware of stress within the family but did not understand it.

After several meetings, the therapist decided to have Tina speak to Isaiah with both Byron and Cynthia present. They agreed that they would be honest with him and respond to all questions to the best of their ability. The therapist guided Tina's parents and grandmother in developmentally appropriate language to use regarding gender and social transition, for the purposes of the first discussion with Isaiah. The therapist anticipated that the disclosure would be met with confusion, fear, and grief from Isaiah, and prepared the family members to support Isaiah through these feelings as they emerged, both in the office and once they returned home. The therapist told Isaiah that he had been speaking with his parents and grandmother. Tina then shared with him that she thought that some of his recent behavior and mood change might be related to the tension in their home right now, and that she was sorry that she had not initially felt comfortable telling him about the source of that stress. She went on to share with him about her transgender identity and desire to transition socially to a male gender

identity. Primarily, the family wanted him to know about Tina's gender transition and did not want him to feel alone or responsible for this change. Each family member shared their love for Isaiah and made very clear that this would always continue regardless of stress within the family.

The following few sessions included Isaiah and Tina, as the therapist decided that it was important to work through feelings between them that had surrounded the disclosure, particularly the inherent dishonesty in hiding one's gender identity for so long from one's child. The therapist opened this discussion initially by having Tina share some of her history with her son. Tina told Isaiah that she had realized that something was different about her early in childhood but did not identify what it was until later in life. She shared that she thought that having grown up in a very conservative, rural community had led her to hide away this aspect of herself for so long, but that eventually she had become less and less comfortable living as a woman. Through his initial individual sessions with the therapist, Isaiah had learned that this was a safe arena in which to air his emotions. Isaiah was initially angry. He was indeed angry that his mom had not shared this with him earlier in his life. Tina was able to tolerate this anger from her son, and able to reflect that she had postponed disclosure partly out of fear that it would harm him somehow. What further emerged was that Isaiah was very fretful. His primary worries were related to the family breaking up, as well as how others might perceive his "mom" or their family and his feeling a duty to protect her. He asked her many questions about what physical transition would look like, and how this might change his relationship with his mother, and what he would call her, fearing that she would "shave her head and show up to school one day as his 'dad' instead of his 'mom.'" He did not share with Tina and the therapist at the time any worries he might have had about his own well-being. After Tina reassured him that the gender transition would be gradual and would take his well-being fully into account, Isaiah seemed less preoccupied in the weeks that followed.

Once Isaiah and Tina were able to communicate about some of his initial feelings regarding her disclosure to him, individual sessions with Isaiah resumed. Isaiah related to the therapist privately that he remained somewhat distressed about the conversation he had had with his mother about her social and medical gender transition. He was glad that she had shared this with him but continued to be upset that she had kept this secret from him for so long. His fears continued to emerge, related to several areas including fear of embarrassment and shame in how others might treat his mother and him because of the gender transition, fear of problems developing between his parents and that they might divorce, and fear of how he was going to disclose and manage this change in his family among his friends who already had known his family. He worried that his family was now altered, "broken," and "was going to fall apart."

What followed was a period of intensifying emotions that Isaiah shared with his therapist, though he was notably reflective about the context of these emotions. During one session, Isaiah shared that he had overheard a cousin making a negative comment about his mother, after having learned about her gender transition. Isaiah recalls getting very angry. Although never having been physically aggressive, Isaiah thought about hitting his cousin. Before he could respond, another cousin said to the overtly hostile cousin: "Be nice to him. He can't help who his parents are." Isaiah said that his anger then shifted into shame and embarrassment. He ran home, in tears. He did not share the experience with any of his immediate family members because he worried this would upset them or cause problems within the family. Instead, he decided to keep it to himself. However, the memory would come up whenever there were extended family gatherings, which were frequent within this family, causing Isaiah to feel increasingly out of place.

This experience reinforced in him the idea that his immediate family was "different" and troubled, and he also became very uncertain of who did and did not know about "the secret." When school resumed several weeks later, he found himself trying to distance himself, by making

jokes and teasing anyone that could be construed as "gay" or gender nonconforming. As time had gone on, he shared with his therapist that he had privately found himself begrudging his mother for "having ruined his life." Isaiah's therapist interpreted Isaiah's struggles through the lens of internalized transphobia and hiding and investigated the degree to which Isaiah was sharing his feelings with his family, and thereby gaining their support. As it turned out, Isaiah was uncomfortable sharing his angst with his immediate family because he thought his discomfort might cause further rifts within his family, which he continued to see as fragile, or cause harm to his mother who would think that it was her fault. In further discussion, Isaiah reported that at home no one had been talking about Tina's gender identity or transition, which had contributed to his notion that these were "secrets."

Based on these systemic factors, the family was referred to a skilled family therapist experienced in working with transgender individuals and their families, while Isaiah continued to work with his individual therapist as well. The family therapist spoke with the family and realized the family's desire to avoid the issue of the gender transition that had been openly discussed previously, and felt that she could be the most helpful initially by educating Isaiah and the rest of the family about what to anticipate with the social and medical aspects of Tina's transition. Over time, the family worked together in therapy on understanding the transitioning parenting roles, the parents' relationship with each other, the role of the grandmother in the household, and how Isaiah's dyadic relationship with each of them would persist, albeit with shifts in term of his mother's gender identity. Tina would remain Tina and his parent, as there was more to her than her gender. This was comforting to Isaiah.

Specific attention was paid to how the family had been able to come together when faced with external stress as related to racial issues and Tina's gender minority status. Isaiah tended to step in and protect his parents and this role was even more pronounced due to a development of distance between Tina and Byron since the initial disclosure. Guided by their family therapist, Tina and Isaiah were eventually able to speak about specific instances of stigma and shame related to transitioning, seeking support from each other instead of keeping secrets out of fear of harming one another. Isaiah was able to become more open with his family members about worries he had regarding Tina's upcoming transition instead of keeping them secret.

As time went on, at the suggestion of their family therapist, Tina entered individual therapy. Eventually, Tina took on the name Teondre and requested the use of male pronouns. He subsequently starting testosterone therapy through an area gender clinic. The family came up with a transitional, androgynous nickname "T" by which Tina/Teondre was known publicly. Their hope was that this would be a small step to help members of their community to adjust to Teondre's new identity. The family therapist helped the family plan and role-play meetings between the adults in the family and stakeholders in the community, which helped the family to be more comfortable sharing Teondre's transition more broadly. Through the process of them coming out as a family with a transgender parent, they faced a spectrum of acceptance and rejection. They were able to rely on each other for support and make decisions together about how to modify their community involvement.

Over the course of a year of ongoing individual therapy with his own therapist, Teondre was able to manage his own personal angst related to his gender transition and confront the fact that the relationship with Byron had changed long ago. Their relationship had remained amicable though it shifted from one of intimate partners to one of close friends. They began arguing over Byron's suggestion that Teondre's personality was changing through the course of the social and medical transition. Teondre, on the other hand, felt that Byron had become uncomfortable with his "outness" when his transgender identity became harder to hide as his body features became more masculinized with hormone treatment. Unfortunately, Teondre and Byron were unable to reconcile these changes in their relationship, and they eventually separated and divorced, sharing custody of Isaiah and maintaining a co-parenting relationship with each other. Family therapy ceased at this point, though both Teondre and Isaiah remained in individual therapy. Isaiah continued to describe his relationships with both Teondre and Byron as close despite the separation and divorce.

Throughout this period, Isaiah had been continuing his own individual therapy sessions. He was able to discuss with his therapist the angst he experienced throughout Teondre's social and physical transformation into a male. He struggled through the changes in superficial matters such as relational terms for Teondre, and also deeper matters such as perceived loss of his nurturing mother, mitigated for him by his grandmother's presence. Isaiah came to appreciate the degree to which his family was open with him about the entire process of Teondre's gender transition, guided at that point by their family therapist. He was relieved that Teondre's behavior and appearance did not change as immediately and drastically as he had initially envisioned, instead occurring gradually over time, which gave him time to adjust. Similarly, Isaiah was appreciative of his parents' communication with him regarding changes in their relationship and ultimate divorce. He told his therapist that he had been able to identify the shift in his parents' relationship before they divorced but was not as bothered by it as he thought he would be. After his parents separated, both remained very involved in his life, and he spent equal time with each parent. He continued to refer to Byron as "dad" and Teondre as "T," which did not bother Teondre. Eventually, Isaiah came to refer to Teondre as "papi," which he says is a name one of his friends has for his father, which he found to be a more endearing term that he thought better represented his close relationship with Teondre.

Isaiah's peer group shifted at school, at least partly related to his papi's transition, though he never found himself lacking friends. Outside of school, Isaiah was very involved in their church. During the family's coming-out process they had started attending a church that was fully inclusive of its LGBTQ members, affirming them in its doctrines, as well as allowing them into positions of leadership within the church family. Isaiah attended church, though he did not consider himself particularly religious at this time; he considered himself "a Christian" and found meaningful his church's message of "serving others and freedom and forgiveness." He considered that he might think further about bigger questions regarding faith and spirituality in the future. He gradually became less involved with sports and more involved with altruistic endeavors, such as working with his church, feeding the homeless in their community, and immigrant and refugee family outreach in the area, many of whom had been displaced by war in their home countries. Isaiah remained in therapy until he, his therapist, and his parents felt that he had made sufficient progress such that he was able to manage ongoing events without changes in his mood and behavior.

Isaiah felt that through the process of his papi's transition he had been able to learn to communicate his feelings, which he had never really been faced with having to do before. He also noted that he developed a new appreciation for "the big picture" and found meaning in helping those in need. Isaiah realized that he came not from a "broken" family but a "special" family. Isaiah had grown thinking a lot about issues of identity and, at the time his treatment ended, he identified as a cisgender, heterosexual, Christian, African-American male. He used the pronouns he/him/his. His earlier anxious despair was well resolved. He left therapy as he transitioned to college. Isaiah, as other children of transgender-parent families, has had the opportunity to explore new avenues of resilience as he works through the meaning of his loved one's transition (Dierckx, Mortelmans, Motmans, & T'Sjoen, 2017).

## Research Addressing Vulnerabilities and Resilience in Gender Queer Parents and Their Children

In 2015, an estimated 18% of transgender people were parents according to the U.S. Transgender Survey, a comprehensive survey of over 27,000 trans people (James et al., 2016). Research that specifically explores the experiences of children of transgender parents lags behind such research on children of sexual minority parents. Early research questions addressed the popular concern at the time that having a transgender parent may confuse a child's own gender identity development or lead to major psychiatric problems, although neither hypothesis has been supported by the literature (Freedman, Tasker, & Di Ceglie, 2002). Further research clearly has been needed to understand the strengths and vulnerabilities of families that include a transgender parent.

Parental gender transition is often an emotional and central event in a family's narrative. Many gender diverse people disclose and transition to their gender identity while seeking to maintain their station within their local community, such as their occupation, family structure, and peer group (Hines, 2006). Transgender parents have tended to manage such disclosure and transition with primary importance given to their children's well-being, and to minimize the conflict that can arise with their partner due to shifting parental gender roles and partnering dynamics (Haines et al., 2014). After disclosure, families must find a way to manage stigma in their interface with their community, as well as changes in the relationships in the family. In the period following disclosure, children may feel deceived by their parent/s, confused about gender identity and sexual orientation, or afraid of abandonment by the family (Haines et al., 2014). A recent study engaged in extensive qualitative interviews with transgender parents, their co-parents, and their children (Dierckx et al., 2017). Themes were identified that seemed to influence the psychological adjustment of the family's children: these included the family's communication, continuity or breakup of the family, acceptance of the co-parent, and meaning attributed to the transgender parent's transition. The children in these families tended to look to the non-trans co-parent to learn how to respond to trans parent's transition, while co-parents faced a conflict between being supportive to their partner and trying to minimize the impact of the transition on the children (Dierckx et al., 2017). In two-parent homes in which one parent is transitioning, the relationship between the parents may tend to shift from intimacy to friendship, and may ultimately lead to parental separation (Hines, 2006). Some children may have the temperament, resilience, and other factors that help them to openly discuss these complicated matters, while others may not. These were themes at play in Isaiah's therapeutic process of coming to terms with his transgender father's coming-out process.

A child's adjustment may differ significantly from both parents, other family members, friends, and trusted members of their community. The child must navigate changes which often include physical changes in the parent, changing pronouns and names, and also how the child understands roles and other aspects of their relationship with the transitioning parent. Tabor (2019) conceptualized this challenge that children face as "role-relational ambiguity." Children might struggle due to their own experiences with the parent and preconceived notions of sexuality and gender which have been internalized. The transitioning parent often maintains similar roles in the child's life even as the gender changes (Tabor, 2019). The restructuring and redefining of relationships impacts the entire family and therefore requires support for all members of the family. One recent survey (von Doussa, Power, & Riggs, 2017) found that transgender parents were often concerned about the potential disruption of their transition on family functioning (see chapter "Transgender-Parent Families"). Many of those parents surveyed reported that health services were ill equipped to assist their families to communicate with each other regarding the gender transition. Additionally, transgender parents may have a number of legal questions related to their parenthood, for example, the impact of their transition on legal parenthood and child custody (Stotzer, Herman, & Hasenbush, 2014). This may be compounded by little to no support by family of origin and their community, putting them in a place of legal uncertainty if their status were to be challenged (Pfeffer, 2012). Riggs, Power, and Von Doussa (2016) suggest that support, or lack of support, from the family of origin impacts the self-esteem and emotional well-being of transgender and gender diverse parents. This vulnera-

bility and stress experienced by the parents is likely to impact the children, as understood by "linked lives" theory (Gilligan et al., 2018).

Children tend to be protective of their parents – in essence, they are protecting themselves by keeping the family together. In her work with transgender-parent families, Hines (2006) noted: "Reciprocal caring between parent and child, however, may mean that the child cares for the parent by not revealing the full extent of what is happening in his or her emotional life" (p. 365). A therapist may need to assess how well the child understands his parents' situation, and the resulting distress at the child's particular stage of development, and help the parents anticipate other issues which may arise at other stages of development. Depending on the age and psychological awareness of the child, s/he may not have the language to communicate complicated feelings about their parent and family's situation, even if s/he has an awareness of the situation itself, as powerfully captured in Isaiah's story.

## Core Considerations for Therapy

The vignettes and theoretical considerations in this chapter serve to inform therapeutic work with the children of LGBTQ parents. The therapist should stay mindful of the fact that the definition of relationships in LGBTQ-parent families may not begin to capture the real or fantasized meaning of these relationships for the child or for the parent(s). Over time, the therapist should inquire about how the child thinks about these varying relationships, as well as the meaning of each of them to the child (Corbett, 2001). Whether the child is adopted or born with known or unknown donors and/or a surrogate or gestational carrier into an LGBTQ family, the child's fantasies and yearnings about these people with whom they have biological and nonbiological ties may evolve and impact their relationships with those closest to them (Ehrensaft, 2008a, 2008b; see chapter "Gay Men and Surrogacy"; see chapter "LGBTQ Adoptive Parents and Their Children"). It is not a reflection of the love the children have for the parents who are raising them, or their loyalty and devotion to them, but is rather a desire to know more about the people with whom they have biological ties. This desire will be different for each child and each family, but the clinician's awareness of this dynamic is important.

If transparency and the permission to talk about their biological origins do not exist between children and their parents, children may suppress their curiosity and desire to know more about these people. Foreclosing on the possibility of exploring this part of their heritage may impact both the child and the parents. In his description of a clinical case where this issue was relevant, Corbett (2001) wrote:

> As opposed to their (parents') fears that their (child's) fantasies would prove overstimulating or separate them as a family, they were able to entertain the opposite—the possibility of minds opening onto and into their collective fantasies in such a way as to bring them together in a family. (p. 610)

Helping the child speak to questions and feelings that emerge at different developmental stages about their biological origins can help the child to traverse normal developmental challenges without closing off access to real or imagined relationships. The ability of the family to openly discuss these complicated relationships may be helpful in the child's process of identity development (Ehrensaft, 2008a, 2008b).

## The Therapist's Office and Therapeutic Space

Creating a safe therapeutic space by developing trust through curiosity and validation can support both the parent(s) and the child(ren) in developing comfort in sharing both their individual narrative and the narrative of the family. As demonstrated in both case vignettes, each therapist started by developing rapport with the child and investigating their own understanding of their situation, irrespective of the additional information they had obtained from the family and their own preconception of what might lie beneath the patient's angst. Each voice is

important to understand how an individual's experience may be similar to and different from that of the other. The historical experiences of the parents, as well as the current experiences of the parents and the children in the community in which they live, should be considered during the course of evaluation and treatment.

## Helping Families Manage Stigma and Anxiety

The impact of parents' internalized homophobia, transphobia, stigma, shame, heterosexism, and microaggressions before, during, and after their coming out as LGBTQ individuals may have implications for their parenting style. The children's experiences of microaggressions, and overt and subtle experiences of homophobia, transphobia, and stigmatization at each developmental stage, may have implications for their ability to negotiate relationships inside the family with relationships outside of the family. The therapist should inquire about such experiences and offer support and psychoeducation. The therapist can help to separate out the parent's feelings and experiences from those of the child, and model for the parents how to discuss difficult issues with their children in a developmentally appropriate manner. If parents can manage their own anxiety, children are likely to feel more secure. They will be more likely to sense that their parents are willing and able to discuss experiences they are having both in the home and outside the home. This was demonstrated in the joint sessions between Isaiah and Tina/Teondre and Melissa with her mothers and Zack and Robert. By extension, if parents have difficulty with managing this anxiety, it may result in the children being more fearful and feeling that it is not permissible to discuss their worries with their parents or with others. They may internalize the anxiety as being a communication of something negative about themselves, and as they get older it may result in feelings of shame and stigma similar to their parents and may impact the child's self-esteem (Fisher, Wallace, & Fenton, 2000), as captured in Melissa's case.

## Holding Secrets

Holding secrets may cause children to become isolated and experience shame rather than integrate a positive sense of self and the capacity to be fully integrated. Although parents may feel that discussing issues of homophobia, transphobia, and heterosexism that the child may face may not be in the child's best interest, the opposite may be true. Corbett (2001) wrote about the treatment of the son of a lesbian couple:

> We (therapist and parents) worked toward the understanding that, while we wish to protect our children from pain, anxiety, and hate, we are in fact helpless to stop those feelings from entering into our child's lives, and furthermore a life without pain and loss would be an impossibly distorted one. (p. 607)

## Helping Families to Identify Stigma and Support and to Find Strength

LGBTQ parents may have experienced "hate" directed toward them or their community. They may now need to help their children to live in a world where they may experience hate directed toward their parents and may themselves experience discrimination. It is important to gain an understanding of the community in which the family resides and appreciate the stressors the family faces. The therapist should identify individual relationships and places where the family members can talk freely about their lives and their family, and in what environments they feel that they must maintain secrecy due to fears for themselves and their family (Telingator & Patterson, 2008). An appreciation of how and where each member of the family has found support and experienced stigma is essential. An understanding of cultural, religious, ethnic, racial, and class issues for each individual member of a family is critical.

Many factors impact the health and well-being of children other than the family structure. It is important to note that family diversity extends far beyond identifying the gender (often in the literature limited to gender binaries) of the parents. Cenegy, Denney, and Kimbro (2018) note that children of same-sex couple families are "more

often racial minorities, their households socio-economically disadvantaged, and their parents are in worse health, and they are more likely to have experienced a divorce or separation when compared with children in different-sex married couple families" (p. 213). Parks, Hughes, and Matthews (2004) highlight the fact that racial and ethnic minority groups learn the norms and values of both majority and minority cultures. As children born into a racial and/or ethnic minority status, their initial experience of being a minority is often supported by family and community and with open dialogues about having a stigmatized status. Thus, their early experiences of negotiating a stigmatized identity with family and community support may help to mitigate impact of the stigma, and they may find a source of strength from this shared identity from their families and communities. This may contrast with the isolation that an LGBTQ individual may experience at whatever developmental stage they begin to understand their sexual and/or gender minority status. Although there may be a shared racial/ethnic background, the sexual identity and/or gender identity may vary vastly from familial expectations. Racial and ethnic LGBTQ minorities deal with a double minority status and the bias and stigma that may be associated with these dual minority identities.

In the case of Melissa, she was born into a Caucasian family with privilege, who were able to choose the school and community in which she was raised. Melissa was both comfortable with her parents' sexuality and was living in a community in which it was safe to be an adolescent with lesbian parents. Although it was a difficult process for Melissa to sort out her own sexuality from that of her parents, she was able to use her therapy to work through what she thought and felt were both parental and societal expectations of her sexuality, and to identify what her own attractions were to begin to explore this aspect of her identity. Further, although Melissa's parents experienced anxiety about her well-being, they had done their own work to understand and integrate their sexual identity and were living as "out" lesbians. Robert and Zack as well were out to family, friends, at work, and in their community. Melissa's family had support in the school and in their community.

They were friends with other lesbian and gay families who they could discuss the struggles they faced openly as lesbian parents.

In contrast, Isaiah was born to a lower middle class African-American family, in a generally conservative racially tense urban Midwestern backdrop, which contributed to a more challenging coming-out process for his transgender father. Isaiah was faced with his family's transition when he was an adolescent. No one in the family had previously experienced the work needed to actively understand a gender minority identity and the impact of this transition on a family. Nevertheless, with the help of effective individual and family therapy, he was able to adapt to this transition and overcome his fears of how this transition might affect him and his family. It is important for the clinician to be mindful of the individual circumstances of each family they encounter, and to formulate a treatment plan that incorporates their immediate and long-term needs. Assessing the children's and the parents' safety and visibility in their community, work, and school settings is essential.

The life of every family is embedded in a sociocultural framework that informs both the developmental life cycle of the parents, and the child. The societal constructs of what is "normal" and what is "not normal" are dictated by the majority. As our culture evolves and the impact of this evolution influences societal norms, society will need to continue to learn how to incorporate people who are diverse in their gender identity, gender expression, and sexual orientation. This change over time is likely to have a positive impact on those who are part of a sexual/gender minority group, as well as the family members who may or may not be part of that minority group. In the meantime, the freedom to discuss the impact of homophobia, heterosexism, transphobia, stigma, and shame within one's family may help to improve communication, strengthen family bonds, and ultimately strengthen the resilience of the child and the family. For the families who run into developmental challenges, therapists can ideally create a safe space in which to freely discuss these complex matters.

# References

Balsam, K. F., Molina, Y., Beadnell, B., Simoni, J., & Walters, K. (2011). Measuring multiple minority stress: The LGBT People of Color Microaggressions Scale. *Cultural Diversity and Ethnic Minority Psychology, 17*, 163–174. https://doi.org/10.1037/a0023244

Bergman, K., Rubio, R., Green, R.-J., & Padrón, E. (2010). Gay men who become fathers via surrogacy: The transition to parenthood. *Journal of GLBT Family Studies, 6*, 111–141. https://doi.org/10.1080/15504281003704942

Biblarz, T. J., & Savci, E. (2010). Lesbian, gay, bisexual, and transgender families. *Journal of Marriage and Family, 72*, 480–497. https://doi.org/10.1111/j.1741-3737.2010.00714.x

Blake, L., Carone, N., Slutsky, J., Raffanello, E., Ehrhardt, A. A., & Golombok, S. (2016). Gay father surrogacy families: Relationships with surrogates and egg donors and parental disclosure of children's origins. *Fertility and Sterility, 106*, 1503–1509. https://doi.org/10.1016/j.fertnstert.2016.08.013

Bos, H. M. W., & Van Balen, F. (2008). Children in planned lesbian families: Stigmatisation, psychological adjustment and protective factors. *Culture, Health & Sexuality, 10*, 221–236. https://doi.org/10.1080/13691050701601702

Carone, N., Baiocco, R., Manzi, D., Antoniucci, C., Caricato, V., Pagliarulo, E., & Lingiardi, V. (2018). Surrogacy families headed by gay men: Relationships with surrogates and egg donors, fathers' decisions over disclosure and children's views on their surrogacy origins. *Human Reproduction, 33*, 248–257. https://doi.org/10.1080/02646830412331298350

Cenegy, L., Denney, J., & Kimbro, R. (2018). Family diversity and child health: Where do same-sex couple families fit? *Journal of Marriage and Family, 80*, 198–218. https://doi.org/10.1111/jomf.12437

Corbett, K. (2001). Nontraditional family romance. *Psychoanalytic Quarterly, 70*, 599–624. https://doi.org/10.1002/j.2167-4086.2001.tb00613.x

Cox, N., Dewaele, A., Van Houtte, M., & Vincke, J. (2010). Stress-related growth, coming out, and internalized homonegativity in lesbian, gay, and bisexual youth. An examination of stress-related growth within the minority stress model. *Journal of Homosexuality, 58*, 117–137. https://doi.org/10.1080/00918369.2011.533631

Dierckx, M., Mortelmans, D., Motmans, J., & T'Sjoen, G. (2017). Resilience in families in transition: What happens when a parent is transgender? *Family Relations, 66*, 399–411. https://doi.org/10.1111/fare.12282

von Doussa, H., Power, J., & Riggs, D. (2017). Family matters: Transgender and gender diverse peoples' experience with family when they transition. *Journal of Family Studies*. Advance online publication. https://doi.org/10.1080/13229400.2017.1375965

Ehrensaft, D. (2008a). When baby makes three or four or more: Attachment, individuation, and identity in assisted-conception families. *Psychoanalytic Study of the Child, 63*, 3–23. https://doi.org/10.1080/00797308.2008.11800797

Ehrensaft, D. (2008b). Just Molly and me, and donor makes three: Lesbian motherhood in the age of assisted reproductive technology. *Journal of Lesbian Studies, 12*, 161–178. https://doi.org/10.1080/10894160802161331

Engel, G. L. (1977). The need for a new medical model: A challenge for biomedicine. *Science, 196*(4286), 129–136. https://doi.org/10.1126/science.847460

Erera, P. I., & Segal-Engelchin, D. (2014). Gay men choosing to co-parent with heterosexual women. *Journal of GLBT Family Studies, 10*, 449–474. https://doi.org/10.1080/1550428X.2013.858611

Farr, R. H. (2017). Does parental sexual orientation matter? A longitudinal follow-up of adoptive families with school-age children. *Developmental Psychology, 53*, 252–264. https://doi.org/10.1037/dev0000228

Fava, G. A., & Sonino, N. (2007). The biopsychosocial model thirty years later. *Psychotherapy and Psychosomatics, 77*(1), 1–2. https://doi.org/10.1159/000110052

Fisher, C., Wallace, S., & Fenton, R. (2000). Discrimination distress during adolescence. *Journal of Youth and Adolescence, 29*, 679–695. https://doi.org/10.1023/A:1026455906512

Flier, J. S., Underhill, L. H., & McEwen, B. S. (1998). Protective and damaging effects of stress mediators. *The New England Journal of Medicine, 338*(3), 171–179. https://doi.org/10.1056/NEJM199801153380307

Fredriksen-Goldsen, K. I., Simoni, J. M., Kim, H.-J., Lehavot, K., Walters, K. L., Yang, J., … Muraco, A. (2014). The health equity promotion model: Reconceptualization of lesbian, gay, bisexual, and transgender (LGBT) health disparities. *American Journal of Orthopsychiatry, 84*, 653–663. https://doi.org/10.1037/ort0000030

Freedman, D., Tasker, F., & Di Ceglie, D. (2002). Children and adolescents with transsexual parents referred to a specialist gender identity development service: A brief report of key developmental features. *Clinical Child Psychology and Psychiatry, 7*, 423–432. https://doi.org/10.1177/1359104502007003009

Frosch, C. A., & Mangelsdorf, S. C. (2001). Marital behavior, parenting behavior, and multiple reports of preschoolers' behavior problems: Mediation or moderation? *Developmental Psychology, 37*, 502–519. https://doi.org/10.1037/0012-1649.37.4.502

Gartrell, N., & Bos, H. (2010). US National Longitudinal Lesbian Family Study: Psychological adjustment of 17-year-old adolescents. *Pediatrics, 126*, 28–36. https://doi.org/10.1542/peds.2009-3153

Gartrell, N., Bos, H., & Koh, A. (2018). National Longitudinal Lesbian Family Study: Mental health of adult offspring. *The New England Journal of Medicine, 379*(3), 297–299. https://doi.org/10.1056/NEJMc1804810

Gilligan, M., Karraker, A., & Jasper, A. (2018). Linked lives and cumulative inequality: A multigenerational family life course framework. *Journal of Family Theory Review, 10*, 111–125. https://doi.org/10.1111/jftr.12244

Goffman, E. (1963). *Stigma: Notes on the management of spoiled identity*. London, UK: Penguin.

Goldbach, J., & Gibbs, J. (2017). A developmentally informed adaptation of minority stress for sexual minority adolescents. *Journal of Adolescence, 55*, 36–50. https://doi.org/10.1016/j.adolescence.2016.12.007

Goldberg, A. E. (2007). (How) does it make a difference? Perspectives of adults with lesbian, gay, and bisexual parents. *American Journal of Orthopsychiatry, 77*, 550–562. https://doi.org/10.1037/0002-9432.77.4.550

Goldberg, A. E. (2010). *Lesbian and gay parents and their children: Research on the family life cycle*. Washington, DC: American Psychological Association.

Goldberg, A. E., Downing, J. B., & Moyer, A. M. (2012). Why parenthood, and why now? Gay men's motivations for pursuing parenthood. *Family Relations, 61*, 157–174. https://doi.org/10.1111/j.1741-3729.2011.00687.x

Goldberg, A. E., Kinkler, L. A., Richardson, H. B., & Downing, J. B. (2012). On the border: Young adults with LGBQ parents navigate LGBTQ communities. *Journal of Counseling Psychology, 59*, 71–85. https://doi.org/10.1037/a0024576

Golombok, S. (2000). *Parenting: What really counts?* London, UK: Routledge.

Golombok, S., Blake, L., Slutsky, J., Raffanello, E., Roman, G., & Ehrhardt, A. (2018). Parenting and the adjustment of children born to gay fathers through surrogacy. *Child Development, 89*, 1223–1233. https://doi.org/10.1111/cdev.12728

Golombok, S., Mellish, L., Jennings, S., Casey, P., Tasker, F., & Lamb, M. E. (2014). Adoptive gay father families: Parent–child relationships and children's psychological adjustment. *Child Development, 85*, 456–468. https://doi.org/10.1111/cdev.12155

Haines, B. A., Ajayi, A. A., & Boyd, H. (2014). Making trans parents visible: Intersectionality of trans and parenting identities. *Feminism & Psychology, 24*, 238–247. https://doi.org/10.1177/0959353514526219

Halfon, N., & Hochstein, M. (2002). Life course health development: An integrated framework for developing health policy and research. *Milbank Quarterly, 80*, 433–479. https://doi.org/10.1111/1468-0009.00019

Hatzenbuehler, M. (2009). How does sexual minority stigma "get under the skin"? A psychological mediation framework. *Psychological Bulletin, 135*, 707–730. https://doi.org/10.1037/a0016441

Hines, S. (2006). Intimate transitions: Transgender practices of partnering and parenting. *Sociology, 40*, 353–371. https://doi.org/10.1177/0038038506062037

James, S. E., Herman, J. L., Rankin, S., Keisling, M., Mottet, L., & Anafi, M. (2016). *The report of the 2015 U.S. Transgender Survey*. Retrieved from National

Center for Transgender Equality website: https://transequality.org/sites/default/files/docs/usts/USTS-Full-Report-Dec17.pdf

Johnson, M. K., Crosnoe, R., & Elder, G. H., Jr. (2011). Insights on adolescence from a life course perspective. *Journal of Research on Adolescence, 21*, 273–280. https://doi.org/10.1111/j.1532-7795.2010.00728.x

Katz-Wise, S., Rosario, M., Calzo, J., Scherer, E., Sarda, V., & Austin, S. (2017). Associations of timing of sexual orientation developmental milestones and other sexual minority stressors with internalizing mental health symptoms among sexual minority young adults. *Archives of Sexual Behavior, 46*, 1441–1452. https://doi.org/10.1007/s10508-017-0964-y

Kaufman, G., & Raphael, L. (1996). *Coming out of shame: Transforming gay and lesbian lives.* New York, NY: Doubleday.

Kuvalanka, K. A., Leslie, L. A., & Radina, R. (2014). Coping with sexual stigma: Emerging adults with lesbian parents reflect on the impact of heterosexism and homophobia during their adolescence. *Journal of Adolescent Research, 29*, 241–270. https://doi.org/10.1177/0743558413484354

Kuvalanka, K., & Goldberg, A. (2009). "Second generation" voices: Queer youth with lesbian/bisexual mothers. *Journal of Youth and Adolescence, 38*, 904–919. https://doi.org/10.1007/s10964-008-9327-2

Lamb, M. (2012). Mothers, fathers, families and circumstances: Factors affecting children's adjustment. *Applied Developmental Science, 16*, 98–111. https://doi.org/10.1080/10888691.2012.667344

Leblanc, A. J., Frost, D. M., & Wight, R. G. (2015). Minority stress and stress proliferation among same-sex and other marginalized couples. *Journal of Marriage and Family, 77*, 40–59. https://doi.org/10.1111/jomf.12160

Meyer, I. H. (1995). Minority stress and mental health in gay men. *Journal of Health & Social Behavior, 36*, 38–56. https://doi.org/10.2307/2137286

Meyer, I. H. (2003). Prejudice, social stress, and mental health in lesbian, gay, and bisexual populations: Conceptual issues and research evidence. *Psychological Bulletin, 129*, 674–697. https://doi.org/10.1037/0033-2909.129.5.674

Mink, M. D., Lindley, L. L., & Weinstein, A. A. (2014). Stress, stigma, and sexual minority status: The intersectional ecology model of LGBTQ health. *Journal of Gay & Lesbian Social Services, 26*, 502–521. https://doi.org/10.1080/10538720.2014.953660

Norton, W., Hudson, N., & Culley, L. (2013). Gay men seeking surrogacy to achieve parenthood. *Reproductive Biomedicine Online, 27*(3), 271–279. https://doi.org/10.1016/j.rbmo.2013.03.016

Pachankis, J. E., Cochran, S. D., & Mays, V. M. (2015). The mental health of sexual minority adults in and out of the closet: A population-based study. *Journal of Consulting & Clinical Psychology, 83*, 890–901. https://doi.org/10.1037/ccp0000047

Parks, C. A., Hughes, T. L., & Matthews, A. K. (2004). Race/ethnicity and sexual orientation: Intersecting identities. *Cultural Diversity and Ethnic Minority Psychology, 10*, 241–254. https://doi.org/10.1037/1099-9809.10.3.241

Pearlin, L. I., Schieman, S., Fazio, E. M., & Meersman, S. C. (2005). Stress, health, and the life course: Some conceptual perspectives. *Journal of Health & Social Behavior, 46*, 205–219. https://doi.org/10.1177/002214650504600206

Pearlin, L. I., & Skaff, M. (1996). Stress and the life course: A paradigmatic alliance. *The Gerontologist, 36*, 239–224. https://doi.org/10.1093/geront/36.2.239

Perlesz, A., Brown, R., Lindsay, J., McNair, R., De Vaus, D., & Pitts, M. (2006). Family in transition: Parents, children and grandparents in lesbian families give meaning to 'doing family'. *Journal of Family Therapy, 28*, 175–199. https://doi.org/10.1111/j.1467-6427.2006.00345.x

Pistella, J., Salvati, M., Ioverno, S., Laghi, F., & Baiocco, R. (2016). Coming-out to family members and internalized sexual stigma in bisexual, lesbian and gay people. *Journal of Child and Family Studies, 25*, 3694–3701. https://doi.org/10.1007/s10826-016-0528-0

Pfeffer, C. (2012). Normative resistance and inventive pragmatism: Negotiating structure and agency in transgender families. *Gender & Society, 26*, 574–602. https://doi.org/10.1177/0891243212445467

Pyne, J., Bauer, G., & Bradley, K. (2015). Transphobia and other stressors impacting trans parents. *Journal of GLBT Family Studies, 11*, 107–126. https://doi.org/10.1080/1550428X.2014.941127

Ray, V., & Gregory, R. (2001). School experiences of the children of lesbian and gay parents. *Family Matters, 59*, 28–34.

Riggs, D., Power, J., & Von Doussa, H. (2016). Parenting and Australian trans and gender diverse people: An exploratory survey. *International Journal of Transgenderism, 17*(2), 59–65. https://doi.org/10.1080/15532739.2016.1149539

Rosario, M., Scrimshaw, E. W., & Hunter, J. (2004). Ethnic/racial differences in the coming out process of lesbian, gay, and bisexual youths: A comparison of sexual identity development over time. *Cultural Diversity & Ethnic Minority Psychology, 10*, 215–228. https://doi.org/10.1037/1099-9809.10.3.215

Ryff, C. D., & Singer, B. (1996). Psychological well-being: Meaning, measurement, and implications for psychotherapy research. *Psychotherapy and Psychosomatics, 65*, 14–23. https://doi.org/10.1159/000289026

Savin-Williams, R. C. (2008). Then and now: Recruitment, definition, diversity, and positive attributes of same-sex populations. *Developmental Psychology, 44*, 135–138. https://doi.org/10.1037/0012-1649.44.1.135

Settersten, R. (2015). Relationships in time and the life course: The significance of linked lives. *Research in Human Development, 12*(3–4), 217–223. https://doi.org/10.1080/15427609.2015.1071944

Stein, M. T., Perrin, E. C., & Potter, J. (2004). A difficult adjustment to school: The importance of family constellation. *Journal of Developmental and Behavioral Pediatrics, 25*(5), S65–S68. https://doi.org/10.1097/00004703-200410001-00013

Stotzer, R. L., Herman, J. L., & Hasenbush, A. (2014). *Transgender parenting: A review of existing research.* Retrieved from Williams Institute website: https://williamsinstitute.law.ucla.edu/wp-content/uploads/transgender-parenting-oct-2014.pdf

Sue, D. W., Capodilupo, C. M., Torino, G. C., Bucceri, J. M., Holder, A. M. B., Nadal, K. L., & Esquilin, M. (2007). Racial microaggressions in everyday life: Implications for clinical practice. *American Psychologist, 62*, 271–286. https://doi.org/10.1037/0003-066X.62.4.271

Tabor, J. (2019). Mom, dad, or somewhere in between: Role-relational ambiguity and children of transgender parents. *Journal of Marriage and Family, 81*, 506–519. https://doi.org/10.1111/jomf.12537

Telingator, C. J., Patterson, C. (2008). Children and adolescents of lesbian and gay parents. *Journal of the American Academy of Child & Adolescent Psychiatry, 47*, 1364–1368. https://doi.org/10.1097/CHI.0b013e31818960bc

Telingator, C. J., Patterson, C., Jellinek, M. S., & Henderson, S. W. (2008). Children and adolescents of lesbian and gay parents. *Journal of the American Academy of Child & Adolescent Psychiatry, 47*, 1364–1368. https://doi.org/10.1097/CHI.0b013e31818960bc

Tornello, S. L., & Patterson, C. J. (2015). Timing of parenthood and experiences of gay fathers: A life course perspective. *Journal of GLBT Family Studies, 11*, 35–56. https://doi.org/10.1080/1550428X.2013.878681

Tornello, S. L., & Patterson, C. J. (2018). Adult children of gay fathers: Parent–child relationship quality and mental health. *Journal of Homosexuality, 65*, 1152–1166. https://doi.org/10.1080/00918369.2017.1406218

Udell, W., Sandfort, T., Reitz, E., Bos, H., & Dekovic, M. (2010). The relationship between early sexual debut and psychosocial outcomes: A longitudinal study of Dutch adolescents. *Archives of Sexual Behavior, 39*, 1133–1145. https://doi.org/10.1007/s10508-009-9590-7

Webster, C., & Telingator, C. (2016). Lesbian, gay, bisexual, and transgender families. *Pediatric Clinics of North America, 63*, 1107–1119. https://doi.org/10.1016/j.pcl.2016.07.010

# Reflectivity, Reactivity, and Reinventing: Themes from the Pedagogical Literature on LGBTQ-Parent Families in the Classroom and Communities

April L. Few-Demo and Valerie Q. Glass

In this chapter, we examine how scholars who teach in university settings have written about the incorporation of LGBTQ-parent family content into social science and community outreach curricula during the period of 1990 through 2018. We conducted a content analysis of their pedagogical strategies to provide a critical framework for presenting LGBTQ-parent family content, to better engage resistance to intersectional inclusivity, and to lay a sustainable groundwork that reflects civility, compassion, and the goals of social justice.

Social mores and political climates may have an influence on how students and instructors interact with one another in the classroom and in communities. Additionally, the social context can temper student receptivity to course content that highlights the experiences of LGBTQ-parent families and LGBTQ individuals. This chapter is written by two family social scientists in a time when the existence of LGBTQ-parent families is being rendered invisible by the Trump administration in the United States (USA) and the legal protections of LGBTQ persons and their families

are being eroded. In 2016, of the 6,121 hate crime incidents reported, 1,076 were based on sexual orientation bias and 124 were based on gender identity bias (Human Rights Campaign, n.d.-a, n.d.-b; Itsowitz, 2017). These numbers reflect a 2% and 9% increase, respectively (Dashow, 2017). In January 2017, many website pages and links regarding LGBTQ-parent families disappeared from the websites of the White House and federal agencies in the USA (Itsowitz, 2017). In May 2017, the Department of Health and Human Services (HHS) announced a plan to roll back regulations interpreting the Affordable Care Act's nondiscrimination provisions that once protected transgender people (Itsowitz, 2017). In October 2017, the Justice Department released a sweeping "license to discriminate" against LGBTQ persons, allowing federal agencies, government contractors, government grantees, and even private businesses to engage in illegal discrimination, as long as they could cite religious reasons for doing so (Human Rights Campaign, n.d.-a, n.d.-b; Itsowitz, 2017). Consistent with this rollback of legal protections for LGBTQ persons and their families, there is evidence that LGBTQ-parent families remain understudied in family science (Eeden-Moorefield, Few-Demo, Benson, & Lummer, 2018).

Pedagogical research has identified the importance of bringing in diverse, minority experiences and voices into classrooms (e.g., Martinez, 2014). Graduate and undergraduate students that are

A. L. Few-Demo (✉)
Department of Human Development and Family Science, Virginia Tech, Blacksburg, VA, USA
e-mail: alfew@vt.edu

V. Q. Glass
Department of Marriage and Family Therapy, Northcentral University, San Diego, CA, USA
e-mail: vglass@ncu.edu

© Springer Nature Switzerland AG 2020
A. E. Goldberg, K. R. Allen (eds.), *LGBTQ-Parent Families*,
https://doi.org/10.1007/978-3-030-35610-1_26

enrolled in courses involving social and behavioral sciences, human services, medicine, social work, and the law will ultimately interact with many family constellations throughout their professional careers. Being able to provide the tools of critical thinking, self-reflexivity, social equity, and adaptation in the areas of LGBTQ-parent families is essential to both attending to power inherent in these types of careers and recognizing the unique intersections of one's own identity and those of others. Pedagogy is what an educator brings to the environment, the underlying sense or feel of the learning experience (Sciame-Giesecke, Roden, & Parkison, 2009). By valuing LGBTQ parents and their families, recognizing the intersections of LGBTQ-parent families, and applying a queer lens to the process of educating students, students will begin to better understand and embrace family differences in their future professional endeavors (Goldberg & Allen, 2018).

It is a politically charged time to be teaching about LGBTQ-parent families. As family social scientists who are passionate about providing an intersectional and queer approach in teaching about LGBTQ-parent families, we recognize the challenges and rewards to teaching complex issues regarding sexual orientation and gender identity. We engage in and espouse *transformational pedagogy*. Transformational pedagogy challenges students to unpack current beliefs and constructions about the world around them. Stone (1994) states transformational pedagogies offer "an alternative epistemological worldview" (p. 224) that is achieved through relational dialog and exploring the world through the lenses of others. Transformational pedagogy, sensitized by an intersectional and queer lens, is critical pedagogy. Giroux (1994) defined critical pedagogy as "pedagogy [that] signals how questions of audience, voice, power, and evaluation actively work to construct particular relations between teachers and students, institutions and society, and classrooms and communities" (p. 30). Critical pedagogy is one that "illuminates the relationship among knowledge, authority, and power" (Giroux, 1994, p. 30). In teaching about LGBTQ-parent families, we recognize that this relationship among knowledge, authority, and power does not merely exist within the

discursive corpus of literature of LGBTQ-parent families but also within the corpus of the academy and in relationships among and between instructors, students, and higher administration. Transformational pedagogy involves fostering dynamic relationships between instructors, students, and a shared body of knowledge – in this case, LGBTQ family studies literature – to promote student learning and personal growth (Slavich & Zimbardo, 2012).

Transformational pedagogy also may involve cultivating *cultural humility* (Mosher et al., 2017). Cultural humility is increasingly used as an interdisciplinary, transformative educational pedagogy when training future helping professionals. Mosher et al. (2017) described cultural humility as (a) a lifelong motivation to learn from others; (b) critical self-examination of cultural awareness; (c) interpersonal respect; (d) developing mutual partnerships that address power imbalances; and (e) and an other-oriented stance, open to new cultural information. Cultural humility is increasingly used as an interdisciplinary, transformative educational pedagogy when training future helping professionals. For instance, Ortega and Faller (2011) stated that:

> a cultural humility approach advocates for incorporating multicultural and intersectional understanding and analyses to improve practice, since together these concepts draw attention to the diversity of the whole person, to power differences in relationships (especially between workers and families), to different past and present life experiences including microaggressions, and to potential resources or gaps. (p. 32)

Teaching students to be critically reflective of the events in their lives and their own social positioning locally and globally is a lifelong learning experience that the instructor cultivates through discussions, application of curriculum content, and presentation of materials on diverse families. Cultural humility allows both the instructor and student to contemplate differences and similarities while respecting the multiplicity of LGBTQ parent-headed family experiences. Learning, then, is conceptualized as more than gathering knowledge; it is about understanding and changing personal social biases, social change, and sometimes, social justice (Stone, 1994).

Thus, the purpose of this chapter is to provide a thematic review of the pedagogical scholarship on teaching about LGBTQ family experience through a critical framework of the three emerging themes which resulted from our content analysis of nearly two decades of pedagogical scholarship on LGBTQ-parent family content. The three emergent themes were: *reflectivity* (i.e., a consideration of which stage we may be in based on personal self-reflectivity and disclosure), *reactivity* (i.e., strategies for resolving student resistance or disclosure), and *reinventing* (i.e., processes for helping students explore the world through a feminist, inclusive lens [Allen, 2000], and strategies for building empathy and sustainability). Our analysis of the literature was sensitized by both intersectionality and queer theories. We argue that these three themes and the lessons within are representative of transformative pedagogy. Our goals are to provide a model of education that promotes both critical thinking and cultural humility and provides a collection of pedagogical resources for educators who are working with students in a variety of social, medical, and behavioral science disciplines.

## Our Theoretical Framework

The goal of critical pedagogy is the "transformation of society" (Rodriguez & Huemmer, 2019, p. 135). Intersectionality and queer theories are poised to help instructors achieve this goal in their teaching and in their students' learning. We drew from these theories to ground our coding of the sample of articles that highlighted practices of integrating LGBTQ-parent content. Critical transformational pedagogy is utilized as it pertains specifically to the combination of queer theory and intersectional theory within pedagogy. The following section presents these theories.

## Intersectionality

Bowleg (2012) defined intersectionality as a theoretical framework that "posits that multiple social categories (e.g., race, ethnicity, gender, sexual orientation, socioeconomic status) inter-

sect at the micro level or individual experiences to reflect interlocking systems of privilege and oppression at the macro, social-structural level (e.g., racism, sexism, heterosexism)" (p. 1267). Intersectionality employs a critical analysis of the multiple identities in which people affiliate; the social positioning of diverse groups which reflects power, privilege, and marginalization; and people's interactions with institutions and policies that provide opportunities or constraints (Collins, 1990; Collins & Bilge, 2016; Crenshaw, 1993). An intersectional lens is appropriate for the craft of teaching LGBTQ content because it allows us to complicate and transcend discursively binary understandings of gender, sexuality, and other social locations (Coston & Kimmel, 2012, p. 97). Students are challenged to acknowledge the vast diversity of human expression, performativity of behaviors (Butler, 2001), and social conditions. In other words, this lens provides the intellectual (and emotional) space for those in a classroom to talk about different ethnicities, cultures, genders, and sexualities, and how the lives (and life chances) of individuals and groups are impacted by institutionalized systems of racism, sexism, heterosexism, and colonialism. For instance, this kind of framework encourages students to be introduced to thinking about pervasive oppression(s) experienced and inequities that are sustained by institutional design and policies (e.g., Jim Crow laws; differential sentencing experienced by different racial groups in the criminal justice system; Don't Ask, Don't Tell policy; child separation created by current immigration policies).

In the classroom setting, intersectionality takes students' understanding of identity a step further by looking at the multiple constructions around one person's identity. Teaching intersectionality is interdisciplinary and takes into account the multiple elements within one's environment that might have an influence on gender or sexual orientation identities (e.g., laws, politics, social norms and expectations, and inequities across personal and professional growth) (Craven, 2019). One way that Craven (2019) teaches intersectionality theory in the classroom is to have students explore, through a written assignment, gender within a country or culture different than their own. This assignment challenges students to consider the intersections of gender and culture. An example of using both intersectionality and queer theories to discuss LGBTQ-parent families may include the following. Imagine that there are two parents and two children. One of the parents identifies as lesbian and the other as pansexual. One parent identifies as a cisgender female and the other defines herself as genderfluid. One parent identifies as African American and the other parent is biracial (Latinx and White). Both parents grew up living in poverty and currently struggle with finances. This family would have to consider the "intersections" of their multiplicative minority statuses – their ethnicities, their minority gender identities, their sexual orientations, and their socioeconomic backgrounds. An instructor using intersectionality theory may ask students: *What does racism look like to this couple when they are in the LGBTQ community? What does heterosexism look like in their cultural, racial, or ethnic communities? How does this family's unique social positioning influence this family's ability to access resources, educational and work opportunities that might foster social mobility, and to negotiate daily microaggressions?* The instructor might present this example as a case study or as an opportunity for students to investigate historical case law, civil law, family law, and LGBTQ rights, social movements, and advocacy groups. The "intersections" of their multiple social locations provide opportunities for students to critically contemplate discrimination, privilege, and stigma.

## Queer Theory

Queer theory problematizes the notion that socially created identities privileged by cisgenderism, cissexism, heterosexism, and transphobia are "more natural" than identities that are more fluid, contingent, homonormative, transcendent, gender expansive, and/or nonbinary. A queer theoretical approach provides an analytic tool that places emphasis on the social location of the intertwined social categories of gender and sexuality that are uniquely situated within the matrix

of oppression (Few-Demo, Humble, Curran, & Lloyd, 2016; Kuvalanka, Goldberg, & Oswald, 2013). For example, a queer lens allows students to contemplate how federal and state legislation and institutional policies have denied LGBTQ people certain rights and privileges in the USA (e.g., health insurance and health care policies that discriminate against transgender individuals by limiting and denying gender affirming treatments; sodomy laws; state religious freedom legislation). Therefore, queer theory interrogates how institutions, cultural values, and policy sustain oppression, inequities, and opportunities for those whose lived experiences are not aligned with heteronormative expectations (Oswald, Blume, & Marks, 2005; Oswald, Kuvalanka, Blume, & Berkowitz, 2009; Shlasko, 2005).

Both queer theory and intersectionality are rooted in feminist thought and bring a liberatory end for those who are disempowered and oppressed (Allen, Lloyd, & Few, 2009). These two fields of thinking also invite the added responsibility of the teacher, researcher, and/or practitioner to place the histories of marginalized groups in the center of analysis. Whereas queer theory highlights the intersection of sexuality and gender, intersectionality theory provides a broader scale of analysis for how other social categories interacting with sexuality and gender produce different social locations and positioning within a multidimensional matrix of oppression(s). Intersectionality and queer theories can influence the development of pedagogical strategies to assist students with the examination of the role of oppression and power dynamics in families, communities, and cultures (Moradi & Grzanka, 2017). From this orientation, we posit that we cannot holistically explore family relationships without interrogating power and our roles within that dynamic (Louis, Mavor, La Macchia, & Amiot, 2014).

## Critical Transformative Pedagogy

Critical transformative pedagogy, which embraces queer theory and intersectionality, provides a platform for students and instructors to "dive deep" into power relations, difference, and social justice. The ultimate goal of an instructor using a critical transformative pedagogy is to lead students to become critical thinkers, to adopt a sense of cultural humility, and to evolve into social justice advocates. The act of integrating sexual and/or gender minority families or solely focusing on these families in a family science course is a political act inspired by critical thought (Giroux, 1994). Critical transformative pedagogy directly relates to teaching content on LGBTQ-parent families. In learning about families with one or more sexual or gender minority members, students wrestle with social representations, sexual politics, and oppressions and privileges experienced by these families. Two components of executing a critical transformative pedagogy involve developing relevant scaffolding activities to set the groundwork for practicing critical thinking skills.

**Scaffolding critical thinking**  One method that instructors can use is scaffolding. Scaffolding can lead to building critical thinking skills that justify the importance of building communities that are more equitable. Scaffolding refers to the implementation of a variety of instructional techniques used to help students (or a child) achieve mastery of a specific task and to progress into independent learners (Puntambekar & Hübscher, 2005; Vygotsky, 1978). Scaffolding activities begin with simple tasks and eventually lead students toward understanding more complex abstractions (Hale, 2018). Accessible tasks that can help encourage critical thinking may begin first with having students learn definitions and key concepts. The next step may be to encourage students to apply these definitions and concepts to visual media involving LGBTQ-parent families (e.g., video clips, movies) and asking students how they might personally relate to stories shared to foster empathy and perspective-taking.

Bauer and Clancy (2018) discussed their experiences scaffolding topics about social justice within their political science courses. They discussed empathetic scaffolding which presents an idea (e.g., concept, historical fact), asks questions, and foments conversations to situate the construct into a more personal frame. The authors shared that their discussions about immigration involve providing specific facts, laws, and statistics about immigration. Then, they connected these facts and statistics to the human element with autobiographies or documentaries, bringing in that first-person experience. A similar scaffolding process could be put into place when discussing LGBTQ-parent families. An initial stage of educating on this topic could be starting with statistics, legal changes, historical shifts, and social perspectives. A scaffolding step might be to invite LGBTQ parents to discuss their person situation, their identity, or their experiences with the class. A third step in the scaffolding process would be to generate dialog that helps students to personally connect to the speaker and the presented materials (Bauer & Clancy, 2018). Examples of scaffolding questions in this scenario could be: *What are some challenges you have experienced as child in your family that you found to be similar or different than the speaker's family?* or *Is there something unique about your family that you thought about as you listened to the speaker?*

**Queering critical thinking skills**  Critical thinking is the process of taking the facts in, engaging with the information, and being able to reflect on the information (Forbes, 2018). Critical thinking involves the putting together of ideas and at times generating a new way of looking at what is presented. For example, taking a queer theory approach to teaching about LGBTQ-parent families evokes critical thinking naturally (Dozono, 2017). Queer theory challenges students to explore the world from the lens of gender and sexual minorities and shift from the more dominate cisgender and heteronormative lens. For example, Dozono (2017) shared that by teaching history with a queer critical thinking lens, students shifted from thinking about LGBTQ individuals within history to thinking about how society has responded to LGBTQ individuals throughout history. Teaching about LGBTQ-parent families from a queer lens is about trying to think through viewing family from a less common lens. Abstract critical thinking may be guided by having students divide into small groups to process historical events that highlight discrimination or inequities, to be self-reflective about microaggressions experienced and committed, and/or strategies to become an ally and coalition-builder.

In summary, queer theory and intersectionality provide a framework and a language for presenting a discussion on pedagogy and LGBTQ-parent families. This chapter is informed by these constructs. Critical transformational pedagogy is a learning theory that is informed by queer theory and intersectionality. Through these lenses, we provide a framework for educators who are seeking to challenge students' thinking, create change in their social communities, and generate space for critical thinking.

## Our Content Analysis Method

We conducted a content analysis of articles that provided advice for including content about LGBTQ individuals and LGBTQ-parent families in family science, psychology, education, women and gender studies, and helping professions (counseling, marital and couple therapy) courses and curricula. We cast a broad net, for we were aware that Eeden-Moorefield et al. (2018) found only seven pedagogy-focused articles published in mainstream family science journals during 2000–2015. We chose the period of 1990–2018 because it is in the 1990s that feminist and queer scholars were breaking cisnormative barriers in publishing, and it is in the later years that family scholars begin writing about incorporating LGBTQ content in teaching. We acknowledge that in family science, feminist pioneers reinterpreted the experiences of women and families in both private and public spheres during this period. A few of the feminist family science foremothers who sensitized the family science discipline to the intersections of gender, sexuality, race, ethnicity, and class were Patricia Bell-Scott, Katherine Allen, Alexis Walker, Linda Thompson, Donna Sollie, Sally Lloyd, and Edith Lewis. Through the years and in different venues, these feminist family scholars have found intellectual spaces to teach academicians about how to "do" inclusive pedagogy, work that included diverse families such as LGBTQ-parent families (e.g., Allen, 1995; Hull, Bell-Scott, & Smith, 1982).

We used EBSCO database to search for articles that were published during 1990–2018 and that provided advice for including content on LGBTQ individuals and LGBTQ-parent families in family science, psychology, education, and helping professions curricula. We used the following keywords and combined phrases to identify articles: LGBT and pedagogy/curriculum, LGBT and student resistance, LGBT and family science and pedagogy, sexual orientation and pedagogy, lesbian and gay and teaching, transgender and teaching, queer and teaching, LGBTQ and pedagogy/curriculum, LGBTQ topics and pedagogy, bisexual and teaching, same sex and teaching/curriculum, and disclosure and pedagogy. The journals that included at least one pedagogical or training curriculum article on LGBT topics which included family or was family-centered were: *Family Relations, Journal of Family Theory & Review, Teaching Sociology, Journal of Feminist Family Therapy, Journal of Marital and Family Therapy, Multicultural Education, International Journal of Qualitative Studies in Education, Romanian Journal of Experimental Applied Psychology, British Journal of Social Work, College English, College Teaching, Journal of Educational Research, Teaching in Psychology,* and *Diversity & Democracy: Civic Learning for Shared Futures.* We identified 21 theoretical and empirical pedagogy-focused articles and four articles explicitly related to working with LGBTQ individuals and LGBTQ-parent families in curricular training for the helping professions. Our list of articles is by no means exhaustive, and is limited, as we tried to include pedagogical articles that had explicit or tangential mention of LGBT families content, LGBT familial experiences content, family or social science courses or helping professions, or were written by family scholars. (See Appendix A for a list of pedagogical articles, chapters, and books.) We limited our review to those articles that place learning in the classroom. We both read each article twice and coded the articles in our sample separately. We compared our independent coding schemes to identify overlapping, incongruent, and congruent codes. Examples of some initial codes included: reflexivity, resistance, modeling, strategies, disclosure, and mentoring. Through an iterative process of collapsing codes and achieving high intercoder agreement, our content analysis resulted in three major themes: reflectivity, reactivity, and reinventing.

## Pedagogical Themes in Teaching About LGBTQ-Parent Families

### Reflectivity

In 1995, Katherine Allen presented groundbreaking reflections on the use of "self" as a pedagogical tool in the classroom. Allen (1995) stated that "by disclosing important aspects of my identity, I invite and model ways for students to understand their own experiences with social locations such as gender, race, class, and sexual orientation" (p. 136). By presenting an authentic self, particularly when elements of one's identity are oppressed and invisible, instructors can open up the perceptions or stigmas that exist for students. Teaching brings with it a sense of transparency where instructors can share experiences of power and privilege, as they have experienced them within the context of their own intersecting identities, with their students. For example, an instructor who is a White lesbian parent may share her experiences of sexism and homophobia while challenging students to consider how differences in religion, race, gender, financial status, and culture may influence LGBTQ-parent families. Once students learn to situate themselves and others in social context through scaffolding exercises, an instructor can guide a class discussion about how groups, such as LGBTQ-parent families, as social entities interact with the constraints and privileges that social institutions sanction in both historical and contemporary contexts (Kuvalanka et al., 2013).

A transformative pedagogy compels instructors to realize that our authentic selves are tied inextricably to larger macrosystemic contexts which create the tides of sociopolitical discourse that ebb and flow with notions of inclusivity and exclusivity (Allen, 2000; Few-Demo et al., 2016).

How we situate ourselves today is very different than how we would have approached writing about our reflectivity than a decade ago and most likely would be a decade from now. Research has explored climate challenges related to incorporating LGBTQ-parent families into coursework and pedagogy (Kuvalanka et al., 2013). The larger political and campus climates seem to be an unpredictable reality that plays a major role in the pedagogical decisions of instructors (Kuvalanka et al., 2013).

Reflectivity involves both the reflectivity of the instructor and inspiring the reflectivity in the students. Instructors can use their own process as one way to model reflectivity. Instructors can also encourage student reflectivity by having students explore their own identity. The intersectionality of LGBTQ-parent families can include race, ethnicity, religion, culture, financial status, education, gender, disability, and the list is continuous (Few-Demo et al., 2016; Goldberg & Allen, 2018; Kuvalanka et al., 2013). Our sample of pedagogical scholarship indicates that having students explore personal intersections in their own families and the multiple ways in which students differ from others with regard to their intersections can expose them to new ways of seeing their own families and the identities that play a role in their decisions, resiliencies, and challenges (Ortega & Faller, 2011). For example, an instructor can invite a student panel to discuss their experiences in nonheteronormative family structures or facilitate a discussion for students to learn about one another's family background. Other strategies that instructors have used to spark reflectivity include inviting panels of LGBTQ individuals to speak to classes and showing videos of LGBTQ people that have relevance to courses with family-related content (Fletcher & Russell, 2001: Kuvalanka et al., 2013; Quilty, 2015; Simoni, 1996). If the goal is to help students make a personal connection to LGBTQ-parent content in visual materials, it is important to make sure that the videos and/or social media are contemporary, meaning that the content reflects present-day issues faced by LGBTQ-parent families and provides variation in how LGBTQ-parent families are represented.

Students may be drawn into contemporary political issues and/or current events that are particularly salient rather than issues that students may mistakenly believe "are over and done" or are invisible due to a relative lack of national attention despite still being discriminatory in nature (e.g., workplace discrimination; transfer of wealth barriers; adoption and fostering children). Instructors should preview videos to ensure that stereotypic tropes of LGBTQ identities are not promoted or presented as representative for all LGBTQ identities, as well as to identify the moments in the video to help students unpack group representation and seek both similarities and differences in life stories. There should also be a time to debrief students about their experiences watching the videos, as well as to discuss their reactions to stories shared in LGBTQ student panels.

**Situating our authentic selves** A common subtheme across the pedagogical literature between 2000 and 2018 that had a focus on LGBTQ individuals and LGBTQ-parent families in curricula was that both instructors and students should engage in scaffolding feminist self-reflective exercises that foster (a) principles of inclusivity; (b) the interrogation of normativity as opposed to "normal" behaviors; (c) an examination of contradictory personal belief systems; (d) an awareness of how power operates in the form of interlocking oppressions, disparities, and inequities caused by heterosexism, homophobia, transphobia, and cisgenderism; and (e) a gradual adaptation and embrace of more inclusive and expansive dialogs, behaviors, and beliefs (Few-Demo et al., 2016; Jaekel, 2016; Kuvalanka et al., 2013; Lewis, 2011; McGeorge & Carlson, 2011; Quilty, 2015; Tasker & Granville, 2011; see chapter "Losing a Child: Death and Hidden Losses in LGBTQ-Parent Families"). As noted by Few-Demo (2014):

> For a feminist family studies instructor, the presentation of social inequalities or injustice using a neutral stance or tone is antithetical to feminist principles; for such a strategy may give the impression that inequalities that are real and salient in

people's lives can be deemphasized or swept over in the curriculum.…Feminist pedagogy allows for a multiplicity of viewpoints and political orientations to be the center of analysis for a classroom. (p. 5)

If LGBTQ-parent families are to be incorporated into traditional heteronormative curricula effectively and with authenticity, then core themes of power, structure, agency, and intersectionality, and how these themes play out in family relationships and larger social systems must be wrestled with intrapersonally and interpersonally in the classroom. For example, the first author, April Few-Demo, identifies as a cisgender, heterosexual, middle-class, Black feminist who uses an intersectional lens to frame her research, outreach, and teaching. She teaches courses on human sexuality, family theories, and family relationships in a Human Development and Family Science (HDFS) department at a Mid-Atlantic predominantly White institution (PWI). In addition to the typical HDFS curriculum, April was trained in feminist, queer, and intersectionality theories and scholarship. Her interest in queer theory and studying the lives of queer individuals has been inspired by her family members, colleagues, and (former) doctoral students. These individuals shared their life experiences and research interests with her, and made her reexamine her own privilege, agency, and power as a cisgender, heterosexual minority woman. For instance, it became clear to her that having power is quite a contingent, nuanced possession; the extent to how much privilege one possesses is determined by the interplay of one's own minority and majority statuses. The second author, Valerie Glass, identifies as a White woman, a lesbian, cisgender, and a single parent. Valerie teaches many courses on the undergraduate and graduate levels that utilize queer, intersectional, and feminist lenses. Teaching critical thought and challenging students' understanding of power and privilege is a professional passion and continues to evolve. For instance, Valerie's use of "self" in her classes includes using her own experiences of being an LGBTQ parent, an LGBTQ child, and a part of LGBTQ communities, working in professional positions with LGBTQ families, or having

LGBTQ family and friends as part of her social circle, and she uses these experiences as educational tools (Allen, 1995) and teaching moments. Reflecting on our own journeys and assumptions as human beings and the thought processes we have gone through in unpacking those assumptions not only enriches our curriculum about all families that do not fit into the heteronormative identities, but allows for students to embrace where they are in this journey (Holloway & Gouthro, 2011).

Reflectivity also includes being aware of one's current and past biases (Fletcher & Russell, 2001; Wentling, Windsor, Schilt, & Lucal, 2008). Reflectivity may be accomplished by keeping a pedagogical journal of teaching experiences and student interactions (Allen, 2000). This iterative continual reflection allows for a "safe space" for discussion, helps an instructor to time student exposure to certain content, and assists in the determination of "readiness" of students to internalize challenges to heteronormative beliefs about family (Ortega & Faller, 2011). Both instructors and students can engage in an iterative continual reflection process by journaling about their reactions to readings and class discussions. For example, instructors may decide to either continue to include or exclude a specific reading or reflective exercise based on student reactions – which can be either positive, neutral, or negative – or student difficulty in mastering key concepts. Students can take ownership of learning content by being made responsible for leading a discussion in class in a flipped classroom. In the flipped classroom, students are provided with information before the class and use the time in class to practice and apply concepts through interaction with peers and teachers (Gomez-Lanier, 2018). After the class, instructors can direct the students to reflect upon the feedback they have received and use this to further their learning.

An excellent classic exercise to help students uncover implicit biases as well as those present in students' own family systems is presented by Allen, Floyd-Thomas, and Gillman (2001). Students are presented with a series of questions that are meant to elicit a personal connection to the investigation of how race, sexuality, and gender influence familial and personal behaviors, attitudes, and social networks. This exercise requires a student to reflect upon how one participates and/or witnesses discrimination in daily life and interactions. Students become aware of their agency, privilege, and oppressions. Reflectivity leads to the practice of active listening, a critical interpersonal skill for both instructor and students to learn. Situating self and reflecting on that place can model for students how to place themselves in larger social contexts and how to continue to grow as professionals.

The stage should be set to allow space for multiple voices and experiences (Fletcher & Russell, 2001). This involves making those that are in different places, different experiences, and different backgrounds feel comfortable in engaging in conversation about LGBTQ topics without feeling attacked. In April's experience, it is important to set the stage by encouraging students to participate in establishing ground rules for discussion. She routinely reminds students to be thoughtful and intentional with their words, saying, "because you never know what the person sitting next to you is going through," which allows students to be empathetic and reflective of the power of words. Students are tasked to defend their positions about LGBTQ topics with social, behavioral, and/or medical science. April has found it has been useful to help students in human sexuality courses to understand that inserting anecdotes, cultural practices, and beliefs, into a scientific debate is like comparing apples and oranges, and that the two incompatible objects should not occupy the same debate. In this way, students learn when it is appropriate to insert specific content or information and how to analyze contradictory information or "apples" effectively.

**Mentoring** We propose that our second sub-theme, mentoring, is an active exercise in self-reflectivity. Similar to modeling a sense of self-disclosure, mentoring can be a tool for building critical thought and understanding difference (Lucey & White, 2017). Articles in our review indicated the necessity of forming a community of mentors for LGBTQ students (Linley et al., 2016; Mulcahy, Dalton, Kolbert, & Crothers,

2016), but this community can also assist instructors as not being the lone actor responsible for supporting LGBTQ-parent content (as noted in the Student Resistance subtheme). Faculty members and peers can be meaningful mentors for students. Mentoring can be set up in a formal way by applying specific goals and directions. Perhaps, pairing mentors and mentees who have experienced similarities in their paths or expressed similar interests. By doing so, effective strategies can be generated or mirrored to diminish discrimination. Mentoring also can be informal as instructors present and model the atmosphere of respect and challenge. The idea of mentoring takes pedagogy outside of the classroom (e.g., community outreach; conference symposia and workshops). Class projects that are connected to community centers or groups who service LGBTQ-parent families can be both subversive and overt experiential learning (Fletcher & Russell, 2001). Examples may include assignments that involve a service learning component, volunteerism or internship, or required participation in programming designed to educate about LGBTQ issues and resources.

## Reactivity

Reactivity is the second most common theme found in the articles that we reviewed. We define reactivity as involving both emotional and intellectual responses by faculty and students when confronted with content that may be adverse or challenging to their core beliefs (Allen et al., 2001). Students often hold values that are congruent with previous experiences interacting with those topics (Allen & Farnsworth, 1993; Mezirow, 1990, 2003). Scholars in our sample recognized the strategies used by instructors in response to and for resolving student resistance to LGBTQ-related content and the ways in which instructors made decisions about self-disclosure.

**Student resistance** Resistance can manifest in many different forms. At times, student resistance can feel like apathy or ambivalence (Holloway & Gouthro, 2011). At other times, stu-

dents might be very vocal about competing positions or even silent. Considering social equity can be painful because it requires a repositioning of power and privilege that may be a new tool for some (Tharp, 2015). Resistance can come in the form of treating everyone as if they are human and no one is different (Tharp, 2015). This resistance discounts the unique experience of LGBTQ-parent families specifically because of the lack of recognition of the cultural context and social constructs that could challenge LGBTQ-parent families on a daily basis (Ben-Ari, 2001; Eichstedt, 1996; Few-Demo et al., 2016; Simoni, 1996). This resistance also serves to deny that these challenges exist and that the resisting person has to recognize these inequities and their role in them.

Exploring the genesis of this reactive resistance with students using an intersectional and queer lens provides an opportunity for instructors to demonstrate how the power of heteronormative majority discourses sustains implicit biases in ourselves, families, and institutions. For example, this resistance may be ingrained and supported in one's own academic department. Kuvalanka et al. (2013) noted that some forms of diversity may be supported more than others by colleagues and on the university campus. For instance, students may find it easier to relate to people who identify as cisgender and gay or lesbian rather than those who affiliate with more fluid notions of gender identity (e.g., transgender, two-spirit, pangender, intersex) and sexual orientation (e.g., asexuality, pansexual) that transcend binary constructions of being. Scholars have documented that content that covers transgender families and individuals provides an opportunity for students to become aware of how steeped bias is in everyday language such as inappropriate pronoun usage for individuals whose notions of gender and being are expansive (Case, Stewart, & Tittsworth, 2009; Kuvalanka et al., 2013; Lovaas, Baroudi, & Collins, 2002; Wentling et al., 2008).

Resistance may occur because colleagues and students see the discussion of diversity as taboo, irrelevant, or impolite (Jaekel, 2016). Kumashiro (2000) argued that resistance may occur when "learning anything that reveals our complicity with racism, homophobia, and other forms of oppression" (p. 43). Using intersectionality and/or queer theory to address student resistance can be perilous work. These theories not only highlight racial, ethnic, gender, and sexual oppression, but also one's own complicity in sustaining power and privilege. For example, students display this complicity when they respond to exemplars of LGBTQ-parent families with phrases such as "I do not know if I can work with LGBTQ families because I am not familiar with any LGBTQ person and do not know much about it" or "it is against my religion." Instructors can assist these students to move gradually beyond this foreclosed status by incorporating activities that help identify and deconstruct sources that undergird these attitudes and discover ways in which inclusivity does not have to compromise belief systems.

**Self-disclosure decisions** Our review revealed self-disclosure as an important decision-making process for instructors who teach content about LGBTQ individuals and LGBTQ-parent families. Instructors wrestle with either the personal choice to reveal their gender and/or sexual orientation identities or wrestle with what to do when a student self-discloses an identity (Allen, 1995; Eichstedt, 1996; Fletcher & Russell, 2001; Goldstein, 1997; Kuvalanka et al., 2013; Liddle, 1997; Linley et al., 2016; Wallace, 2002). Instructor self-disclosure can be both rewarding and affirming for instructors and students alike (Allen, 1995). For example, some studies indicate that an instructor (or student) who reveals a minority gender and/or sexual identity in the classroom creates an empowering, safe space for the instructor and students to discuss LGBTQ content; and that being out in the classroom facilitates (intersectional and queer) critical thinking among students, provides a positive role model for students, and communicates a genuine authenticity and transparency (Fletcher & Russell, 2001; Gates, 2011; Johnson, 2009; Liddle, 2009; Orlov & Allen, 2014). However, there is also evidence that instructor self-disclosure of a minority sexual or gender identity can come at a cost to instructors. Instructors have

reported as being punished for this act of transparency, resulting in poor student evaluations and student resistance that decries instructor delegitimacy and bias (Orlov & Allen, 2014; Russ, Simonds, & Hunt, 2002; Sand, 2009; Sapon-Shevin, 2004; Sapp, 2001). Therefore, we suggest that instructors who teach "incendiary" topics should invest in conducting midsemester teaching evaluations in order to determine how information is being processed by students and the extent of achieved mastery, identify if there are students who need and are seeking a queer role model, and develop strategies to address discomfort or reactivity expressed by students. Taking the temperature of the room can help an instructor to weigh the decision to self-disclose or not.

## Reinventing and Sustainability

Students and instructors are socially constructed products of their own environments (Giroux, 1994). In other words, we are influenced by the transmission of family and cultural norms and values and the social consequences of either conforming or breaking these norms and values. Our social interactions contribute to our sense of self and belonging in the world (Blumer, 1969). In transforming traditional curriculum on family, scholars in our sample advocated for reinventing how we think about diverse families, how we study diverse families, and how we connect our pedagogy to spaces outside of the classroom. Reinventing involves moving aside notions of heteronormativity and cisnormativity from the "center" of our curriculum and pedagogical strategies and creating an intellectual discourse that is authentically inclusive and noncontroversial (Allen, 2000; Few-Demo et al., 2016; Goldberg & Allen, 2018). All of the articles in our sample advocated for curricula that are inclusive of the experiences of LGBTQ-identified people and LGBTQ-parent families. In their implications, discussion, and future directions sections, scholars in our sample suggested that instructors be strategic in their risk-taking and strive to cultivate a critical consciousness within students that extends beyond the classroom. We also encourage active sustainability of this inclusive critical consciousness beyond the classroom. This goal can be achieved by being attentive to the representation of specific groups across an undergraduate or graduate curriculum (Few-Demo et al., 2016) and/or community workshops so that curricular messaging does not support or promote monolithic identities or experiences, but challenges stereotypes and misinformation.

## Discussion and Final Thoughts

In reviewing articles that discuss teaching about LGBTQ individuals and LGBTQ-parent families, we have noted a literature with practical advice, challenges, and trends that are remarkably consistent over the decades. We would like to highlight a few considerations to continue the decades-long conversation that these scholars have provided for those interested in incorporating LGBTQ-parent families into their pedagogy and curriculum. These considerations are often implicit in this scholarship, but it is our hope that we stimulate further study on these topics. We humbly offer that there is further work to be done on language and identity politics in the classroom, student activists in the classroom, spotlighting teachable moments, and linking our pedagogical goals beyond the classroom and into our communities.

## Language and Identity Politics

Even in choosing to use the descriptor "LGBTQ-parent families," we privilege our acknowledgment of certain identities over others; thus, these other identities are rendered invisible or are marginalized. Language provides a powerful construction about identity, belonging, and authenticity. There have been historical shifts in the language we use, and by extension, so has the meaning of labels and identities shifted (Goldberg & Allen, 2018). Pedagogy about LGBTQ-parent families should include discussions of labels and how identities can change

over time and the influence of these labels (Goldberg & Allen, 2018). The declaration and overlapping of other "identities" (e.g., asexuality, pansexuality, relationship anarchist, demisexuality, polyamorous families, mixed orientation families) are becoming more common in public spaces. The prevalence of these "new" diverse identities as ascribed identities not only has an impact on family roles, but also on how we represent these families in our classes, research, and other public spaces. Instructors who are attentive to intersectionality and queer theories should facilitate students' ability to position themselves within language and be critical perspective takers (Jaekel, 2016). Consider how common it is for students to say "Moms and Dads" or to discuss heteronormative examples in family-related or human sexuality courses. An accessible means to address language that reflects heteronormativity and cisgenderism is to develop exercises that will allow students to analyze ways that they talk about LGBTQ individuals and LGBTQ-parent families (Boucher, 2011; Fletcher & Russell, 2001; Goldberg & Allen, 2018). Using broad generalizations in one's language about LGBTQ-parent families will play a role in constructions of thought (Fletcher & Russell, 2001) about these families. Avoiding generalizations and encouraging students to look at the meaning behind their own generalizations widens students' mindsets and enables them to examine intersectionality within LGBTQ-parent families.

## Student Activists in the Classroom

Most literature about student reactions to LGBTQ content often focuses on student resistance (e.g., Allen et al., 2001; Eichstedt, 1996; Goldstein, 1997; Jaekel, 2016; Lovaas et al., 2002; Robinson & Ferfolja, 2001; Simoni, 1996; Wallace, 2002; Wentling et al., 2008; Zacko-Smith & Smith, 2010). Less represented in the pedagogical literature are the students in the classroom who embody passionate activism for LGBTQIA topics (Linder, 2018; Louis et al., 2014; Moradi & Grzanka, 2017). These students may identify personally with the topics around LGBTQ families or be passionate about creating a particular social climate related to LGBTQ individuals and LGBTQ-parent families. The personal drive motivating these student activists can bring a welcomed energy, creating an inclusive climate in the classroom that cannot be achieved by the instructor alone. Moreover, the responsibility of sustaining an inclusive climate becomes the responsibility of students and not the instructor's alone. The other side of the coin is that student activists can sometimes stifle or silence other voices and perspectives in the classroom or become frustrated with instructors if content is perceived as lacking (Goldberg & Allen, 2018). This is not to say that all perspectives have equal value or all perspectives are based on facts supported by research. In addition, we see this side of the coin not so much as a negative but more so as opportunities for teachable moments to distinguish between beliefs and facts (Allen, 1995). Intersectional and queer theories complicate present understandings or popular stances by positioning present-day narratives in historical context. The instructor's challenge is to develop activities that provide challenging information and mentoring to student activists while developing a climate that invites multiple voices and creates new allies (Allen et al., 2001).

Linder (2018) described activism as "the commitment of transforming systems for comprehensive change" (p. 1). Instructors can integrate discussions on intersectionality, power, and privilege to encourage a more complex understanding of perspectives by multiple stakeholders, even within the group to which students ascribe. Intersectionality and queer theories question the notion of monolithic group goals, needs, and representations. Instructors can encourage student activists to find platforms for their activism outside of the classroom by directing students to university policies or pledges, connecting students with supportive campus units, and by integrating experiential learning activities to focus on LGBTQ experiences. Finally, instructors also can provide flexibility in assignments to allow students to deploy activism as part of the course.

## Implications for Practice: Teachable Moments

Given the time in which we have written this chapter, we are particularly sensitized to the political climate where laws and policies that protect LGBTQ individuals and families are being challenged. Teachable moments can be invoked by social and political climates into the classroom in the form of critical debate among students (Fournier-Sylvester, 2013). Family studies courses provide unique opportunities for students to discuss real-time family policies that impact LGBTQ-parent families differentially than families who fall outside of this initialism and heterosexual-parent families. For instance, health insurance policies, adoption, work–family balance policies, elder care, end-of-life decisions, divorce, inheritance, civil and criminal laws provide contexts for students to explore power, privilege, discrimination, and implicit biases. These contexts also provide opportunities for students to identify and practice deconstructing subtle and overt heteronormative language and assumptions in the law. Teaching students how to methodically and logically question what is "normal" and what is "equitable" is imparting social justice values. Critical thinking contributes to teaching students that self-aware, conscientious, and equitable communities are possible and attainable (Fletcher & Russell, 2001).

## Ethical Considerations Beyond the Classroom

We began this review of articles using an intersectional and queer theoretical lens to describe our sample of articles, which happen to embody elements of transformational pedagogy. We would be remiss if we did not connect the knowledge offered by the scholars whose work we include in our sample to communities outside of the classroom. Classroom experiences are a microcosm for the development of ideas and skills that will play a role in what students will take into their personal and professional lives. Classroom spaces are provided to assist students in critical thinking, techniques, and self-reflection that is a necessary component to their professional growth. Taking a critical stance that is informed by feminist intellectual traditions is to take on a responsibility to demonstrate the necessity of social justice to future professionals who will attend to the safety and quality care of LGBTQ-parent families. In order to extend our pedagogical stance from the classroom into our communities, we suggest that instructors consider adopting a social justice framework identified by some accredited programs (Holloway & Gouthro, 2011) or integrating ethical provisions that mandate professionals affirm and support diverse families, in our case, LGBTQ-parent families, into their curriculum (Dentato et al., 2016; McGeorge, Carlson, & Maier, 2016). A discussion of professional ethical provisions also presents an opportunity for students to wrestle with notions of cultural humility (Mosher et al., 2017).

In conclusion, our review primarily reflects the perspective of instructors and their experiences incorporating content about LGBTQ individuals and LGBTQ-parent families into their curriculum. We have identified three themes in this pedagogical literature – reflectivity, reactivity, and reinventing. We end our rumination hoping that our final thoughts spark an interest in investigating how students may internalize our efforts to implement notions of inclusivity beyond the classroom – in their close relationships, families, and communities.

# Appendix A

## Pedagogy Articles

Allen, K. R. (1995). Opening the classroom closet: Sexual orientation and self-disclosure. *Family Relations, 44*, 136–141.

Allen, K. R., Floyd-Thomas, S. M., & Gillman, L. (2001). Teaching to transform: From volatility to solidarity in an interdisciplinary family studies classroom. *Family Relations, 50*, 317–325.

Case, K. A., Stewart, B., & Tittsworth, J. (2009). Transgender across the curriculum: A psychology for inclusion. *Teaching of Psychology, 36*, 117–121.

Eichstedt, J. L. (1996). Heterosexism and gay/lesbian/bisexual experiences: Teaching strategies and exercises. *Teaching Sociology, 24*, 384–388.

Few-Demo, A. L., Humble, Á. M., Curran, M. A., & Lloyd, S. A. (2016). Queer theory, intersectionality, and LGBT-parent families: Transformative critical pedagogy in family theory. *Journal of Family Theory & Review, 8*, 74–94.

Fletcher, A. C., & Russell, S. T. (2001). Incorporating issues of sexual orientation in the classroom: Challenges and solutions. *Family Relations, 50*, 34–40.

Goldstein, T. (1997). Unlearning homophobia through a pedagogy of anonymity. *Teaching Education, 9*, 115–124.

Hackman, H. W. (2012, Winter). Teaching LGBTQI issues in higher education: An interdependent framework. *Diversity & Democracy: Civic Learning for Shared Futures, 15*, 2–4.

Jaekel, K. (2016). What is normal, true, and right: A critical discourse analysis of students' written resistance strategies on LGBTQ topics. *International Journal of Qualitative Studies in Education, 29*, 845–859.

Kuvalanka, K. A., Goldberg, A. E., & Oswald, R. F. (2013). Incorporating LGBTQ issues into family courses: Instructor challenges and strategies relative to perceived teaching climate. *Family Relations, 62*, 699–713.

Liddle, B. J. (1997). Coming out in class: Disclosure of sexual orientation and teaching evaluations. *Teaching of Psychology, 24*, 32–35.

Linley, J. L., Nguyen, D., Brazelton, G. B., Becker, B., Renn, K., & Woodford, M. (2016). Faculty as sources of support for LGBTQ college students. *College Teaching, 64*, 55–63.

Lovaas, K. E., Baroudi, L., & Collins, S. M. (2002). Transcending heteronormativity in the classroom: Using queer and critical pedagogies to alleviate trans-anxieties. In E. P.

Cramer (Ed.), *Addressing homophobia and heterosexism on college campuses* (pp. 177–189). Binghamton, NY: Harrington Park Press.

McGeorge, C. R., Carlson, T. S., & Maier, C. A. (2016). Are we there yet? Faculty members' beliefs and teaching practices related to the ethical treatment of lesbian, gay, and bisexual clients. *Journal of Marital and Family Therapy, 43*, 322–337.

Mulcahy, M., Dalton, S., Kolbert, J., & Crothers, L. (2016). Informal mentoring for lesbian, gay, bisexual, and transgender students. *Journal of Educational Research, 109*, 405–412.

Quilty, A. (2015). Empowering realities: LGBTQ empowerment through a programme based on critically engaged, queer pedagogy. *Romanian Journal of Experimental Applied Psychology, 6*, 36–48.

Robinson, K. H., & Ferfolja, T. (2001). 'What are we doing this for?' Dealing with lesbian and gay issues in teacher education. *British Journal of Sociology of Education, 22*, 121–133.

Simoni, J. M. (1996). Confronting heterosexism in the teaching of psychology. *Teaching of Psychology, 23*, 220–226.

Wallace, D. L. (2002). Out in the academy: Heterosexism, invisibility, and double consciousness. *College English, 65*, 53–66.

Wentling, T., Windsor, E., Schilt, K., & Lucal, B. (2008). Teaching transgender. *Teaching Sociology, 36*, 49–57.

Zacko-Smith, J. D., & Smith, G. P. (2010, Fall). Recognizing and utilizing queer pedagogy. *Multicultural Education, 18*, 2–9.

## Pedagogy-Related Chapters and Books

Goldberg, A. E., & Allen, K. R. (Eds.). (2013). *LGBT-parent families: Innovations in research and implications for practice.* New York, NY: Springer.

Harbeck, K. M. (Ed.). (1992). *Coming out of the classroom closet: Gay and lesbian students, teachers and curricula.* Binghamton, NY: Teachers College Press.

Jennings, K. (Ed.). (1995). *One teacher in 10: Gay and lesbian educators tell their stories.* Boston, MA: Alyson.

Kumashiro, K. (2002). *Troubling education: Queer activism and antioppressive pedagogy.* New York, NY: Routledge-Falmer.

Meyer, E. (2007). But I'm not gay: What straight teachers need to know about queer theory. In N. Rodriguez & W. Pinar (Eds.), *Queering straight teachers: Discourse and identity in education.* New York, NY: Peter Lang.

Oswald, R. (2010). Teaching about marriage inequality: A classroom simulation. In L. A. De Reus & L. B. Blume (Eds.), *Social, economic, and environmental justice for all families* (pp. 27–49). Ann Arbor, MI: Groves Conference on Marriage and Family.

Rodriguez, N., & Pinar, W. (Eds.). (2007). *Queering straight teachers: Discourse and identity in education.* New York, NY: Peter Lang.

Savin-Williams, R. C. (1993). Personal reflections on coming out, prejudice, and homophobia in the academic work place. In L. Diamant (Ed.), *Homosexual issues in the workplace* (pp. 225–241). Washington, DC: Taylor & Francis.

## Helping Professions Training and Curricula

Ben-Ari, A. T. (2001). Homosexuality and heterosexism: Views from academics in the helping professions. *British Journal of Social Work, 31*, 119–131.

Edwards, L. L., Robertson, J. A., Smith, P. M., & O'Brien, N. B. (2014). Marriage and family training programs and their integration of lesbian, gay, and bisexual identities. *Journal of Feminist Family Therapy, 26*, 3–27.

Godfrey, K., Haddock, S. A., Fisher, A., & Lund, L. (2006). Essential components of curricula for preparing therapists to work effectively with lesbian, gay, and bisexual clients: A

Delphi study. *Journal of Marital and Family Therapy, 32*, 491–504.

Goodwin, A. M., Kaestle, C. E., & Piercy, F. P. (2013). An exploration of feminist family therapists' resistance to and collusion with oppression. *Journal of Feminist Family Therapy, 25*, 233–256.

McGeorge, C., & Carlson, T. S. (2011). Deconstructing heterosexism: Becoming an LGB affirmative heterosexual couple and family therapist. *Journal of Marital and Family Therapy, 37*, 14–26.

# References

Allen, K. R. (1995). Opening the classroom closet: Sexual orientation and self-disclosure. *Family Relations, 44*, 136–141. https://doi.org/10.2307/584799

Allen, K. R. (2000). A conscious and inclusive family studies. *Journal of Marriage and Family, 62*, 4–17. https://doi.org/10.1111/j.1741-3737.2000.00004.x

Allen, K. R., & Farnsworth, E. B. (1993). Reflexivity in teaching about families. *Family Relations, 42*, 351–356. https://doi.org/10.2307/585566

Allen, K. R., Floyd-Thomas, S. M., & Gillman, L. (2001). Teaching to transform: From volatility to solidarity in an interdisciplinary family studies classroom. *Family Relations, 50*, 317–325. https://doi.org/10.1111/j.1741-3729.2001.00317.x

Allen, K. R., Lloyd, S. A., & Few, A. L. (2009). Reclaiming feminist theory, method, and praxis for family studies. In S. A. Lloyd, A. L. Few, & K. R. Allen (Eds.), *Handbook of feminist family studies* (pp. 3–17). Thousand Oaks, CA: Sage.

Bauer, K., & Clancy, K. (2018). Teaching race and social justice at a predominantly white institution. *Journal of Political Science Education, 14*, 72–85. https://doi.org/10.1080/15512169.2017.1358175

Ben-Ari, A. T. (2001). Homosexuality and heterosexism: Views from academics in the helping professions. *British Journal of Social Work, 31*, 119–131.

Blumer, H. (1969). *Symbolic interactionism: Perspective and method*. Englewood Cliffs, NJ: Prentice-Hall.

Boucher, M. J. (2011). Teaching 'trans issues': An intersectional and systems-based approach. *New Directions for Teaching & Learning, 2011*, 65–75. https://doi.org/10.1002/tl.434

Bowleg, L. (2012). The problem with the phrase women and minorities: Intersectionality-an important theoretical framework for public health. *American Journal of Public Health, 102*, 1267–1273. https://doi.org/10.2105/AJPH.2012.300750

Butler, J. (2001). *Gender trouble: Feminism and subversion of identity*. Hoboken, NJ: Taylor & Francis.

Case, K. A., Stewart, B., & Tittsworth, J. (2009). Transgender across the curriculum: A psychology for inclusion. *Teaching of Psychology, 36*, 117–121.

Collins, P. H. (1990). *Black feminist thought: Knowledge, consciousness, and the politics of empowerment*. London, UK: Unwin Hyman.

Collins, P. H., & Bilge, S. (2016). *Intersectionality*. Cambridge, UK: Polity Press.

Coston, B., & Kimmel, M. (2012). Seeing privilege where it isn't: Marginalized masculinities and the intersections of privilege. *Journal of Social Issues, 68*, 97–111. https://doi.org/10.1111/j.1540-4560.2011.01738.x

Craven, S. (2019). Intersectionality and identity: Critical considerations in teaching introduction to women's and gender studies. *Frontiers: A Journal of Women Studies, 40*, 200–228. https://doi.org/10.5250/fronjwomestud.40.1.0200

Crenshaw, K. (1993). Demarginalizing the interaction of race and sex: A Black feminist critique of antidiscrimination doctrine, feminist theory, and anti-racist politics. In D. Weisberg (Ed.), *Feminist legal theory: Foundations* (pp. 383–411). Philadelphia, PA: Temple University Press.

Dashow, J. (2017, November 13). *New FBI data shows increased reported incidents of anti-LGBTQ hate crimes in 2016*. Retrieved from https://www.hrc.org/blog/new-fbi-data-shows-increased-reported-incidents-of-anti-lgbtq-hate-crimes-i

Dentato, M. P., Craig, S. L., Lloyd, M. R., Kelly, B. L., Wright, C., & Austin, A. (2016). Homophobia within schools of social work: The critical need for affirming classroom settings and effective preparation for service with the LGBTQ community. *Social Work Education, 35*, 672–692. https://doi.org/10.1080/02615479.2016.1150452

Dozono, T. (2017). Teaching alternative and indigenous gender systems in world history: A queer approach. *History Teacher, 50*, 425–448. Retrieved from http://www.societyforhistoryeducation.org/pdfs/M17_Dozono.pdf

Eeden-Moorefield, B., Few-Demo, A. L., Benson, K., & Lummer, S. (2018). A content analysis of LGBT family research in top family journals 2000–2015. *Journal of Family Issues, 39*, 1374–1395. https://doi.org/10.1177/0192513X17710284

Eichstedt, J. L. (1996). Heterosexism and gay/lesbian/bisexual experiences: Teaching strategies and exercises. *Teaching Sociology, 24*, 384–388.

Few-Demo, A. L. (2014). Intersectionality as the "new" critical approach in feminist family studies: Evolving racial/ethnic feminisms and critical race theories. *Journal of Family Theory & Review, 6*, 169–183. https://doi.org/10.1111/jftr.12039

Few-Demo, A. L., Humble, A., Curran, M., & Lloyd, S. (2016). Queer theory, intersectionality, and LGBT-parent families: Stretching and challenging family theories. *Journal of Family Theory and Review, 8*, 74–94. https://doi.org/10.1111/jftr.12127

Fletcher, A. C., & Russell, S. T. (2001). Incorporating issues of sexual orientation in the classroom:

Challenges and solutions. *Family Relations, 50*, 34–40. https://doi.org/10.1111/j.1741-3729.2001.00034.x

Forbes, K. (2018). Exploring first year undergraduate students' conceptualizations of critical thinking skills. *International Journal of Teaching & Learning in Higher Education, 30*, 443–442. Retrieved from http://www.isetl.org/ijtlhe/

Fournier-Sylvester, N. (2013). Daring to debate: Strategies for teaching controversial issues in the classroom. *College Quarterly, 16*, 1–7. Retrieved at https://scinapse.io/papers/321379127

Gates, T. G. (2011). Coming out in the social work classroom: Reclaiming wholeness and finding the teacher within. *Social Work Education, 30*, 70–82. https://doi.org/10.1080/02615471003721202

Giroux, H. A. (1994). *Disturbing pleasures: Learning popular culture.* New York, NY: Routledge.

Goldberg, A. E., & Allen, K. R. (2018). Teaching undergraduates about LGBTQ identities, families, and intersectionality. *Family Relations, 67*, 176–191. https://doi.org/10.1111/fare.12224

Goldstein, T. (1997). Unlearning homophobia through a pedagogy of anonymity. *Teaching Education, 9*, 115–124.

Gomez-Lanier, L. (2018). Building collaboration in the flipped classroom: A case study. *International Journal for the Scholarship of Teaching & Learning, 12*, 1–9. https://doi.org/10.20429/ijsotl.2018.120207

Hale, M. (2018). Thwarting plagiarism in the humanities classroom: Storyboards, scaffolding, and a death fair. *Journal of the Scholarship of Teaching and Learning, 18*, 86–110. https://doi.org/10.14434/josotl.v18i4.23174

Holloway, S. M., & Gouthro, P. A. (2011). Teaching resistant novice educators to be critically reflective. *Discourse: Studies in The Cultural Politics of Education, 32*, 29–41. https://doi.org/10.1080/01596306.2011.537069

Human Rights Campaign. (n.d.-a). *Trump's timeline of hate.* Retrieved from https://www.hrc.org/timelines/trump

Hull, G., Bell-Scott, P., & Smith, B. (Eds.). (1982). *All the women are White, all the Blacks are men, but some of us are brave.* New York, NY: Feminist Press.

Human Rights Campaign. (n.d.-b). *New FBI data shows increased reported incidents of anti-LGBT hate crimes.* Retrieved from https://www.hrc.org/blog/new-fbi-data-shows-increased-reported-incidents-of-anti-lgbtq-hate-crimes-i

Itsowitz, C. (2017, January 20). *LGBT rights page disappears from White House web site.* Retrieved from https://www.washingtonpost.com/local/2017/live-updates/politics/live-coverage-of-trumps-inauguration/lgbt-rights-page-disappears-from-white-house-web-site/?noredirect=on&utm_term=.408ba6446450

Jaekel, K. (2016). What is normal, true, and right: A critical discourse analysis of students' written resistance strategies on LGBTQ topics. *International Journal of Qualitative Studies in Education, 29*, 845–859. https://doi.org/10.1080/09518398.2016.1162868

Johnson, S. (2009). Between a rock and a hard place. *Feminism & Psychology, 19*, 186–189. https://doi.org/10.1177/0959353509102195

Kumashiro, K. K. (2000). Toward a theory of anti-oppressive education. *Review of Educational Research, 70*, 25–53. https://doi.org/10.2307/1170593

Kuvalanka, K. A., Goldberg, A. E., & Oswald, R. F. (2013). Incorporating LGBTQ issues into family courses: Instructor challenges and strategies relative to perceived teaching climate. *Family Relations, 62*, 699–713. https://doi.org/10.1111/fare.12034

Lewis, M. M. (2011). Body of knowledge: Black queer feminist pedagogy, praxis, and embodied text. *Journal of Lesbian Studies, 15*, 49–57. https://doi.org/10.1080/10894160.2010.508411

Liddle, B. J. (2009). Coming out in class: Disclosure of sexual orientation and teaching evaluations. *Teaching of Psychology, 24*, 32–35.

Linder, C. (2018). Power-conscious and intersectional approaches to supporting student activists: Considerations for learning and development. *Journal of Diversity in Higher Education, 12*, 17–26. https://doi.org/10.1037/dhe0000082

Linley, J. L., Nguyen, D., Brazelton, G. B., Becker, B., Renn, K., & Woodford, M. (2016). Faculty as sources of support for LGBTQ college students. *College Teaching, 64*, 55–63. https://doi.org/10.1080/87567555.2015.1078275

Louis, W. R., Mavor, K. I., La Macchia, S. T., & Amiot, C. E. (2014). Social justice and psychology: What is, and what should be. *Journal of Theoretical and Philosophical Psychology, 34*, 14–27. https://doi.org/10.1037/a0033033

Lovaas, K. E., Baroudi, L., & Collins, S. M. (2002). Transcending heteronormativity in the classroom: Using queer and critical pedagogies to alleviate trans-anxieties. In E. P. Cramer (Ed.), *Addressing homophobia and heterosexism on college campuses* (pp. 177–189). New York, NY: Harrington Park Press.

Lucey, T. A., & White, E. S. (2017). Mentorship in higher education: Compassionate approaches supporting culturally responsive pedagogy. *Multicultural Education, 24*, 11–17.

Martinez, S. (2014). Teaching a diversity course at a predominantly White institution: Success with statistics. *Journal of College Student Development, 55*, 75–78. https://doi.org/10.1353/csd.2014.0005

McGeorge, C., & Carlson, T. S. (2011). Deconstructing heterosexism: Becoming an LGB affirmative heterosexual couple and family therapist. *Journal of Marital and Family Therapy, 37*, 14–26. https://doi.org/1752-0606.2009.00149.x

McGeorge, C. R., Carlson, T. S., & Maier, C. A. (2016). Are we there yet? Faculty members' beliefs and teaching practices related to the ethical treatment of lesbian, gay, and bisexual clients. *Journal of Marital and Family Therapy, 43*, 322–337. https://doi.org/10.1111/jmft.12197

Mezirow, J. (1990). How critical reflection triggers transformative learning. In J. Mezirow (Ed.), *Fostering critical reflection in adulthood: A guide to transformative and emancipatory learning* (pp. 1–20). San Francisco, CA: Jossey-Bass.

Mezirow, J. (2003). Transformative learning as discourse. *Journal of Transformative Education, 1,* 58–63. https://doi.org/10.1177/1541344603252172

Moradi, B., & Grzanka, P. R. (2017). Using intersectionality responsibly: Toward critical epistemology, structural analysis, and social justice activism. *Journal of Counseling Psychology, 64,* 500–513. https://doi.org/10.1037/cou0000203

Mosher, D. K., Hook, J. N., Captari, L. E., Davis, D. E., DeBlaere, C., & Owen, J. (2017). Cultural humility: A therapeutic framework for engaging diverse clients. *Practice Innovations, 2,* 221–233. https://doi.org/10.1037/pri0000055

Mulcahy, M., Dalton, S., Kolbert, J., & Crothers, L. (2016). Informal mentoring for lesbian, gay, bisexual, and transgender students. *Journal of Educational Research, 109,* 405–412. https://doi.org/10.1080/00220671.2014.979907

Orlov, J. M., & Allen, K. R. (2014). Being who I am: Effective teaching, learning, student support, and societal change through LGBQ faculty freedom. *Journal of Homosexuality, 61,* 1025–1052. https://doi.org/10.1080/00918369.2014.870850

Ortega, R. M., & Faller, K. C. (2011). Training child welfare workers from an intersectional cultural humility perspective: A paradigm shift. *Child Welfare, 90,* 27–49.

Oswald, R., Blume, L., & Marks, S. (2005). Decentering heteronormativity: A model for family studies. In V. L. Bengtson, A. C. Acock, K. R. Allen, P. Dilworth-Anderson, & D. M. Klein (Eds.), *Sourcebook of family theory & research* (pp. 143–165). Thousand Oaks, CA: Sage.

Oswald, R. F., Kuvalanka, K. A., Blume, L., & Berkowitz, D. (2009). Queering "the family". In S. A. Lloyd, A. Few, & K. Allen (Eds.), *Handbook of feminist family studies* (pp. 43–55). Thousand Oaks, CA: Sage.

Puntambekar, S., & Hübscher, R. (2005). Tools for scaffolding students in a complex learning environment: What have we gained and what have we missed? *Educational Psychologist, 40,* 1–12. https://doi.org/10.1080/13562517.2012.752726

Quilty, A. (2015). Empowering realities: LGBTQ empowerment through a programme based on critically engaged, queer pedagogy. *Romanian Journal of Experimental Applied Psychology, 6,* 36–48.

Robinson, K. H., & Ferfolja, T. (2001). 'What are we doing this for?' Dealing with lesbian and gay issues in teacher education. *British Journal of Sociology of Education, 22,* 121–133.

Rodriguez, N. S., & Huemmer, J. (2019). Pedagogy of the depressed: An examination of critical pedagogy in higher ed's diversity-centered classrooms post-trump. *Pedagogy, Culture & Society, 27,* 133–149. https://doi.org/10.1080/14681366.2018.1446041

Russ, T. L., Simonds, C. J., & Hunt, S. K. (2002). Coming out in the classroom … an occupational hazard?: The influence of sexual orientation on teacher credibility and perceived student learning. *Communication Education, 51,* 311–324. https://doi.org/10.1080/03634520216516

Sand, S. (2009). To reveal or not to reveal, that is the question. *Lesbian & Gay Psychology Review, 10,* 23–26.

Sapon-Shevin, M. (2004). Being out, being silent, being strategic: Troubling the difference. *Journal of Gay & Lesbian Issues in Education, 2,* 73–77. https://doi.org/10.1300/J367v02n02_07

Sapp, J. (2001). The interconnection between personal liberation and social change: Coming out in the classroom as a transformative act. *Multicultural Education, 9,* 16–22.

Sciame-Giesecke, S., Roden, D., & Parkison, K. (2009). Infusing diversity into the curriculum: What are faculty members actually doing? *Journal of Diversity in Higher Education, 2,* 156–165. https://doi.org/10.1037/a0016042

Shlasko, G. D. (2005). Queer (v.) pedagogy. *Equity & Excellence in Education, 38,* 123–134. https://doi.org/10.1080/10665680590935098

Slavich, G. M., & Zimbardo, P. G. (2012). Transformational teaching: Theoretical underpinnings, basic principles, and core methods. *Educational Psychology Review, 24,* 569–608. https://doi.org/10.1007/s10648-012-9199-6

Simoni, J. M. (1996). Confronting heterosexism in the teaching of psychology. *Teaching of Psychology, 23,* 220–226.

Stone, L. (1994). Toward a transformational theory of teaching. In L. Stone (Ed.), *The education feminist reader* (pp. 221–228). New York, NY: Routledge.

Tasker, F., & Granville, J. (2011). Children's views of family relationships in lesbian-led families. *Journal of GLBT Family Studies, 7,* 182–199. https://doi.org/10.1080/1550428X.2011.540201

Tharp, D. S. (2015). Using critical discourse analysis to understand student resistance to diversity. *Multicultural Education, 23,* 2–8.

Vygotsky, L. (1978). *Mind in society: The development of higher psychological processes.* Cambridge, MA: Harvard University Press.

Wallace, D. L. (2002). Out in the academy: Heterosexism, invisibility, and double consciousness. *College English, 65,* 53–66.

Wentling, T., Windsor, E., Schilt, K., & Lucal, B. (2008). Teaching transgender. *Teaching Sociology, 36,* 49–57. https://doi.org/10.1177/0092055X0803600107

Zacko-Smith, J. D., & Smith, G. P. (2010, Fall). Recognizing and utilizing queer pedagogy. *Multicultural Education, 18,* 2–9.

# Part IV

# Methodology

# Multilevel Modeling Approaches to the Study of LGBTQ-Parent Families

JuliAnna Z. Smith, Abbie E. Goldberg, and Randi L. Garcia

One of the most central pursuits of family theory and research is to better understand and explore the dynamics of interpersonal family relationships. Understanding these relationships is furthered by collecting information on multiple family members (Jenkins et al., 2009). There is a growing body of LGBTQ research that draws from the experiences of multiple family members (Carone, Lingiardi, Chirumbolo, & Baiocco, 2018; Farr, 2017; Goldberg & Garcia, 2015, 2016; Pollitt, Robinson, & Umberson, 2018). Unfortunately, by their very nature, family members' experiences are interdependent, and this interdependence complicates the analysis of data from multiple family members (Atkins, 2005; Bolger & Shrout, 2007; Jenkins et al., 2009; Sayer & Klute, 2005). With the right analysis strategy, this interdependence can also be a rich source of information about family processes.

Data interdependence precludes the use of many statistical methods that assume the errors are independent, such as ordinary least squares (OLS) regression or standard analysis of variance (ANOVA). Several statistical methods that take into account the dependency in family members' outcomes are available to researchers and have become the standard in family research journals. Many of the most commonly used approaches, however, are easiest to employ when one distinguishes family members on the basis of some characteristic meaningful to the analyses (Sayer & Klute, 2005). For example, in parent/child dyads, one can easily distinguish dyad members on the basis of whether they are the parent or child (Shih, Quiñones-Camacho, Karan, & Davis, 2019). In research on heterosexual couples, partners are most commonly distinguished on the basis of gender (assuming a binary male/female conception of gender; Claxton, O'Rourke, Smith, & DeLongis, 2012; Kuo, Volling, & Gonzalez, 2017; Perry-Jenkins, Smith, Wadsworth, & Halpern, 2017; Raudenbush, Brennan, & Barnett, 1995). Such approaches to distinguishing partners on the basis of gender, however, are clearly not useful to researchers of same-sex couples. In some cases, same-sex partners may be distinguished on the basis of some other characteristic, such as biological versus nonbiological parent (Goldberg & Perry-Jenkins, 2007; Goldberg & Sayer, 2006), where that distinction is relevant to the analyses. In other cases, however, no such

J. Z. Smith (✉)
Independent Methodological Consultant, Amherst, MA, USA

A. E. Goldberg
Department of Psychology, Clark University, Worcester, MA, USA
e-mail: agoldberg@clarku.edu

R. L. Garcia
Department of Psychology, Smith College, Northampton, MA, USA
e-mail: rgarcia@smith.edu

A. E. Goldberg, K. R. Allen (eds.), *LGBTQ-Parent Families*,
https://doi.org/10.1007/978-3-030-35610-1_27

meaningful distinctions can be made – for example, in many analyses of same-sex nonparent couples or same-sex adoptive parents, wherein neither partner is the biological parent. In these instances, alternate statistical models must be employed.

This chapter discusses the challenges faced by researchers analyzing data from multiple family members, with a focus on couples. It addresses advances in research methods using multilevel modeling (MLM). MLM, which is a fairly straightforward extension of the more familiar OLS multiple regression, provides one of the more versatile and accessible approaches available to model couple and family data (Sayer & Klute, 2005). As such, it is becoming a common method for LGBTQ-parent family researchers to examine data collected from two (or more) individuals nested within a couple or family (e.g., Carone et al., 2018; Farr, 2017; Goldberg & Smith, 2017). We begin by discussing the role of MLM in family research, in general, and in dyadic (or paired) data, more specifically. Next, we consider some of the common difficulties encountered by scholars examining LGBTQ-parent family data. We then describe the basic multilevel models available to researchers analyzing (a) cross-sectional and (b) longitudinal dyadic data. Next, we address the application of these models to analyses of multiple informant data, when multiple family members provide reports of the same outcome. In addition, we present some considerations that researchers using these statistical methods should take into account.

## Multilevel Modeling in Family Research

The use of MLM became more common in family journals at the end of the last decade (e.g., Kretschmer & Pike, 2010; Soliz, Thorson, & Rittenour, 2009), a trend that has continued, particularly in research on heterosexual couples (e.g., Kuo et al., 2017; Perry-Jenkins et al., 2017). Yet the adoption of MLM by researchers who study LGBTQ couples and families was initially

somewhat slower. In part, this is because the area of LGBTQ couples and families was relatively new in the 2000s, and much of the early research was qualitative and exploratory as opposed to quantitative (see Goldberg, 2010, for a review). In addition, those studies that used quantitative methods tended to rely on fairly small sample sizes of LGBTQ couples and families (e.g., Goldberg & Sayer, 2006; Patterson, Sutfin, & Fulcher, 2004), thereby decreasing power and the ability to detect effects. Small sample sizes may lead researchers to use methods other than maximum likelihood methods, an estimation technique used in multilevel modeling, which perform best with large samples (Raudenbush, 2008). An additional barrier to using multilevel modeling with same-sex couples is when members of couples or dyads are not clearly distinguishable from one another on the basis of some central characteristic such as gender (i.e., members are "indistinguishable" or "exchangeable"). This scenario requires methods designed to take this indistinguishability into account. Treating dyad members as indistinguishable requires the use of MLM approaches that may be less familiar to many family researchers, including LGBTQ-focused researchers, given the field's overall focus on the (binary gender) based distinguishable model.

In comparison to MLM, structural equation modeling (SEM), an alternate method for the analysis of dyadic data, provides more flexibility in many areas, such as the ability to place constraints on estimates of all parameters of the model, a wider range of model fit indices, and a more sophisticated analysis of the effects of measurement error for latent variables (Ledermann & Kenny, 2017). Unfortunately, SEM is much more complex, can be challenging to learn, requires specialized software, and requires much larger sample sizes (over 200 cases, and therefore dyads, when analyzing latent variables) (Ledermann & Kenny, 2017). In addition, Ledermann and Kenny (2017) suggest that SEM is often more straightforward for the analysis of data from distinguishable dyads, whereas MLM is often more straightforward for indistinguishable members. Further, MLM is available in most software packages. Consequently, we will focus on MLM, although later in the chapter, we will briefly describe some types of analyses that can only be done in an SEM framework. For further discussion and helpful comparisons of the advantages of MLM versus SEM in examining dyadic data, see Ledermann and Kenny (2017), as well as Hong and Kim (2019).

A fairly large body of work discusses the application of MLM to heterosexual couples using models for distinguishable dyads (Bolger & Shrout, 2007; Hong & Kim, 2019; Ledermann & Kenny, 2017; Raudenbush et al., 1995; Sayer & Klute, 2005). Much less work is available on its application to indistinguishable couples (Kenny, Kashy, & Cook, 2006; Ledermann & Kenny, 2017). There is a clear need to bring together recent advances in several areas: (a) the analyses of indistinguishable dyads; (b) advances in longitudinal analyses of indistinguishable dyads (Kashy, Donnellan, Burt, & McGue, 2008); (c) the analyses of mixed samples, such as analyses including female couples, male couples, and heterosexual couples (Ledermann, Rudaz, & Grob, 2017; West, Popp, & Kenny, 2008); (d) multiple informant models (Georgiades, Boyle, Jenkins, Sanford, & Lipman, 2008); and (e) the important limitations to using MLM (Hong & Kim, 2019; Ledermann & Kenny, 2017), especially when examining dyads and other small groups (Raudenbush, 2008). Consequently, this chapter focuses on multilevel modeling approaches to analyzing dyadic data when couple members can be considered indistinguishable. While these approaches are valuable for the study of same-sex couples, they are also useful in the study of twins, friends, roommates, and other types of relationships where members cannot be distinguished from each other based on some meaningful characteristic (Kenny et al., 2006). For this reason, the information presented in this chapter may be useful and relevant to family scholars more generally.

Family theorists from a wide range of perspectives, including family systems theory, life course theory, social exchange theory, symbolic interaction theory, conflict theory, and social ecological theory, have long been interested in the relationships between family members and how those relationships affect family members. For example, family systems theory views individuals as part, not only of a family, but also of multiple, mutually influencing family subsystems (Cox & Paley, 1997). Individuals' experiences and their dyadic relationships with other family members affect not only those directly involved but other individuals and relationships within the family system as well. Life course theory examines changes in the intertwined lives of family members over the life span (Bengtson & Allen, 1993). Finally, ecological theory posits the importance of understanding the family as a central social context that influences all of the individuals within it (Bronfenbrenner, 1988). Research examining data from multiple family members allows researchers to start to tease apart these complex family relationships. For example, Georgiades et al. (2008) examined multiple family members' reports of family functioning ($N = 26,614$ individuals in 11,023 families). Using MLM enabled them to distinguish shared perceptions of family functioning from unique individual perceptions.

Collecting information from more than one individual per family allows for the examination of the association between family members' scores (Bolger & Shrout, 2007). Multilevel modeling provides a means of disentangling the variability in the outcome. The variability in the outcome (i.e., the variance) is due to two sources: within-family variability and between-family variability. MLM methods provide a means for separating the variability in the outcome into these two sources, as well as appropriately testing both family-level and individual-level predictors of that variability.[1] It is not surprising, therefore, that MLM has become widely used in family research (e.g., Kretschmer & Pike, 2010; Kuo et al., 2017; Perry-Jenkins et al., 2017). The

---

[1]It should be noted, however, that one should be wary of the inference tests of the parameter estimates of variance components based on models examining dyadic data, as they are known to be low powered due to the small number of individuals per group/dyad (Maas & Hox, 2005; Raudenbush, 2008). The fixed effects, however, are quite reliable.

nature of family research has subsequently led to adaptations of MLM approaches to suit the specialized needs of this field. This has occurred, most notably, in the area of modeling couple data (or dyadic data more generally), starting with the early models to examine cross-sectional (Barnett, Marshall, Raudenbush, & Brennan, 1993) and longitudinal (Raudenbush et al., 1995) data, and developing to address more specific needs in family research, such as the examination of diary data (Bolger & Shrout, 2007) or the complex interactions between partners in the Actor–Partner Interdependence Model (APIM; Campbell & Kashy, 2002; Cook & Kenny, 2005; Garcia, Kenny, & Ledermann, 2015).

## Key Issues in Analyzing Data from LGBTQ Couples and Families

### The Issue of Dependence

It is important to clarify why special statistical methods may be required when analyzing data from multiple family members. One of the central assumptions underlying conventional statistical methods such as OLS regression and standard ANOVAs is that the residuals (errors) are independent. This assumption is untenable in the case of dyadic or family data. Partners who are in a relationship are likely to have outcome scores that are similar, and this similarity or dependency must be taken into account when performing statistical analyses. Failure to take into account dependence in the outcome scores results in inaccurate estimates of the standard errors leading to both Type I and Type II errors, depending on the direction of the dependence and level of predictor variable (Griffin & Gonzalez, 1995; Kenny et al., 2006; Kenny & Judd, 1986). In addition, failure to account for dependency in the outcome can also lead to incorrect estimates of effect sizes (Kenny et al., 2006).

There are a number of reasons why family members' outcomes may be associated (Kenny et al., 2006). For example, partners may have chosen each other at least partly on the basis of

shared interests in community involvement (mate selection). Alternately, a small family income may affect the financial confidence of all of the members of a particular family (shared context). Similarly, family members who live together are likely to be affected by each other's moods and behavior (mutual influence), perhaps even in the negative direction (e.g., individual time spent on housework). Statistical methods such as paired sample t-tests and repeated-measures ANOVA do adjust the estimates for the dependency in the outcome and can be used to answer many basic research questions. For example, a researcher may investigate if lesbian mothers and their teen daughters have mean differences in the level of conflict they report in their relationship. MLM provides a means of better understanding the relationship between those two family members' reports on the same outcome, breaking down the variance into that which occurs within families and that which occurs between families. In addition, it enables the examination of the effects of both individual-level (e.g., age or stress level) and family-level (e.g., number of children or family income) variables (Kenny et al., 2006; Sayer & Klute, 2005). In other words, instead of treating the dependence between family members' reports as a nuisance to be adjusted for, MLM enables researchers to treat this dependence as interesting in its own right and to explore predictors of it.

### The Issue of Distinguishability

When studying same-sex couples, researchers are often faced with an additional methodological difficulty. For example, most analyses of heterosexual couples within family studies distinguish between the two members of the couple on the basis of a binary distinction between male and female genders (Claxton et al., 2012; Kuo et al., 2017; Perry-Jenkins et al., 2017; Raudenbush et al., 1995). In research on same-sex couples, distinguishing partners by gender is not an option. In some instances, same-sex partners should be distinguished on the basis of some other characteristic, if that distinction is important for the analyses conducted. For example, in Abbie Goldberg's work on lesbian couples who used alternative insemination to become parents ($N = 29–34$ couples), she distinguished between the biological mothers and the nonbiological mothers and found differential predictors of relationship quality and mental health across the transition to parenthood (Goldberg & Sayer, 2006; Goldberg & Smith, 2008a). Other distinguishing features that may be relevant to analyses might be work status (e.g., working/not working, in single-earner couples), primary/secondary child caregiver status, or diseased/not diseased (O'Rourke et al., 2010).

It is important that the distinction between dyad members is justified by the research questions being asked and the analyses being conducted and is thereby meaningful in a substantive sense. As it is always possible to find some distinguishing feature, however arbitrary, it is important to carefully evaluate whether the distinguishing feature is in fact relevant.[2] There are, for example, times when distinguishing partners within heterosexual couples based on gender may not be relevant to the analyses being conducted (Atkins, 2005; Kenny et al., 2006). The use of a particular distinguishing feature should be supported by the theoretical frameworks guiding the research, by prior research findings suggesting that this is a meaningful distinction, and by empirical investigation of the data being examined (Kenny et al., 2006). Kenny and Ledermann (2010) contend that distinguishability must be supported empirically. In other words, if dyad members are to be treated as distinguishable in the analyses, distinguishability analyses should be conducted to give empirical support for this decision. Kenny et al. (2006) describe an

Omnibus Test of Distinguishability conducted using SEM that examines the means, variances, covariances, effect estimates, and intercepts in a model in order to show that the data support distinguishing dyad members. MLM techniques can also be used to test for distinguishability, although distinguishability in predictor variable means and variances cannot be assessed using MLM (Kenny et al., 2006).

There are also methods that can be used within the context of multilevel modeling to empirically support the use of a particular feature to distinguish between dyad members. Consider, for example, Goldberg and Smith's (2008b) analyses of social support and well-being in lesbian inseminating couples, where partners were distinguished by whether or not they were the biological mother of the child. The MLM approach for distinguishable dyads provides separate parameter estimates for the two partners based on the distinguishing feature (in our example, biological mother or nonbiological mother). Researchers can test whether these estimates are statistically significantly different from each other, by fitting a second model, in which these two separate parameter estimates are constrained to be equal. Model comparison tests are then used to determine which model is a better fit to the data. If there is no significant decrement in model fit, then there is not enough of a difference in the partners' estimates to justify the estimation of two separate parameters. If there is a decrement in model fit, this supports the decision to treat partners as being meaningfully distinguished on the basis of the selected distinguishing feature (i.e., in this case, biological versus nonbiological mother).

Even when there are theoretical and empirical reasons to distinguish between partners, it is possible that researchers will find that only some parameter estimates differ between them. Those parameters that are not found to be significantly different can then be constrained to be equal, creating a more parsimonious model. Such an approach was used in Goldberg and Smith's (2008a) examination of changes in the anxiety of lesbian inseminating couples over time ($N = 34$

---

[2]One question that is worth considering, for researchers, is whether partners in so-called heterosexual or different-sex couples actually identify as male and female. Assumptions about gender identity are routinely made in family research – and should perhaps be revisited and avoided by explicitly asking parents or partners about their self-identified gender, with a range of possible gender identity options.

couples). Their analyses revealed that while the effect of some factors such as neuroticism did not significantly differ for biological and nonbiological lesbian mothers, other factors did have a differential effect on biological and nonbiological mothers. Work hours and proportional contribution to housework were related to higher levels of anxiety only for biological mothers, while high infant distress and low instrumental social support were related to greater increases in anxiety only in nonbiological mothers. Such differential findings strongly supported the decision to distinguish partners on the basis of whether or not they were the biological mother.

## MLM Approaches to Analyzing Data from Indistinguishable Dyads

As noted, in many cases in LGBTQ couple research, a salient, distinguishing feature will not be available for researchers. Having a distinguishing feature allows the researcher to assign each member to a group based on that distinction and then examine these separate groups in the analyses. As a result, some researchers may be tempted to deal with the lack of a distinguishing feature on which to assign dyad members to groups by randomly assigning members to one of the two groups (e.g., partner A and partner B) and then treating them as if they were distinguishable or by using an arbitrary characteristic to distinguish them (see Kenny et al., 2006). The problem with such an approach is that it can lead to erroneous findings. The assignment to a group is purely arbitrary and, yet, findings will differ depending on how the individuals are assigned. For example, when examining couple data, one of the first questions a researcher may want to consider is "How correlated are partners' scores?" Once the researcher has distinguished between the two partners and assigned them to separate groups, the researcher can simply examine the correlation between the two partners' scores. Unfortunately, however, the estimate of this correlation will differ depending on the way in which partners were assigned to groups (see Kenny et al., 2006, for a more detailed discussion of this issue).

## Cross-sectional Model for Indistinguishable Dyads

Multilevel modeling provides a relatively simple extension of OLS regression, which takes into account the nesting of data within families or couples. In this statistical approach, the variance in the outcome is partitioned into the variance that occurs *within* couples (how partners differ from each other) and the variance that occurs *between* couples (how couples differ from each other). Predictors, both those that vary by couples (such as number of children and length of relationship) and by partner (such as age or mental health status), can then be added to explain this variance. In the model for the cross-sectional analysis of dyadic data, the multilevel model generally used to examine individuals who are nested within groups (such as students within classrooms, workers within organizations, or patients within hospitals) is commonly adapted to deal with the fact that dependence in dyads can be negative (because there are exactly two members in each group). For example, one common adaptation is in the specification of the error structure (i.e., using compound symmetry), whereby the dyad members' residuals (errors) are modeled as correlated as opposed to including a random dyad intercept in the model as would be the more traditional MLM specification. Group/dyad variance can only be positive and thus, the random intercept model can only handle positive dependence, but in a correlated errors model it can accommodate negative dyadic dependence as well as positive dependence. The random intercept model is described in detail below.

The MLM approach to indistinguishable dyads is actually a simpler model, in terms of the number of parameters to be estimated, than the one more commonly used model for distinguishable dyads (Kenny et al., 2006). Several studies of same-sex couples have used this approach (e.g., Goldberg & Smith, 2008b, 2009b, 2017; Kurdek, 1998). For example, in his early pioneering work in the field, Lawrence Kurdek (2003) used this approach to analyze differences between gay and lesbian cohabiting partners' relationship beliefs, conflict resolution strategies, and level of perceived social support variables in a sample of 80 gay male and 53 lesbian couples.

| | FAMID | MEMBER | FAMSUP | A1AGE | P1AGE | A1EDUC | P1EDUC | A1PINC | P1PINC |
|---|---|---|---|---|---|---|---|---|---|
| 1 | 1 | 1 | 3.10 | 43 | 43 | 5 | 5 | $9.50 | 2.10 |
| 2 | 1 | 2 | 1.45 | 43 | 43 | 5 | 5 | $2.10 | 9.50 |
| 3 | 2 | 1 | 3.50 | 40 | 53 | 5 | 6 | $9.00 | 14.00 |
| 4 | 2 | 2 | 1.95 | 53 | 40 | 6 | 5 | $14.00 | 9.00 |
| 5 | 3 | 1 | 2.85 | 36 | 37 | 5 | 6 | $4.50 | 9.50 |
| 6 | 3 | 2 | 3.50 | 37 | 36 | 6 | 5 | $9.50 | 4.50 |
| 7 | 4 | 1 | 1.85 | 38 | 41 | 4 | 2 | $6.60 | 3.85 |
| 8 | 4 | 2 | 3.55 | 41 | 38 | 2 | 4 | $3.85 | 6.60 |

**Fig. 1** Example of a Level-1 (within-couples) data file for the analysis of cross-sectional dyadic data

**Fig. 2** Example of a Level-2 (between-couples) data file for the analysis of cross-sectional dyadic data

| | FAMILYID | lesbian | PrivAdop | PubAdopt | IntAdopt |
|---|---|---|---|---|---|
| 1 | 1 | 1 | 1 | 0 | 0 |
| 2 | 2 | 1 | 1 | 0 | 0 |
| 3 | 3 | 1 | 0 | 0 | 1 |
| 4 | 4 | 1 | 1 | 0 | 0 |
| 5 | 5 | 1 | 1 | 0 | 0 |
| 6 | 6 | 1 | 0 | 1 | 1 |
| 7 | 7 | 1 | 0 | 0 | 1 |
| 8 | 8 | 1 | 1 | 0 | 0 |

The most basic model is an unconditional model, with no predictors at either level; this is often referred to as a random intercept model (Raudenbush & Bryk, 2002). This model provides estimates for the grand mean of the outcome across all couples as well as estimates for the two sources of variability: within-couples and between-couples. We calculate the proportion of variance that is due to between-group differences, or the intraclass correlation coefficient (ICC), from these two estimates of variability: the between-couples variance divided by the total variance (the sum of the within-couples and between-couples variances).[3] The ICC provides two central pieces of information: (a) the extent of the dependence within couples on the outcome and (b) the proportion of variance that lies between couples versus the proportion that lies within couples. Any ICC larger than a few percentage points indicates a degree of dependence on the data that cannot be overlooked and justifies the use of MLM.

It is easiest to understand multilevel models if one looks at the levels separately. In the cross-sectional model for dyads, Level 1 provides the within-couple model, in which individual responses are nested within couples, while Level 2 provides the between-couples model. Examining the structure of the data for the two levels, as required by the software program HLM, can help one better understand the distinction between these levels; see Figs. 1 and 2 (Raudenbush, Bryk, & Congdon, 2004). In Eq. (1) of the unconditional model, the intercept, $\beta_{0j}$, represents average outcome score for each couple, and $r_{ij}$ represents the deviation of each member of the couple from the couple average. This intercept is treated as randomly varying; that is, it is allowed to take on different values for each couple. The intercepts that are estimated for each

---

[3]The ICC is simply the estimate of the error correlation in the dyadic model that parameterizes the dependence within couples by way of a residual correlation as opposed to a between-couples variance term. The ICC estimates from these two approaches will be the same when maximum likelihood estimation is used in both models.

couple are treated as an outcome variable at Level 2. The intercept in the Level-2 equation, Eq. (2), $\gamma_{00}$, provides an estimate of the average outcome score across couples and $u_{0j}$ represents the deviation of each couple from the overall average across all couples.

Level 1 (*within* couples; Eq. 1):

$$Y_{ij} = \beta_{0j} + r_{ij} \tag{1}$$

Level 2 (*between* couples; Eq. 2):

$$\beta_{0j} = \gamma_{00} + u_{0j} \tag{2}$$

where $Y_{ij}$ represents the outcome score of partner $i$ in dyad $j$, where $i = 1, 2$ for the two members of the dyad. In addition to the above "fixed effect" estimate (e.g., the $\gamma_{00}$), estimates of the variance of the "random effects" both within and between couples are provided (e.g., the variance of the $r_{ij}$'s and the $u_{0j}$'s). Predictors can then be added to the model, with those that vary within couples (e.g., partners' ages) added at Level 1 (Eq. 3):

$$Y_{ij} = \beta_{0j} + \beta_{1j} \left( \text{Age} \right)_{ij} + r_{ij} \tag{3}$$

and those that vary between couples (e.g., length of time in a relationship together) added at Level 2 (Eq. 4):

$$\beta_{0j} = \gamma_{00} + \gamma_{01} \left( \text{Relationship duration} \right)_{j} + u_{0j} \tag{4}$$

We can add a variable at Level 2 that provides us with a way to tease out important group differences in the couple averages, such as the type of couple. For example, in Abbie Goldberg's research on lesbian, gay male, and heterosexual adoptive couples, this multilevel modeling approach is used to provide estimates of means for each group (on reports of love, conflict, and ambivalence), as well as to test for differences in these means (Goldberg, Smith, & Kashy, 2010). To examine group means, a dichotomous variable is created that indicates the type of couple (e.g., gay male or heterosexual), which is then entered at Level 2. The intercept provides the mean level of the outcome for the reference group (lesbian, in this case), while the coefficient for the predictor (e.g., gay male) indicates the difference between that group and the reference group. An

alternative parameterization of the effects of couple type suggested by West et al. (2008) is described below.

## Considering Partner Effects

Personal relationship theory, which examines the predictors, processes, and outcomes of close relationships, has shown the importance of considering the role of partner characteristics in dyadic research (Kenny & Cook, 1999). It may not be immediately evident how such a model can be used to examine partner effects – that is, the association between one partner's predictor with the other partner's outcome score. It is helpful to think of these associations within the context of the Actor–Partner Interdependence Model (APIM; Campbell & Kashy, 2002; Cook & Kenny, 2005). Using this approach, one simultaneously considers the respondent's value on a predictor, such as age, as well as the respondent's partner's value on this predictor in relation to the outcome. For example, Fergus, Lewis, Darbes, and Kral (2009) found that in examining the HIV risk of gay men ($N = 59$ couples), it was important to consider not only individuals' own integration into the gay community, but also their partners' integration. In the MLM approach, both of these predictors are entered into the model at Level 1 (Kenny et al., 2006).

Level 1 (within couples; Eq. 5):

$$\begin{aligned} Y_{ij} = \beta_{0j} + \beta_{1j} \left( \text{Actor race} \right)_{ij} \\ + \beta_{2j} \left( \text{Partner race} \right)_{ij} + r_{ij} \end{aligned} \tag{5}$$

Level 2 (between couples; Eq. 6):

$$\begin{aligned} \beta_{0j} &= \gamma_{00} + u_{0ij} \\ \beta_{1j} &= \gamma_{10} \\ \beta_{2j} &= \gamma_{20} \end{aligned} \tag{6}$$

The APIM goes further, however, suggesting that it is necessary not only to consider both actor and partner characteristics as main effects, but also to consider the interaction between them (Garcia et al., 2015). The interaction term models the specific pairing of the two individuals in the couple. For example, the effect of parents' disciplinary style on the child's behavior may vary as a function of their partners' disciplinary style. In such a case, it would be important to test an interaction between actors' disciplinary style and partners' disciplinary style. Whenever the theoretical framework guiding the analyses and past research suggest the potential importance of such an interaction and sample size permits its inclusion, it is crucial that the interaction term be included (Cook & Kenny, 2005).

## Modeling (Binary) Gender and Sexual Orientation Using the APIM Approach

Research in the field of personal relationships extended the APIM approach specifically to address the role of gender and sexual orientation (particularly in the area of partner preferences; West et al., 2008). West et al. (2008) argue for the need to include same-sex couples in research on the effects of partner gender (using a binary approach to gender). In addition, they contend that both actor gender and partner gender should be considered in analyses that examine data from both heterosexual (distinguishable) and same-sex (indistinguishable) couples. They propose what they term a "factorial method" that considers respondent gender, partner gender, and "dyad gender" (i.e., the difference between same-gender and different-gender respondents, where dyad gender is the interaction between actor and partner gender). They point out that examining group differences between female, male, and heterosexual couples without taking into account the gender differences within heterosexual couples may lead to an inadequate understanding of the data, as it conflates the scores for men and women within heterosexual couples. West and colleagues provide an example in which findings from a group difference approach (i.e., looking only at differences between female, male, and heterosexual couples) showed that female and male same-sex couples placed less importance on the social value of a partner (e.g., appeal to friends,

similar social class background, financial worth) than heterosexual couples ($N = 784$ female couples, 969 male couples, and 4292 heterosexual couples). When within-dyad gender differences are taken into account, however, the results showed that it was not that lesbians and gay men placed less emphasis on the social value of a partner than heterosexuals, but that heterosexual *women* placed much more emphasis on the social value of a partner than gay men and heterosexual men, with lesbians placing slightly more emphasis on the social value than gay men.

Randi Garcia et al. (2015) delve further into the role of moderators in the APIM. Specifically, they describe many patterns of moderation effects that can be tested when adding moderators to the indistinguishable and distinguishable dyad APIMs, and they discuss modeling techniques using both MLM and SEM.

## Examining Change Over Time in Indistinguishable Dyads

To get a better grasp of longitudinal multilevel models for dyadic data, it is useful to understand how change is modeled in a basic (nondyadic) multilevel model. The cross-sectional approach to dyads considered individuals nested within dyads, modeling individuals at Level 1 and couples at Level 2. When examining change over time, we are looking at multiple time points nested within each individual. Level-1 models change within individuals, while Level-2 models differences in change between individuals. There are essentially two MLM approaches to modeling change over time within dyads: (a) a 2-level model in which trajectories of change for both dyad members are modeled at Level 1, while between-dyad differences in change are modeled at Level 2 (Raudenbush et al., 1995); and (b) a 3-level model in which change over time within each individual is modeled at Level 1, individuals within dyads at Level 2, and between-dyad differences at Level 3 (Atkins, 2005; Kurdek, 1998; Simpson, Atkins, Gattis, & Christensen, 2008).

While conceptually, the 3-level approach might appear to make perfect sense, there is a statistical problem in terms of the random effects. That is, while it is a 3-level model in terms of the data structure, it is only a 2-level model in terms of the within-level variation. Consequently, most articles on dyadic multilevel modeling recommend the 2-level approach (Bolger & Shrout, 2007; Raudenbush et al., 1995; Sayer & Klute, 2005). Even proponents of the 3-level model admit to a reduction in power and related changes in findings when using this model in comparison to the 2-level model most easily used for distinguishable dyads[4] (Atkins, 2005). Deborah Kashy has developed an extension of the 2-level multilevel model generally used to examine change in distinguishable dyads, which can be applied in the case of indistinguishable dyads (Kashy et al., 2008). While Kashy's initial work was on twin research, more recent work has extended the use of this model to lesbian and gay male parents (Farr, 2017; Goldberg et al., 2010; Goldberg & Garcia, 2016; Goldberg & Smith, 2009a, 2011). For example, in a study of female, male, and heterosexual adoptive parents, this approach was used to examine preadoptive factors on relationship quality (love, conflict, and ambivalence) across the transition to adoptive parenthood (Goldberg et al., 2010; $N = 44$ female couples, 30 male couples, and 51 heterosexual couples). Parents who reported higher levels of depression, greater use of avoidant coping, lower levels of relationship maintenance behaviors, and less satisfaction with their adoption agencies before the adoption reported lower relationship quality at the time of the adoption. The effect of avoidant coping on relationship quality varied by gender. The use of a longitudinal model enabled Goldberg et al.

(2010) to examine change in relationship quality across this transition as well: Parents who reported higher levels of depression, greater use of confrontative coping, and higher levels of relationship maintenance behaviors prior to the adoption reported greater declines in relationship quality.

The longitudinal model for indistinguishable dyads is very similar to the distinguishable dyad model in which trajectories for both dyad members are modeled at Level 1, with separate intercepts and slopes modeled for each member of the dyad (Raudenbush et al., 1995). The two partners' intercepts are allowed to covary, as are their rates of change (slopes). Due to the inability to distinguish between dyad members in the indistinguishable case, however, parameter estimates for the average intercept and average slope (the fixed effects) are pooled across partners as well as dyads (Kashy et al., 2008). In addition, drawing from approaches to modeling indistinguishable dyads in structural equation modeling (Olsen & Kenny, 2006; Woody & Sadler, 2005), this approach constrains the estimates of intercept and slope (if random) variance to be equal for partners.[5] Similar to the distinguishable model, two (redundant) dummy variables, P1 and P2, are used to systematically differentiate between the two partners. In other words, if the outcome score is from partner 1, P1 = 1, and otherwise P1 = 0; and, if the outcome score is from partner 2, P2 = 1, and otherwise P2 = 0. At Level 1 of the model (in which there are no predictors aside from Time), an intercept and slope for time for each partner is modeled:

Level 1 (within couples; Eq. 7):

$$Y_{ijk} = \beta_{01j}(P1) + \beta_{11j}(P1 * \text{Time})_{1jk} + \beta_{02j}(P2) + \beta_{12j}(P2 * \text{Time})_{2jk} + r_{ijk} \quad (7)$$

where $Y_{ijk}$ represents the outcome score of partner $i$ in dyad $j$ at time $k$, and $i = 1, 2$ for the two members of the dyad.

---

[4]The overtime model is more difficult to use for indistinguishable dyads than for distinguishable dyads because the elements of the covariance matrix of random effects need to be fixed to be equal across dyads in the indistinguishable case. Not all statistical software packages allow this custom specification.

---

[5]Estimates of within-person and between-person intercept-slope covariances are also constrained to be equal across members.

In this model, intercepts and slopes can vary between dyads. The inability to distinguish between dyad members would make it meaningless to have separate parameter estimates for member 1 and member 2; therefore, the parameter estimates for the fixed effects are aggregated across dyad members. In the Level-1 equation (Eq. 7), $\beta_{01j}$ and $\beta_{02j}$ represent the intercepts, for partners 1 and 2 in couple $j$, and estimate the level of depressive or anxious symptoms at the time of the adoption. Likewise, $\beta_{11j}$ and $\beta_{12j}$ represent the slopes for the two partners. These slopes estimate the change in the outcome over the transition to adoptive parenthood. Unlike the distinguishable model, however, the estimates for the intercepts and slopes are then pooled ($\beta_{0ij}$ and $\beta_{1ij}$) creating only two Level-2 equations, one for the intercept and one for the slope.

Level 2 (between couples; Eq. 8):

$$\beta_{0ij} = \gamma_{00} + u_{0ij}$$
$$\beta_{1ij} = \gamma_{10} + u_{1ij}$$
(8)

As these two equations show, the intercepts are pooled not only between but *within* dyads (i.e., across both $i$ and $j$) to estimate the fixed effect, $\gamma_{00}$, which is the average intercept (or the average level of the outcome when Time = 0), and similarly, the slopes for time are pooled both between and within dyads to estimate the average slope, $\gamma_{10}$ (or the average rate of change in the outcome across all partners).

The variance components are also pooled both between and within dyads. At Level 2, the variance in the intercept, Var($u_{0ij}$), represents the variability in the outcome at the time of the adoptive placement, and the variance in the slopes, Var($u_{1ij}$), represents the variability in how depressive or anxious symptoms change over time. The third variance component, Var($r_{ijk}$), is the variance of the Level-1 residuals (or the difference between the observed values of the outcome and the predicted values from the fitted trajectories). The variance of the Level-1 residuals is constrained to be equal for both partners and across all time points. In addition to the variances, several covariances commonly estimated in dyadic growth models can also be included in this model. For example, the covariance between the two slopes

estimating change for each person uniquely shows the degree of similarity in partners' pattern of change, to name one such covariance.[6]

## Considerations When Modeling Change Over Time

When modeling change, the reliability of the change trajectories will be greatly improved with a greater number of assessment points (Raudenbush & Bryk, 2002; Willett, 1989). In addition, the use of more assessment points allows researchers to examine more complex patterns of change. For example, research on heterosexual-parent couples has shown relationship quality and many mental health outcomes such as depression to follow curvilinear trajectories particularly across the transition to parenthood (Perry-Jenkins, Smith, Goldberg, & Logan, 2011). Such patterns cannot be captured with only three time points.

----

[6] In addition to the variances, Kashy et al.' (2008) model for analyzing longitudinal data from indistinguishable dyads provides estimates for several covariances. Dyadic growth models often include three covariances. First, the covariance between the intercepts estimates the degree of similarity in partners' outcome scores at the time of the adoption. Second, the covariance between the slopes estimates the degree of similarity in partners' patterns of change. Third, a time-specific covariance assesses the similarity in the two partners' outcome scores at each time point after controlling for all of the predictors in the model.

Two additional covariances are estimated using Kashy et al.' (2008) approach. An intrapersonal covariance between the intercept and slope can be estimated to examine, for example, if having higher depressive symptoms at the time of adoption is related to greater increases in depressive symptoms over time. An interpersonal covariance between the intercept and slope can also be estimated to examine, for example, if partners of individuals with high initial stress experience greater increases in stress over time. As some software such as SPSS does not allow for estimation of these covariances, these are not always included in the models (Goldberg et al., 2010; Goldberg & Smith, 2009a; Goldberg & Smith, 2011). As these covariance estimates are less important, and less likely to affect findings, the use of models with and without them may well be adequate for most research. In fact, identical patterns of results have been found with and without the covariance constraints in the existing published literature (Goldberg et al., 2010; Goldberg & Smith, 2009a; Goldberg & Smith, 2011).

Note that the software program HLM does not allow for either variances or covariances to be constrained.

While more time points are preferable, it is possible to fit the change models to examine change between two time points (i.e., a latent difference score). Goldberg and Smith (2009a) used this approach to examine changes in perceived parenting skill in lesbian, gay male, and heterosexual adoptive couples after the adoption of their first child. Examination of change between only two time points is essentially a difference score. While not ideal, the use of multilevel modeling to generate difference scores provides better estimates of change than observed difference scores, as it provides some correction for measurement error, and takes into account level as well as amount of change (O'Rourke et al., 2010; Sayer & Klute, 2005). (Note that SEM would accommodate further modeling of measurement error; Iida, Seidman, & Shrout, 2018.) For an example of using MLM to examine change between two time points in distinguishable dyads, see Goldberg and Sayer's (2006) examination of change in relationship quality in 29 lesbian inseminating couples across the transition to parenthood.

Additional data preparation is necessary to estimate change between two time points. With only two time points at Level 1, there would be too few degrees of freedom to estimate two fixed effects (an intercept and rate of change) and the residuals (or error) around the fitted regression line, unless additional information on the outcome was available and introduced into the modeling procedure. This additional information can be provided, however, by dividing the outcome measure into two parallel scales with comparable variance and reliability, allowing for the estimation of error (Raudenbush et al., 1995; Sayer & Klute, 2005).[7] In addition, the use of parallel scales provides a limited

measurement component to the multilevel model and consequently a somewhat more accurate measure of both error and latent change scores. Future research, however, is needed to examine the reliability of the estimates for change from such models.

## Multiple Informants

In family research, one often attains multiple reports of the same outcomes. For example, a researcher examining the behavior of children of lesbian mothers may have both mothers report on the child's behavior. While structural equation modeling provides the best available method of handling data from multiple reporters, multilevel modeling may also be used to examine these data. By using reports from both parents, researchers can introduce a limited measurement component to the model. While this is a new area for LGBTQ research, it is a growing area in family research. A particularly interesting study was conducted by Georgiades et al. (2008) who used MLM to examine reports of family functioning gathered from multiple family members ($N = 26,614$ individuals in 11,023 families). While using reports from multiple members of the family provided a better measure of family functioning, the use of MLM enabled the researchers to distinguish shared perceptions of family functioning from unique individual perceptions, as well as to examine predictors of these perceptions.

Dyadic models such as those presented in this chapter can also be employed to examine reports from multiple informants. In the simplest application, MLM provides a composite score across multiple reporters, while taking into account the degree of association between dyad members' reports. This approach was used by Meteyer and Perry-Jenkins (2010) to examine change in fathers' involvement in childcare across the transition to parenthood in a sample of 98 heterosexual couples. The authors used a multilevel model with a single intercept and slope at Level 1 for each couple. The level of father involvement is estimated as this single intercept based

---

[7] Parallel scales are generally created based on the items' variance. First, the variances of all of the items in the scale are determined. The items are then assigned to each of the two scales on the basis of their variance. In other words, the item with the most variance would be assigned to scale A. The item with the second highest variance would go in scale B. The item with the third highest variance would also go in scale B. The items with the next highest variance would go in scale A, as would the next, and so forth.

on both mothers' and fathers' reports of father involvement; similarly, the single rate of change in involvement is based on both parents' reports of father involvement.

For indistinguishable dyads, this approach simply involves use of the indistinguishable model presented earlier in this chapter. For example, Goldberg and Smith (2017) examined the relationship between parents' involvement in children's schools and children's well-being as reported by both parents in a sample of 106 female, male, and heterosexual couples with adopted children. In the dyadic, cross-sectional model, the composite score for the dyad (dyad average; i.e., child well-being) is represented by the Level-1 intercept. MLM also estimates the correlation between the parents' scores, indicating the strength of the relationship between parents' reports within couples. Recall that in the MLM models, variance in the reports is partitioned into two sources: that which lies *between* dyads and that which lies *within* dyads. Predictors were then entered to explain this variance. At Level 1 (i.e., within couple), individual-level predictors included parent–school relationships at T1 (school involvement, parent–teacher relationship quality, parent–school contact about child problems, and perceived acceptance by other parents) and adoption-specific school experiences at T1 (parent input about classroom inclusion and parent–teacher conflicts related to adoptive family status). At Level 2 (i.e., between couple), couple and family-level variables (i.e., variables that varied between rather than within couples) were entered. These included family type (e.g., same-sex or heterosexual couple) and demographic control variables, such as child gender, child age, and private versus public school. Goldberg and Smith found that parent–school involvement was negatively related to later internalizing symptoms in children; providing input to teachers about inclusion and parent–teacher conflicts related to adoption were both positively related to later internalizing symptoms in children. Perceived acceptance by other parents was negatively related to later child internalizing and externalizing symptoms. School-initiated contact about child problems

more strongly predicted higher externalizing symptoms among children in same-sex parent families than among children in heterosexual parent families.

With distinguishable dyads, the two-intercept model makes it easy to examine differential predictors of the two respondents' reports. For example, in the case of parent and child reports of child well-being, the model would include separate estimates for child reports and parent reports at Level 1. Predictors, such as family income, would be entered at Level 2. This model provides separate parameter estimates for the effect of income on parents' and children's reports. It is then possible to test whether these estimates are statistically different by constraining the two estimates to be the same and conducting model comparison tests (as discussed early in the section on distinguishability). This approach was used by Kuo, Mohler, Raudenbush, and Earls (2000), to examine the relationship between demographic risk factors and reports of children's exposure to violence ($N = 1,880$ children and 1776 parents). The researchers also used the traditional method of conducting analyses separately on fathers' and children's reports and found the results for individual parameter estimates to be very similar. However, it is only possible to statistically test for the differences between informants using the MLM (or SEM) approach, as the two reports must be modeled simultaneously.

Conducting similar analyses is not feasible in MLM using the indistinguishable model, as that model does not provide separate parameter estimates of the effects of a couple-level (Level-2) predictor on the two partners' reports (as the two partners are not distinguished). The APIM could, however, be used to examine differential effects of characteristics that vary for individuals. For example, one could examine the effects of individuals' own characteristics and their and partners' characteristics on individuals' reports.

An alternate approach for distinguishable dyads is to examine discrepancies between the reports of the two dyad members (Lyons, Zarit, Sayer, & Whitlach, 2002). Coley and Morris (2002) use this approach to examine discrepancies in mothers' and fathers' reports of father involvement in 228 low-income families. Specifically, reports of the outcome are regressed onto dummy indicators for the mother (−0.5) and father (0.5).

Discrepancy model: Level 1 (Eq. 9):

$$Y_{ij} = \beta_{0j} + \beta_{1j} \left( \text{indicator} \right) + r_{ij} \qquad (9)$$

In this model, the intercept represents the *average* of the two parents' reports of father involvement, and the slope represents the *discrepancy* between the two reports, as there is exactly 1.0 unit between indicators. Predictors for the average and the discrepancy can then be added at Level 2. Coley and Morris (2002) found that parental conflict, fathers' nonresidence, and fathers' age, as well as mothers' education and employment, predicted larger discrepancies between fathers' and mothers' reports. Use of the discrepancy approach, however, requires the ability to differentiate between dyad members.

## Beyond Basic Multilevel Moldels

While MLM provides many valuable approaches for the analysis of dyadic data, some analyses can only be done in SEM or are more easily done in SEM (by those already familiar with SEM), which we discuss only briefly. For example, mediation is most easily examined using SEM or using multilevel SEM (MSEM; Ledermann, Macho, & Kenny, 2011). Although, SEM is the preferred approach to examining mediation, strategies for examining mediation do exist within MLM framework. Kenny, Korchmaros, and Bolger (2003) provide a crude approach that consists of estimating the paths in separate models and then analyzing the results of the separately estimated models. In addition, Bauer, Preacher, and Gil (2006) developed an approach in which the data are restructured in order to test all effects.

In addition, SEM provides the ability to examine other models, such as the dyadic latent congruence model and the mutual influence model (which is similar to the APIM, but considers reciprocal effects), and to conduct confirmatory factor analyses using dyadic data and examine measurement invariance across distinguishable dyad members (Ledermann & Kenny, 2017). Common Fate Models (CFM; Galovan, Holmes, & Proulx, 2017; Iida et al., 2018; Kenny et al., 2006) and Common Fate Growth Models (CFGM; Ledermann & Macho, 2014) provide a better means to examine variables at the couple or family level than the MLM multiple informant model discussed above. (See Iida et al. (2018) for an excellent discussion comparing the uses of APIM, common fate, and a dyadic score model within an SEM framework.) Goldberg and Garcia (2016) used a CFGM in a sample of 181 couples with adopted children (56 female couples, 48 male couples, and 77 heterosexual couples). Specifically, they used the two parents' reports of their child's play as indicators of the child's behavior, as a family-level latent variable, and investigated parent-reported gendered play of children across three time points. Using this approach, they found that regardless of family type, the parent-reported gender-typed behavior of boys, but not girls, significantly changed over time (i.e., boys' behavior became more masculine).

The basic cross-sectional model and a longitudinal growth model can also be fit in SEM (although the growth model requires the same time intervals between measurements for all dyads). Hong and Kim (2019) present APIMs using MLM and SEM, showing how the estimates are essentially identical. However, Hong and Kim also prefer SEM over MLM, given the looser underlying assumptions regarding measurement and factor loadings in SEM, and the better selection of model fit indices available.

In an attempt to make dyadic SEM more accessible to researchers, Stas, Kenny, Mayer, and Loeys (2018) have made a simplified form of SEM analysis available through a web application *APIM_SEM* that allows one to easily fit basic APIMs for both distinguishable and indistinguishable dyads using one or two predictors and controlling for covariates. The free web application is available at http://datapp.ugent.be/shiny/apim_sem/.

## Limitation of Dyadic Multilevel Modeling Due to Small Number of Families per Group

While multilevel modeling provides a useful method for examining family data, it also has important limitations. Most importantly, MLM is a large sample statistical approach; it is at its best when examining a large number of groups (like families) with a large number of individuals per group. Having too few groups or two few individuals per group (such with dyads) presents a power issue, as there is not enough information to reliably detect effects and can lead to a lack of precision in certain parameter estimates (Maas & Hox, 2005; Raudenbush, 2008).

### Number of Families Required

Given the limited number of individuals in families and dyads, a large number of groups (at least 100) are required to obtain accurate estimates of the fixed effects, such as the intercept, rate of change, and the predictors, as well as their standard errors (Raudenbush, 2008). While there are alternative estimation procedures that provide more accurate estimates when there are a small number of units (groups or dyads) at the highest level (Level 2 for the models presented here) with many people per group, these alternatives cannot address the problem of the small number of individuals per dyad.

While having a sample of at least 100 dyads will provide accurate parameter estimates of the fixed effects and their standard errors, other parameter estimates lack precision due to the small number of individuals per dyad, specifically the estimates of the Level-2 variance components may be inaccurate (e.g., the amount of variability between dyads; Raudenbush, 2008). Consequently, researchers should not rely on statistical tests regarding the amount of variability when deciding whether or not to enter predictors into their model. In addition, the MLM estimates of individual scores for each dyad (the estimated Bayesian coefficients) are unreliable. This is of greatest concern with cross-sectional models, as

well-fitting longitudinal models with assessments across multiple time points (i.e., more than two) allow for more accurate estimation. The unreliability of the estimates of variance should also raise concern with the accuracy of estimates of the ICC which is derived from the variance estimates.

### Noncontinuous Outcomes

Another important limitation to having a small number of individuals per family or dyad is that these models should only be applied to the analysis of continuous outcomes (Raudenbush, 2008; but see Ledermann & Kenny, 2017, for a different perspective). When examining outcomes that are not continuously and normally distributed, such as categorical or count data, MLM cannot provide accurate estimates when there are only a few number of individuals per group, even if there are a large number of these small groups. When there are a large number of dyads, SEM or a generalized version of MLM would be the preferred approach to analyzing dichotomous or count data (or any other outcome that requires a link function to transform the outcome scores). Simulations have shown that generalized linear mixed models (GLMM) can provide reliable estimates in samples larger than 100 couples when the correlations within dyads are positive (Spain, Jackson, & Edmonds, 2012). Loeys and Molenberghs (2013) showed generalized estimating equations (GEE) to be a reliable and accessible alternative to GLMM (using a robust variance estimate), reporting that simulations demonstrated that GEE produce more reliable estimates than GLMM in smaller samples and when the within-dyad correlations are negative. Loeys and Molenberghs still recommend a sample size of more than 50 dyads to test an APIM, however. (For an excellent primer on GEE, see Loeys, Cook, De Smet, Wietzker, & Buysse, 2014.)

Goldberg, Smith, McCormick, and Overstreet (2019) use a GEE approach in their examination of predictors of health behaviors and outcomes in 141 parents in same-sex couples (76 women in 43 couples and 65 men in 39 couples). They found that parenting stress and internalized homophobia were most commonly associated with health behaviors and outcomes, but functioned differently in women and men. Women with high stress had greater odds of exercising at least 3 days a week, but women with high internalized homophobia had lower odds of exercising that much, while the effects were vice versa in men. In addition, men were more likely to report depression than women; and, men with low internalized homophobia more often slept less than 7 hours a week and reported greater alcohol intake than those with high internalized homophobia. Among all parents, those with multiple children and those who were unmarried had lower odds of exercising at least 3 days a week, while those with high stress had greater odds of depression and of a chronic health condition.

## Future Directions

While there are still many areas requiring further development in the application of multilevel modeling to the examination of family data, the most important need in the area of LGBTQ family research is the need to make existing methods more available to researchers. In order to use MLM approaches to dyadic data analysis, researchers must learn both the basics of MLM and the inner workings of dyadic models. While multilevel modeling is increasingly being taught in departments such as family studies, human development, sociology, and psychology, they are still unavailable to students in many programs. Most researchers who study LGBTQ couples, parents, and families will need to seek out training beyond the courses they were offered in their graduate program. There are several training workshops analyzing dyadic data available across the country – many of these include SEM as well as MLM approaches. There are also, however, many useful resources available on the web (see Appendix A).

If researchers who study LGBTQ couples, parents, and families are unable to employ the statistical methods appropriate for their data and research questions, it hinders the development of the field. Researchers who are unfamiliar with the appropriate statistical methods to analyze their data are unable to publish, particularly in the leading journals in fields such as family studies, psychology, and others. In addition, they are often unable to capitalize on the richness of datasets. Currently, the greatest need in this area is to provide statistical training in methods such as multilevel modeling to junior and senior researchers and to facilitate collaborations between LGBTQ family researchers who lack this training and both established and emerging methodologists in the field of dyadic data analysis.

## Appendix A: Online Resources for Dyadic Data Analysis

Overview of Dyadic Data Analysis
   http://www.davidakenny.net/dyad.htm
Materials and Syntax to Accompany Kenny et al.
   (2006), *Dyadic Data Analysis*
   http://www.davidakenny.net/kkc/kkc.htm
Multilevel Listserv
   https://www.jiscmail.ac.uk/cgi-bin/webadmin
   ?A0=multilevel

## References

Atkins, D. (2005). Using multilevel models to analyze couple and family treatment data: Basic and advanced issues. *Journal of Family Psychology, 19*, 86–97. https://doi.org/10.1037/0893-3200.19.1.98

Barnett, R. C., Marshall, N. L., Raudenbush, S. W., & Brennan, R. T. (1993). Gender and the relationship between job experiences and psychological distress: A study of dual-earner couples. *Journal of Personality and Social Psychology, 64*, 794–806. https://doi.org/10.1037/0022-3514.64.5.794

Bauer, D. J., Preacher, K. J., & Gil, K. M. (2006). Conceptualizing and testing random indirect effects and moderated mediation in multilevel models: New procedures and recommendations. *Psychological Methods, 11*, 142–163. https://doi.org/10.1037/1082-989X.11.2.142

Bengtson, V. L., & Allen, K. R. (1993). The life course perspective applied to families over time. In P. G. Boss, W. J. Doherty, R. LaRossa, W. R. Schumm, S. K. Steinmetz, P. G. Boss, & S. K. Steinmetz (Eds.),

*Sourcebook of family theories and methods: A contextual approach* (pp. 469–504). New York, NY: Plenum Press.

Bolger, N., & Shrout, P. E. (2007). Accounting for statistical dependency in longitudinal data on dyads. In T. D. Little, J. A. Bovaird, & N. A. Card (Eds.), *Modeling contextual effects in longitudinal studies* (pp. 285–298). Mahwah, NJ: Lawrence Erlbaum Associates.

Bronfenbrenner, U. (1988). Interacting systems in human development. In N. Bolger, A. Caspi, G. Downey, & M. Moorehouse (Eds.), *Persons in context: Developmental processes* (pp. 25–49). New York, NY: Cambridge University Press.

Campbell, L. J., & Kashy, D. A. (2002). Estimating actor, partner, and interaction effects for dyadic data using PROC MIXED and HLM5: A user-friendly guide. *Personal Relationships, 9*, 327–342. https://doi.org/10.1111/1475-6811.00023

Carone, N., Lingiardi, V., Chirumbolo, A., & Baiocco, R. (2018). Italian gay father families formed by surrogacy: Parenting, stigmatization, and children's psychological adjustment. *Developmental Psychology, 54*, 1904–1916. https://doi.org/10.1037/dev0000571

Claxton, A., O'Rourke, N., Smith, J. Z., & DeLongis, A. (2012). Personality traits and marital satisfaction within enduring relationships: An intra-couple concurrence and discrepancy approach. *Journal of Social and Personal Relationships, 29*, 375–396. https://doi.org/10.1177/0265407511431183

Coley, R., & Morris, J. (2002). Comparing father and mother reports of father involvement among low-income minority families. *Journal of Marriage and Family, 64*, 982–997. https://doi.org/10.1111/j.1741-3737.2002.00982.x

Cook, W. L., & Kenny, D. A. (2005). The actor-partner interdependence model: A model of directional effects in developmental studies. *International Journal of Behavioral Development, 29*, 101–109. https://doi.org/10.1080/01650250444000405

Cox, M. J., & Paley, B. (1997). Families as systems. *Annual Review of Psychology, 48*, 243–267. https://doi.org/10.1146/annurev.psych.48.1.243

Farr, R. H. (2017). Does parental sexual orientation matter? A longitudinal follow-up of adoptive families with school-age children. *Developmental Psychology, 53*, 252–264. https://doi.org/10.1037/dev0000228

Fergus, S., Lewis, M. A., Darbes, L. A., & Kral, A. H. (2009). Social support moderates the relationship between gay community integration and sexual risk behavior among gay male couples. *Health Education & Behavior, 36*, 846–859. https://doi.org/10.1177/1090198108319891

Galovan, A. M., Holmes, E. K., & Proulx, C. M. (2017). Theoretical and methodological issues in relationship research: Considering the common fate model. *Journal of Social and Personal Relationships, 34*, 44–68. https://doi.org/10.1177/0265407515621179

Garcia, R. L., Kenny, D. A., & Ledermann, T. (2015). Moderation in the actor–partner interdependence model. *Personal Relationships, 22*, 8–29. https://doi.org/10.1111/pere.12060

Georgiades, K., Boyle, M. H., Jenkins, J. M., Sanford, M., & Lipman, E. (2008). A multilevel analysis of whole family functioning using the McMaster Family Assessment Device. *Journal of Family Psychology, 22*, 344–354. https://doi.org/10.1037/0893-3200.22.3.344

Goldberg, A. E. (2010). *Lesbian and gay parents and their children: Research on the family life cycle.* Washington, DC: American Psychological Association.

Goldberg, A. E., & Garcia, R. (2015). Predictors of relationship dissolution in lesbian, gay, and heterosexual adoptive couples. *Journal of Family Psychology, 29*, 394–404. https://doi.org/10.1037/fam0000095

Goldberg, A. E., & Garcia, R. L. (2016). Gender-typed behavior over time in children of lesbian, gay, and heterosexual parents. *Journal of Family Psychology, 30*, 854–865. https://doi.org/10.1037/fam0000226

Goldberg, A. E., & Perry-Jenkins, M. (2007). The division of labor and perceptions of parental roles: Lesbian couples across the transition to parenthood. *Journal of Social and Personal Relationships, 24*, 297–318. https://doi.org/10.1177/0265407507075415

Goldberg, A. E., & Sayer, A. G. (2006). Lesbian couples' relationship quality across the transition to parenthood. *Journal of Marriage and Family, 68*, 87–100. https://doi.org/10.1111/j.1741-3737.2006.00235.x

Goldberg, A. E., & Smith, J. Z. (2008a). The social context of lesbian mothers' anxiety during early parenthood. *Parenting: Science & Practice, 8*, 213–239. https://doi.org/10.1080/15295190802204801

Goldberg, A. E., & Smith, J, Z. (2008b). Social support and well-being in lesbian and heterosexual preadoptive couples. *Family Relations, 57*, 281–291. https://doi.org/10.1111/j.1741-3729.2008.00500.x

Goldberg, A. E., & Smith, J. Z. (2009a). Perceived parenting skill across the transition to adoptive parenthood: A study of lesbian, gay and heterosexual couples. *Journal of Family Psychology, 23*, 861–870. https://doi.org/10.1037/a0017009

Goldberg, A. E., & Smith, J. Z. (2009b). Predicting non-African American lesbian and heterosexual preadoptive couples' openness to adopting an African American child. *Family Relations, 58*, 346–360. https://doi.org/10.1111/j.1741-3729.2009.00557.x

Goldberg, A. E., & Smith, J. Z. (2011). Stigma, support and mental health: Lesbian and gay male couples across the transition parenthood. *Journal of Counseling Psychology, 58*, 139–150. https://doi.org/10.1037/a0021684

Goldberg, A. E., & Smith, J. Z. (2017). Parent-school relationships and young adopted children's psychological adjustment in lesbian-, gay-, and heterosexual-parent families. *Early Childhood Research Quarterly, 40*, 174–187. https://doi.org/10.1016/j.ecresq.2017.04.001

Goldberg, A. E., Smith, J. Z., & Kashy, D. (2010). Preadoptive factors predicting lesbian, gay and heterosexual couples relationship quality across the transition parenthood. *Journal of Family Psychology, 24*, 221–232. https://doi.org/10.1037/a0019615

Goldberg, A. E., Smith, J. Z., McCormick, N. M., & Overstreet, N. M. (2019). Health behaviors and outcomes of parents in same-sex couples: An exploratory study. *Psychology of Sexual Orientation and Gender Diversity, 6*(3), 318–335. https://doi.org/10.1037/sgd0000330

Griffin, D., & Gonzalez, R. (1995). Correlational analysis of dyad-level data in the exchangeable case. *Psychological Bulletin, 118*, 430–439. https://doi.org/10.1037/0033-2909.118.3.430

Hong, S., & Kim, S. (2019). Comparisons of multilevel modeling and structural equation modeling approaches to actor–partner interdependence model. *Psychological Reports, 122*, 558–574. https://doi.org/10.1177/0033294118766608

Iida, M., Seidman, G., & Shrout, P. E. (2018). Models of interdependent individuals versus dyadic processes in relationship research. *Journal of Social and Personal Relationships, 35*, 59–88. https://doi.org/10.1177/0265407517725407

Jenkins, J. M., Cheung, C., Frampton, K., Rasbash, J., Boyle, M. H., & Georgiades, K. (2009). The use of multilevel modeling for the investigation of family process. *European Journal of Developmental Science, 3*, 131–149. https://doi.org/10.3233/DEV-2009-3204

Kashy, D. A., Donnellan, M. B., Burt, S. A., & McGue, M. (2008). Growth curve models for indistinguishable dyads using multilevel modeling and structural equation modeling: The case of adolescent twins' conflict with their mothers. *Developmental Psychology, 44*, 316–329. https://doi.org/10.1037/0012-1649.44.2.316

Kenny, D. A., & Cook, W. (1999). Partner effects in relationship research: Conceptual issues, analytic difficulties, and illustrations. *Personal Relationships, 6*, 433–448. https://doi.org/10.1111/j.1475-6811.1999.tb00202.x

Kenny, D. A., & Judd, C. M. (1986). Consequences of violating the independence assumption in analysis of variance. *Psychological Bulletin, 99*, 422–431. https://doi.org/10.1037/0033-2909.99.3.422

Kenny, D. A., Kashy, D., & Cook, W. (2006). *Dyadic data analysis*. New York, NY: Guilford Press.

Kenny, D. A., Korchmaros, J. D., & Bolger, N. (2003). Lower level mediation in multilevel models. *Psychological Methods, 8*, 115–128. https://doi.org/10.1037/1082-989X.8.2.115

Kenny, D. A., & Ledermann, T. (2010). Detecting, measuring, and testing dyadic patterns in the actor–partner interdependence model. *Journal of Family Psychology, 24*, 359–366. https://doi.org/10.1037/a0019651

Kretschmer, T., & Pike, A. (2010). Associations between adolescent siblings' relationship quality and similarity and differences in values. *Journal of Family Psychology, 24*, 411–418. https://doi.org/10.1037/a0020060

Kuo, M., Mohler, B., Raudenbush, S. L., & Earls, F. J. (2000). Assessing exposure to violence using multiple informants: Application of hierarchical linear model.

*Journal of Child Psychology and Psychiatry, 41*, 1049–1056. https://doi.org/10.1111/1469-7610.00692

Kuo, P. X., Volling, B. L., & Gonzalez, R. (2017). His, hers, or theirs? Coparenting after the birth of a second child. *Journal of Family Psychology, 31*, 710–720. https://doi.org/10.1037/fam0000321

Kurdek, L. A. (1998). Relationship outcomes and their predictors: Longitudinal evidence from heterosexual married, gay cohabiting, and lesbian cohabiting couples. *Journal of Marriage and the Family, 60*, 553–568. https://doi.org/10.2307/353528

Kurdek, L. A. (2003). Differences between gay and lesbian cohabiting couples. *Journal of Social and Personal Relationships, 20*, 411–436. https://doi.org/10.1177/02654075030204001

Ledermann, T., & Kenny, D. A. (2017). Analyzing dyadic data with multilevel modeling versus structural equation modeling: A tale of two methods. *Journal of Family Psychology, 31*, 442–452. https://doi.org/10.1037/fam0000290

Ledermann, T., & Macho, S. (2014). Analyzing change at the dyadic level: The common fate growth model. *Journal of Family Psychology, 28*, 204–213. https://doi.org/10.1037/a0036051

Ledermann, T., Macho, S., & Kenny, D. A. (2011). Assessing mediation in dyadic data using the actor-partner interdependence model. *Structural Equation Modeling, 18*, 595–612. https://doi.org/10.1080/10705511.2011.607099

Ledermann, T., Rudaz, M., & Grob, A. (2017). Analysis of group composition in multimember multigroup data. *Personal Relationships, 24*, 242–264. https://doi.org/10.1111/pere.12176

Loeys, T., Cook, W., De Smet, O., Wietzker, A., & Buysse, A. (2014). The actor–partner interdependence model for categorical dyadic data: A user-friendly guide to GEE. *Personal Relationships, 21*, 225–241. https://doi.org/10.1111/pere.12028

Loeys, T., & Molenberghs, G. (2013). Modeling actor and partner effects in dyadic data when outcomes are categorical. *Psychological Methods, 18*, 220–236. https://doi.org/10.1037/a0030640

Lyons, K. S., Zarit, S. H., Sayer, A. G., & Whitlach, C. J. (2002). Caregiving as a dyadic process: Perspectives from caregiver and receiver. *Journal of Gerontology: Psychological Sciences, 57*, 195–204. https://doi.org/10.1093/geronb/57.3.P205

Maas, C. J. M., & Hox, J. J. (2005). Sufficient sample size for multilevel modeling. *Methodology, 1*, 86–92. https://doi.org/10.1027/1614-2241.1.3.86

Meteyer, K., & Perry-Jenkins, M. (2010). Father involvement among working-class, dual-earner couples. *Fathering, 8*, 379–403. https://doi.org/10.3149/fth.0803.379

O'Rourke, N., Kupferschmidt, A. L., Claxton, A., Smith, J. Z., Chappell, N., & Beattie, B. L. (2010). Psychological resilience predicts depressive symptoms among spouses of persons with Alzheimer disease over time. *Aging and Mental Health, 14*, 984–993. https://doi.org/10.1080/13607863.2010.501063

Olsen, J. A., & Kenny, D. A. (2006). Structural equation modeling with interchangeable dyads. *Psychological Methods, 11*, 127–141. https://doi.org/10.1037/1082-989X.11.2.127

Patterson, C. J., Sutfin, E. L., & Fulcher, M. (2004). Division of labor among lesbian and heterosexual parenting couples: Correlates of specialized versus shared patterns. *Journal of Adult Development, 11*, 179–189. https://doi.org/10.1023/B:JADE.0000035626.90331.47

Perry-Jenkins, M., Smith, J. Z., Goldberg, A., & Logan, J. N. (2011). Working-class jobs and new parents' mental health. *Journal of Marriage and Family, 73*, 1117–1132. https://doi.org/10.1111/j.1741-3737.2011.00871.x

Perry-Jenkins, M., Smith, J. Z., Wadsworth, L., & Halpern, H. (2017). Work-place policies and new parents' mental health in the working-class. *Community, Work and Family, 20*, 1–24. https://doi.org/10.1080/13668803.2016.1252721

Pollitt, A. M., Robinson, B. A., & Umberson, D. (2018). Gender conformity, perceptions of shared power, and marital quality in same- and different-sex marriages. *Gender and Society, 32*, 109–131. https://doi.org/10.1177/0891243217742110

Raudenbush, S., Bryk, A., & Congdon, R. (2004). *HLM6: Hierarchical linear and nonlinear modeling*. Chicago, IL: Scientific Software International.

Raudenbush, S. W. (2008). Many small groups. In J. de Leeuw, E. Meijer, J. de Leeuw, & E. Meijer (Eds.), *Handbook of multilevel analysis* (pp. 207–236). New York, NY: Springer. https://doi.org/10.1007/978-0-387-73186-5_5

Raudenbush, S. W., Brennan, R., & Barnett, R. (1995). A multivariate hierarchical model for studying psychological change within married couples. *Journal of Family Psychology, 9*, 161–174. https://doi.org/10.1037/0893-3200.9.2.161

Raudenbush, S. W., & Bryk, A. S. (2002). *Hierarchical linear models: Applications and data analysis methods*. Thousand Oaks, CA: Sage.

Sayer, A. G., & Klute, M. M. (2005). Analyzing couples and families: Multilevel methods. In V. L. Bengtson, A. C. Acock, K. R. Allen, P. Dilworth-Anderson, & D. M. Klein (Eds.), *Sourcebook of family theory and research* (pp. 289–313). Thousand Oaks, CA: Sage.

Shih, E. W., Quiñones-Camacho, L. E., Karan, A., & Davis, E. L. (2019). Physiological contagion in parent-child dyads during an emotional challenge. *Review of Social Development, 28*(3), 620–636. https://doi.org/10.1111/sode.12359

Simpson, L. E., Atkins, D. C., Gattis, K. S., & Christensen, A. (2008). Low-level relationship aggression and couple therapy outcomes. *Journal of Family Psychology, 22*, 102–111. https://doi.org/10.1037/0893-3200.22.1.102

Soliz, J., Thorson, A. R., & Rittenour, C. E. (2009). Communicative correlates of satisfaction, family identity, and group salience in multiracial/ethnic families. *Journal of Marriage and Family, 71*, 819–832. https://doi.org/10.1111/j.1741-3737.2009.00637.x

Spain, S. M., Jackson, J. J., & Edmonds, G. W. (2012). Extending the actor-partner interdependence model for binary outcomes: A multilevel logistic approach. *Personal Relationships, 19*, 431–444. https://doi.org/10.1111/j.1475-6811.2011.01371.x

Stas, L., Kenny, D. A., Mayer, A., & Loeys, T. (2018). Giving dyadic data analysis away: A user-friendly app for actor–partner interdependence models. *Personal Relationships, 25*, 103–119. https://doi.org/10.1111/pere.12230

West, T. V., Popp, D., & Kenny, D. A. (2008). A guide for the estimation of gender and sexual orientation effects in dyadic data: An actor-partner interdependence model approach. *Personality & Social Psychology Bulletin, 34*, 321–336. https://doi.org/10.1177/0146167207311199

Willett, J. B. (1989). Some results on reliability for the longitudinal measurement of change: Implications for the design of studies of individual growth. *Educational and Psychological Measurement, 49*, 587–601. https://doi.org/10.1177/001316448904900309

Woody, E., & Sadler, P. (2005). Structural equation models for interchangeable dyads: Being the same makes a difference. *Psychological Methods, 10*, 139–158. https://doi.org/10.1037/1082-989X.10.2.139

# Qualitative Research on LGBTQ-Parent Families

Jacqui Gabb and Katherine R. Allen

The wide-ranging networks of intimacy that constitute LGBTQ-parent family life are, akin to the feminist maxim, personal and political. Indeed, the study of lesbian, gay, bisexual, transgender, and queer (LGBTQ)-parent families grew out of feminist activism and scholarship on families that did not fit the heteronormative mainstream of a two generational (parent and child) structure, headed by a male breadwinner and his emotionally sensitive, homemaking wife. Qualitative analyses of LGBTQ-parent families are grounded in a critical feminist perspective where sexuality is overtly considered in the mix, and thus not assumed, tamed, muted, or denied. Furthermore, qualitative investigations of LGBTQ-parent families in general owe their legacy to the reflexive methodologies of memoir, personal narrative, and autoethnography, where individuals who have lived in families apart from the mainstream have first charted the way to describe and account for their own experiences. Over the past decade, qualitative research on LGBTQ-parent families and queer individuals and families of all kinds has burgeoned, to include not just narratives, interviews, and ethnographies, but a variety of strategies, such as diaries, emotion maps, participatory action research, and visual and performative methods—individually or in combination. As we argue in this chapter, qualitative methods in LGBTQ-parent family research have come of age. A great deal of exciting research is being conducted around the globe, making forays into previously unchartered territory.

As queer feminist researchers, we are keenly aware of the need to foreground issues of epistemology within our discussion of methodology, to be ever mindful of the personal, social, and political contexts impacting queer family life. Qualitative research enables us to use our academic voices to evidence the material impact of contemporary precarities (Butler, 2015) and the ways that they are shaping lived experiences and intimacies. Methods, queer or otherwise, are not objective tools that we take into the field to reveal hitherto unknown facts about social life. Methods are dynamic instruments which convey meanings and generate knowledge steeped in the research context. The researcher's standpoint (e.g., identity, race, and social class status; political beliefs; personal biography) and local and global political contexts are all crucial (Allen, 2016; Gabb, 2011a). Therefore, we situate our "inside-out" status (Fuss, 1991) as academic researchers who have been living and researching LGBTQ-parenthood, family life, and relational dissolution over the past 30 years.

J. Gabb (✉)
Faculty of Arts and Social Sciences,
The Open University, Milton Keynes, UK
e-mail: jacqui.gabb@open.ac.uk

K. R. Allen
Department of Human Development and Family
Science, Virginia Tech, Blacksburg, VA, USA
e-mail: kallen@vt.edu

© Springer Nature Switzerland AG 2020
A. E. Goldberg, K. R. Allen (eds.), *LGBTQ-Parent Families*,
https://doi.org/10.1007/978-3-030-35610-1_28

Contemporary studies of families can be characterized as a dynamic interdisciplinary engagement with shifting trends in the patterning of family and intimate networks of care that create and consolidate diverse intra- and intergenerational relationships (Allen & Jaramillo-Sierra, 2015; Gabb & Fink, 2015a; Jamieson, Morgan, Crow, & Allan, 2006). In this chapter, we join our respective disciplinary (sociology and family science) and locational (United Kingdom and United States) perspectives in order to examine the nature of qualitative family research on LGBTQ-parent families, and we address knowledge gaps and potentials as well.

In the United Kingdom, sociologists tend to employ predominantly qualitative research methodologies that allow them to focus on how families as interacting entities are made and remade through "family practices" (Morgan, 1996). In the United States, the growth of research on LGBTQ family issues over the life course can be found in the past decade to complement the rich foundation of qualitative work that has characterized the early years of LGBTQ family research (Allen & Demo, 1995; Biblarz & Savci, 2010). This growth corresponds with the increasingly sophisticated use of quantitative research methods, including meta-analysis (Cao et al., 2017) and large-scale demographic surveys (Fish & Russell, 2018; Gates, 2015; see chapters "Methods, Recruitment, and Sampling in Research with LGBTQ-Parent Families" and "The Use of Representative Datasets to Study LGBTQ-Parent Families: Challenges, Advantages, and Opportunities") as well as the ability of researchers to now distinguish among various sexual orientation and gender identities (e.g., bisexual individuals: Pollitt, Muraco, Grossman, & Russell, 2017; Scherrer, Kazyak, & Schmitz, 2015; and transgender individuals: Liu & Wilkinson, 2017), thereby separating out the components of who is encapsulated under the LGBTQ acronym. US scholars are building on much of the critical and queer theoretical framing found in international settings (e.g., Europe, Australia), attempting to queer family research methods by problematizing the heteronormative foundation that has characterized much of LGBTQ family research (Acosta, 2018;

Fish & Russell, 2018; Goldberg, Allen, Ellawalla, & Ross, 2018; Mizielińska, Gabb, & Stasińska, 2018; Oswald, Kuvalanka, Blume, & Berkowitz, 2009) and warning about the establishment of "a new gay norm" (Moore & Stambolis-Ruhstorfer, 2013).

Another change is that the majority of research is no longer focused mainly on lesbian mother families, as was observed by Biblarz and Savci (2010) in their review of LGBTQ family research in the first decade of the twenty-first century. Extending beyond the parent–child or partnership tie, a great deal of LGBTQ family research now focuses on youth and families with diverse identities and experiences, including new ways of examining the challenges associated with coming out, for LGBTQ homeless youth (Robinson, 2018) and for young adults who are the second sexual minority sibling in their family of origin to come out (see chapter "LGBTQ Siblings and Family of Origin Relationships"). Qualitative LGBTQ-parent family research is also addressing wider social contexts, including school choice for same-sex couples with transracially adopted children (Goldberg, Allen, Black, Frost, & Manley, 2018) and social support networks among Black lesbian couples (Glass, 2014). The qualitative literature has also extended its reach beyond primarily English-speaking countries, with research appearing on other international samples, including South Africa (Breshears & Lubbe-De Beer, 2016), Japan (Ishii, 2018), and Poland (Mizielińska & Stasińska, 2018) for example.

## Conceptual and Methodological Tensions in Qualitative LGBTQ-Parent Research

Despite the richness of this interdisciplinary, international, and increasingly intersectional body of qualitative research, several conceptual and methodological tensions are evident. These tensions reveal that LGBTQ-parent family researchers are continually challenged to not merely produce research that reinforces the heteronormative status quo but to retain a critical perspective on normalizing processes.

## Tensions with Conceptualizing Sexuality, Intimacy, and Family

We know very little about the ordinary experiences of sexuality practices in families per se, while the sexual identities of LGBTQ parents are afforded greater significance. In this chapter, we try to address this schism between sexuality studies and studies of family life by demonstrating how a qualitative multiple methods approach can shed new light on everyday practices of "family sexuality" (Gabb, 2001), enabling us to better understand the multidimensional identities of LGBTQ parents and the absence–presence of sexuality in queer family living. We use the terms "family sexuality" and "family intimacy" to simultaneously locate sexuality and intimacy in the context of everyday family relationships. We recognize the need to tread carefully around issues of sexuality in the context of parent–child relationships and LGBTQ-parent families in particular. Given the taboo nature of even considering sexuality, children, and family, much of social science research tends to "desex" families, with some rare exceptions (e.g., Allen, Gary, Lavender-Stott, & Kaestle, 2018; Fineman, 1995; Gabb, 2004; Malone & Cleary, 2002). We resituate sexuality as part of family life by deploying "families" as interactional units that are created and maintained through sets of relationship practices. This focus on everyday practice facilitates insight on the ways that partner and parenting dynamics are materialized in LGBTQ-parent families. We hope to nudge forward debate on how we can make sense of sexuality in the context of LGBTQ-parent families in light of these conceptual tensions.

## Tensions with Heteronormativity in LGBTQ-Parent Family Research

The recent advances in socio-legal queer partnership and parenthood rights in many parts of the world have helped to break down the homo–hetero binary and distinctions between LGBTQ and hetero parent–families. These rights, however hard won and welcome, have not come without a cost. While cultural studies and queer theorizing have started to critically engage with and critique socio-legal advances, much of the empirical research on LGBTQ parenthood has glossed over the problematic of contemporary equality rights which reinforces the heteronorm and focuses instead on the opportunities presented. Queer parenthood research all too often instantiates gender and sexuality through insufficient attention to everyday experience and the ways in which this queers kinship. Geopolitical (e.g., location of fieldwork) and sociocultural contexts (e.g., demographic sample variables) are used as scene setting rather than being operationalized to pry apart the intersections of public–private intimacies. Parenthood and bloodlines are once again defining families, albeit queer practices of conception now fix the boundaries rather than hegemonic norms associated with how families should function. All of these factors have generated rich insights into contemporary LGBTQ-parent families, but they have also occluded more diverse forms of kinship and the residual inequalities that persist within and across regions and nation states. We engage with these issues of how LGBTQ-parent family research is structured because they inform the qualitative research process; they call attention to the ways in which sexuality and family are interwoven with questions of methodology (Boyce, 2018).

## Tensions in Theorizing Qualitative LGBTQ-Parent Family Research

Tensions are present in how theory is used to guide qualitative LGBTQ-parent research, particularly in terms of mainstream theories (e.g., ecological, life course), which tend to reinstate heteronormativity, in comparison to more critical or postmodern theories (e.g., feminist, minority stress, queer), which may speak to a much smaller audience of scholars and practitioners. A promising direction is to borrow from and integrate mainstream and critical approaches, as in Glass and Few-Demo's (2013) use of symbolic interactionism and Black feminist theories, as well as the development of transfamily theory

(McGuire, Kuvalanka, Catalpa, & Toomey, 2016). While analyses may incorporate a strong theoretical perspective, another tension is the lack of explicit theoretical grounding in many studies of sexual minority parent families, as Farr, Tasker, and Goldberg (2017) found in their analysis of highly cited studies in LGBTQ family research.

## Tensions in the Scholarship of Intersectionality

Scholarship on intersectionality has demonstrated that there are many crucial factors which shape the lives of LGBTQ-parents which typically fall outside the analytical frame of reference (see chapters "Race and Ethnicity in the Lives of LGBTQ Parents and Their Children: Perspectives from and Beyond North America" and "LGBTQ-Parent Families in the United States and Economic Well-Being"; Moore, 2011). Race, ethnicity, religiosity, socioeconomic, and educational disadvantage, for example, inform experience and the data that are generated—even when they are declared absent from the predominantly White, well-educated, professional sample. Issues surrounding race, class, and gender disparities are delimited to just one type of family formation. Surrogacy, for example, seldom falls within the imagination of a working class man; likewise, in vitro fertilization (IVF) and even donor insemination are out of the reach for many socially disadvantaged lesbians. Queer divorce proceedings, which invoke pronatalist rhetoric to advantage the biological mother and write the social mother out of the parenting equation, are rarely integrated into LGBTQ–parent family research (Allen, 2019). Although 15–20% of pregnancies end in miscarriage, loss and bereavement are seldom mentioned as part of family formation (see chapter "Losing a Child: Death and Hidden Losses in LGBTQ-Parent Families"; Craven & Peel, 2014). Qualitative research has the capacity to be inclusive in its scope and to engage with the complexities and unpalatable dimensions of queer lived experience.

## Tensions with Standardizing Qualitative Research in the Publication Process

As the literature on qualitative research in general, and qualitative LGBTQ family research in particular, has come of age, expectations to formalize how qualitative research is reported have increased. On the one hand, having guidelines for best practices in writing up findings is an aid for journal editors, reviewers, and authors to ensure transparency and clearly convey how the research was conducted. Guidelines can be found in most of the major mainstream journals that publish qualitative family research, for example, in family science (Goldberg & Allen, 2015), psychology (Levitt et al., 2018), and gender studies (Chatfield, 2018), to name just a few. These guidelines provide practical suggestions on topics ranging from when to include frequency counts, how to identify the social locations of the researcher, and when to provide graphic or visual portrayals of the linkages among research questions, key themes, and conclusions drawn. For example, most qualitative family research utilizes some variation of grounded theory or thematic analysis. The basic analytic process is to work through the stages of data reduction from open to focused to theoretical coding, in order to produce a storyline that offers a coherent explanation of the nuances and patterns the researchers found in the data (Braun & Clarke, 2006; Charmaz, 2014; Daly, 2007), and it is important to reveal and provide exemplars of how the study was conducted and results found (Goldberg & Allen, 2015; Humble & Radina, 2019).

On the other hand, standardization in the mainstream journals can leave some of the more innovative and groundbreaking projects relegated to book chapters or nonranked journals, venues that may be more willing to take a chance on publishing experimental or experiential methods. Before the groundbreaking ethnographies of gay and lesbian family life were published, such as Krieger's (1983) study of a lesbian community and Weston's (1991) study of chosen kinship, those wanting to study or learn about lesbian and gay families turned to anthologies of personal stories written by and about lesbian parents (Alpert, 1988; Hanscombe & Forster, 1981), for example.

We see the benefits of standardization, but only if they take the form of guidelines that are not prescriptive or designed to iron out the creativity that can come with a critical analysis of lived experience. There are at least two ways in which qualitative family researchers can resist the straightjacket approach of standardization. The first is in heeding advice to insert the researcher's reflexivity throughout the research report. Both Charmaz (2014) and Daly (2007) claim that too often, qualitative researchers leave out their own commitments to the work, or how their values, theories, and choices overtly or covertly structured the process of doing the research and writing up the manuscript. A second is to encourage researchers to put their own lives to the test by engaging in autoethnography, whereby in some reports, they grapple with how their own lived experience has led them to their research interests (Adams & Manning, 2015; Allen, 2019; Gabb, 2018). The embodied vantage point of autoethnography has been a powerful tool for breaking new ground on topics, such as mental illness, abuse, violence, death, and the impact of various forms of xenophobia (e.g., racism, sexism, homophobia) that have, at least in the past, been deemed too sensitive, traumatic, or distasteful to research (see chapter "Losing a Child: Death and Hidden Losses in LGBTQ-Parent Families"). For example, in his recent account of the diverse and novel forms of kinship that characterize contemporary LGBTQ-parent families, Gamson (2015) combines observation, memoir, and ethnographic storytelling techniques to bring the field to life.

## Qualitative Multiple Methods (QMM)

We now turn to a way of framing qualitative family research through the use of qualitative multiple methods (QMM), drawing primarily

from Gabb's[1] research on lesbian parenthood and sexuality,[2] intimacy in same-sex and heterosexual-parent households,[3] and long-term couple relationships.[4] QMM is framed by the theoretical approach of family practices (Morgan, 1996). There may be tensions between the "families we live by" and the "families we live with" (Gillis, 1996), but the routinization of daily practices means that social roles and identities become embedded into the rhythm of family life (Phoenix & Brannen, 2014). Habitual practices are rendered meaningful through wider social structures which in turn shift over time (Smart, 2007). Family practices engage the materiality of sociocultural change by linking together biography and history (Morgan, 2011) and thus serve as a site for both family change and the reproduction of dominant heteronormative myths and sexual scripts (Plummer, 1995).

Next, we illustrate some of the kinds of data that are generated by using different qualitative methods under the conceptual rubric of family practices: diaries, emotion maps, participant observation, autoethnography, semistructured interviews, and photo elicitation. The methods that we detail here are not exhaustive. Indeed, over the past 10 years, there has been a methodological explosion in many fields of social research as qualitative researchers develop

---

[1] All studies were completed in the United Kingdom. The content and scope of these projects were discussed in full with all participants including children living in the household. Children's age and maturity are important factors in making sense of family practices; the age of children is therefore included when citing extracts from their data. Pseudonyms are used for all participants.

[2] *Perverting Motherhood? Sexuality and Lesbian Motherhood* was ESRC-funded doctoral research completed in 1999–2002. Lesbian mothers ($n = 18$) and children ($n = 13$).

[3] *Behind Closed Doors* was an ESRC-funded project (RES-000-22-0854), completed in 2004–2005. Mothers ($n = 9$), fathers ($n = 5$), and children ($n = 10$).

[4] *Enduring Love?* was an ESRC-funded project (ESRC RES-062-23-3056), completed in 2011–2014. Women ($n = 54$), men ($n = 43$), and gender queer ($n = 3$). Seventeen of these couples identify as LGBQ and in four couples, one partner is trans. Due to the focus of this chapter, we will not refer to survey data ($n = 5445$), only qualitative data from couples ($n = 50$).

dynamic tools to probe the lives and experience of people whose voices are ordinarily silenced and/or are pushed to the margins of academic study. Some of these extend interview-based researcher–participant approaches, while others have pushed at the boundaries of participatory action research (PAR) around the co-production of data and use of an array of participatory methods from theatre and dance workshops to creative arts and installations (Fine, 2018). PAR techniques offer an exciting potential for future research on LGBTQ–parent families.

## Diaries

Diary data add a temporal dimension to qualitative research, generating information on every-dayness and routine family processes (Laurenceau & Bolger, 2005). Diaries can elucidate the personal meanings of relating practices. They highlight the "affective currencies" (Gabb, 2008, p. 141), using symbolic phrases, such as "hugs and kisses" and "I love you," as affective shorthand to stand in for more complex emotion work and/or ambivalent feelings. They can facilitate research in that they introduce the research topic to participants at a pace and pitch that feel comfortable to them and provide background information which enables the researcher to tailor subsequent interview questions around the individual family situation. Diaries can include photos, pictures, and mementos of activities completed over the course of the diary period.

## Emotion Maps

Emotion maps use emoticon stickers to situate emotions at the center of research rather than as descriptors of experience (Gabb, 2008). The researcher is taken on a guided tour of the family home, and a household floor plan is produced, which is then reproduced using a paint or word processing or paint package. Several days later, a copy of the floor plan is given out to each participant with a set of colored emoticon stickers,

denoting happiness, sadness, anger, and love/affection. Family members are individually assigned a color. To spatially locate relational encounters, participants then place these different colored emoticon stickers on their household floor plan to indicate where an interaction occurs and between whom. The emotion map method is not reliant on language skills, and so it helps to flatten out intergenerational competencies among parents and children, and because children are familiar with sticker charts, they tend to be extremely adept in completing this method. Emotion maps are particularly useful for practitioners in clinical practice and assessment (Gabb & Singh, 2015).

## Participant Observation

Grounded in the principles of ethnography, observation provides a glimpse of everyday practices of intimacy that are usually recorded in researcher field notes, audio or written format, and accompanying photographs. Observation data can take many forms including the researcher's personal reflections on their own experience (autoethnography), diary writing, photo albums, children's drawings, scrapbooks, memory, and conversations. The researcher's immersion in the field can shed light on the texture of intimate family life, which highlights how the absence–presence of sexuality becomes enacted and the performances of relationships and family that participants chose to make public. Ethnographic research requires entry into private relationships, where researchers often live within the family unit for a sustained period of time. This level of researcher intervention is costly and can be seen to intrude upon people's privacy; hence, ethnographic observations are uncommon in LGBTQ-parent research. Notable exceptions are Mizielińska and Stasińska's (2018) mixed methods study of queer kinship and chosen families in Poland, in which participant observation was a major focus, and Carrington's (2002) ethnography of the day-to-day life of gay and lesbian couples.

## Autoethnography

Autoethnography explicitly engages the researcher's personal experience, whereby "our authorial position remains on the page and writing *through* this situated position places us in dynamic relation to the others whose stories we recount" (Gabb, 2018, p. 1004). Gabb (2018) used her personal experience, as a child who was adopted in the 1960s, to challenge the presupposition of birth motherhood and explore what happens when you start research from the margins, outside the embodied experience of bio-discourses. Allen (2007) used critical reflection to chronicle the unresolved grief that accompanies the ambiguous loss (e.g., psychological presence but physical absence) of losing all contact with her nonbiological child when her former partner "unimaginably" left their family. In writing as a lesbian mother, Gabb (2018) used autoethnography to focus attention on everyday moments that may otherwise pass by unnoticed. This inclusion of everyday experience is part of a wider political project as it renders the experience of marginalized groups as epistemologically valid (Craven & Davis, 2013, p. 27). Everyday moments divert attention away from "fateful" events (Giddens, 1991) onto "ordinary affects" (Stewart, 2007), which can provoke us to double take and think again (Baraitser, 2009).

## Interviews

In qualitative studies of LGBTQ-parent families, semistructured interviews that are derived from guiding research questions have been the method of choice, comprising most of the research cited in this chapter. Individual interviews enable participants to give their version of their own experiences and their interpersonal relationships in a family context. The use of dyadic and multiple family member interviews is a valuable yet still underdeveloped avenue for interview studies (Beitin, 2008; Daly, 2007; Reczek, 2014). Another avenue for further development is the use of open-ended interviews, especially to situate experiences of intimacy and sexuality across the life course, within the participants' own frame of reference and through events they define as significant (Gabb, 2008).

## Visual Methods

The use of visual methods has grown exponentially, leading to journals (e.g., *Visual Methodologies*), information guides (Rose, 2016), and handbooks (Margolis & Pauwels, 2011). This interest parallels the rise of "the visual" in culture and society, promoted through the digital mode of production and dissemination of images more widely. Visual methods are now an ordinary part of the qualitative researcher's toolkit, especially when children's lives and experience are being investigated (Lomax, 2012). Task-centered activities are particularly effective because they avoid the need for eye contact which can reduce imbalances of power (Mauthner, 1997) and are useful for working with adults and children whose first language is not English or with limited language skills.

These creative visual methods can access the more hidden aspects of family experience and have been used in LGBTQ research to explore diverse sexuality and gender identities and experiences (Barker, Richards, & Bowes-Catton, 2012). Visual methods have also been used as an elicitation tool or photo-prompt technique. Discussion of photographs can enable the researcher to approach highly sensitive topics that might otherwise be deemed too risky if tackled through personal experience. Gabb (2008) used photo methods to talk directly about the management of boundaries around children and sexuality and adult–child intimacy more widely. Using an image taken from a parenting handbook depicting a man sharing a bath with a child, she initiated conversation on how men, as fathers, negotiate issues of nudity and bodily contact. This opened up wider discussion on "family rules" and the normative judgments that are invoked to manage perceptions of risk associated with different practices of intimacy.

## Analyzing QMM Research Methods: A Moment's Approach

Qualitative multiple research methods produce a richly textured account of *where, when, how*, and *why* intimacy is experienced in LGBTQ-parent families, thereby using "complex methodological hybridity and elasticity" (Green & Preston, 2005, p. 171). Yet, the sheer volume and complexity of data required a novel approach to analysis. Building upon the everyday practices which underpin a QMM research design, Gabb developed a "moments approach" to analyze such multidimensional data (Gabb & Fink, 2015b). This attends to the ways in which micro and macro networks of relations intersect and overlap through "emotional scenarios" (Burkitt, 2014, p. 20). The approach integrates data by treating materials generated through different methods as "facets" which can be configured to build up a holistic picture of phenomena (Mason, 2011), while simultaneously retaining the paradigmatic nature of each method (Gabb & Fink, 2015b; Moran-Ellis et al., 2006). The moments approach focuses on the ways in which everyday practices, individual experience, and the patterning of social phenomena are constitutive and iterative, and it is this *doing* of relationships which informs all aspects of the research design and analysis. For example, in their research on couple relationships, Gabb and Fink (2015a) have shown how partnerships are sustained through ordinary gestures rather than big shows of affection and/or momentous celebrations. The relationship practice of bringing a partner a regular cup of tea in bed speaks volumes; it is deeply meaningful because of its regularity and the thoughtfulness of the "gift." In interview-only research, such gestures might slip under the analytic radar, precisely because of their ordinariness.

## Conceptualizing and Conducting Qualitative Research on LGBTQ-Parent Families

We now engage with empirical illustrations primarily from Gabb's research on LGBTQ-parent families to reveal how methodological creativity

continues to enrich knowledge. These integrative thematic exemplars serve as both provocation and encouragement to be alive to the dynamic contexts of conducting queer research on queer families.

## Era, Age, and Generation

Qualitative studies of LGBTQ-parenthood that attend to the social-historical *era* in which research is completed, the specificity of experience in terms of the *age* of participants, and the *generational* vantage points from which participants speak reveal how era, age, and generation intersect. For example, lesbian motherhood during the 1970s and 1980s was characterized by women's experience of divorce narratives and custody disputes (Hanscombe & Forster, 1981), resulting in 90% of lesbians in the United Kingdom losing their children (Rights of Women, 1986). Gabb's *Perverting Motherhood* study was completed when the pain and distress of earlier socio-legal contexts still impacted their experience, as Vicky, a lesbian mother who lost custody of her children, explains:

> I wanted to take them with me but I didn't have anywhere to take them to…and my partner convinced me that if we took them they would be tormented at school and taunted about it and all sorts of things like that. And my husband begged me not to take them. And the other thing was, I couldn't face going into a court and fighting for them and being told that I was a bad mother.

The past trauma and present-day emotional scars of Vicky's experience emerged through the face-to-face interview. Qualitative research has the capacity to not simply describe events, it can also foreground feelings; as such, Vicky's story drew attention to the pain and precariousness that shaped experiences of lesbian motherhood at this time. Today, partnership and parenting rights may have increased, but the experience of same-sex relationship dissolution and LGBTQ divorce rates remain relatively high (Office for National Statistics, 2013, 2018). While some former couples manage to reach an amicable settlement, cases of contested custody are increasing, and in such instances, the "biological rights" of the birth mother are all too often recognized formally (in law) and informally (in extended families) above and beyond emotional attachments forged over time between children and the social mother. Allen (2007) also reflected this confluence of era, age, and generation at a time in the United States prior to legal protections for LGBTQ-parent families, charting the emotional devastation and disempowerment of losing her intentional family of "a carefully constructed, deliberate mix of chosen and biological ties" when her partner left and "took her biological son with her" (p. 178).

Gabb (2018) similarly reflected upon her experience of lesbian motherhood over the past 25 years, noting the shifting political and personal landscape that characterizes this period of time. She highlights how lesbians raising sons were previously sometimes challenged by other lesbians who espoused separatism, and children were not always welcome or included in LGBTQ community events. The normalcy of LGBTQ-parenthood today means that "the scene" and personal experiences of parents have effectively changed beyond all recognition. In contrast to a generation ago, young couples (aged 18–34) in the recent *Enduring Love?* study structured their imagined futures together around family plans, with children regularly featuring on their relationship horizon (Gabb & Fink, 2015a). LGBTQ young people spoke about the reproductive and socio-legal options that were available to them and through which ideas of futurity and the couple norm become embedded.

> Stella: I'm excited about parenting with [Partner]. I cannot imagine doing this with anybody else and I think, again, the differences that we bring to our relationship will really complement each other in parenting as well….I know categorically that if I was single I would probably not end up parenting on my own, because I wouldn't want that just for…for myself. It's um…you know, it's because I feel that we can do this together…we want to be mums.

In these interviews with contemporary young couples, then, parenthood is seen as something which is a shared venture and that will consolidate the couple relationship. While earlier iterations of lesbian motherhood were premised on children conceived in former heterosexual rela-

tionships and subsequent families of choice studies explored diverse arrangements of kinship that often eschewed pronatalist discourse and the rhetoric of "compulsory coupledom" (Wilkinson, 2012), these young lesbians freely imagined parenting options and assumed "natural" feelings associated with natal family making (see chapter "Clinical Work with LGBTQ Parents and Prospective Parents"). In the United Kingdom, they grew up knowing that they could form legally sanctioned partnerships (and now marriage), give birth to children, and adopt; notwithstanding the financial burden, from this vantage point, they presented a trouble-free account of LGBTQ-parent family futures.

The other factor that distinguishes the generational narratives presented above is the material circumstances that surround LGBTQ-parent families and the "options" that are available to same-sex couples. Vicky's earlier account of childless motherhood is important because it calls attention to both the emotional range of experience that constitutes LGBTQ-parent families and also the structural factors beyond sexuality that impact upon LGBTQ-parent family making. Because of her limited social capital and lack of financial freedom, for women like Vicky, the "choices" available were overwhelmingly punitive: she could neither afford nor imagine keeping her children. Today, advances in sexuality rights have dramatically changed the queer family landscape, but the ways in which cultural capital and socioeconomic circumstances adversely shape contemporary experiences of LGBTQ parenthood persist. Thus, qualitative research has the capacity to call attention to the lasting and constitutive significance of era, age, and generation in LGBTQ-parent families so that novelty does not overwrite sexuality histories and obfuscate the complexity of lived lives.

## Social Class, Sociocultural Capital, and the Economies of Reproductive Labor

In LGBTQ-parent family research, research remains predominantly middle class (Biblarz & Savci, 2010). Widening the scope of the academic research lens to incorporate socioeconomic diversity is crucial in opening up understandings of LGBTQ-parent families. Working-class parents lack the financial resources and cultural capital to fully achieve the status of respectability (Skeggs, 1997), revealing that family practices are shaped by sets of circumstances and choices (e.g., personal privacy, owning one's own home) that are not always of parents' own making. Accounting for the ways that class positioning, educational advantage, and cultural capital shape perceptions and experiences of parenthood adds a much needed perspective in the otherwise partial LGBTQ-parent family narrative. The inclusion of socioeconomic diversity within the study sample ensures that findings are not steeped in privilege, thereby furthering the marginalization of traditionally stigmatized families. In Gabb and Fink's (2015a) study of couple relationships, the material impact of limited resources shaped young people's imaginations of family and the reality of options that were open to them. The process and practicalities of becoming pregnant as a lesbian were entangled with concerns around money rather than emotional investment in maternal roles and future imaginings of family, as revealed in Fiona's narrative:

> Fiona: It makes me so angry when people just have kids whenever they want. You know, and you see people just, like, popping them out and stuff….I've got to really work hard and save up a lot of money, this is…that's really expensive….It's like, £400, like, to start with, and then it's £200 a year. Well, it's not bad. It's not a lot, but look at IVF and stuff, that's horrendously expensive, and I know people that have gone through, kind of, five, six cycles and got nowhere.

Imagining lesbian parenthood and a future together as a family was similarly troublesome for Chloe and Leanne. In their couple interview, they repeatedly return to financial costs required by planned parenthood. Money and the need to start building up savings appear to be a source of consternation, leading to a somewhat terse exchange on the topic.

> Chloe: I think it will be good to look at it, sort of, logically and go, right, what are the options if we want to have kids? Like, what the different options are, so like adoption or,
>
> Leanne: I'm not adopting.
>
> Chloe: I'm just saying we look at all the options.
>
> Leanne: Yeah, I don't see the point in looking at that, because I'm not doing that….What worries me about having a child is the financial burden of it. It's one of the main things that makes me go "ha ha no thank you."
>
> Chloe: I think it's the initial outlay, because that would be –
>
> Leanne: No, it's the continued outlay.
>
> Chloe: Yes, and also I mean the continued outlay, you can absorb it, and people do, but the initial outlay is what I think, because it's going to cost a lot of money to get some sperm or to get a baby, isn't it? Um, and it's a lot of money, it's a deposit on a house.

Rather than working toward consensus as typical in dyadic interviews, Leanne firmly lays out her boundaries around LGBTQ-parent family planning. Pressures around money are adversely impacting on the options available to these women and their relationship dynamics. This couple demonstrates that equality of rights is not experienced equally. In contemporary studies of LGBTQ parenthood, the de-contextualization of research from diverse socioeconomic circumstances can all too easily result in the characterization of an able neoliberal citizen who can pick from a smorgasbord of choices that have been afforded through advances in legal rights. But choices are not free-floating signifiers of opportunity and agency; they are political and they are defined by context. Demographic factors are not simply variables; they define the research sample and thus the scope of research. Socioeconomic and educational disadvantage (class) remains fundamental in the experience of queer kinship and LGBTQ parenthood.

## Listening to Children

While some queer research has pointed to the incompleteness of LGBTQ-parent family studies when intergenerational perspectives are omitted (Gabb, 2008; Perlesz et al., 2006; Perlesz &

Lindsay, 2003), children's perspectives typically remain excluded (Weeks, Heaphy, & Donovan, 2001). Gabb's (2018) research bucks this trend, interweaving empirical data on LGBTQ-parent families with (auto)ethnographic observation of her own life as a lesbian mother and that of her son, as he grew up and experienced LGBTQ parenthood. For example, Liam (Gabb's son) formed attachments to parents, partners, friends, and his surroundings in ways that challenge heteronormative understandings of "family"; his emotional life world was constituted through "relating practices" which connected him to other people and things, breaking down distinctions between family, kin, humans, animals, and objects that occupy meaningful places in our family existence (Gabb, 2011a). These insights and the extracts below demonstrate why it is crucial to listen to children's voices if we are to fully understand LGBTQ-parent families. They not only provide another piece of the family jigsaw but also add a missing intergenerational perspective. Research with children does not require specialized skills (Harden, Scott, Backett-Milburn, & Jackson, 2000), only a creative methodological imagination.

The youngest children that actively contributed to Gabb's family research were 6 years old. Individual informed consent from all children was achieved by talking each child through the research, in a way that was age appropriate and comprehensible. This consent was subject to ongoing negotiation throughout the duration of the fieldwork, following ethical procedures that have been developed for research with children (Gabb, 2010). Younger children, up to adolescence, often want to speak about their families, and Gabb found that this includes an openness to talk about the impact of their mothers' sexual orientation on their lives. Asking children to describe their families can yield unexpected rewards and generate immensely rich data. For example, children from Gabb's *Perverting Motherhood* study were largely adamant that their families are indistinguishable from any other, as Reece revealed:

> Reece (age 10): We're just like a normal family really but with two women in it instead of a woman and a man really.

> Interviewer: Can you think of any differences between you and other kids?

> Reece: Only that I'm vegetarian and my friends aren't!

While some parents in their 30s–50s used "normal" as a pejorative term, many children used it to describe the ordinariness of families. Some children did, however, appear to perceive their families as different in some ways. What constituted this difference was typically unclear although explanations tended to focus on difficulties in *fitting* the nonbirth mother into traditional understandings of family. That is, the presence of the other mother was an identifiable source of family difference which required explanation, and it was this which made children susceptible to being teased.

Children were not directly asked about similarities and differences between heterosexual-parent and lesbian-parent families; instead, only words and concepts that were familiar to them were used. Questions focusing on their mother(s)' lesbian sexuality were asked only when and if they ventured onto this subject. Taking the cue from them (i.e., listening to the words they used to describe their mothers, their families, etc.), and only referring to lesbianism at their instigation, ensured that anxieties were not created where none previously existed (Gabb, 2005). Asking young children to talk about such sensitive issues would have been hard to approach head-on, but sitting down with these children, usually on their bedroom floor, and unpacking a bag full of drawing paper and sets of pencils and colored crayons, eased the awkwardness of the situation. Schools and playgroups often focus teaching on stories and pictures of home and family life because these experiences feature centrally in children's worlds; thus, the research topic was familiar to young children. Researcher–participant/adult–child imbalances of power were lessened because the activity was completed in their space and on their terms.

To begin, younger children were usually asked to draw a picture of their family which could feature anyone they wanted to include. Some children's pictures were figurative; one child drew vehicles, because he "couldn't draw people" (see

Gabb, 2005). Drawing enabled children to focus on something that captured their imagination while facilitating conversation on the topic. Thus, both researcher and child got something out of the encounter. Once copies of the pictures were made, the originals were all returned to the children, as promised.

Children's silences can speak volumes. A qualitative approach that advances critical discourse analysis is able to incorporate pauses, diversions, and associations as part of children's data, paying careful attention to what is said and unsaid and the way that descriptions are articulated. For example, when James drew his family (see Fig. 1), he did not explicitly identify Jill (his social mother) as the source of difference, but his *train of thought* suggests this may be the case.

> Interviewer: Are you going to draw Jill [other mother] in this picture?
>
> James (age 7): I'm not really sure about that [Interviewer: Why aren't you sure?] I don't know.
>
> Interviewer: Is your family the same as all your friends' families?
>
> James: A bit different [Interviewer: In what ways different?] I don't know, just a bit different.
>
> Interviewer: So can you think of any things that make your family different?
>
> James: I can try and draw Jill, but she's just dyed her hair.

Using "draw and talk" techniques can thus be helpful in focusing analytical attention on children's struggle to publicly account for their families within the heteronormative discourse that is readily available to them and which remains the mainstay of much direct and indirect school curriculum. While creative methods can thus be highly successful with young children (aged 6–12 years old), research encounters with adolescents are typically most successful when framed as gentle conversations. This is, in part, because young people largely feel unheard or marginalized within society and the opportunity of getting their viewpoint listened to and valued is welcomed. For example, Jeffrey spoke eloquently about the politics of sexuality. He was keen to question the distinction between the homo/heterosexual divide and expressed dissatisfaction with the categorization process of sexual identity-based politics.

> Jeffrey (age 19): I don't know why anybody makes a big deal about anything. I mean Gay Pride, why are you proud to be gay. It's nothing to be proud or ashamed of it just is and if everybody thought like that then there would be no bigotry in the world. It's not "oh you're a lesbian we'll treat you different." It's not. Or "we're lesbians so we have to treat you the same" it's just you're you. So what, who cares! It just doesn't make a difference, or at least it shouldn't.

Gabb's findings suggest that Jeffrey is perceptive in seeing the differentiation between homosexual and heterosexual families as more discursive than experiential. A child-centered approach to LGBTQ-parent research adds more than an intergenerational dimension to queer kinship; listening to children refocuses the analytical

**Fig. 1** James (aged 7). "My Family"

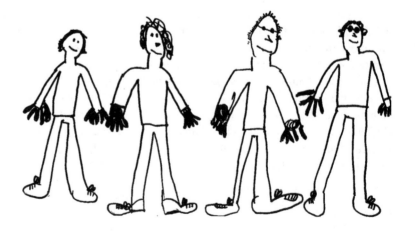

lens onto lived experience rather than sexual identity politics. From a child's point of view, all parents, kin, and significant friendships may constitute family (Allen & Demo, 1995). The shift in emphasis—from adult to children, discursive to experiential—portrays the emotional investments and materiality of what families do. This does not contest the particularities that comprise same-sex families, nor occlude the queering of parental categories in LGBT-parent families (Gabb, 2005), but it does shift the emphasis away from sexuality as *the* defining criterion of these particularities.

## Situating Sexual–Maternal Identities at Home

Locating practices of sexuality and identity formations in the household reveals how these vital data are enmeshed in wider household interactions which constitute the everyday realities of family living. Qualitative data on routine and ordinary interactions reflect the dynamic of LGBTQ-parent families rather than highlights or empirical snapshots. They also shed light on parents' strategies to manage their sexual and maternal identities inside the family home (Malone & Cleary, 2002). Gabb's (2001, 2005) research demonstrates how parents' parental–sexual selves are not experienced as mutually exclusive; they are experienced through sets of circumstances with sexuality and parental responsibility being negotiated around the absence–presence of others, especially children. In the *Perverting Motherhood?* project, this was articulated in open and explicit terms:

> Michelle: Obviously…you don't shag in front of your kids, anyone will tell you that hopefully, but we're quite openly affectionate in front of Rob [son, aged 7].

> Janis: [Bedrooms] become baby-feeding spaces actually! Oh yeah, that's definitely true.…So in a way the bedroom has always kind of a cross between sort of where you go to sleep and where you go and do "it" or whatever, or have a cuddle.

Data such as these substantiate the truism that having a child changes your life, but they do not position maternal and familial identities beyond sexuality; instead, lived experiences of lesbian motherhood illustrate intersections between sexual–maternal feelings and expressions of intimacy (Gabb, 2004) and the need for linguistic management of these shifting identities (Gabb, 2005). Parents talked about sharing their beds with young children and/or opening out intimate/sexual embraces to include them in "a family hug" (Matilda). The presence of the child in these scenarios can be seen to consolidate the synergy of lesbianism and motherhood; conversely, it sanitizes and desexualizes the lesbian relationship by tightly focusing the lens on ideas of responsible and respectable parenthood.

Gabb (2005) found that data generated through semi-structured interviews with mothers talking about the significance of their sexuality on everyday family life produced on one level broadly conflicting accounts. Whether lesbian sexuality was manifestly *on display* (e.g., in their homes) fell into two camps: "It's everywhere!" (Michelle) and "It's not really noticeable!" (Matilda). However, mothers' polarized assertions often belied the commonality of experience that was evident when QMM data were combined together. Observations detailed how "subtle signifiers of lesbian identity" (Valentine, 1996, p. 150) revealed the presence of lesbian sexuality. Coded signs, such as lesbian iconography and media aimed at the queer market, were visible in all homes, here and there, if one knew where to look and what to look for. Images of favorite celebrities, snapshots of family and friends, and iconic pictures of women predominately adorned the walls and shelves of rooms. These observations, documented in field notes, add a deeper layer to interview data on how maternal and sexual identities are experienced.

Visual data shed further light on the opaqueness of LGBTQ-parent family living. In the *Perverting Motherhood?* project, parents and children were asked to take pictures representing their lesbian families. The images that were produced and discussion over why pictures were not taken by some households illustrated the uncertainty about what constitutes lesbian parent family life. Images of people reinforced ideas of "the couple," valorizing normative ideals of the dyadic two-parent family model. Other images were either concerned with household chores or with showing loving relationships—closeness and embodied intimacy that was captured in family embraces. Sexuality was notably absent and the "family displays" (Finch, 2007) that were depicted revealed normative ideals of family rather than understandings of the particularities of lesbian parent family living (Gabb, 2011b). Perhaps, the most insightful depiction was of a bathroom shelf which included three toothbrushes in a pot, two adult, colored blue and green, the third a child's toothbrush depicting a superhero. Simply stated, this signified the "lesbian family"—ordinary, like any other, concerned with mundane everyday life.

Dairies and emotion maps were also and especially useful in generating data on how parents experienced and managed intimacy and sexuality at home. Diary data are typically steeped in temporal referents—clock time, age and generation, personal time, family time, precious time for the self, and the time needed to maintain and manage relationships. Emotion map data chart the emotional geographies of the family household and can be further probed in follow-up interviews. Together, these methods generated significant insight on the spatial–temporal patterning of family sexuality and intimacy. For example, furtive embraces and brief moments of intimacy were fitted into the spatial and temporal cracks of family living, while the immediacy of sexual intimacy and desire was contained by the presence of children, pets, and lodgers.

> Stella (diary): Slowly woke up and we made the time to go back to bed to be intimate which is usually passionate as well as involving laughter. Sometimes its [cat] who makes us laugh as he thinks its family time so joins us on the bed but then realizes he's not going to get attention so plonks himself right in the middle of the bed and we end up moving around. We had a shower together which is a practical thing but a nice treat.

Stella and her partner are one of the younger couples who took part in the *Enduring Love?* Study (Gabb & Fink, 2015a). They spoke at length about their plans to become parents. Children were identified as the marker of permanency, something that was shored up with the bricks and mortar of a soon-to-be purchased family home. For the moment, however, it is their pet cat who generates "family time" and who occupies the (physical and emotional) space of their imagined child. Pets have featured in many of the participating households in Gabb's research projects illustrating the capacity of qualitative research to respond to the messiness of lived lives rather than being overly determined by the unit of analysis (Gabb, 2011a).

The parents' bedroom, a cultural sign of sexuality that personifies "the sexual family" (Fineman, 1995), is a potent yet difficult site to investigate. As the place of parental sex, it marks the child's separation from the mother and signifies the hierarchical difference between parent and child. The double bed thus signifies the real and cultural difference between generationally defined adult (sexual) relations and parent/child (nurturing) relationships (Holloway, 1997, p. 55). It is not surprising that when participants in Gabb's (2004) research talked about their emotion maps and the experiences of intimacy and sex which these depicted, that they worked hard to establish categorical boundaries around codes of conduct "just in case" (Fig. 2).

> Interviewer: Right, so on the bed in your room, there's kind of stickers at one end and stickers at the other end. Is that significant?

> Claire: [Partner] stayed over one night and this [points to emotion map] is because I've got a hug [from son]—but it wasn't sort of a sexual nature or anything like that…it has changed, it does change over the years…things have changed and I think that's the noticeable thing for me is that [teenage son] often comes into my bedroom and has a chat.

Claire identifies the children's freedom to come into her bedroom on demand as a factor

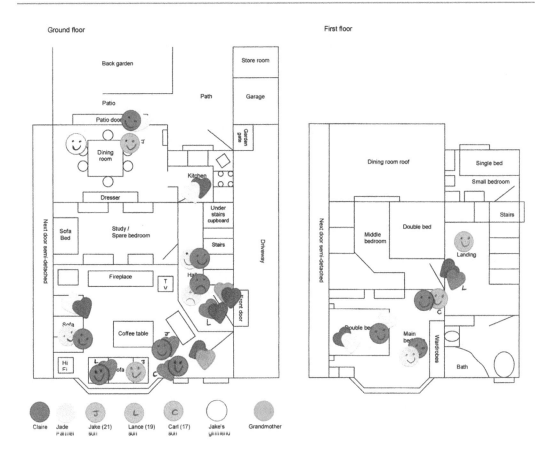

**Fig. 2** Claire's emotion map

that has delimited sex when they were younger. In many ways, then, the maternal bed/room remains a family space rather than a site of adult-sexual intimacy. In discussing her emotion map, she also works hard to differentiate person-specific forms of intimacy, such as how a hug with a partner felt different to one with a child. She points to age as a factor which impacted on the nature, time, and place for parent–child embraces. Talking in the third person, the defensiveness that marked earlier responses is replaced with flexibility including pragmatism around bed-sharing with both pets and children. Later on, in her discussion of photographs which depict parent–child nudity such as those published in parenting handbooks, Claire talked about her experience in comparison. Methods which use third-party scenarios can thus advance understanding of people's

beliefs and opinions and how these translate in everyday family experience, adding another layer of meaning as to how the participant's experience as an individual intersects with sociocultural factors. By combining methods, a dynamic picture emerges, providing multidimensional knowledge to understandings of LGBTQ-parent family lives and how sexual-parental identities are negotiated in everyday practices of intimacy at home.

## Implications and Recommendations

Human sexuality is part of ordinary life, but we need to know more about how the boundaries of intimacy are routinely established and maintained in LGBTQ-parent family households and how these navigate the particularity of circumstances. Race, ethnicity, religiosity, socioeconomic, and educational disadvantage feature to various degrees in LGBTQ-parent study samples, but the ways in which these demographic variables intersect and impact experience are often marginal in LGBTQ-parent family research. The sample size and/or focus on research questions on family formation foreclose in-depth analysis of the structural factors which shape experience. Empirical investigations are providing much needed insight into everyday life in LGBTQ-parent households. Queer theorizing is simultaneously advancing a critique of the heteronormative natal discourses which underpin LGBTQ parenthood. Rigorous development and theory building in empirical research are not yet embedded.

The rise of parental and partnership rights around the globe presents new opportunities for LGBTQ people through the capacity to legitimize hitherto precarious kinship ties, for example. The ways in which these opportunities obfuscate queer alternatives and instantiate heteronormative coupledom and dyadic parenthood need further investigation. We also need to acknowledge into the differences that are obscured under the LGBTQ umbrella. Gender diverse households, transparent families, and bisexual parenthood, for example, are likely to share some experiences with lesbian and gay counterparts, but their location on the sexual margins means that they are also likely to experience different challenges in day-to-day life within their families and outside the household. The burgeoning field of LGBTQ-parent family studies has been accompanied by an expectation to formalize and standardize the reporting of qualitative findings leading to a lessening in researcher creativity. Method is a slow, uncertain, and troubling process (Law, 2004). As queer researchers, we should be mindful of any individual and/or external impetus to neaten the research picture: "life experience is messy, we may do well, in our portrayals of that experience, to hold onto some of that messiness in our writings" (Daly, 2007, pp. 259–260). Social phenomena can be captured only fleetingly in momentary stability because the qualitative

research process aims to open space for the indefinite. Leaving in methodological and emotional uncertainties is not analytical sloppiness; rather, it reflects the ephemera and flux of LGBTQ relationships across the life course (Gabb, 2009).

The integrative themes that we use to frame our analysis in this chapter—generation and era, class and socioeconomic circumstances, listening to children, and sexual and parental identities—reflect some of the key vectors that cut across LGBTQ-parent family research. More than this, collectively, they also point to the need to situate studies of LGBTQ parenthood in the materiality of everyday life. These issues return us to the feminist maxim that we highlighted at the outset of this chapter and which has shaped the work that we have completed over the course of our careers: the personal is political; research is political. Qualitative research on LGBTQ parenthood has the capacity to engage with and advance knowledge which has lasting reach and also celebrates and exploits the research imagination.

## References

Acosta, K. L. (2018). Queering family scholarship: Theorizing from the borderlands. *Journal of Family Theory & Review, 10*, 406–418. https://doi.org/10.1111/jftr.12263

Adams, T. E., & Manning, J. (2015). Autoethnography and family research. *Journal of Family Theory & Review, 7*, 350–366. https://doi.org/10.1111/jftr.12116

Allen, K. R. (2007). Ambiguous loss after lesbian couples with children break up: A case for same-gender divorce. *Family Relations, 56*, 175–183. https://doi.org/10.1111/j.1741-3729.2007.00444.x

Allen, K. R. (2016). Feminist theory in family studies: History, biography, and critique. *Journal of Family Theory & Review, 8*, 207–224. https://doi.org/10.1111/jftr.12133

Allen, K. R. (2019). Family, loss, and change: Navigating family breakup before the advent of legal marriage and divorce. In A. E. Goldberg & A. Romero (Eds.), *LGBTQ divorce and relationship dissolution: Psychological and legal perspectives and implications for practice* (pp. 221–232). New York, NY: Oxford University Press.

Allen, K. R., & Demo, D. H. (1995). The families of lesbians and gay men: A new frontier in family research.

*Journal of Marriage and the Family, 57*, 111–127. https://doi.org/10.2307/353821

Allen, K. R., Gary, E. A., Lavender-Stott, E. S., & Kaestle, C. E. (2018). "I walked in on them": Young adults' childhood perceptions of sex and nudity in family and public contexts. *Journal of Family Issues, 39*, 3804–3831. https://doi.org/10.1177/0192513X18793923

Allen, K. R., & Jaramillo-Sierra, A. L. (2015). Feminist theory and research on family relationships: Pluralism and complexity. *Sex Roles, 73*, 93–99. https://doi.org/10.1007/s11199-015-0527-4

Alpert, H. (Ed.). (1988). *We are everywhere: Writings by and about lesbian parents*. Freedom, CA: Crossing Press.

Baraitser, L. (2009). *Maternal encounters: The ethics of interruption*. London, UK: Routledge.

Barker, M., Richards, C., & Bowes-Catton, H. (2012). Visualizing experience: Using creative research methods with members of sexual and gender communities. In C. N. Phellas (Ed.), *Researching non-heterosexual sexualities* (pp. 57–80). Farnham, UK: Ashgate.

Beitin, B. K. (2008). Qualitative research in marriage and family therapy: Who is in the interview? *Contemporary Family Therapy, 30*, 48–58. https://doi.org/10.1007/s10591-007-9054-y

Biblarz, T. J., & Savci, E. (2010). Lesbian, gay, bisexual, and transgender families. *Journal of Marriage and Family, 72*, 480–497. https://doi.org/10.1111/j.1741-3737.2010.00714.x

Boyce, P. (2018). Knowability. In C. Morris, P. Boyce, A. Cornwall, H. Frith, L. Harvey, & Y. Huang (Eds.), *Researching sex and sexuality* (pp. 18–22). London, UK: Zed Books.

Braun, V., & Clarke, V. (2006). Using thematic analysis in psychology. *Qualitative Research in Psychology, 3*, 77–101. https://doi.org/10.1191/1478088706qp063oa

Breshears, D., & Lubbe-De Beer, C. (2016). Same-sex parented families' negotiation of minority social identity in South Africa. *Journal of GLBT Family Studies, 12*, 346–364. https://doi.org/10.1080/1550428X.2015.1080134

Burkitt, I. (2014). *Emotions and social relations*. London, UK: Sage.

Butler, J. (2015). *Notes towards a performative theory of assembly*. Cambridge, MA: Harvard University Press.

Cao, H., Zhou, N., Fine, M., Liang, Y., Li, J., & Mills-Koonce, W. R. (2017). Sexual minority stress and same-sex relationship well-being: A meta-analysis of research prior to the U.S. nationwide legalization of same-sex marriage. *Journal of Marriage and Family, 79*, 1258–1277. https://doi.org/10.1111/jomf.12415

Carrington, C. (2002). *No place like home: Relationships and family life among lesbians and gay men*. Chicago, IL: University of Chicago Press.

Charmaz, K. (2014). *Constructing grounded theory* (2nd ed.). Thousand Oaks, CA: Sage.

Chatfield, S. L. (2018). Considerations in qualitative research reporting: A guide for authors preparing articles for *Sex Roles*. *Sex Roles, 79*, 125–135. https://doi.org/10.1007/s11199-018-0930-8

Craven, C., & Davis, D.-A. (Eds.). (2013). *Feminist activist ethnography: Counterpoints to neoliberalism in North America*. Lanham, MD: Lexington.

Craven, C., & Peel, E. (2014). Stories of grief and hope: Queer experiences of reproductive loss. In M. F. Gibson (Ed.), *Queering motherhood: Narrative and theoretical perspectives* (pp. 97–110). Bradford, ON: Demeter Press.

Daly, K. J. (2007). *Qualitative methods for family studies & human development*. Thousand Oaks, CA: Sage.

Farr, R. H., Tasker, F., & Goldberg, A. E. (2017). Theory in highly cited studies of sexual minority parent families: Variations and implications. *Journal of Homosexuality, 64*, 1143–1179. https://doi.org/10.1080/00918369.2016.1242336

Finch, J. (2007). Displaying families. *Sociology, 41*, 65–81. https://doi.org/10.1177/0038038507072284

Fine, M. (2018). *Just research in contentious times: Widening the methodological imagination*. New York, NY: Teachers College Press.

Fineman, M. A. (1995). *The neutered mother, the sexual family, and other twentieth century tragedies*. New York, NY: Routledge.

Fish, J. N., & Russell, S. T. (2018). Queering methodologies to understand queer families. *Family Relations, 67*, 12–25. https://doi.org/10.1111/fare.12297

Fuss, D. (1991). *Inside/out: Lesbian theories, gay theories*. New York, NY: Routledge.

Gabb, J. (2001). Desirous subjects and parental identities: Toward a radical theory on (lesbian) family sexuality. *Sexualities, 4*, 333–352. https://doi.org/10.1177/136346001004003004

Gabb, J. (2004). "I could eat my baby to bits"; Passion and desire in lesbian mother-children love. *Gender, Place and Culture, 11*, 399–415. https://doi.org/10.1080/0966369042000258703

Gabb, J. (2005). Lesbian m/otherhood: Strategies of familial-linguistic management in lesbian parent families. *Sociology, 39*, 585–603. https://doi.org/10.1177/0038038505056025

Gabb, J. (2008). *Researching intimacy in families*. Basingstoke, UK: Palgrave Macmillan.

Gabb, J. (2009). Researching family relationships: A qualitative mixed methods approach. *Methodological Innovations Online, 4*(2), 37–52.

Gabb, J. (2010). Home truths: Ethical issues in family research. *Qualitative Research, 10*, 461–478. https://doi.org/10.1177/1468794110366807

Gabb, J. (2011a). Family lives and relational living: Taking account of otherness. *Sociological Research Online, 16*(4), 141–150. https://doi.org/10.5153/sro.2443

Gabb, J. (2011b). Troubling displays: The affect of gender, sexuality and class. In E. Dermott & J. Seymour (Eds.), *Displaying families: A new concept for the sociology of family life* (pp. 38–60). Basingstoke, UK: Palgrave Macmillan.

Gabb, J. (2018). Unsettling lesbian motherhood: Critical reflections over a generation (1990–2015). *Sexualities, 21,* 1002–1020. https://doi.org/10.1177/1363460717718510

Gabb, J., & Fink, J. (2015a). *Couple relationships in the 21st century.* Basingstoke, UK: Palgrave Macmillan.

Gabb, J., & Fink, J. (2015b). Telling moments: Qualitative mixed methods research on personal relationships and family lives. *Sociology, 49,* 970–987. https://doi.org/10.1177/0038038515578993

Gabb, J., & Singh, R. (2015). The uses of emotion maps in research and clinical practice with families and couples: Methodological innovation and critical inquiry. *Family Process, 54,* 185–197. https://doi.org/10.1111/famp.12096

Gamson, J. (2015). *Modern families: Stories of extraordinary journeys to kinship.* New York, NY: New York University Press.

Gates, G. J. (2015). LGBT family formation and demographics. In W. Swan (Ed.), *Gay, lesbian, bisexual, and transgender civil rights: A public policy agenda for uniting a divided America* (pp. 21–34). Boca Raton, FL: CRC Press.

Giddens, A. (1991). *Modernity and self-identity: Self and society in the late modern age.* Cambridge, UK: Polity Press.

Gillis, J. R. (1996). *A world of their own making: Myth, ritual, and the quest for family values.* New York, NY: Basic.

Glass, V. Q. (2014). "We are with family": Black lesbian couples negotiate rituals with extended families. *Journal of GLBT Family Studies, 10,* 79–100. https://doi.org/10.1080/1550428X.2014.857242

Glass, V. Q., & Few-Demo, A. L. (2013). Complexities of informal social support arrangements for Black lesbian couples. *Family Relations, 62,* 714–726. https://doi.org/10.1111/fare.12036

Goldberg, A. E., & Allen, K. R. (2015). Communicating qualitative research: Some practical guideposts for scholars. *Journal of Marriage and Family, 77,* 3–22. https://doi.org/10.1111/jomf.12153

Goldberg, A. E., Allen, K. R., Black, K., Frost, R., & Manley, M. (2018). "There is no perfect school": The complexity of school decision-making among lesbian and gay adoptive parents. *Journal of Marriage and Family, 80,* 684–703. https://doi.org/10.1111/jomf.12478

Goldberg, A. E., Allen, K. R., Ellawalla, T., & Ross, L. E. (2018). Male-partnered bisexual women's perceptions of disclosing sexual orientation to family across the transition to parenthood: Intensifying heteronormativity or queering family? *Journal of Marital and Family Therapy, 44,* 150–164. https://doi.org/10.1111/jmft.12242

Green, A., & Preston, J. (2005). Editorial: Speaking in tongues—Diversity in mixed methods research. *International Journal of Social Research Methodology, 8,* 167–171. https://doi.org/10.1080/13645570500154626

Hanscombe, G. E., & Forster, J. (1981). *Rocking the cradle: Lesbian mothers: A challenge in family living.* Boston, MA: Alyson.

Harden, J., Scott, S., Backett-Milburn, K., & Jackson, S. (2000). Can't talk, won't talk?: Methodological issues in researching children. *Sociological Research Online, 5*(2), 104–115. https://doi.org/10.5153/sro.486

Holloway, W. (1997). The maternal bed. In W. Holloway & B. Featherstone (Eds.), *Mothering and ambivalence* (pp. 54–79). London, UK: Routledge.

Humble, A. M., & Radina, M. E. (Eds.). (2019). *How qualitative data analysis happens: Moving beyond "themes emerged".* New York, NY: Routledge.

Ishii, Y. (2018). Rebuilding relationships in a transgender family: The stories of parents of Japanese transgender children. *Journal of GLBT Family Studies, 14,* 213–237. https://doi.org/10.1080/1550428X.2017.1326015

Jamieson, L., Morgan, D., Crow, G., & Allan, G. (2006). Friends, neighbours and distant partners: Extending or decentring family relationships? *Sociological Research Online, 11*(3), 39–47. http://www.socresonline.org.uk/11/13/jamieson.html

Krieger, S. (1983). *The mirror dance: Identity in a women's community.* Philadelphia, PA: Temple University Press.

Laurenceau, J.-P., & Bolger, N. (2005). Using diary methods to study marital and family processes. *Journal of Family Psychology, 19,* 86–97. https://doi.org/10.1037/0893-3200.19.1.86

Law, J. (2004). *After method: Mess in social science research.* London, UK: Routledge.

Levitt, H. M., Bamberg, M., Creswell, J. W., Frost, D. M., Josselson, R., & Suarez-Orozco, C. (2018). Journal article reporting standards for qualitative primary, qualitative meta-analytic, and mixed methods research in psychology: The APA Publications and Communications Board Task Force Report. *American Psychologist, 73,* 26–46. https://doi.org/10.1037.amp0000151

Liu, H., & Wilkinson, L. (2017). Marital status and perceived discrimination among transgender people. *Journal of Marriage and Family, 79,* 1295–1313. https://doi.org/10.1111/jomf.12424

Lomax, H. (2012). Contested voices? Methodological tensions in creative visual research with children. *International Journal of Social Research Methodology, 15,* 105–117. https://doi.org/10.1080/13645579.2012.649408

Malone, K., & Cleary, R. (2002). (De)sexing the family. Theorizing the social science of lesbian families. *Feminist Theory, 3,* 271–293. https://doi.org/10.1177/146470002762492006

Margolis, E., & Pauwels, L. (Eds.). (2011). *The SAGE handbook of visual research methods.* Los Angeles, CA: Sage.

Mason, J. (2011). Facet methodology: The case for an inventive research orientation. *Methodological Innovations Online, 6*(3), 75–92.

Mauthner, M. (1997). Methodological aspects of collecting data from children: Lessons from three research projects. *Children & Society, 11*, 16–28. https://doi.org/10.1111/j.1099-0860.1997.tb00003.x

McGuire, J. K., Kuvalanka, K. A., Catalpa, J. M., & Toomey, R. B. (2016). Transfamily theory: How the presence of trans∗ family members informs gender development in families. *Journal of Family Theory & Review, 8*, 60–73. https://doi.org/10.1111/jftr.12125

Mizielińska, J., Gabb, J., & Stasińska, A. (2018). Editorial introduction to special issue: Queer kinship and relationships. *Sexualities, 21*, 975–982. https://doi.org/10.1177/1363460717718511

Mizielińska, J., & Stasińska, A. (2018). Beyond the Western gaze: Families of choice in Poland. *Sexualities, 21*, 983–1001. https://doi.org/10.1177/1363460717718508

Moore, M. R. (2011). *Invisible families: Gay identities, relationships, and motherhood among Black women.* Berkeley, CA: University of California Press.

Moore, M. R., & Stambolis-Ruhstorfer, M. (2013). LGBT sexuality and families at the start of the twenty-first century. *Annual Review of Sociology, 39*, 491–507. https://doi.org/10.1146/annurev-soc-071312-145643

Moran-Ellis, J., Alexander, V. D., Cronin, A., Dickinson, M., Fielding, J., Sleney, J., & Thomas, H. (2006). Triangulation and integration: Processes, claims and implications. *Qualitative Research, 6*, 45–59. https://doi.org/10.1177/1468794106058870

Morgan, D. H. J. (1996). *Family connections: An introduction to family studies.* Cambridge, UK: Polity Press.

Morgan, D. H. J. (2011). *Rethinking family practices.* Basingstoke, UK: Palgrave Macmillan.

Office for National Statistics. (2013). *Trends in civil partnerships: How will marriages to same sex couples change statistics?* Newport, UK: ONS.

Office for National Statistics. (2018). *Marriages in England and Wales: 2015. Statistical bulletin.* Newport, UK: ONS.

Oswald, R., Kuvalanka, K., Blume, L., & Berkowitz, D. (2009). Queering "the family". In S. A. Lloyd, A. L. Few, & K. R. Allen (Eds.), *Handbook of feminist family studies* (pp. 43–55). Thousand Oaks, CA: Sage.

Perlesz, A., Brown, R., Lindsay, J., McNair, R., Vaus, D. d., & Pitts, M. (2006). Family in transition: Parents, children and grandparents in lesbian families give meaning to "doing family". *Journal of Family Therapy, 28*, 175–199. https://doi.org/10.1111/j.1467-6427.2006.00345.x

Perlesz, A., & Lindsay, J. (2003). Methodological triangulation in researching families: Making sense of dissonant data. *International Journal of Social Research Methodology, 6*, 25–40. https://doi.org/10.1080/13645570305056

Phoenix, A., & Brannen, J. (2014). Researching family practices in everyday life: Methodological reflections from two studies. *International Journal of Social Research Methodology, 17*, 11–26. https://doi.org/10.1080/13645579.2014.854001

Plummer, K. (1995). *Telling sexual stories: Power, change and social worlds.* London, UK: Routledge.

Pollitt, A. M., Muraco, J. A., Grossman, A. H., & Russell, S. T. (2017). Disclosure stress, social support, and depressive symptoms among cisgender bisexual youth. *Journal of Marriage and Family, 79*, 1278–1294. https://doi.org/10.1111/jomf.12418

Reczek, C. (2014). Conducting a multi family member interview study. *Family Process, 53*, 318–335. https://doi.org/10.1111/famp.12060

Rights of Women Lesbian Custody Group. (1986). *Lesbian mothers' legal handbook.* London, UK: Women's Press.

Robinson, B. A. (2018). Conditional families and lesbian, gay, bisexual, transgender, and queer youth homelessness: Gender, sexuality, family instability, and rejection. *Journal of Marriage and Family, 80*, 383–396. https://doi.org/10.1111/jomf.12466

Rose, G. (2016). *Visual methodologies: An introduction to researching with visual materials.* London, UK: Sage.

Scherrer, K. S., Kazyak, E., & Schmitz, R. (2015). Getting "bi" in the family: Bisexual people's disclosure experiences. *Journal of Marriage and Family, 77*, 680–696. https://doi.org/10.1111/jomf.12190

Skeggs, B. (1997). *Formations of class and gender: Becoming respectable.* London, UK: Sage.

Smart, C. (2007). *Personal life.* Cambridge, UK: Polity Press.

Stewart, K. (2007). *Ordinary affects.* Durham, NC: Duke University Press.

Valentine, G. (1996). (Re)negotiating the "heterosexual street": Lesbian productions of space. In N. Duncan (Ed.), *Body space: Destabilizing geographies of gender and sexuality* (pp. 146–155). London, UK: Routledge.

Weeks, J., Heaphy, B., & Donovan, C. (2001). *Same sex intimacies: Families of choice and other life experiments.* New York, NY: Routledge.

Weston, K. (1991). *Families we choose: Lesbians, gays, kinship.* New York, NY: Columbia University Press.

Wilkinson, E. (2012). The romantic imaginary: Compulsory coupledom and single existence. In S. Hines & Y. Taylor (Eds.), *Sexualities: Past reflections, future directions* (pp. 130–148). Basingstoke, UK: Palgrave Macmillan.

# The Use of Representative Datasets to Study LGBTQ-Parent Families: Challenges, Advantages, and Opportunities

Stephen T. Russell, Meg D. Bishop,
Allen B. Mallory, and Joel A. Muraco

Until recently, LGBTQ-parent families have been largely invisible in surveys of family life. Yet new understandings of LGBTQ-parent families have emerged in the last decades, and the analysis of several national- or population-based data sources has added new perspectives to the knowledge base on LGBTQ-parent families. It was not until the 1990s that scholars, along with the general public, began to recognize LGBTQ-parent families as a legitimate family form that was not going to go away. The growing research literature on LGBTQ-parent families during the 1990s (see Goldberg, 2010) prompted the designers of large-scale family surveys to begin to consider nonheterosexual family forms. Thus, new possibilities emerged with, for example, the US Census (Simmons & O'Connell, 2003) and the National Longitudinal Study of Adolescent to Adult Health (Add Health; e.g., Wainright, Russell, & Patterson, 2004), which began to include the possibility for respondents to identify same-sex partners in families and households.[1]

With the growing visibility of LGBTQ people, a growing number of large-scale datasets in the United States and around the world have been extended to include attention to LGBTQ-parent families, and for the first time, population samples of LGBTQ people are emerging. These studies offer the potential to greatly advance understandings of contemporary families. In this chapter, we consider the use of large-scale secondary data sources (many of which are population-based and nationally or regionally representative) for the study of LGBTQ-parent families. We include a detailed list of large-scale secondary data sources in an appendix at the end of this chapter. We also discuss the advantages and opportunities that such datasets offer, as well as the challenges that define working with secondary data on such an understudied and marginalized population.

Since the last edition of this volume (Russell & Muraco, 2013), there has been a dramatic shift in the zeitgeist related to reproducible research, transparency in data use and analysis, and data

---

S. T. Russell (✉) · M. D. Bishop · A. B. Mallory
Population Research Center, Human Development and Family Sciences, University of Texas at Austin, Austin, TX, USA
e-mail: stephen.russell@utexas.edu; meg.bishop@utexas.edu; amallory@utexas.edu

J. A. Muraco
Student Engagement and Career Development, University of Arizona, Tucson, AZ, USA

[1]We use "LGBTQ-parent families" to be consistent with the nomenclature of this book, acknowledging the complexities of individual personal LGBTQ identities and experiences. As we describe in more detail later in this chapter, the datasets to which we refer often include measures of same-sex partnerships in households, and thus, the personal sexual identities of household members are often unknown. There are no known population studies of transgender-parent families.

© Springer Nature Switzerland AG 2020
A. E. Goldberg, K. R. Allen (eds.), *LGBTQ-Parent Families*,
https://doi.org/10.1007/978-3-030-35610-1_29

archiving (Winerman, 2017). The impact of this shift for representative data of LGBTQ-parent families is substantial: since the last edition, we have located 47 additional representative datasets which allow for identification of LGBTQ-parent families. The identification of these data sources appears to be due both to the increasing inclusion of LGBTQ measures in population data sources and to greater access to data through public data archives and improvement of the quality of documentation of public data. Two large data enclaves that we utilized to locate these sources were the Inter-university Consortium for Political and Social Research (ICPSR; https://www.icpsr. umich.edu/icpsrweb/) archive and the Integrated Public Use Microdata Series (https://www.ipums. org/). However, there are other new advances beyond these archives. For example, the United Kingdom has a data archive similar to ICPSR (https://www.ukdataservice.ac.uk/). Google also recently released a search engine that searches for publicly available data (Castelvecchi, 2018). Some universities maintain data archives (e.g., Harvard:            https://dataverse.harvard.edu/; Princeton:      https://opr.princeton.edu/archive/), and there are also individual efforts to accumulate data for a specific population (e.g., http:// www.lgbtdata.com/).

We consider several types of datasets that hold potential for the study of LGBTQ-parent families (the appendix includes examples of each of these types of datasets). First are population-based, representative surveys of the general population that may be local, regional, or national in scope and are typically designed to allow for generalizations to the larger populations that they represent and that include measures to identify LGBTQ-parent families. Examples are the US Census, which includes information on same-sex couple householders, or the Add Health study, which includes questions about young adult sexual identity and orientation as well as marital or family status. A subgroup group among representative studies are large-scale cohort studies: The 1970 British Cohort Study (BCS) and the 1958 National Child Development Study (NCDS) are unit in that the design of both studies includes a complete population (rather than a "sample" per

se) at a given point in time (all births in one week, followed across childhood and into adulthood). Both studies ask respondents in adulthood about their marital (or marriage-like) relationships and household composition, including information about gender and how study members are related to other householders. Results from these studies are generalizable to similar age cohorts.

A second group of studies are large-scale studies but are not representative of or generalizable to a broader population. Nonrepresentative local, regional, or multi-site samples that provide sufficient numbers of LGBTQ-parent families for study may not be specifically generalizable to a broader population, but may illuminate important associations or processes that characterize LGBTQ-parent family life. An example is the National Longitudinal Lesbian Family Study (NLLFS).

A third group of studies have emerged since the first edition of this chapter was written: population-based studies specific to LGBTQ communities. Several studies, some of which at the time of this writing are still in the field, offer the first population-based, representative samples of LGBTQ and transgender US populations: the California Quality of Life Survey (CQLS), the Generations Study, the TransPop Study, and the National Couples' Health and Time Study.

The potential of these data sources within the context of research on LGBTQ-parent families is important because, historically, research on LGBTQ-parent families developed from and was grounded in a particular set of very different methodological approaches and disciplines. Early questions about child adjustment (with particular attention to sexual orientation, gender identity, and psychological adjustment) in LGBTQ-parent families emerged from the fields of psychology, child development, and family studies, fields that were already attuned to diverse family forms (Patterson, 1992). Further, studies based on small samples of distinct populations that are not population-based were typical in those fields: Early studies were based largely on community or regional samples (Patterson, 2006). These studies focused on child adjustment and the well-being of mothers, both because these constructs were central in these fields and because scholars were responding to fears that lesbians were mentally unwell and would therefore negatively influence their children (Goldberg, 2010). Over time, LGBTQ-parent research extended to include parenting, family processes, and the well-being of LGBTQ parents (Goldberg, 2010). As this body of work grew, it attracted the attention of other fields of study relevant to families and children, including demography, sociology, economics, and health. Thus, new studies from the population sciences provide a vantage point for understanding LGBTQ-parent families that were population-based and generalizable and that allowed comparisons with heterosexual-parent families (see Biblarz & Savci, 2010, for a review).

Today there are a number of large-scale datasets available that afford the possibility of studying LGBTQ-parent families; however, most have rarely or never been used for this purpose (e.g., the Survey of Income and Program Participation [SIPP]). Some nationally representative studies of families and households in the United States have begun to include questions about the LGBTQ identity status of adult householders, many of whom have children (e.g., the Survey of Income and Program Participation (SIPP), the Panel Study of Income Dynamics (PSID), and the US Census). Other large-scale studies began as population-based, longitudinal studies of children: As the study members have grown up and been followed into adulthood, many have become LGBTQ parents themselves. For instance, it is possible with the Add Health study to follow those who reported same-sex attractions or relationships in adolescence into adulthood, affording the opportunity to study their coupling and parenting in adulthood. The prospective birth cohort studies such as the NCDS and the BCS make it possible to identify same-sex couple and parent households when cohort members are adults (Lau, 2012; Strohm, 2010).

Finally, the analysis of representative data of LGBTQ-parent families has been invoked in the promotion of civil rights for LGBTQ people (e.g., Gates, 2013), yet misinterpretation of data has perpetuated misinformation about LGBTQ

families. A critical example emerged recently, when findings regarding the well-being of children of LGBTQ parents were inaccurately reported from the New Family Structures Study (NFSS) and used to support legal cases against marriage for same-sex couples (see Manning, Fettro, & Lamidi, 2014, for a discussion). After the original report was published, over 150 social scientists endorsed a letter rejecting the academic integrity and intellectual merit of the study (Gates, 2012b; Perrin, Cohen, & Caren, 2013; Umberson, Cavanagh, Glass, & Raley, 2012), and reanalyses of the data using the NFSS have invalidated the initial findings (Cheng & Powell, 2015). The controversy surrounding the misuse of the NFSS underscores the responsibility of primary investigators, as well as reviewers and publishers, to attend to the political implications of studies of LGBTQ parenting and families.

In this chapter, we review findings based on some of these existing data sources while identifying challenges as well as advantages of using population-based representative datasets to study LGBTQ-parent families. Given the growing number of large-scale representative studies that now allow for the study of LGBTQ-parent families, we identify a number of areas of research that are largely understudied but from which much could be learned in the coming years.

## Challenges in Using Secondary Data to Study LGBTQ-Parent Families

There are a number of challenges in any research based on analyses of existing secondary data sources, some of which are further complicated in studies of LGBTQ-parent families. We consider challenges associated with conceptual breadth as well as measurement inclusion in existing studies. The use of secondary data is relatively new among researchers of LGBTQ-parent families, in part because measures for identifying LGBTQ people and LGBTQ-parent families have only recently been included in secondary data sources and also in part due to the origins of the study of LGBTQ-parent families in disciplines where secondary data analysis was less common. Thus, we also briefly review other basic challenges and suggest strategies to address these challenges.

## Conceptual Challenges

At the most basic level, scholars who use secondary datasets must negotiate the discrepancies between their research questions and available data (Hofferth, 2005; Russell & Matthews, 2011). Unless the researcher was directly involved with the data collection process, it is unlikely that full information will be available to address their precise questions. However, they may find that sufficient data exists to partially address their questions or to allow an adjustment of the question based on available data. Most datasets that are focused on broad populations have been developed by economists and sociologists who may not be concerned with many of the constructs that are important to family scholars and psychologists, such as individual or family histories and processes (Russell & Matthews, 2011). Thus, the researcher undoubtedly will be required to be flexible with the conceptual design and creative in posing research questions that can be addressed with available data. At a fundamental level, this is a conceptual problem but one that typically plays out as problems with measurement (what is measured and how).

The most obvious example of this conceptual challenge is that most of what is known from nationally representative studies are based on families in same-sex couple households rather than couples or individuals who specifically identify themselves as lesbian, gay, bisexual, or transgender. For example, since 1990, the US Census has included the option that a primary householder may report an "unmarried partner." It is difficult to imagine how one could construct a single question to accurately ascertain LGBTQ-parent family status, and we know of no study that does this. Rather, researchers must combine multiple questions to identify households with children in which the parents are same-sex partners and householders or engage in same-sex sexual practices or behaviors. Measures of self-

identification as LGBTQ on large-scale surveys continue to be relatively rare; however, participant gender and the gender of their partner/s may be available (Gates & Romero, 2009).

Another conceptual challenge for using secondary data sources to study LGBTQ-parent families is that many of the important constructs in this field are LGBTQ-specific and are unavailable in population-based studies. Thus, important questions specific to LGBTQ-parent families may be missing. For example, how and why do LGBTQ couples decide to have children? How do same-sex couples manage historically gendered parenting roles (Goldberg, 2012; Goldberg, Smith, & Perry-Jenkins, 2012)? What is the impact of LGBTQ-specific minority stress (the experiences of stigma, prejudice, or discrimination due to LGBTQ status; Meyer, 2003) on parenting options, processes, and family life (Chapman et al., 2012)? These questions have been addressed using samples of LGBTQ-parent families, but not population-based samples.

Overall, most of the research literature on LGBTQ-parent families concern constructs that are generalizable to all populations: child adjustment, parent relationship quality, and parenting practices. Yet for questions about LGBTQ-specific dimensions of social or family life (e.g., LGBTQ-specific discrimination; methods for becoming parents and related decision-making), secondary data sources designed for the general population may simply not be suitable.

## Measuring LGBTQ-Parent Families

In terms of measurement, there are a number of challenges specific to the availability of measures in secondary data sources. Research based on any one data source must be interpreted in light of other studies, yet there is variability across studies in the specific measures that can be used to identify LGBTQ-parent families. For example, several federally initiated surveys such as the Behavioral Risk Factor Surveillance System (BRFSS) surveys are administered by states, and although some states have begun to include measures that would allow the study of LGBTQ individuals and thus LGBTQ parents and families, the measures are not consistent across states.

Within BRFSS, for example, Massachusetts is unusual because it includes measures since 2000 (some that differ across the years) for same-sex sexual behavior as well as sexual identity (whether one identifies as lesbian, gay, or bisexual); beginning in 2007, a measure for transgender identity was included (Behavioral Risk Factor Surveillance System, 2011). As of the 2016 survey, 26 states included the BRFSS sexual and gender identity optional module as part of their survey, leading to a number of studies that account for presence of children in household studies of LGBTQ individuals (Boehmer, Clark, Lord, & Fredman, 2018; Cranney, 2016; Fredriksen-Goldsen, Kim, Barkan, Muraco, & Hoy-Ellis, 2013; Gonzales & Henning-Smith, 2017). Yet, no one, to our knowledge, has used this dataset to directly examine LGBTQ-parent families. One challenge is that not all participating states include the same measures, which hinders cross-state comparison and prevents the study of how state characteristics—such as state laws, policies, or practices affect LGBTQ-parent families.

There are also a number of measurement challenges particularly relevant for longitudinal studies of LGBTQ-parent families. Sometimes the measures used in prospective studies change over the span of the study (measures for young children will not be identical to those for adolescents and adults; Russell & Matthews, 2011). For repeated cross-sectional studies, there are challenges when measures are changed. For example, the US Census maintains that, as a result of flaws in the way they classified same-sex households in 1990,[2] the data from 1990 and 2000 cannot be compared (Smith & Gates, 2001). In addition to data errors that result from classifications, some argue that there has been notable change over only a few decades in the diversity of sexual self-

identity labels: Some individuals or couples may prefer, for example, the term "queer" to "gay" or "lesbian" (Morandini, Blaszczynski, & Dar-Nimrod, 2016; Russell, Clarke, & Clary, 2009). Further, individuals and couples may change their preferred identity label over time. The existing variability in measures across studies may only be compounded by changes over time in the ways that LGBTQ parents self-label and disclose their identities and family statuses to researchers.

Finally, as the legal basis for LGBTQ family relationships has been in flux, definitions and measures have shifted (and likely will continue to shift). For example, since the first edition of this chapter in 2013, three times as many countries now allow marriage for same-sex couples (10 countries in 2013; 30 countries as of this writing). As legal statuses change, personal meanings change as well. Prior to the legalization of marriage of same-sex couples, couples mostly cohabited, yet in the most recently available data, close to two out of five same-sex couple are married. Same-sex couples are still more likely to cohabit, yet they marry and divorce at rates similar to different-sex couples (Gates, 2015). Beyond marriage, there are other ways that couple and family life is shifting demographically, with implications for the meanings—and measures—of households, parents, and families. For example, "living apart together" (LAT) relationships (non-residential partnerships) are gaining visibility in Western countries, and LGBTQ people are more likely to be living in these forms of family (Gabb & Fink, 2017; Strohm, Seltzer, Cochran, & Mays, 2009). Such family structural diversity has implications for how individuals and families are captured in population samples (i.e., LAT individuals are often recorded as "single") and thus who may be included or excluded when we study LGBTQ-parent families.

To address these challenges, it is crucial at a most basic level to carefully sort out the opportunities and limitations of the match between one's research question and the data available through secondary sources. For example, one could use the National Health Interview Survey (NHIS) to examine same-sex couple household

---

[2] In the 1990 US Census, when the responding householder identified two persons of the same sex as being spouses, or legally married, the Census Bureau administratively changed the reported gender of the spouse in most cases. Thus, same-sex couple households were undercounted and reported as heterosexual married couple households.

access to health care (the NHIS collects respondents' gender and the gender of others in the household and their relationship to the respondent). However, if one's theory of health-care access and utilization relies on arguments about homophobic discrimination in the health-care setting, the absence of data for householders' sexual identities is crucial. Having a clear understanding of the alignment between one's research question and the secondary dataset will help formulate a strong case for a study's rationale and ultimately for persuading reviewers that the opportunity the data affords outweighs any limitations. In the example above, it may be an important first step for the field to simply document differences in health-care access and utilization based on householder couple status. The researcher must be flexible and creative in matching the research question to available data (Russell & Matthews, 2011). In addition to the need for conceptual and analytic flexibility and creativity with regard to measurement, we turn to several other basic challenges and suggestions for addressing them.

## Methodological Challenges

Becoming familiar with a large and complex existing dataset is time-consuming, and researchers often overlook the "costs" of learning. One must understand a study's design, data structure, and distinct methodological characteristics that may influence analyses (Hofferth, 2005). Studies often employ complex sampling designs which require specialized statistical analytic techniques: Researchers may need to learn methods for adjusting for complex sample designs (e.g., nested samples or cluster designs) or methods for the use of weighted data responses (Russell & Matthews, 2011). There is a common perception that using existing data simply circumvents a data collection phase of research; however, recoding existing variables into useful constructs is time-consuming (after 20 years of experience, the first author has found it necessary to estimate the time it will take and multiply by four!). At the same time,

there are often opportunities for learning: Many large-scale studies have user groups or conferences designed to allow researchers to network with one another.[3] These networks offer possibilities for collaboration or the sharing of strategies for analysis, as well as for learning about others' questions and research efforts. Although when working with publicly available data there is a possibility of having one's idea "scooped" (i.e., taken, tested, and published before one is able to do so oneself), participating in scholarly networks of study users can keep one abreast of developments by other scholars in the field.

## Professional Challenges

Finally, a unique challenge in using secondary data is potential professional costs. In many fields and at many institutions, for various reasons, original data collection may be more highly valued. In some fields, original data has value in itself. At the same time, in research-intensive institutions where grant funding is an important marker of career success, the higher costs and thus larger extramural grants required to collect data may be valued above analyses of secondary data. As research-focused institutions place greater demand on researchers to receive external funding, it is important to acknowledge that grants for secondary data analyses tend to require less overall time and staff. The challenge of acquiring grant funding for LGBTQ-parent research using secondary data analysis may therefore be a disincentive for junior scholars concerned with meeting academic tenure requirements. Yet despite these challenges, the availability and access to a growing number of secondary data sources offers a new array of research possibilities for studying LGBTQ-parent families.

---

[3]For example, Add Health, MIDUS, NCDS, and other datasets offer online searchable databases of publications and other uses of data. User seminars and conferences are held for a number of large-scale studies; for example, the US National Center for Health Statistics holds a National Conference on Health Statistics, offering hands-on education sessions on the full range of data systems they offer.

## Advantages of Secondary Data for Studies of LGBTQ-Parent Families

Having discussed some of the challenges, we now describe the potential advantages of using large-scale or population-based secondary datasets for the study of LGBTQ-parent families. Important advantages include generalizability to broad populations, large sample sizes (including sufficient numbers of underrepresented populations and power for statistical analyses), and the ability to conduct comparative analyses with populations of heterosexual-parent families. Some data sources allow for additional advantages: They may be longitudinal, include data from multiple reporters, allow insights about multiple contexts and processes of development, or allow cross-historical or cross-national comparisons (Russell & Matthews, 2011). An obvious practical advantage is low cost and ease of access (Hofferth, 2005) compared to the labor-intensive work of sample selection and data collection to begin a new study of LGBTQ-parent families.

First, the possibility for making generalizations to broader populations of LGBTQ-parent families is a crucial advantage that can advance this field of study. For example, the 2000 US Census counted 594,391 same-sex couples (Simmons & O'Connell, 2003); of those same-sex couples, about a quarter reported a child under the age of 18 living in their household (Gates & Ost, 2004). Never before had there been a true census of LGBTQ-parent families (or more accurately, households headed by parenting same-sex couples): For the first time, researchers asserted that they had "identified same-sex couples in every state and virtually every county in the United States" (Sears, Gates, & Rubenstein, 2005, p. 1) and provided population estimates of the proportion of households headed by same-sex couples who are parenting in every state (the proportion of same-sex couples out of all households ranged from .27% to .80%). Notably, the same statistics have also been challenged because, with data only available for relationships among adult householders

and thus on couples, they dramatically undercount the total number of single LGBTQ people and single LGBTQ-parent families in the United States. Yet, these results were groundbreaking for establishing the presence of these families for policy makers and planners. The results have also been instrumental in challenging stereotypes about LGBTQ-parent families, for example, that they are typically White, affluent, coastal, and urban. Indeed, these data have established that, although same-sex couples without children are more likely to reside in California and Vermont, same-sex couples with children are more likely to reside in rural states (Mississippi, Wyoming, Alaska, Idaho, and Montana; Gates, 2013, Gates & Ost, 2004). Yet California is where gay and lesbian adoptive and foster families are most likely to live (Gates, Badgett, Macomber, & Chambers, 2007). Further, same-sex couples of color are more likely to have children compared to their White counterparts (Bennett & Gates, 2004; Black, Sanders, & Taylor, 2007; Carpenter & Gates, 2008; Gates, 2012a; 2013).

Second, large sample sizes are beneficial because they allow for both the study of small and often marginalized subpopulations and statistical power for complex analyses (Russell & Matthews, 2011). Obviously, LGBTQ people and LGBTQ-parent families are present in all large-scale studies: The question is whether data are obtained to acknowledge them or whether they are invisible. Given their very small proportion within the total population, only huge studies will yield sufficient numbers of LGBTQ-parent families to allow for statistical analyses. For example, over 20,000 adolescents were included in the in-home portion of the Add Health study collected in 1994–1995; over 17,000 of their parents completed surveys. Wainright et al. (2004) were among the first investigators to use these data to investigate the well-being of adolescents growing up in same-sex parent households. They investigated psychosocial adjustment, school outcomes, and romantic relationships for 44 adolescents determined to be parented by same-sex couples based on parent reports of their gender and the gender of their partner (all were mothers; there were too few two-father families for inclusion in the study). Compared to a matched group of adolescents from heterosexual-parent families, no differences were found in adolescent adjustment (Wainright et al., 2004).

The Add Health study was the first of its kind based on a nationally representative sample to allow comparisons across family types, yet even with over 17,000 responding parents in that study, only 44 adolescents parented by female same-sex couples were identified. It is important to note that these low numbers may also be explained by heteronormative assumptions in the design of the household measures in the original waves of the Add Health study that (a) did not ask the sexual orientation/identity of responding parents, (b) gave preference to female parents on the parent survey, and (c) precluded the possibility for adolescents to indicate on the adolescent-reported household roster that an adult living in the household could be the same-sex partner of a parent.

Add Health data have since been utilized for a number of studies examining children of mothers in same-sex couples. Wainright and Patterson (2006) found that regardless of family type, adolescents whose mothers described closer relationships with their children reported less delinquent behavior and substance use. Further, Wainright and Patterson (2008) found that regardless of family type, adolescents whose mothers described closer relationships with their children reported higher-quality peer relations and more friends in school. These findings support the assertion that the quality of the parent-adolescent relationship better predicts adolescent outcomes than family type (Wainright & Patterson, 2006, 2008). Future studies should examine whether such findings remain true for children of male same-sex couples.

An additional benefit of very large samples is the possibility to study differences among LGBTQ-parent families based on demographics such as race/ethnicity, class, age, and gender. Gates (2013) reports that among same-sex couples in the United States, people of color are twice as likely as their White counterparts to have children under 18 living at home: 41% of non-White women in same-sex couples have children under 18 living at home, compared to 23% of their White counterparts. Among non-White men in same-sex couples, 20% have children living at home relative to 8% of their White counterparts (see Bennett & Gates, 2004; Black et al., 2007; Carpenter & Gates, 2008; Gates & Romero, 2009). Some studies have also begun to measure socioeconomic diversity among LGBTQ-parent families, displacing stereotypes of affluence and reporting higher rates of poverty relative to their heterosexual counterparts (Cenegy, Denney, & Kimbro, 2018; Gates, 2013; Schneebaum & Badgett, 2018; Sears & Badgett, 2012). These findings are groundbreaking in identifying more diversity in LGBTQ-parent families than has been represented in the existing literature, which has been largely derived from community-based samples of LGBTQ-identified parents who, until recently, consisted of primarily White lesbian mothers.

Another advantage to the use of population-based data sources is that some utilize longitudinal designs (Russell & Matthews 2011). Some, like the General Social Survey (GSS) and the National Health Interview Survey (NHIS), collect data longitudinally by collecting representative data across time (but do not follow the same participants prospectively from year to year); few if any published studies based on these data have examined LGBTQ-parent families. Other datasets, such as Add Health, the National Child Development Study (NCDS), and the British Cohort Study (BCS), allow for the study of individuals across time so that hypotheses concerning human development and change can be explored. The members of the Add Health and both the NCDS and BCS cohorts are now adults or young adults, many of whom are becoming parents. These datasets offer unique opportunities to study characteristics from the early life course (childhood and adolescence) that may be associated with the well-being of LGBTQ adults and their children or the adult lives of children who were parented in same-sex households; again, we are aware of no studies that have taken this approach.

Other benefits of large-scale survey studies (e.g., Fragile Families, https://fragilefamilies. princeton.edu/) include perspectives from multiple reporters such as children and parents, which allow for more than one perspective on family life. Finally, another potential advantage is the ability to conduct cross-historical or cross-national comparisons (Russell & Matthews, 2011). For example, a component of the GSS, the International Social Survey Program, was specifically developed to allow for cross-cultural comparisons between the United States, Australia, Great Britain, and West Germany. Such surveys may allow for future comparisons of LGBTQ-parent families across multiple countries.

## New LGBTQ-Focused Population Studies

Several methodological innovations have allowed for in-depth study of LGBTQ individuals and families drawing from general population samples. As marketing and research samples have grown in size and online methods of data collection have been developed, new possibilities have emerged for reaching LGBTQ populations (see chapter "Methods, Recruitment, and Sampling in Research with LGBTQ-Parent Families"). In one of the first examples to use two-phase sampling, LGBTQ participants in the California Health Interview Survey (CHIS) were recontacted for participation in the California Quality of Life Survey (CQLS) which included all participants of CHIS who reported their sexual identity as gay, lesbian, or bisexual or as having had same-sex sexual activity and who agreed to participate in future surveys on the CHIS (Strohm et al., 2009). The CQLS was designed to include questions specific to LGBTQ individuals and families.

More recently, the first nationally representative probability study of LGBTQ adults, the Generations Study (http://www.generations-study.com/), and the first nationally representative probability study of transgender health, the Transpop Study (http://www.transpop.org/), were begun. These interdisciplinary study teams are composed of scientists across fields including psychology, sociology, demography, human development and family sciences, and public health—a testament to a

growing recognition of the importance of diverse perspectives in the study of LGBTQ lives. These projects will allow for some of the first nationally representative evidence from the United States about the lives and health of LGBTQ and transgender adults and provide more accurate estimates related to stigma and health.

Lastly, researchers are in the process of collecting data for the National Couples' Health and Time Study (http://u.osu.edu/kamp-dush.1/about-me/), which will provide the first representative sample of same-sex couples' family functioning, experiences of stigma, and coping. This dataset will address several critical gaps in prior LGBTQ-couple data, including limitations to analysis of dyadic data, a lack of detailed information about family functioning and stress mechanisms, and limited ethnic/racial diversity.

## Implications for Future Research

There is a rich tradition of population-based survey research in the social and behavioral sciences that has provided a baseline for scientific and public understanding of the social and economic health and development of families, yet for generations, LGBTQ people and families were invisible. Developments in recent decades have changed that. More large-scale surveys now include possibilities to identify, study, and understand LGBTQ-parent families. Such large-scale representative studies are one path for building scientific understanding of LGBTQ-parent families. The appendix includes descriptions of relevant data sources, some of which to our knowledge have never been used for the study of LGBTQ-parent families. To compile our appendix, we used five sources: (a) our knowledge of available datasets, (b) Inter-university Consortium for Political and Social Research (ICPSR), (c) UK data archive; (d) a search of EBSCO host for articles using representative data since the publication of the first edition of this book, and (e) a search of Integrated Public Use Microdata Series (IPUMS) data for national census data. The search had two main criteria: The data had to be representative of a population (i.e., national, state, regional) and have the potential to identify same-sex parents or lesbian, gay, bisexual, trans, or queer parents.

In addition to the challenges and opportunities we have discussed, we note some areas in the study of LGBTQ-parent families that have been particularly underexamined and for which the use of secondary data sources may provide important new possibilities. Gay fathers are fewer in number than their female counterparts, which may help to explain why they have been under-represented in existing studies of LGBTQ-parent families. In 1990, one in five female same-sex couples was raising children compared to one in twenty male same-sex couples (Gates & Ost, 2004). By 2000, one in three female same-sex couples and one in five male same-sex couples were raising children (Gates & Ost, 2004). Data from the American Community Survey from 2014 to 2016 found that 8% of male same-sex couples were raising children while 24% of female same-sex couples were raising children (Goldberg & Conron, 2018). Although datasets such as the National Longitudinal Lesbian Family Study (NLLFS) exist to expand research on same-sex female couples, no existing data source is comparable for the study of male same-sex couples raising children (Gartrell et al., 1996). The NLLFS is not population-based and thus is not representative of all lesbian-parent families; however, it is a large sample that includes a birth mother and a co-mother with at least one child from whom data have been collected five times (before the child was born and then when the child was 2, 5, 10, and 17). Data from the NLLFS have allowed researchers to explore the lives of lesbian mothers to debunk common myths. Results find, for example, that the development of psychological well-being in children of lesbian mothers over a 7-year period from childhood to adolescence is the same for those with known and unknown donors (Bos & Gartrell, 2010); no similar information exists about the children of gay fathers using known and unknown donors. Although some studies are beginning to address the importance of examining gay male parenting (e.g., Golombok et al., 2014; Green, Rubio, Rothblum, Bergman, & Katuzny, 2019;

Carneiro, Tasker, Salinas-Quiroz, Leal, & Costa, 2017; see chapters "Gay Men and Surrogacy" and "LGBTQ Adoptive Parents and Their Children"), more attention to gay male parenting is warranted, especially using longitudinal data.

Further, there are few, if any, studies based on population-representative data sources that examine bisexual- or transgender-parent families (there are few existing studies of bisexual or transgender persons and family life in general; see chapter "What Do We Now Know About Bisexual Parenting? A Continuing Call for Research", for a review of bisexual-parent family research, and see chapter "Transgender-Parent Families", for a review of trans-parent family research). Of the sources included in the appendix, the Behavioral Risk Factor Surveillance System (BRFSS, select states), British Cohort Study (BCS), and the National Child Development Studies (NCDS) include measures that allow identification of transgender people. Even though these sources are largely untapped, they afford unprecedented opportunities for scholarship. Lastly, little is known about LGBTQ-parent families and socioeconomic status; much of the existing research focuses on middle-class LGBTQ-parent families (see chapter "LGBTQ-Parent Families in the United States and Economic Well-Being"). Yet studies using new sources of population data have shown, for example, that it is socioeconomic status rather than same-sex family structure that is associated with children's economic well-being (Brown, Manning, & Payne, 2016) and that LGBTQ parents in middle and upper socioeconomic classes are more protected from discrimination (Cenegy et al., 2018).

In conclusion, we have identified challenges as well as opportunities for scholars who may pursue the study of LGBTQ-parent families through analysis of secondary data sources or large-scale surveys. There are many new possibilities for the study of LGBTQ-parent families (and even more possibilities to study LGBTQ individuals). To date, findings from such studies have been groundbreaking. Not only have they demonstrated, for example, that child and family well-being do not differ in LGBTQ-parent and heterosexual-parent families (Bos, Knox,

Rijn-van Gelderen, & Gartrell, 2016; Gartrell, Bos, & Koh, 2018; Rosenfeld, 2010; Wainright et al., 2004; Wainright & Patterson, 2006, 2008), but also they have dispelled myths about who LGBTQ parents are and where they live (Gates, 2013; Gates & Ost, 2004; Gates & Romero, 2009) and have shown simply—yet radically— that LGBTQ-parent families are everywhere (Simmons & O'Connell, 2003; see chapter "LGBTQ-Parent Families in Community Context"). There are remarkable possibilities waiting in these data sources. They are opportunities to propel the field of LGBTQ-parent families, and thus our understanding of all contemporary families, forward.

**Acknowledgments** The authors acknowledge support for this research from the Priscilla Pond Flawn Endowment at the University of Texas at Austin. This work was supported by grant P2CHD042849, Population Research Center, and by grant T32HD007081, Training Program in Population Studies, both awarded to the Population Research Center at The University of Texas at Austin by the Eunice Kennedy Shriver National Institute of Child Health and Human Development. The research was also supported by a predoctoral training grant, F31MH115608, awarded to Allen Mallory in the Population Research Center at the University of Texas at Austin by the National Institute of Mental Health. The content is solely the responsibility of the authors and does not necessarily represent the official views of the National Institutes of Health.

# Appendix: Secondary Data Opportunities

*American Community Survey*
Representative of US population; http://www.census.gov/acs/www/

*American National Election Studies 2016 Time Series Study*
Nationally representative sample of people in the United States over 18 in 2016; https://www.icpsr.umich.edu/icpsrweb/ICPSR/series/3

*Annual Population Survey (UK) 2013–2017*
Nationally representative longitudinal study of the United Kingdom; https://beta.ukdataservice.ac.uk/datacatalogue/studies/study?id=6721

*Behavioral Risk Factor Surveillance System*
Representative at state level; http://www.cdc.gov/brfss/

*Brazil 2010 Census*
Representative of Brazilian population in 2010; https://ww2.ibge.gov.br/english/estatistica/populacao/censo2010/default.shtm

*British Cohort Study*
All infants ($N = 17{,}200$) born during a one-week period in England, Scotland, Wales, and Northern Ireland in April 1970; https://beta.ukdataservice.ac.uk/datacatalogue/studies/study?id=5558

*British Household Panel Survey: Waves 1–18, 1991–2009*
Nationally representative household survey of the United Kingdom collected for eighteen waves between 1991 and 2009; https://discover.ukdataservice.ac.uk/catalogue/?sn=5151&type=Data%20catalogue

*California Health Interview Survey: Adult*
Representative of the state of California; http://www.chis.ucla.edu/about.html

*California Quality of Life Survey*
Gay, lesbian, and bisexual individuals in the state of California; https://britecenter.org/current-projects/ca-quality-of-life-survey/

*Canadian Community Health Survey*
Nationally representative sample of Canada that is collected annually; http://www23.statcan.gc.ca/imdb/p2SV.pl?Function=getSurvey&SDDS=3226#a2

*Census for Puerto Rico*
Representative of Puerto Rican residents; https://usa.ipums.org/usa-action/variables/SSMC#availability_section

*Census for Spain 2001 and 2011*
Representative of Spain residents in 2001 and 2011; https://international.ipums.org/international-action/variables/SAMESEX#codes_section

*Civil Union Study 2000–2002*
Population-based study of about 500 individuals in Vermont from 2000 to 2001; https://www.icpsr.umich.edu/icpsrweb/ICPSR/studies/31241

*Early Childhood Longitudinal Program-B*
Nationally representative of 14,000 children born in the United States in 2001; https://nces.ed.gov/ecls/

*Early Childhood Longitudinal Program-K*

Nationally representative longitudinal study of children from kindergarten to the eighth grade from the fall and the spring of kindergarten (1998–1999), the fall and spring of first grade (1999–2000), the spring of third grade (2002), the spring of fifth grade (2004), and the spring of eighth grade (2007); https://nces.ed.gov/ecls/

*Early Childhood Longitudinal Program-K 2011*

Nationally representative US sample selected from both public and private schools attending both full-day and part-day kindergarten in 2010–2011; https://nces.ed.gov/ecls/

*Fragile Families (wave 15)*

National weights make the data of 16 of the 20 cities representative of births in the 77 US cities with populations over 200,000. Wave 15 was collected between 2014 and 2017; https://fragilefamilies.princeton.edu/

*General Lifestyle Survey (2000–2011)*

Previously known at the General Household Survey (GHS), a continuous nationally representative survey of people in Great Britain living in private households. Closed in 2011; https://discover.ukdataservice.ac.uk/catalogue/?sn=6716&type=Data%20catalogue

*General Social Survey*

Representative of US population; http://www.norc.org/GSS+Website/About+GSS/

*Generations*

Nationally representative longitudinal sample of LGB individuals in the United States, starting in 2016; http://www.generations-study.com/

*How Couples Meet and Stay Together (Waves 1–5)*

Nationally representative longitudinal sample of 4002 people in the United States collected from 2009 to 2015; https://www.icpsr.umich.edu/icpsrweb/ICPSR/studies/30103/variables?q=same+sex

*Longitudinal Study of Generations*

Representative longitudinal study of families in Los Angeles collected for eight waves between 1971 and 2005; https://www.icpsr.umich.edu/icpsrweb/ICPSR/studies/22100/variables?q=partner

*Midlife in the United States*

National sample of over 7000 adults ages 25–74, at wave 1, in the United States with multiple waves: wave 1 (1995–1997), wave 2 (2004–2009), a refresher (2011–2014), and wave 3 (2013–2014)—there is an African American subsample from Milwaukee at wave 2 (2005–2006) and wave 3 (2016–2017); https://www.icpsr.umich.edu/icpsrweb/ICPSR/series/203

*National Adult Tobacco Survey*

Representative of the states of the United States; https://www.cdc.gov/tobacco/data_statistics/index.htm

*National Alcohol Survey*

Nationally representative sample of 5000 US adults quinquennially; http://arg.org/resources-tools/databases/

*National Child Development Study*

All infants ($N = 17,500$) born during a one-week period in England, Scotland, and Wales in March 1958; http://www.cls.ioe.ac.uk/page.aspx?&sitesectionid=724&sitesectiontitle=National+Child+Development+Study

*National Couples' Health and Time Study*

Representative of same-sex couples in the United States; data collection ongoing; https://projectreporter.nih.gov/project_info_description.cfm?aid=9596545&icde=43649856

*National Crime Victimization Survey*

Nationally representative biennial sample of 49,000 households comprising about 100,000 persons; https://www.bjs.gov/index.cfm?ty=dcdetail&iid=245

*National Epidemiological Survey of Alcohol and Related Conditions I and II*

Nationally representative longitudinal sample with data collection beginning on 2001; https://pubs.niaaa.nih.gov/publications/arh29-2/74-78.htm

*National Epidemiological Survey of Alcohol and Related Condition III*

Nationally representative US sample of 36, 309 individuals collected 2013–2014; https://www.niaaa.nih.gov/research/nesarc-iii

*National Health and Nutrition Examination Survey*

Nationally representative US sample of about 5000 persons each year; https://www.cdc.gov/nchs/nhanes/index.htm

*National Health and Social Life Survey*

National probability sample of people between aged 18 and 59 in the United States collected in 1992; https://www.icpsr.umich.edu/icpsrweb/ICPSR/studies/6647/variables?q=parenting

*National Health Interview Survey*

Representative of US population; http://www.cdc.gov/nchs/nhis/about_nhis.htm

*National Household Education Survey*

National sample of household members in the United States between 1991 and 2016; https://nces.ed.gov/nhes/

*National Household Survey on Drug Abuse (1996) Renamed the National Survey on Drug Use and Health*

Nationally representative household survey of the United States; https://pdas.samhsa.gov/#/

*National Intimate Partner and Sexual Violence Survey*

Nationally representative survey of people in the United States and individual states in 2010; https://www.icpsr.umich.edu/icpsrweb/NACJD/studies/34305?archive=NACJD&q=nisvs&permit%255B0%255D=AVAILABLE&x=0&y=0

*National Longitudinal Lesbian Family Study*

Recruitment occurred in Boston; Washington, DC; and San Francisco; http://www.nllfs.org/about/

*National Longitudinal Study of Adolescent Health*

Representative of US population; http://www.cpc.unc.edu/projects/addhealth/about

*National Social Life, Health, and Aging Project*

National household sample of 4440 people born between 1920 and 1947 in the United States between 2005 and 2006; https://www.icpsr.umich.edu/icpsrweb/ICPSR/studies/20541/summary

*National Survey of America's Families 1999 and 2002*

Nationally representative sample of 42,360 households with members under 65 in the United States in 1999; https://www.icpsr.umich.edu/icpsrweb/ICPSR/studies/3927/summary

*National Survey of Children's Health*

Nationally representative of the US population, with survey data collected annually as of 2016; http://childhealthdata.org/learn/NSCH/data

*National Survey of Families and Households*

Nationally representative longitudinal sample of 13,007 people in the United States collected for three waves: wave 1 (1987–1988), wave 2 (1992–1994), and wave3 (2001–2002); https://www.icpsr.umich.edu/icpsrweb/ICPSR/series/193

*National Survey of Family Growth*

Prior to 2002, the sample was representative of women 15–44 living in the United States. Starting with the sixth wave in 2002, the population became representative of all people 15–44 living in the United States; www.cdc.gov/nchs/data/nhsr/nhsr036.pdf

*National Survey of Sexual Attitudes and Lifestyles, 2000*

Nationally representative of the United Kingdom collected 1990–1991, 1999–2001, and 2010–2012; https://discover.ukdataservice.ac.uk/catalogue/?sn=8178&type=Data%20catalogue#documentation

*National Trans Discrimination Survey*

The largest survey of trans individuals in the United States. Participants were about 28,000 respondents from all fifty states, the District of Columbia, American Samoa, Guam, Puerto Rico, and US military bases overseas, and data was collected in 2015; http://www.ustranssurvey.org/reports#USTS

*New Family Structures Study*

Nationally representative of the United States, with data collected from about 3000 adults between 2011 and 2012; https://www.icpsr.umich.edu/icpsrweb/ICPSR/studies/34392

*NLSY 79*

Nationally representative US sample of 12,686 14–22 years old when they were first surveyed in 1979. These individuals were interviewed annually through 1994 and are currently interviewed on a biennial basis; https://www.bls.gov/nls/nlsy79.htm

*NLSY 97*

Nationally representative longitudinal sample of approximately 9000 12 to 16 years beginning in 1996 who are interviewed on an annual basis; https://www.bls.gov/nls/nlsy97.htm

*Northern Ireland Life and Times Survey (pre1998 Called the Young Life and Times Survey)*

Nationally representative of Ireland collected beginning in 1998; https://discover.ukdataservice.ac.uk/catalogue/?sn=4587&type=Data%20catalogue

*Pairfam*

Nationally representative longitudinal sample of more than 12,000 persons of the three birth cohorts 1971–1973, 1981–1983, 1991–1993 and their partners that is collected annually; http://www.pairfam.de/en/

*Project on Human Development in Chicago Neighborhoods*

Representative longitudinal study of people living in Chicago between 1994 and 1995 and at subsequent waves between 1997–1999 and 2000–2001; https://www.icpsr.umich.edu/icpsrweb/ICPSR/series/206

*Survey of Income and Program Participation*

Representative of US population; http://www.census.gov/sipp/intro.html

*The National Child Development Study: Partnership Histories (1974–2013)*

All adults born in Great Britain in one week in 1958. Studied longitudinally beginning in 1974; https://discover.ukdataservice.ac.uk/catalogue/?sn=6940&type=Data%20catalogue

*TransPop*

Representative of trans individuals in the United States; data collection ongoing; http://www.transpop.org/)

*United States Census (2010)*

Representative of US population; http://2010.census.gov/2010census/index.php

*Welfare, Children, and Families: A Three-City Study*

Low income families in Boston, Chicago, and San Antonio; http://web.jhu.edu/threecitystudy/index.html.

*Youth and Development Study*

Random population sample of ~25,000 Dutch residents with children under 18 years old; https://www.narcis.nl/dataset/RecordID/oai%3Aeasy.dans.knaw.nl%3Aeasy-dataset%3A61653/id/1/Language/NL/uquery/OJO/coll/dataset

*Youth Development Study, 1988–2011*

Representative longitudinal study of ninth graders in St. Paul Public School District in Minnesota between 1987 and 1988 and subsequent waves until 2011 including participant parents and participant children; https://www.icpsr.umich.edu/icpsrweb/ICPSR/studies/24881/summary

# References

Bennett, L., & Gates, G. J. (2004). *The cost of marriage inequality to children and their same-sex parents*. Washington, DC: Human Rights Campaign Foundation. Retrieved from https://tinyurl.com/y586fwta

Biblarz, T. J., & Savci, E. (2010). Lesbian, gay, bisexual, and transgender families. *Journal of Marriage and Family, 72*, 480–497. https://doi.org/10.1111/j.1741-3737.2010.00714.x

Black, D. A., Sanders, S. G., & Taylor, L. J. (2007). The economics of lesbian and gay families. *Journal of Economic Perspectives, 21*, 53–70. https://doi.org/10.1257/jep.21.2.53

Boehmer, U., Clark, M. A., Lord, E. M., & Fredman, L. (2018). Caregiving status and health of heterosexual, sexual minority, and transgender adults: Results from select U.S. regions in the Behavioral Risk Factor Surveillance System 2015 and 2016. *The Gerontologist*, Advance online publication. https://doi.org/10.1093/geront/gny109

Bos, H. M., Knox, J. R., van Rijn-van Gelderen, L., & Gartrell, N. K. (2016). Same-sex and different-sex parent households and child health outcomes: Findings from the National Survey of Children's Health. *Journal of Developmental & Behavioral Pediatrics, 37*, 179–187. doi:https://doi.org/10.1097/dbp.0000000000000288

Bos, H. M. W., & Gartrell, N. K. (2010). Adolescents of the U.S. National Longitudinal Lesbian Family Study: The impact of having a known or an unknown donor on the stability of psychological adjustment. *Human Reproduction, 26*, 630–637. https://doi.org/10.1093/humrep/deq359

Brown, S. L., Manning, W. D., & Payne, K. K. (2016). Family structure and children's economic well-being:

Incorporating same-sex cohabiting mother families. *Population Research and Policy Review, 35*, 1–21. https://doi.org/10.1007/s11113-015-9375-8

Carneiro, F. A., Tasker, F., Salinas-Quiroz, F., Leal, I., & Costa, P. A. (2017). Are the fathers alright? A systematic and critical review of studies on gay and bisexual fatherhood. *Frontiers in Psychology, 8*, 1636–1648. https://doi.org/10.3389/fpsyg.2017.01636

Carpenter, C., & Gates, G. (2008). Gay and lesbian partnerships: Evidence from California. *Demography, 45*, 573–590. https://doi.org/10.1353/dem.0.0014

Castelvecchi, D. (2018, September). Google unveils search engine for open data. *Nature, 561*, 161–162. Retrieved from https://www.nature.com/articles/d41586-018-06201-x

Cenegy, L. F., Denney, J. T., & Kimbro, R. T. (2018). Family diversity and child health: Where do same-sex couple families fit? *Journal of Marriage and Family, 80*, 198–218. https://doi.org/10.1111/jomf.12437

Chapman, R., Wardrop, J., Freeman, P., Zappia, T., Watkins, R., & Shields, L. (2012). A descriptive study of the experiences of lesbian, gay and transgender parents accessing health services for their children. *Journal of Clinical Nursing, 21*, 1128–1135. https://doi.org/10.1111/j.1365-2702.2011.03939.x

Cheng, S., & Powell, B. (2015). Measurement, methods, and divergent patterns: Reassessing the effects of same-sex parents. *Social Science Research, 52*, 615–626. https://doi.org/10.1016/j.ssresearch.2015.04.005

Cranney, S. (2016). The LGB Mormon paradox: Mental, physical, and self-rated health among Mormon and non-Mormon LGB individuals in the Utah behavioral risk factor surveillance system. *Journal of Homosexuality, 64*, 731–744. https://doi.org/10.1080/00918369.2016.1236570

Fredriksen-Goldsen, K. I., Kim, H. J., Barkan, S. E., Muraco, A., & Hoy-Ellis, C. P. (2013). Health disparities among lesbian, gay, and bisexual older adults: Results from a population-based study. *American Journal of Public Health, 103*, 1802–1809. https://doi.org/10.2105/ajph.2012.301110

Gabb, J., & Fink, J. (2017). *Couple relationships in the 21st century: Research, policy, practice.* Cham, Switzerland: Springer Nature.

Gartrell, N., Bos, H., & Koh, A. (2018). National Longitudinal Lesbian Family Study-Mental health of adult offspring. *The New England Journal of Medicine, 379*, 297–299. https://doi.org/10.1056/nejmc1804810

Gartrell, N., Hamilton, J., Banks, A., Mosbacher, D., Reed, N., Sparks, C. H., & Bishop, H. (1996). The National Lesbian Family Study: 1. Interviews with prospective mothers. *American Journal of Orthopsychiatry, 66*, 272–281. https://doi.org/10.1037/h0080178

Gates, G. (2012a, January). Family formation and raising children among same-sex couples. *National Council of Family Relations, 51*, 1–4. Retrieved from https://escholarship.org/uc/item/5pq1q8d7

Gates, G. J. (2012b). Letter to the editors and advisory editors of *Social Science Research. Social Science Research, 41*, 1350–1351. https://doi.org/10.1016/j.ssresearch.2012.08.008

Gates, G. J. (2013). *LGBT parenting in the United States.* Los Angeles, CA: The Williams Institute, UCLA School of Law. Retrieved from https://tinyurl.com/yda3aq3e

Gates, G. J. (2015). Marriage and family: LGBT individuals and same-sex couples. *The Future of Children, 25*, 67–87. https://doi.org/10.1353/foc.2015.0013

Gates, G. J., Badgett, M. V. L., Macomber, J. E., & Chambers, K. (2007). *Adoption and foster care by gay and lesbian parents in the United States.* Los Angeles, CA: The Williams Institute, UCLA School of Law. https://doi.org/10.1037/e690872011-001

Gates, G. J., & Ost, J. (2004). *The gay and lesbian atlas.* Washington, DC: Urban Institute.

Gates, G. J., & Romero, A. (2009). Parenting by gay men and lesbians: Beyond the current research. In E. Peters & C. M. Kamp Dush (Eds.), *Marriage and family: Perspectives and complexities* (pp. 227–246). New York, NY: Columbia University Press.

Goldberg, A. E. (2010). *Lesbian and gay parents and their children: Research on the family life cycle.* Washington, DC: American Psychological Association.

Goldberg, A. E. (2012). *Gay dads: Transitions to adoptive fatherhood.* New York, NY: NYU Press.

Goldberg, A. E., Smith, J. Z., & Perry-Jenkins, M. (2012). The division of labor in lesbian, gay, and heterosexual new adoptive parents. *Journal of Marriage and Family, 74*, 812–828. https://doi.org/10.1111/j.1741-3737.2012.00992.x

Goldberg, S. K., & Conron, K. J. (2018). Demographic characteristics of lesbian, gay, bisexual, and transgender adults in the United States: Evidence from the 2015–2017 Gallup Daily Tracking Survey. In W. Swan (Ed.), *The Routledge handbook of LGBTQIA administration and policy* (pp. 41–74). New York, NY: Routledge.

Golombok, S., Mellish, L., Jennings, S., Casey, P., Tasker, F., & Lamb, M. E. (2014). Adoptive gay father families: Parent–child relationships and children's psychological adjustment. *Child Development, 85*, 456–468. https://doi.org/10.1111/cdev.12155

Gonzales, G., & Henning-Smith, C. (2017). Health disparities by sexual orientation: Results and implications from the Behavioral Risk Factor Surveillance System. *Journal of Community Health, 42*, 1163–1172. https://doi.org/10.1007/s10900-017-0366-z

Green, R. J., Rubio, R. J., Rothblum, E. D., Bergman, K., & Katuzny, K. E. (2019). Gay fathers by surrogacy: Prejudice, parenting, and well-being of female and male children. *Psychology of Sexual Orientation and Gender Diversity.* Advance online publication. https://doi.org/10.1037/sgd0000325

Hofferth, S. L. (2005). Secondary data analysis in family research. *Journal of Marriage and Family, 67*, 891–907. https://doi.org/10.1111/j.1741-3737.2005.00182.x

Lau, C. Q. (2012). The stability of same-sex cohabitation, different-sex cohabitation, and marriage. *Journal of Marriage and Family, 74*, 973–988. https://doi.org/10.1111/j.1741-3737.2012.01000.x

Manning, W. D., Fettro, M. N., & Lamidi, E. (2014). Child well-being in same-sex parent families: Review of research prepared for American Sociological Association Amicus Brief. *Population Research and Policy Review, 33*, 485–502. https://doi.org/10.1007/s11113-014-485-502.

Meyer, I. H. (2003). Prejudice, social stress, and mental health in lesbian, gay, and bisexual populations: Conceptual issues and research evidence. *Psychological Bulletin, 129*, 674–697. https://doi.org/10.1037/0033-2909.129.5.674

Morandini, J. S., Blaszczynski, A., & Dar-Nimrod, I. (2016). Who adopts queer and pansexual sexual identities? *The Journal of Sex Research, 54*, 911–922. https://doi.org/10.1080/00224499.2016.1249332

Patterson, C. J. (1992). Children of lesbian and gay parents. *Child Development, 63*, 1025–1042. https://doi.org/10.2307/1131517

Patterson, C. J. (2006). Children of lesbian and gay parents. *Current Directions in Psychological Science, 15*, 241–244. https://doi.org/10.1111/j.1467-8721.2006.00444.x

Perrin, A. J., Cohen, P. N., & Caren, N. (2013). Are children of parents who had same-sex relationships disadvantaged? A scientific evaluation of the no-differences hypothesis. *Journal of Gay & Lesbian Mental Health, 17*, 327–336. https://doi.org/10.1080/19359705.2013.772553

Rosenfeld, M. J. (2010). Nontraditional families and childhood progress through school. *Demography, 47*, 755–775. https://doi.org/10.1353/dem.0.0112

Russell, S. T., Clarke, T. J., & Clary, J. (2009). Are teens "post-gay"? Contemporary adolescents' sexual identity labels. *Journal of Youth and Adolescence, 38*, 884–890. https://doi.org/10.1007/s10964-008-9388-2

Russell, S. T., & Matthews, E. (2011). Using secondary data to study adolescence and adolescent development. In K. Trzesniewki, M. B. Donnellan, & R. E. Lucas (Eds.), *Obtaining and analyzing secondary data: Methods and illustrations* (pp. 163–176). Washington, DC: American Psychological Association.

Russell, S. T., & Muraco, J. (2013). The use of representative datasets to study LGBT-parent families: Challenges, advantages and opportunities. In A. E. Goldberg & K. R. Allen (Eds.), *LGBT-parent families: Innovations in research and implications for practice* (pp. 343–348). New York, NY: Springer.

Schneebaum, A., & Badgett, M. L. (2018). Poverty in U.S. lesbian and gay couple households. *Feminist Economics, 25*, 1–30. https://doi.org/10.1080/13545701.2018.1441533

Sears, B., & Badgett, L. (2012). *Beyond stereotypes: Poverty in the LGBT community*. The Williams Institute, UCLA School of Law. Retrieved from https://williamsinstitute.law.ucla.edu/williams-in-the-news/beyond-stereotypes-poverty-in-the-lgbt-community/

Sears, R. B., Gates, G., & Rubenstein, W. B. (2005). *Same-sex couples and same-sex couples raising children in the United States: Data from Census 2000*. Los Angeles, CA: The Williams Institute, UCLA School of Law. Retrieved from http://www.law.ucla.edu/Williamsinstitute/publications/USReport.pdf

Simmons, T., & O'Connell, M. (2003). Married-couple and unmarried-couple households: 2000. *Census 2000 Special Reports*. Washington, DC: U.S. Census Bureau.

Smith, D. M., & Gates, G. J. (2001). Gay and lesbian families in the United States: Same-sex unmarried partner households. *A Human Rights Campaign Report*. Washington, DC. Retrieved from http://www.urban.org/url.cfm?ID=1000494

Strohm, C. Q. (2010). *The stability of same-sex cohabitation, different-sex cohabitation, and marriage* (Report No. PWP-CCPR-2010-013). Retrieved from California Center for Population Research website: http://papers.ccpr.ucla.edu/papers/

Strohm, C. Q., Seltzer, J. A., Cochran, S. D., & Mays, V. M. (2009). "Living apart together" relationships in the United States. *Demographic Research, 21*, 177–214. https://doi.org/10.4054/DemRes.2009.21.7

Umberson, D., Cavanagh, S., Glass, J., & Raley, K. (2012, June 26). Texas professors respond to new research on gay parenting. *Huffington Post*. Retrieved from https://www.huffingtonpost.com/debra-umberson/texas-professors-gay-research_b_1628988.html

Wainright, J. L., & Patterson, C. (2008). Peer relations among adolescents with female same-sex parents. *Developmental Psychology, 44*, 117–126. https://doi.org/10.1037/0012-1649.44.1.117

Wainright, J. L., & Patterson, C. J. (2006). Delinquency, victimization, and drug, tobacco, and alcohol use among adolescents with female same-sex parents. *Journal of Family Psychology, 20*, 526–530. https://doi.org/10.1037/0893-3200.20.3.526

Wainright, J. L., Russell, S. T., & Patterson, C. (2004). Psychosocial adjustment, school outcomes, and romantic attractions of adolescents with same-sex parents. *Child Development, 75*, 1886–1898. https://doi.org/10.1111/j1467-8624.2004.00823.x

Winerman, L. (2017). Trends report: Psychologists embrace open science. *Monitor on Psychology, 48*, 90. Retrieved from http://www.apa.org/monitor/2017/11/trends-open-science.aspx

# Methods, Recruitment, and Sampling in Research with LGBTQ-Parent Families

Emma C. Potter and Daniel J. Potter

While the field of lesbian, gay, bisexual, transgender, and queer (LGBTQ) parenting is subject to ideological, political, and moral debates, it is also not immune from methodological debate. Common methodological debates center on limited sample sizes (see Moore & Stambolis-Ruhstorfer, 2013)—even with the use of larger datasets (see Rosenfeld, 2010, 2013). As social scientists, our scientific and theoretical conclusions are only as good as the methods by which we collect and analyze our data. Methodological debates make clear that transparency— to openly discuss the issues and best practices—around the decisions and execution of methods is of vital importance. The purpose of this chapter is to give an in-depth look at methods, recruitment strategies, and sampling techniques of research related to LGBTQ-parent families.

E. C. Potter (✉)
Department of Psychology, University of Virginia, Charlottesville, VA, USA
e-mail: ecp3f@virginia.edu

D. J. Potter
Houston Education Research Consortium, Rice University, Houston, TX, USA
e-mail: dpotter@rice.edu

## Chapter Overview

In our view, two major lines of method-related conversations have recently emerged. The first line is the need for more research on underrepresented populations in LGBTQ research. Historically, LGBTQ-parent research has had varying success in sampling diverse LGBTQ people and their families (Biblarz & Savci, 2010; Goldberg, 2010; Patterson, 2000; van Eeden-Moorefield, Few-Demo, Benson, Bible, & Lummer, 2018), with much of the research heavily reflecting experiences of White, middle- to upper-class LGBTQ-parent families who live in a select handful of urban locales in the United States. Despite these common perceptions of who LGBTQ families are and where they live, US Census data show a more diverse picture of these families—families with racial and ethnic minority diversity, more likely to live in the South, and from across the economic spectrum (Gates, 2013). The field of LGBTQ-parent research continues to work toward centering the experiences of those often minimized in research (Bermúdez, Muruthi, & Jordan, 2016), and researchers *can* successfully engage LGBTQ people from all walks of life (see Battle, Pastrana, & Harris, 2017a, 2017b, 2017c; Chung, Oswald, & Wiley, 2006; Mays, Chatters, Cochran, & Mackness, 1998; Moore, 2011; Orel, 2014; see chapter "LGBTQ-Parent Families in Community Context"; Oswald & Lazarevic, 2011). This

© Springer Nature Switzerland AG 2020
A. E. Goldberg, K. R. Allen (eds.), *LGBTQ-Parent Families*,
https://doi.org/10.1007/978-3-030-35610-1_30

chapter highlights the growing possibilities and paths to successfully engaging and reflecting diverse LGBTQ-parent families in research.

The second method-related issue has to do with conducting more research that utilizes nationally representative data. This need stems from the continued methodological conversations related to survey research (Ridolfo, Miller, & Maitland, 2012), limited sample size critiques (Schumm & Crawford, 2018), and group comparisons (see Rosenfeld, 2010, 2013). Some of the more well-known studies on LGBTQ-parent families have tended to use convenience or purposive sampling (Gartrell et al., 1996), and while this method is understandable for trying to study smaller groups in the population, it often limits the diversity in the types of families included in the study. We acknowledge the utility of expanding the use of nationally representative data and advocate for *further expansion* of sexual orientation and gender identity measures to be included in national datasets. We put forward ideas of how such measurement can be improved related to this point. But, we also intend to use this chapter to argue that nationally representative data using simple random sampling strategies may not always be the most meaningful form of data. Thus, this chapter works toward a narrative that argues for better measurement, innovative recruitment strategies, and alternative sampling techniques that may better serve the field of LGBTQ-parent research.

With these methodological concerns in mind (i.e., diversity in LGBTQ-parent families and calls for more nationally representative data), this chapter is composed of five major sections. First, we provide a brief overview of the state of LGBTQ-parent research from a methodological perspective using existing content analyses and reviews. The second section discusses issues and measurement of identities and other pertinent factors for LGBTQ scholars to consider in their use of qualitative and quantitative methods. Third, we shift the discussion to recruitment with LGBTQ-parent populations. Here, we detail some of the opportunities and challenges in recruiting LGBTQ-parent families for research. Fourth, we turn our attention to issues of sampling

in survey and qualitative research. Lastly, we end with future research methods and implications for practice and provide practical resources for readers and researchers.

## State of LGBTQ-Parent Research Methods

LGBTQ-parent family research remains a relatively new frontier in family research (Allen & Demo, 1995), and the field has grown substantially over the last 20 years. Yet, discipline-specific reviews (Biblarz & Savci, 2010; Moore & Stambolis-Ruhstorfer, 2013) and content analyses (Hartwell, Serovich, Grafsky, & Kerr, 2012; Sullivan & Losberg, 2003; Tasker & Patterson, 2007; van Eeden-Moorefield et al., 2018) estimate that LGBTQ research accounted for only about 2% of total academic social science scholarship (see van Eeden-Moorefield et al., 2018). A growing proportion of *LGBTQ research* has examined LGBTQ parents (increasing from an estimated 13.5% of LGBTQ research studies in Sullivan and Losberg (2003) to 28.8% in van Eeden-Moorefield et al. (2018)), although, admittedly, far fewer studies have focused on trans- or queer-identified parents. Among those articles on LGBTQ parents, most academic focus has been on child outcomes (Tasker & Patterson, 2007), family formation (Goldberg, 2010; Tasker & Delvoye, 2015), and relationship dynamics (Biblarz & Savci, 2010; Vaccaro, 2010; Veldorale-Griffin, 2014).

Researchers in social work (Sullivan & Losberg, 2003), marriage and family therapy (Hartwell et al., 2012), sociology (Moore & Stambolis-Ruhstorfer, 2013), psychology (Rostosky & Riggle, 2017; Tasker & Patterson, 2007), and family science (van Eeden-Moorefield et al., 2018) have examined the state of LGBTQ research (building on the tradition set by Allen and Demo (1995)). From a methodological standpoint, content analyses and reviews have detailed the use of both quantitative and qualitative research in LGBTQ-parent studies. van Eeden-Moorefield et al. (2018) and Hartwell et al. (2012) found that quantitative methods were used in 41.8% and 39.3% of LGBTQ studies, compared to qualitative methods (34% and 13.3%, respectively). van Eeden-Moorefield et al. (2018) also provided a much needed examination of the form of data collection; they reported that the most common forms included interviews (35.8%), surveys (35.0%), secondary data analysis (14.6%), and content analyses (4.9%). Quantitative methods in LGBTQ research have often been comparative (Moore & Stambolis-Ruhstorfer, 2013; van Eeden-Moorefield et al., 2018), and some have utilized large national datasets (Tasker & Patterson, 2007). The use of other methodologies (e.g., clinical, theoretical, mixed method) varies according to field. For example, Hartwell et al. (2012) found, unsurprisingly, that 43.9% of therapy-related publications on LGBTQ individuals were clinical or theoretical, while Farr, Tasker, and Goldberg (2016) found that among the top 30 cited articles in social sciences (e.g., psychology, sociology, and education), only 27% of articles explicitly employed theory in the research design.

While survey research has been the most frequent form of data collection in recent decades, such quantitative methods are not considered the only methodological path forward in LGBTQ research (van Eeden-Moorefield & Chauveron, 2016). That is, while quantitative methodologies are more often used (Hartwell et al., 2012; Sullivan & Losberg, 2003; Tasker & Patterson, 2007; van Eeden-Moorefield et al., 2018), one methodology does not dominate the other in the field of LGBTQ studies. Scholars of LGBTQ research readily acknowledge the value of both qualitative (e.g., in-depth interviews, content analysis, discourse analysis) and quantitative research (e.g., survey questionnaires, Likert scale). The field of LGBTQ studies is unique in its appreciation and acknowledgment of how qualitative work can validate, enhance, clarify, and expand quantitative work and vice versa (Sullivan & Losberg, 2003; van Eeden-Moorefield & Chauveron, 2016). Some of the most valuable theoretical advances in LGBTQ research are owed to qualitative work (Moore & Stambolis-Ruhstorfer, 2013; Rostosky & Riggle, 2017; Tasker & Patterson, 2007; van Eeden-

Moorefield & Chauveron, 2016). Qualitative work has and continues to reveal important processes, mechanisms, and structure or social forces that shape everyday life and outcomes for LGBTQ individuals. Such insights accentuate the limitations in existing quantitative (even big data) approaches and push the field to produce higher-quality, more contextualized quantitative research (van Eeden-Moorefield & Chauveron, 2016). Indeed, LGBTQ family studies have been *strengthened* by the use of different methodologies (Biblarz & Savci, 2010).

## Measurement in Research

The operationalization of a construct—that is, how we measure the thing we are interested in studying—is a crucial component of all research. Capturing this complexity and appropriately incorporating identity into research are the struggles constantly faced by researchers. In this part of the chapter, we focus particularly on measurement issues related to a person's identities (e.g., sexual, gender, racial/ethnic, socioeconomic) in the context of qualitative and quantitative research. A person's multidimensional identities serve an important role in research, as each dimension as well as the amalgamation of dimensions can shape the social positions of an individual within larger societal structures of power and opportunity (Few-Demo, Humble, Curran, & Lloyd, 2016). Measurement of social and personal identities is ever-evolving, and we acknowledge that our brief conversation in this chapter is not exhaustive and encourage readers to seek out and investigate emerging and innovative ways of measuring identity in social science research.

## Identities

When it comes to gender and sexual identity, qualitative research excels at permitting space for self-definition, which can be clarified by member checking or elaborated on with coding. Open-ended, narrative-based inquiries allow for participants to describe, define, and elaborate on their identities in the midst of interviews (Blackwell et al., 2016). Qualitative research has provided the field with important insights into identity language and identity complexities, and the challenge for researchers is to reconcile qualitative approaches to examining identity with quantitative measurement.

Measurement of sexual identity has long been a topic of conversation with some of the most prominent groundwork put forward by Kinsey, Pomeroy, and Martin (1948) and later Laumann, Gagnon, Michael, and Michaels (2000). Current recommendations for quantitatively measuring sexual identity involve a multipronged measure: sexual orientation (cognitive label of sexual identity), sexual attraction (attraction toward opposite- or same-sex individuals), and sexual behavior (past and present sexual activity) (The Williams Institute, 2009). Recommendations on measuring gender identity include two measures: sex assigned at birth and current self-reported gender identity (The Williams Institute, 2014). Despite guidelines for measuring sexual and gender identity, few large-scale surveys adhere to the multipronged approach (Patterson, Jabson, & Bowen, 2017). For those few large-scale surveys that ask about sexual identity, most rely on a singular sexual orientation question (e.g., "Which best describes you: heterosexual/straight, gay or lesbian, bisexual, or other?") (Ridolfo et al., 2012).

Choices around the measurement of sexual identity have several implications and raise practical and theoretical questions for researchers (Oswald, Blume, & Marks, 2005). A multipronged approach to measuring sexual identity raises issues related to the challenge of turning the latent into the observed. The creation of condensed and regimented measures has served the field of LGBTQ studies by helping make identity observable and, thus, measurable. But, as a result, it is not surprising that most research on LGBTQ-parent families has focused on the experiences of those whose identities can be more easily categorized than those who identify as bisexual (Tasker & Delvoye, 2015), queer (Ross et al., 2008), or trans (Veldorale-Griffin, 2014). Software capable of running more advanced statistical methods (e.g., latent class analysis, cluster analysis,

structural equation modeling) along with theoretical advances (e.g., queer, intersectionality) do, however, hold many promises to helping scholars address these measurement challenges.

## Intersections of Identity

Black feminist scholars laid the groundwork for our understanding about intersections of identities (Alimahomed, 2010; Bowleg, 2008; Few-Demo et al., 2016). Sexual and gender identity are not fully understood in isolation from other factors like race, class, or age. Measurement of racial and ethnic identities is a continued area of debate (Cokley, 2007), but for the purposes of this chapter, we will focus on the role of power structures (i.e., the "-isms" of racism, heterosexism, ageism, etc.) in shaping the lived experiences of underrepresented LGBTQ-parent populations. In considering experiences of people of color, it is important to note that "LGBT" has historically been a White marker of sexual identity (Ridolfo, Miller, & Maitland, 2012; Ward, 2008) and an erasive term for queer people of color. Such terminology is not universally used or embraced by subgroups in the population. Researchers who want to create space for underrepresented, racial and ethnic minority LGBTQ parents should note if and how their terminology and norms (Ward, 2008) offer space for identities previously left out of research. Examples include, but are not limited to, "queer," "same-gender-loving" (Harris & Battle, 2013), and "Latinx" (pronounced "Lah-*teen*-ecks") (Garcia, 2017). We encourage readers to engage with the materials (see "Website Examples") provided at the end of the chapter for examples of language used to discuss sexual identity.

Contrastingly, researchers that consider structural and social forces of discrimination and oppression *within* LGBTQ communities have also worked to develop tools to center intersecting identities in research. Again, qualitative research is most poised to comprehensively examine issues of race and/or ethnicity as it intersects with sexual and/or gender identity (DeBlaere, Brewster, Sarkees, & Moradi, 2010), but scholars have developed quantitative measures to examine race, gender, and sexual orientation with particular focus on microaggressions (Balsam, Molina, Beadnell, Simoni, & Walters, 2011; Lewis & Neville, 2015; Sarno, Mohr, Jackson, & Fassinger, 2015). Recent work has focused on racial microaggressions and led to the development of the LGBT People of Color Microaggressions Scale (Balsam et al., 2011), Conflict in Allegiance Scale (Sarno et al., 2015), and the Gendered Racial Microaggressions Scale (Lewis & Neville, 2015). Such scales and measures seek to capture LGBTQ experiences that acknowledge how *other* identities shape their interactions with their communities (e.g., "I have to educate White LGBT people about race issues," "I feel unwelcomed by people from my own racial or ethnic background"; Balsam et al., 2011), feeling as though they belong (e.g., "I feel angry at the way LGBT community treats members of my cultural group"; Sarno et al., 2015), or, specifically, confronting Black women stereotypes (e.g., "I have been made to feel exotic as a Black woman," "I have been accused of being angry when speaking calm"; Lewis & Neville, 2015). The development of scales and measures to assess power structures and identity provides opportunity for scholars to include and expand this type of intersectionality into quantitative research, thereby working to more fully describe the complexity and context of identity work (Few-Demo et al., 2016).

Socioeconomic status (SES) or social class is also important in LGBTQ-parent research (Diemer, Mistry, Wadsworth, López, & Reimers, 2013). SES shapes many components of LGBTQ family life (Goldberg, 2010), often offering protection (e.g., high SES affords gay fathers with high-status occupations the ability to pursue surrogacy) (see chapter "Gay Men and Surrogacy") or exposing vulnerabilities (e.g., low SES prohibits same-sex couples from pursuing expensive paths to parenthood) (Oswald & Culton, 2003). Social class can serve as an index for one's "power, prestige, and control over resources" (Diemer et al., 2013, p. 79), and scholars' explicit consideration of class or socioeconomic status (rather than its use as a covariate) can provide

insights into the relationships and mechanisms that income, occupation, and education play in the lives of LGBTQ parents. For example, Schneebaum and Badgett's (2019) explicit consideration of income, poverty status, and education among different- and same-sex couples (both lesbian and gay) examined the myth of gay affluence. In their study, Schneebaum and Badgett (2019) found that while same-sex couples were more likely to report higher education and that education levels kept poverty rates among same-sex couples low, same-sex couples were still more likely than different-sex couples to be poor after controlling for education and rate of employment. The ways that education, employment, and income operate in LGBTQ-parent families warrant further investigation (see chapter "LGBTQ-Parent Families in the United States and Economic Well-Being").

Paths to parenthood and family formation also uniquely shape experiences of LGBTQ parents. LGBTQ individuals become parents through varying means: divorce or termination of previous heterosexual relationship, adoption, and assisted reproductive technologies (Goldberg, 2010). The paths that LGBTQ individuals take to parenthood shape family processes and connections to children (e.g., biological, legal, and symbolicties). For example, Gartrell et al.'s (1999) study of 84 lesbian families created through donor insemination revealed unique processes and anxieties related to co-mothers' ability to bond with nonbiological children. Paths to parenthood also determine LGBTQ parents' interactions with different institutions (Goldberg, Weber, Moyer, & Shapiro, 2014). For example, Goldberg (2012) documented the ways in which gay fathers navigated the adoption system and how interactions with adoption agencies shaped their transition to parenthood. As paths to and context of parenthood continue to evolve for LGBTQ individuals, researchers will want to acknowledge (i.e., make space for) and explicitly investigate how family formation type produces different lived experiences for parents and children (Potter & Potter, 2017).

Furthermore, age and context also shape LGBTQ parents' lives on both intrapersonal and interpersonal levels (Orel, 2014). Age (both ontological and sociohistorical) shapes LGBTQ parents' experiences and opportunities (Elder, 1978) in leading their lives and creating their families (Cohler, 2005). Belonging to a certain age cohort shapes one's experiences, and from a methodological standpoint, researchers should consider if and how different processes impact LGBTQ individuals at different points in their life and context. Important upcoming and ongoing research is working to tackle some of these questions (e.g., Ilan Meyer's generation website at the end of this chapter under "Website Examples"; see Moore's (2018b) ongoing work with older LG people of color).

## Recruitment: Trends, Challenges, and Opportunities

Often researchers interested in studying LGBTQ-parent families cannot find data to sufficiently answer their question using preexisting data sources, in which case the researchers must either abandon their study or gather their own data (see chapter "The Use of Representative Datasets to Study LGBTQ-Parent Families: Challenges, Advantages, and Opportunities"). If a researcher is required to collect their own data, the quality and composition of one's dataset rely on successful recruitment and sampling strategies—no matter the analytic methodology. In this section, we discuss forms of recruitment, highlighting strategies scholars have successfully used, particularly in the recruitment and study of underrepresented individuals in LGBTQ-parent research. Our focus is on recruitment efforts for researchers creating their own datasets, and we intend this discussion to provide insights into the tools used in recruitment, promising future directions, and the increased reliance on the Internet for recruitment.

## Engaging "Hard-to-Reach" Populations

Historically, LGBTQ populations were not only hard-to-reach given the geographic dispersion and small numbers, but many individuals did not desire to be identified; anti-gay stigma and social and legal discrimination contributed to people's unwillingness to participate (Hughes, Emel, Hanscom, & Zangeneh, 2016; Meyer & Wilson, 2009). Improvements in social climate, inclusion in some national data collection, policy changes, and ease of access (Internet-based studies) have impacted if and how researchers reach LGBTQ individuals. In general, social and technological changes have improved researchers' ability to reach traditionally hard-to-reach populations (Potter & Allen, 2016); however, including underrepresented voices in research requires consideration of the community being studied (Moore, 2018a; Oswald & Culton, 2003). In research on LGBTQ-parent families, conversations around hard-to-reach LGBTQ populations often take the form of figuring out how to most effectively and respectfully recruit LGBTQ-parent families living in rural settings as well as LGBTQ-parent families of color. Below, we briefly discuss the strategies and successes scholars have had in conducting research with these underrepresented groups.

Research on rural queer life has demonstrated that rurality and sexuality are not mutually exclusive (Oswald & Lazarevic, 2011). Metronormativity in LGBTQ research has reproduced the image of LGBTQ communities according to White, male, upper-class, and cosmopolitan ideals (Halberstam, 2005; Stone, 2018). While large, urban locales on either coast of the United States have served as "gay meccas" (Oswald & Culton, 2003), demographic research demonstrates LGBTQ-parent families are more prevalent in southern states, far from the bright lights of coastal cities (The Williams Institute, 2014). In their study of 527 LGBTQ adults living in nonmetropolitan areas, Oswald and Culton (2003) found that informal social networks in rural communities were often strong, but vulnerable; sources of support and tapping into such informal networks without insider knowledge proved difficult. When studying rural LGBTQ life, community (i.e., local history and local knowledge), rural identity, and trust are key to successful recruitment (Lavender-Stott, Grafsky, Nguyen, Wacker, & Steelman, 2018; Oswald & Lazarevic, 2011).

For sociologist Mignon Moore, engaging queer communities of color required making investments (both financial and personal), establishing trust, and activating personal networks (Moore, 2011, 2018a; see chapter "Race and Ethnicity in the Lives of LGBTQ Parents and Their Children: Perspectives from and Beyond North America"). Pioneering studies with queer communities of color beyond Moore (2011) have examined complex caregiving in Black families (Mays et al., 1998), generation status among queer Korean women (Chung et al., 2006), and social and economic justice issues for Latinx, African American, and Asian American communities (Battle et al., 2017a, 2017b, 2017c). Researchers have demonstrated that engaging and activating queer communities of color are not only possible but also realistic. For example, Martinez et al. (2014) recruited 14 Spanish-speaking Latino same-sex male couples in only 4 weeks using ads in mobile apps, concluding that their population was "not so 'hard-to-reach' after all" (p. e113).

It is important to recognize, however, the remaining political opposition, anti-gay stigma, and legal discrimination that continue to play a role in how LGBTQ individuals and parents can live openly (Goldberg, 2012; Goldberg, Gartrell, & Gates, 2014; Veldorale-Griffin, 2014). But perhaps the biggest recruitment challenges to accessing hard-to-reach populations have shifted from contending with LGBTQ outness and stigma to issues of researcher trust, accountability, and community building. With the appropriate methods and resources, scholars may be more effective in reaching LGBTQ parents.

## Forms of Recruitment

Recruitment, often condensed to one to three sentences in a manuscript, is a time-consuming and vital part of the research process. Recruitment processes and considerations remain more opaque than transparent at times, often obscured in favor of reporting on data (Charmaz, 2014). Yet, divulging one's exact methods of recruitment risks exposing LGBTQ individuals and

their families to recruitment overburden or fatigue. Researchers may need to consider how to avoid creating or perpetuating a recruitment pipeline in which numerous researchers rely on a select few groups, email Listservs, or organizations for potential participants (e.g., a popular LGBTQ-parenting group or organization). This hypothetical pipeline risks identifying, overwhelming, or pushing away participants. Furthermore, repeated sampling of the same people over and over again risks participant fatigue and misrepresentation of LGBTQ experiences. This next section discusses different recruitment methods, reflects on emerging use of online technology in recruitment, and highlights special considerations for LGBTQ-parent scholars. Our discussion of recruitment strategies is not intended to be prescriptive but instructive.

In Table 1, we articulate active, passive, and mediated recruitment and illustrative examples (an expansion of a framework set forward by Gelinas et al. (2017)). By *active*, we refer to recruitment strategies in which researchers directly interact with individuals who may be suitable candidates for research—that is, a targeted approach. By *passive*, we refer to recruitment strategies that involve public distribution of materials with the intention that potential participants initially engage with recruitment materials rather than the researcher (Gelinas et al., 2017). By *mediated*, we refer to recruitment strategies that involve the process of accessing the target population through a gatekeeper. Gatekeepers are often an individual or organization with connections to eligible participants (Korczynski, 2003). Recruitment can be online (i.e., via the Internet, social media, online Listservs) or off-line (i.e., via personal contact, paper flyers, events). We advocate for researchers to take a both/and, not an either/or approach to their recruitment forms.

**Active** The medium (format) of active recruitment strategies can vary. Direct engagement with participants can occur through mail campaigns, direct online messaging, and direct personal contact. Active recruitment demands the most time and energy from researchers but may be the most valuable form of recruitment. Researchers can

**Table 1** Illustrative examples of active, passive, and mediated forms of recruitment separated by online and off-line activities

|  | Online | Off-line |
|---|---|---|
| **Active**<br>*(personal networks, attendance at events, approaching eligible candidates directly)* | Direct messaging potential participants with information on study (via email, social media)<br>Emailing members of personal network who may be eligible for study | Attending an LGBTQ event and talking to potential participants about the study<br>Mailing letters directly to potential participants |
| **Passive**<br>*(posting flyers, posting online, placing advertisements, posting to public forums)* | Posting information or advertisements on publicly open social media site (e.g., Craigslist, public Twitter, or Facebook accounts)<br>Paid advertisements on websites | Posting flyers on a bulletin board in businesses, buses, or libraries<br>Creation of a website and reliance on algorithm tags to show site to potentially eligible participants<br>Paid advertisements on television, radio, or print resources |
| **Mediated**<br>*(organizations, groups (social, therapy, support), restricted access Listservs)* | Information sent out through the administrator of an email Listserv<br>Administrator or member of support group posting information about study to their support group | Recruitment of potential participants through doctor referrals to the study, organization-approved announcements, or personal gatekeeper providing referrals to study<br>Personal referrals from participants<br>Personal referrals from personal networks |

seek out events hosted by LGBTQ organizations or centers, gay pride events, or LGBTQ-friendly establishments (Alimahomed, 2010; Chung et al., 2006; Moore, 2011, 2018a; Orel, 2014; Potter & Allen, 2016). Such activities can improve visibility for researchers, provide the means to reach out to participants directly, and help establish credibility and connection to potential participants (Moore, 2018a). Moore's detailed account of her experiences of engaging with queer communities of color in New York and Los Angeles showcased that her repeated engagement—rather than a one-off visit—with queer communities of color was not only a time-consuming and stressful process but also meaningful to her and her eventual participants. She credits her engagement with these communities as key to her success in recruiting participants for her work (Moore, 2018a).

Active recruitment can occur in other contexts or situations. A researcher's profession may facilitate direct engagement with eligible or potentially eligible candidates for a study. For example, those who work in clinical settings may have direct access to potential participants. Direct recruitment can also occur through social media whereby researchers can use publicly available data (i.e., publicly visible social media profiles) to identify eligible candidates. Researchers have utilized publicly available data to gain direct access to same-sex couples in other ways. In their comparison of same-sex couples to different-sex couples, Solomon, Rothblum, and Balsam (2004) accessed publicly available records on same-sex civil union partnerships to identify their potential participant pool and mailed letters directly to participants. Researchers have creatively utilized resources of publicly available data to identify potential participants or gatekeepers, but this approach deserves careful consideration and acknowledgment around the sensitivity of study. We will briefly discuss the implications of recruitment strategies later.

**Passive** Flyers, once the exemplar form of recruitment, play an important but diminished role in recruitment, particularly in off-line settings. Passive recruitment strategies are increasingly becoming digital (via social media pages and profiles) which give researchers a passive online presence. Researchers using social media should be intentional about their use of each platform—each has its own nuanced uses. Figure 1 differentiates users' intended use of some of the most popular social media platforms. As shown

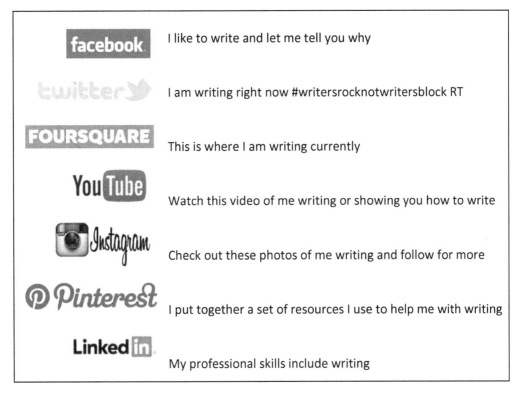

**Fig. 1** The figure above lists some of the most popular social media sites on the left with a descriptor on the right. Each of these descriptors is an illustrative example of the kinds of ideas generally communicated on each platform. The choice of social media platforms is often for different motivations. The illustrative sentences above aim to demonstrate how each social media platform differs from another. The most common and appropriate social media platforms to utilize for research recruitment include Facebook, Twitter, and Instagram. Figure adapted from the University of Rochester Medical Center

in Fig. 1, each platform serves a slightly different purpose in a virtual environment, and theoretically, any platform could be utilized, but Facebook, Twitter, and Instagram are most often used for recruitment (Guillory et al., 2018; Martinez et al., 2014; Saines, 2017; Wilson, Gosling, & Graham, 2012).

Facebook or Twitter account pages can serve as the "face" of the study through which online recruitment could occur (e.g., Abbie Goldberg's Transition to Adoptive Parenthood Project, or TAPP, under "Website Examples"). Facebook pages' "About" sections and Twitter "biographies" are especially useful spaces to provide study details and materials (e.g., links to copies of informed consent, online surveys, eligibility screenings). Social media posts serve as virtual flyers on virtual bulletin boards; images catch the eye, improving the chances that potential participants will even see the research (Kosinski, Matz, Gosling, Popov, & Stillwell, 2015). Indeed, posts with images improve visibility of posts—by between 200% (QuickSprout, 2019) and 313% percent on Twitter (Newberry, 2017); posts with videos are 10 times more likely to have user engagement (Window, 2018). Additionally, the use of hashtags ("#") connected to a word or phrase (e.g., #LGBTQ) creates a searchable, clickable link on Twitter (Hiscott, 2013). Researchers, or research assistants, who become acquainted with the tools and opportunities in social media can use it to assist in recruitment in meaningful ways.

Passive recruitment strategies also include paid advertisements off-line (e.g., television, local radio, print magazines) and online (ads on websites). The use of no-cost Facebook tools limits visibility of posts or pages to only friends or subscribers. For those with a small budget, low-cost ways to advertise include Facebook post "boosts" (DeMers, 2018). Boosts magnify visibility of posts to a bigger, targeted audience that can be designated by researchers (e.g., parents aged 35–50 with children under the age of 18 living in the Midwest; Demers, 2018). Those with larger budgets can opt to pay for more traditional ads placed in online or off-line media. Common outlets for advertisements reported in research include Facebook, Parenting.com, Gay Parent Magazine, Human Rights Campaign, CYFERnet, and Grindr.

**Mediated**  The most common form of mediated LGBTQ recruitment is through LGBTQ organizations, whether brick and mortar locations or online Listservs. Gatekeepers (i.e., LGBTQ organizations or individuals) can serve a vital role in recruitment (Moore, 2018a) and have been an important part of research involving LGBTQ youth (see chapter "The Use of Representative Datasets to Study LGBTQ-Parent Families: Challenges, Advantages, and Opportunities"), parents (Veldorale-Griffin, 2014), grandparents (Orel, 2014), or family members (e.g., PFLAG, for parents of LGBTQ children; COLAGE, for children of LGBTQ parents; Goldberg & Allen, 2013). We provide a database tool to assist in locating LGBTQ-oriented organizations (see resources at the end of this chapter).

When it comes to LGBTQ *parents*, however, recruitment through LGBTQ organizations may not be as fruitful as expected (Compton, 2018; Veldorale-Griffin, 2014). LGBTQ parents often have differing needs and services that may differ from the initiatives, goals, and missions of LGBTQ community centers. Engagement with LGBTQ-oriented community centers and organizations is an important endeavor, but reliance on community centers may (a) be inappropriate according to their mission/population served, (b)

ask too much of an organization or members (resources may already be stretched too thin), or (c) perpetuate the use of samples lacking racial and ethnic diversity for reasons discussed earlier in the chapter.

Researchers have utilized other groups and services. Adoption agencies have served as gatekeepers by offering study information to non-heterosexual and heterosexual clients who could contact the researcher if they wished (Goldberg, 2012). Groups with values on inclusivity and community can also serve as gatekeepers. For example, researchers have been able to serve LGBTQ youth by reaching out to community homeless shelters or temporary housing. Other scholars have utilized general parent support programs, owing some of their recruitment success to heterosexual parents who provided information about ongoing research to sexual minority parents (Compton, 2018).

Recruitment using email Listservs continues to increase and has become a mainstay in LGBTQ research. In partnership with the Human Rights Campaign, Goldberg (2012) was able to utilize the HRC's FamilyNet Listserv (accessed 15,000/month) to recruit prospective same-sex adoptive parents. Email Listservs may emerge as the most often utilized form of mediated online recruitment for researchers who work with LGBTQ-parent families. With the click of a button, a researcher has the ability to reach hundreds, even thousands of potential participants.

With mediated recruitment, however, researchers need to establish and maintain a relationship with the gatekeepers—particularly when working with underrepresented populations. Researchers' successes in reaching underrepresented populations often stem from personal connections and/or their understanding of the needs of their community. For example, Juan Battle and colleagues (see Social Justice Sexuality Project in "Website Example") linked their research to issues of social justice specific to LGBTQ communities of color such as employment, criminal justice, health, and housing. Others have used culturally sensitive practices and incentives or cultural brokers (persons with similar identities to the population—or perhaps can speak the language) and gatekeepers (Gatlin & Johnson, 2017). For example, in their study of 25 queer women of Korean heritage, Chung et al. (2006) served as a broker to gain access to a private and seemingly closed queer Korean community. Chung et al. credited the first author's racial or ethnic membership as it afforded her knowledge of private networks of queer women and the ability to offer to conduct interviews in Korean.

## Issues in Recruitment: Internet Use in the United States

Access to online and mobile technology continues to rise in the United States, and recruitment through online means is only expected to rise (Gatlin & Johnson, 2017) given its cost-effectiveness and efficiency of reaching hard-to-reach populations (Gelinas et al., 2017). Such increased reliance and use of online recruitment methods have historically run the risk of excluding potential participants from research, in that Internet recruitment limited participant pools to those individuals with access to a computer, decreasing the diversity of the potential sample's race, class, and geography (rural vs. urban) (Zickuhr & Smith, 2012).

The risk of excluding certain types of participants from research has declined in recent years due to a narrowing *digital divide* in the United States or the disparity in who has access to the Internet and its resources (Anderson & Rainie, 2014; Norris, 2001; Rainie, 2016). In 2016, "limits to access to Internet" made up only 7% of the reasons given for Internet avoidance (or nonuse). The most common response explaining Internet avoidance was "just not interested" or "not sure how to use" (Rainie, 2016). Today, 90% of adults in the United States report Internet usage. Unsurprisingly, the youngest adults (aged 18–29) report the highest levels of Internet usage followed by 30–49-year-olds and 50–64-year-olds (99%, 96%, and 89%, respectively; Rainie, 2017). Internet usage is consistent across race in the United States (90% of Whites, 86% of Blacks, and 90% of Hispanics; Rainie, 2017). More than half of individuals with disabilities use the Internet and nearly three-quarters of Spanish-speaking individuals use the Internet in the United States (Rainie, 2017). Differences by gender have all but disappeared, and a majority of adults in the United States report Internet usage regardless of socioeconomic status (ranging from a low of 81% for households earning under $30,000/year and a high of 99% for households earning more than $150,000/year; Rainie, 2017).

Increases in access to the Internet may be partially due to the rise in smartphone ownership in the US (with access to the Internet and social media), which is reflected in the fact that Internet access through smartphones increased between 2013 and 2015 while broadband access leveled out or decreased (Rainie, 2017). Smartphone access reflects the same patterns as with Internet usage with youngest adults reporting the most adoption (92%) and no differences across race (77% of Whites, 72% of Blacks, and 75% of Hispanics; Rainie, 2017). Smartphone and Internet access is becoming a mainstay for most families in the United States. The decreasing digital divide in the United States indicates that the Internet provides a promising avenue for recruitment of LGBTQ parents and suggests that potential samples recruited through the Internet may be less biased or selective than in the past.

## Use of Social Media for Recruitment

One major limitation to most forms of recruitment (e.g., events, organizations, email Listservs) is reliance on potential participants to be engaged with a community or group. Not all individuals who identify as LGBTQ can or desire to be involved in an LGBTQ community group. Social media recruitment can help overcome this limitation by reaching those who may not ever connect to or access LGBTQ community resources. Additionally, social media outreach is an efficient form of broadcasting; as a medium, social media are designed to reach a wide audience.

**Social Media Users** A majority of American adults continue to utilize social media from all walks of life (Pew Research Institute, 2018). As of 2018, 68% of all US adults reported using Facebook (Smith & Anderson, 2018). Women, those with higher incomes and those living in more suburban or urban areas, are slightly more likely to use social media, but there were no significant differences with usage based on race or ethnicity (67% of Whites, 73% of Hispanics, and 70% of African Americans use social media today; Pew Research Institute, 2018). Social media does, however, have different meanings across racial and ethnic groups (Anderson, Toor, Rainie, & Smith, 2018). Anderson et al. (2018) found that half of Black or African Americans and nearly half of Hispanics report using social media in order to engage with racial identity-based activism. Adults from historically marginalized groups reported viewing social media as an important tool to discuss issues not receiving attention in mainstream media. Fewer White adults did not see social media in this way (32% reporting usage for identity-based activism). Researchers may want to consider the intentions of the platform and its users when designing studies and recruitment materials, especially for underrepresented populations.

**Connecting with LGBTQ Parents** Research suggests social media are promising ways to reach LGBTQ parents because parents are online, particularly on Facebook. Social media usage rates for parents align with usage rates for nonparents (74% parents vs. 70% nonparents). Among Internet users, 74% of parents report using Facebook (81% mothers, 66% fathers; Duggan, Lenhart, Lampe, & Ellison, 2015), and 59% of parents reported that they found parenting information while on social media (Duggan et al., 2015). Moreover, parental social media engagement is not only passive absorption of information; 42% of parents reported they had received emotional support, and 31% reported using social media to ask parenting questions (Duggan et al., 2015). In all, researchers interested in accessing LGBTQ parents may find social media to serve as a favorable inlet or means of access to parents that may not be connected to specific groups or communities. Therefore, social media can serve to connect researchers to participants that may otherwise not be reached (Heldman, Schindelar, & Weaver, 2013).

## Use of a Website

A website is increasingly becoming a mainstay in research. LGBTQ-parent research is no exception to this trend. A dedicated website performs several important functions for researchers and participants. There are, however, no established standards in the creation of a website. In this next section, we articulate three key ideas to consider and refer to illustrative examples that are provided at the end of this chapter.

**Rapport Building and Communicating Science** The content of a website serves to convey information about the research and researcher. A carefully crafted website can help establish researcher authenticity (Gatlin & Johnson, 2017). For example, Kate Kuvalanka (transkids.info) discussed her research team's makeup and motivations on their website:

> Trans*Kids Project was initiated by a mother of a transgender child…. We will be tracking [caregiver and child well-being and identity] so that we may learn from these youth … and also identify ways to better support them and their families.

Potential participants can learn more about the researcher, research partnerships, and intentions of the study through a website. Research websites can also give insights about the interview or survey process. For example, Samantha Tornello's website for her study on Gender Diverse Parenting (www.genderdiverseparents.com) includes information about "clinical or negative" questions on the survey to help participants understand the use of certain measures in research. Crafting the content of a website is also an exercise in communicating science to a general audience. Too technical or research-oriented language or too much content can overwhelm participants. Researchers may avoid such a fate by piloting their website content with members of their target populations (Miner, Bockting, Romine, & Raman, 2012). Consider each page as an opportunity to establish authenticity and rapport and provide relevant information.

**Tool in Research** A research website can serve specific functions. Websites may act as information kiosks—centralized locations for contact and study information. Websites can also be utilized in the research process to connect potential participants to eligibility screenings or survey questionnaires. Websites can also provide potential participants with electronic versions of informed consent that participants can review in their own time and at their own pace (King, O'Rourke, & DeLongis, 2014). Ilan Meyer and his colleagues' Generations study website (www.generations-study.com) offers electronic copies of informed consent. Practically speaking, a website can alleviate some time commitment and make access to the study easier for participants.

**Design** The design and aesthetic of a website must also be considered. With the rise in smartphone ownership, researchers should work to ensure their websites (and materials or survey) are desktop- and mobile-friendly with clearly marked menus and navigation (Thorlacius, 2007). Several website creation companies specialize in hosting and displaying content on multiple devices (e.g., Squarespace, Wix, Weebly, WordPress). In addition, the style and graphics in a website should work to establish credibility and reflect the population under study. A simple design with selective graphics avoids information overload and conveys integrity to an audience (Lin, Yeh, & Wei, 2013). Recruitment and website materials should also be representative or reflect identities of the desired sample. Consider creating multiple versions of recruitment materials tailored to the audience (Gatlin & Johnson, 2017) or the use of imagery that does not involve photographs of individuals (e.g., cartoon, stick figures). Researchers should aim to be intentional in their recruitment and website images and design.

## Further Considerations in Recruitment

LGBTQ parents and their families reside in vulnerable political and social spaces (given the lack of legal protections and discrimination in some states). Increased reliance and use of online recruitment may introduce new issues surrounding trust and privacy. Next, we discuss how to better ensure participant privacy and researcher trustworthiness in online and off-line settings.

In online settings, sensitive approaches to participants and responsible data management can better ensure participant privacy. Practically speaking, researchers can responsibly manage data through the use of secure servers (encrypted data entry, e.g., https://) in addition to storing data in secure on- and off-line locations. However, privacy is an issue with regard to when and how researchers approach potential participants in an online setting. Online or public displays of LGBTQ parenthood (via blogs, social media posts, social media accounts) do not indicate a desire to take part in research. In projecting their lives online, some accounts or blogs serve as a political space for LGBTQ parents—a space of advocacy and activism. For other LGBTQ parents, online displays may be incidental or unintentional advocacy (Blackwell et al., 2016). LGBTQ parents may experience burnout from having their lives serve as a form of advocacy or may not intend for publicly available posts to signal a willingness to participate in research. With this in mind, researchers should work to approach or contact LGBTQ parents in ways that are transparent and avoid what Gelinas et al. (2017) refer to the as the researcher "creepiness" factor.

Researchers should also work to create a transparent online presence and, when possible, work to gain access to populations through gatekeepers. Gelinas et al. (2017) have documented troubling researcher behavior in which researchers have posed as individuals on dating sites or as members of a support group. This behavior perpetuates systems of oppression and exploitation. Researchers working with sexual minority populations *have* been successful when they were transparent about their research. For example, Martinez et al. (2014) quickly recruited participants after posting clear and purposeful ads on gay-specific social media and dating apps. Furthermore, researchers can work with gatekeepers to earn access to target populations over time.

In off-line settings (perhaps in combination with online engagement), researchers can consider developing community partnerships. For example, Wright et al. (2017) identified community partners in sections of health, housing, research, and aging for LGBT elders. Community partnerships must be healthy in order to be productive, and there are several common pitfalls researchers should be aware of when deciding to enter a partnership (Wright et al., 2017). Healthy community partnerships require trust, respect, and a learning mindset. First, researchers should recognize the limits of their reputation, perceived prestige in the academic world, or external funding sources in the realm of community partnerships. Most community groups or organizations will not be acquainted or interested in a researcher's resume or curriculum vitae and may hesitate to join in a partnership due to external funding or institutional history (i.e., past experiences working with a university in which outcomes or expectations were not met). Researchers should not expect trust to be given, but must seek to earn trust from community partners.

Our advice on working with community partners is to strive for repeated and respectful engagement. It is important to have regular check-in meetings (not only at major or minor milestones in the research project) to ensure the partnership continues to serve the partners' needs and mission. Regular and repeated updates ensure engagement and reliable lines of communication. There are challenging consequences to the breakdown of communication; partners may feel neglected, out of the loop, or exploited. In addition, a partnership thrives in the context of respect. The health of a community partnership can be tarnished far easier than it can be nurtured. One of the best ways to build and ensure respect is to embrace a learning mindset—a mindset that recognizes the researcher is in a position to learn from the community partner and the partner can learn from the researchers—for every member on the research team (Minkler, 2012). A researcher never needs to be the smartest person in the room to be an effective agent for change. Researchers can consider using a learning mindset to mitigate the potential differential in power and resources between institutions and community partners.

## Sampling Techniques

For many researchers—specifically, those who use secondary datasets—sampling is rarely considered. Researchers rely on existing data and data documentation for a general explanation of data collection procedures, and such data availability has rapidly expanded. For other researchers, the issue of sampling presents a fundamental hurdle to their research goals and ambitions. In a review of the literature, van Eeden-Moorefield et al. (2018) found that out of 123 studies looking at LGBTQ families, only two used data from a simple random sample. The other 121 studies used some form of purposive sampling including quota, snowball, and convenience sampling. In this section, we entail a discussion of a variety of sampling strategies, highlighting the pros and cons of each approach (see Table 2) with the intention of justifying a variety of sampling options. Research in the field of survey methodology largely shapes this discussion, and as such, it is heavily quantitative. We briefly discuss issues related to sampling in qualitative research. We conclude with an overview of more recent and innovative sampling tools and strategies that are emerging in social science.

### Simple Random Sampling

In the context of primary data collection (i.e., collecting one's own data), a simple random sample is considered the gold standard when it comes to producing a sample capable of providing inferential statistics (Weathington, Cunningham, & Pittenger, 2017). Each case in a researcher's

**Table 2** Pros and cons of different sampling strategies

| Strategy | Pros | Cons | Example(s) |
|---|---|---|---|
| Simple random | Provides data that could be used to generate estimates about the LGBTQ population more broadly | Requires resources beyond levels of most organizations and individuals<br>Without sufficiently sized sample, runs the risk of producing unreliable, inaccurate, and improperly designed to describe population<br>Done poorly can render research irrelevant and potentially harmful | *2016 Gallup Poll* (Gates, 2017) |
| Stratified | In theory, prohibitively large sample size not required and while producing generalizable data<br>Ensures groups from the population are in the sample, if the group is a strata<br>Ideally suited for studying subgroups | Requires development of sampling frames with the necessary elements to develop the desired strata<br>Vast majority of sampling frames do not contain the elements required to develop the desired strata, so its current utility is minimal | N/A |
| Purposive | Researchers can actively control their sample, ensuring the study will collect data on the group of interest<br>Generally cheaper and quicker than a probability sampling technique while generating the same amount of data<br>Unprecedented amounts of data | Since purposive sampling is non-probabilistic, it is exceedingly difficult to use data collected from these samples to make generalizations or inferences | *Atlantic Coast Families Study* (Fulcher, Sutfin, & Patterson, 2008)<br>*National Longitudinal Lesbian Family Study* (Gartrell, Rodas, Deck, Peyser, & Banks, 2006) |
| Quota | Can be used to develop a sample reflective of the larger populations on targeted characteristics | Samples derived in this fashion are often not reflective on characteristics that were not of interest to the researcher or were originally unobservable | *NYC Stress Exposure and Coping* (Meyer, Schwartz, & Frost, 2008) |
| Snowball | Useful for studying special or hard-to-reach populations<br>More diverse set of cases<br>Relies on respondents | Exceedingly difficult to use data collected from these samples to make generalizations or inferences<br>Relies on respondents, may result in less diverse samples | *Gay Male-Parented Families* (Panozzo, 2015) |
| Convenience | Selecting people based on their accessibility and proximity to the researcher<br>Often the easiest form of sampling | Sample is likely to have the least variety<br>Samples are least likely to provide valid reflections of a larger group or population<br>Sample may fail to reflect the subgroup it was designed to study | Common sampling strategy |
| Theoretical | Flexible strategy of sampling that guides researchers to pursue pertinent cases<br>Sampling contributes to the development of grounded theory | Sample is not likely to provide generalizable results<br>Sampling poses obstacles to researchers as they cannot anticipate core categories or may have trouble identifying cases | *Fathers with Families* (Carroll, 2018) |

sampling frame has the same nonzero probability of selection, producing a sample that can be used to make inferences and generalizations about its population. Despite its usefulness for creating generalizable findings (Weathington et al., 2017), research specifically targeting LGBTQ individuals and their families has rarely taken this approach. Researchers have tended to shy away from using simple random sampling to study LGBTQ populations because they make up a small percentage of the total population.

According to a 2016 Gallup Poll, about 4.1% of Americans, aged 18 and older, identified as LGBTQ (Gates, 2017). While this estimate translates to over ten million adults, it is still a relatively small proportion of the entire US population, and notably, the LGBTQ population density varies by region, state, and urbanicity (U.S. Census Bureau, 2018). Using simple random sampling for the specific purpose of studying LGBTQ parents presents many challenges, particularly around acquiring a sufficient sample size to allow for valid and robust estimates. For example, Gallup researchers used a random sampling procedure with telephone interviews, and in order to identify roughly 49,000 individuals who identified as LGTBQ, Gallup conducted more than 1.6 million interviews (Gates, 2017). Admittedly, studies of LGBTQ-parent families may not require 49,000 respondents, but the ratio of targeted individuals to the total sample size illustrates the magnitude of the undertaking required. For example, consider a more reasonable or feasible sample size of 1000 LGBTQ persons: the total sample size required in simple random sampling to achieve that target number would be over 32,000 individuals. For 100 LGBTQ individuals, the sample would need to be more than 3200 individuals. While some organizations, like Gallup, are in a position where they can invest the money, people, and time (the sampling used by Gallup took over 4 years to collect), for most researchers, the magnitude of this type of collection is beyond their resources.

## Stratified Random Sampling

While simple random sampling may be the gold standard for most research endeavors, it is not always the most ideal sampling strategy (Weathington et al., 2017), particularly for research aimed at small and/or hard-to-reach

groups in the US population (Sullivan & Losberg, 2003). Many groups in the population are considered to be small or hard-to-reach, and researchers have worked tirelessly to develop the most efficient method for balancing the desire to capture these individuals in their study while also producing representative data that can be used to make inferences about a larger population (Tourangeau, Edwards, Johnson, Wolter, & Bates, 2014). One successful strategy (and listed by some as a superior technique to simple random sampling) has been to use stratified random sampling (Tourangeau, Le, Nord, & Sorongon, 2009).

Rather than random sample from the entire population, stratified random sampling first divides the population (i.e., the sampling frame) into subgroups, known as strata, based on key characteristics (primarily the characteristics the researcher is interested in). Once the strata have been defined, simple random sampling is done *within each strata* to produce the final sample. In this way, the key characteristics of interest are guaranteed to be sufficiently represented in the sample while simultaneously preserving the necessary information on the probability of sampling to allow for generalizable and inferential statistics to be estimated. While stratified random sampling has been used in a variety of national studies (e.g., Early Childhood Longitudinal Study, Kindergarten Cohort 2010–2011; High School Longitudinal Study of 2009), it *has not* typically been applied by researchers designing a study of LGBTQ people and families, because stratification requires that the researcher has information on the stratifying characteristic for all members of the sampling frame. That is to say, while researchers are able to stratify on race/ethnicity, language spoken in the home, and poverty status because those details are often *now* standard elements contained in available sampling frames, an individual's sexual identity has rarely, if ever, appeared as an element in sampling frames. While some researchers have called for surveys to universally ask about sexual orientation as a way of improving the accuracy and usefulness of health statistics in other settings

(Semlyen & Hagger-Johnson, 2017), no similar call or availability of such sampling frames in other fields exists.

## Purposeful Sampling Techniques

Purposeful sampling—an umbrella term to capture a variety of strategies and not any single specific sampling technique—differs from simple or stratified random sampling in calculating the probability for a case to be selected for a sample and the generalizability of resulting data (Shadish, Cook, & Campbell, 2002). Both simple random and stratified random sampling allow the researcher to calculate a probability that each case was selected into the sample. Using the calculated selection probability, the researcher creates a sampling weight, which when applied produces results that are said to be generalizable to the population from which the sample was selected. Purposive sampling techniques, generally, do not provide the opportunity to calculate the probability for selecting any particular case, meaning sampling weights cannot be computed nor applied. This makes the results difficult to generalize beyond the specific sample from which the data were collected. Researchers choosing purposive sampling techniques should remain ever aware of its limits, particularly in the context of conducting survey research.

Purposive sampling limitations in quantitative research have been detailed for many years (Neyman, 1934) and continue to be echoed by survey methodologists today (Banks, 2011). Yet, not all researchers intend their study to generalize to the larger population. Instead, they intend to provide insights into the lives and experiences of a special group (even if they exist throughout the population), sometimes in a unique or limited context. These are the types of studies for which purposive sampling can excel and have been used strategically and effectively by researchers studying LGBTQ people and their families (see Table 2). While being non-probability samples, these studies highlight the benefits that doing research with purposive sampling can provide.

Purposeful sampling's largest benefit to researchers is that it provides data on the exact group they are interested in studying and often with unprecedented amounts of data. For example, the National Longitudinal Lesbian Family Study (NLLFS) (Gartrell et al., 1996) provided data on over 150 lesbian-parented families, offering insights into parenting practices, stresses, household division of labor, disciplinary practices, schooling expectations and aspirations, children's development, and plentiful other topics which had previously been largely unknown or understood at only an anecdotal level. This does not mean researchers should take findings from the NLLFS, whether they are positive or negative, and generalize them onto the broader population of LGBTQ families, parents, and individuals. But purposive sampling provided data and insights into a group of families to enable fuller understanding and appreciation of the diverse family systems that exist.

## Quota Sampling

Quota sampling is similar to stratified random sampling, in that the researcher can define which characteristics are ensured to be included in a sample; however, unlike stratified sampling, quota sampling does not rely on a sampling frame. It can be used to effectively develop a sample reflective of the larger populations on the characteristics the researcher is interested in studying *and* that are observable. For example, quota sampling *could* be used to create a sample of men who belong to historically underserved racial/ethnic groups and sexual minority groups, but would not capture the spectrum of diversity in this population along with other characteristics. That is, quota sampling could be used to create a sample that is reflective of the targeted population along the two targeted characteristics (i.e., race/ethnicity and sexuality), but would not be reflective of this population in terms of its *other* characteristics (e.g., socioeconomic status, health status). Quota sampling can be a useful strategy for research on LGBTQ-parent families because of its ability to produce a sample of specific interest to the researcher but still has limits that are important to consider (Yang & Banamah, 2014).

## Snowball Sampling

Snowball sampling is a unique strategy for developing a sample and differs from other techniques because it relies on actual respondents to enact. In snowball sampling, the researcher identifies and selects the first cases into their sample (Charmaz, 2014; Kosinski et al., 2015). Once a case is part of the sample, the researchers ask the participant to nominate other possible individuals to contact for the study. In this way, the sample grows out of the researcher's recruiting efforts *and* the respondents' social networks. This has been a particularly useful sampling strategy for studying small or hard-to-reach populations. For example, Panozzo (2015) relied on gay father participants to refer or vouch for the study to other gay fathers (though it should be noted that this still risks producing a sample composed of very similar participants). More technical discussions of snowball sampling are available (Noy, 2008), but in general, this approach to sampling has been heavily used in qualitative research and with general success in LGBTQ research (van Eeden-Moorefield et al., 2018).

## Convenience Sampling

Convenience sampling creates a sample by selecting cases based on their accessibility and proximity to the researcher. As the name would suggest, these are the most convenient cases—the "easiest" to gather. From a quantitative standpoint, convenience sampling has many shortcomings that limit its usefulness (see Table 2). From a qualitative standpoint, convenience sampling may yield less data-rich cases to research as well. Still, in certain situations, convenience sampling may be considered acceptable depending on the needs and intent of a study (Koerber & McMichael, 2008). In LGBTQ research, researchers may often contend with institutional-,

community-, and individual-level obstacles in reaching their target population. For example, researchers working in rural settings face the obstacles of lower population density. Thus, researchers may use convenience sampling in which they "venture to places where people are likely to have key insights on a chosen topic and then proceed to recruit and sample available participants within those settings" (Abrams, 2010, p. 542). This approach is likely to be cheaper and quicker than most any alternative. While the efficiency of convenience sampling can be luring, its implementation deserves careful consideration.

## Theoretical Sampling

Theoretical sampling—a foundational method in grounded theory research—is a markedly different form of sampling in which researchers are "seeking pertinent data to develop emerging theory" (Charmaz, 2006, p. 96). Theoretical sampling involves comparison of cases and data from the onset of data collection. As such, the researcher is engaged in a sampling process rather than marking a single sampling decision and executing that choice. Theoretical sampling "directs [researchers)] where to go" (Charmaz, 2006, p. 100) in terms of data collection so that the researcher is able to produce meaningful theoretical development. Theoretical sampling is not preoccupied with representativeness or generalizability, but is focused on the development of theoretical insights or theory development. For example, Carroll (2018) used theoretical sampling in addition to observational data to "select interviewees who could advance theoretical concepts" (Carroll, 2018, p. 108). Theoretical sampling shaped her targeted recruitment of 56 gay fathers (i.e., gay fathers of color, single gay fathers, gay fathers not connected to a parent support group) who would have often been left out of research that utilized other sampling methods. Carroll's (2018) sampling served to shape her theorizing process (Charmaz, 2006). Thus, theoretical sampling may be a fruitful endeavor and result in meaningful contributions to LGBTQ-parent research by highlighting voices and experiences of under-represented subgroups (e.g., asexual parents; see chapter "Asexuality and Its Implications for LGBTQ-Parent Families") in LGBTQ-parent populations.

## New and Innovative Techniques and Platforms

Survey methodology and sampling techniques are experiencing a bit of a renaissance. Until recently, the fields of survey methodology mainly suggested avoiding the use of email and the Internet for data collection. Yet, the standard practices of collecting large amounts of data have given way to novel approaches for using social media and big data to collect data and disentangle social patterns. Indeed, digital spaces are creating new platforms for survey and data collection (King et al., 2014). Online survey research panels, as well as many competing online survey tools, such as SurveyMonkey, Amazon MTurk, Zoho, and SurveyGizmo, have provided researchers with multiple new venues for data gathering. In other ways, the novel efforts of sampling today are relocations of prior techniques to new platforms. For example, snowball sampling techniques are being developed for use on social networking sites, such as Facebook, in which a study participant can send along the information about a research project through their personal networks to other eligible participants or post it to their own boards and chatrooms. This type of virtual snowball has the potential to open up previously closed networks and grow the accessible size of networks that were previously seen as small or generally agreed upon as difficult to identify (Baltar & Brunet, 2012).

While new tools and digital spaces hold much promise, researchers will want to embrace these new frontiers in sampling with necessary appreciation for what these methods will and will not provide. For example, utilizing Facebook and other social media platforms may provide researchers with access to undeniably large amounts of data (in terms of sample size, variables collected, time period covered); however, lots of data are not a substitute for "good" data. In other words, data from thousands, perhaps even hundreds of thousands, of respondents do not guarantee the data are representative or high quality (Kosinski et al., 2015). As "big data" becomes an increasingly present source of information in social science research, conscientious efforts to monitor its quality and true applicability to answering important questions related to LGBTQ-parent families will need to be continually monitored.

In this section, we have outlined the pros and cons to different survey sampling techniques and briefly highlighted some qualitative sampling techniques. While we encourage researchers to advocate for the inclusion of sexual orientation and gender identity questions in large, national datasets, not every research question requires nationally representative data to answer. There are certain research objectives that can be met with nonrepresentative data, and as researchers design their study, the key is ensuring appropriate alignment between the research questions and the data. Such consideration can determine the sampling method that produces the most credible, relevant, and robust results.

## Future Research Directions

Decisions around recruitment and sampling shape research in various ways. In this section, we posit promising future directions for research that may engage LGBTQ-parent families in new ways. We have provided a discussion on the state of the field of LGBTQ research, recruitment strategies, and sampling techniques that can help researchers achieve the goals of engaging underrepresented populations and create more and better data moving forward. We propose that future research can take different theoretical and methodological approaches. One such way to engage underrepresented LGBTQ parents is to call greater attention to the experiences of currently marginalized groups through research (Bermúdez et al., 2016). Frameworks that move away from White, middle-class perspectives or take a strength-based approach may serve to engage new participants. Researchers may choose to focus on invisible or structural mechanisms that specifically shape the lives of LGBTQ parents but often get left out of research. For example, future questions could examine intergenerational and cultural mechanisms in parenting. How is LGBTQ parenting shaped by intergenerational transmission of cultural values and family practices, particularly among multigenerational households? Perhaps researchers could consider the role of kinscripts (Stack & Burton, 1994, p. 34), familism (Sayegh & Knight, 2011), or familial piety (Yang & Yeh, 2005) among LGBTQ parents. The consideration of different theoretical frameworks outside parenting division of labor, minority stress, or social exchange theory can serve to provide a space for underrepresented LGBTQ-parent families and explore understudied mechanisms.

Methodologically speaking, the increased adoption of community-based participatory research may also move the field of LGBTQ-parent research forward. Such an approach does not rely on researchers articulating the problems facing LGBTQ parents. Instead, researchers may work with parent communities to identify challenges and problems in a collaborative effort (Gatlin & Johnson, 2017). Designing and building a research project in concert with members of the community may activate private or previously hesitant LGBTQ communities to engage in research. Such a framework demands tremendous resources, but the resulting programs, community partnerships, knowledge, or potentially innovative interventions that come from such an approach warrant pursuit.

We posit three methodological undertakings that hold promise for examining within group variation among LGBTQ-parent families. First, the field of LGBTQ-parent research can develop new measures through the use of various quantitative techniques. The use of latent class analysis, mixture regression, structural equation modeling, and cluster analysis to examine constructs related to racial and sexual identity holds much promise (Fish & Russell, 2018). Such pursuits should hinge on intersectionality, and the groundwork

has already been laid (Balsam et al., 2011; Lewis & Neville, 2015; Sarno et al., 2015). Furthermore, scholars should take on the important and needed exercise of testing and validating new measures.

Second, we encourage multi-method research—combinations of qualitative methods (e.g., examination of historical artifacts and in-depth interviews) or quantitative methods (e.g., participant survey and census data). This can contextualize research and readily allows for examination of systems of power, privilege, and oppression. Duncan and Hatzenbuehler (2014) provide a relevant example in their examination of youth in Massachusetts. They triangulated neighborhood-level assault data with LGBT youth suicide ideation and identified "mechanisms through which LGBT assault hate crimes contribut [ed] to elevations in suicidality" (Duncan & Hatzenbuehler, p. 276).

Lastly, LGBTQ-parent research can be advanced through the adoption and explicit use of mixed method research (e.g., mixture of qualitative and quantitative as a part of research design). Both qualitative and quantitative methods serve LGBTQ-parent studies well. Some scholars have included quantitative surveys in combination with their qualitative interviews (Goldberg, 2012; Orel, 2014), but few (2–5% of articles) LGBTQ-parent scholars have explicitly considered a mixed method design, research questions, and publication (i.e., a publication where both methods are detailed in the same article as opposed to splitting a mixed method study into two separate publications, one qualitative and one quantitative; Hartwell et al., 2012; van Eeden-Moorefield et al., 2018). The field is relatively new and continuing to emerge as a promising way of examining complex problems (Teddlie & Tashakkori, 2010). As a relatively new form of research (compared to quantitative and qualitative), the epistemologies and frameworks of mixed method research continue to evolve, and LGBTQ-parent researchers have an opportunity to lead and shape the future of mixed method research.

Methodological and epistemological debates abound in any field of research, and recently, scholars in LGBTQ research have posed interesting new ideas about the way methods can evolve. Fish and Russell (2018) posit that a way forward involves adopting a queer methodology, in which norms and traditional measures of research are problematized. Few-Demo et al. (2016) posit that integrating queer theory and intersectionality in theory can transform the methods of all family research. We acknowledge these critical and valuable conversations that have the potential to transform the entire field of family research. Their ideas invite inclusive and innovative ways to integrate new epistemologies and methods in order to shed new light on LGBTQ-parent families.

## Practical Implications and Recommendations

Discussions and decisions regarding methods, recruitment, and sampling have implications beyond research integrity and rigor: they open up new possibilities of thinking about scholarship, intervention, and policy initiatives that impact LGBTQ-parent families in different ways–particularly the possibilities of queer-, bisexual-, and trans-parent families that so rarely appear in research. Important conversations about how to conduct and improve LGBTQ-parent research methods have largely focused on the United States, but new conversations are emerging on LGBTQ research in international contexts (Fish & Karban, 2015; Peterson, Wahlström, & Wennerhag, 2018). The methods utilized in the field of LGBTQ-parent research have been vital in ensuring hard-fought victories in court cases and fighting for protections against discrimination in workplace, housing, and healthcare. At the beginning of the chapter, we argued that methods matter because the consequences of our research carry weight. As researchers work toward using data and information to improve the lives, examine the strengths, and advance the understanding of LGBTQ-parent families and parenting processes, there are pertinent conversations to be had about methodological approaches. What we hope is made clear in this chapter is that researchers working with LGBTQ parents should not strive to adopt one method in an effort to create a "gold standard" in LGBTQ research. Rather it is important that researchers strive to thoroughly consider their methodological choices and match their research questions with the most appropriate method. Furthermore, researchers should work to expand the academic space where they can justify and argue their choices in research. Useful guidelines on how to approach this in journal article format are available (Fish & Russell, 2018; Goldberg & Allen, 2015; see chapter "Qualitative Research on LGBTQ-Parent Families", and chapter "The Use of Representative Datasets to Study LGBTQ-Parent Families: Challenges, Advantages, and Opportunities"). Engaging in these practices makes the field less vulnerable to criticism and opposition. Lastly, it is important that researchers avoid becoming complacent in their methodology, as this can result in the perpetuation of stale research. By encouraging researchers to give more intentional consideration to the methods and recruitment strategies being used for studies of LGBTQ parent families, we hope to see the field serves as an incubator for new methodological and substantive advances that can further our understanding of these and all families.

## Practical Resources for Methods, Recruitment, and Sampling

### Find an LGBT Center

CenterLink: The Community of LGBT Centers
This resource provides a list of lesbian, gay, bisexual, trans, and queer community centers that are a part of the CenterLink network. While not exhaustive, this search tool can provide researchers with connection to available community centers. The CenterLink network extends across and beyond the United States.
Website: https://www.lgbtcenters.org/LGBT Centers

## Website Examples

The following examples include links to research studies conducted in the area of LGBTQ kids/youth, parents, and older adults. We provide these as a resource from which to learn and design future research websites.

Title: Gender Diverse Parents Study
Lead Investigator: Samantha Tornello, PhD
Institution: Pennsylvania State University—State College
Website: http://www.genderdiverseparents.com/

Title: Generations: A Study of the Life and Health of LGB People in a Changing Society
Lead Investigator: Ilan Meyer, PhD
Institution: University of California—Los Angeles
Website: http://www.generations-study.com/

Title: The Social Justice Sexuality Project
Lead Investigator: Juan Battle, PhD
Institution: The City University of New York
Website: http://socialjusticesexuality.com/

Title: Transition to Adoptive Parenthood Project (TAPP)
Lead Investigator: Abbie Goldberg, PhD
Institution: Clark University
Website: https://wordpress.clarku.edu/agoldberg/research/transition-to-ladoptive-parenthood-project-tapp/lhttps://wordpress.clarku.edu/agoldberg/research/transition-to-ladoptive-parenthood-project-tapp/
Facebook: https://www.facebook.com/The-Transition-to-Adoptive-Parenthood-Project-TAPP-210464812313047/

Title: Trans*Kids
Lead Investigator: Katherine Kuvalanka, PhD
Institution: University of Miami—Ohio
Website: transkids.info

## References

Abrams, L. S. (2010). Sampling 'hard to reach' populations in qualitative research: The case of incarcerated youth. *Qualitative Social Work, 9*, 536–550. https://doi.org/10.1177/1473325010367821

Alimahomed, S. (2010). Thinking outside the rainbow: Women of color redefining queer politics and identity. *Social Identities, 16*, 151–168. https://doi.org/10.1080/13504631003688849

Allen, K. R., & Demo, D. H. (1995). The families of lesbians and gay men: A new frontier in family research. *Journal of Marriage and Family, 57*, 111–127. https://doi.org/10.2307/353821

Anderson, J., & Rainie, L. (2014). *The future of the internet*. Retrieved from http://www.pewinternet.org/2014/03/11/digital-life-in-2025/

Anderson, M., Toor, S., Rainie, L., & Smith, A. (2018). *Activism in the social media age*. Retrieved from http://www.pewinternet.org/2018/07/11/activism-in-the-social-media-age/

Balsam, K. F., Molina, Y., Beadnell, B., Simoni, J., & Walters, K. (2011). Measuring multiple minority stress: The LGBT People of Color Microaggressions Scale. *Cultural Diversity & Ethnic Minority Psychology, 17*, 163–174. https://doi.org/10.1037/a0023244

Baltar, F., & Brunet, I. (2012). Social research 2.0: Virtual snowball sampling method using Facebook. *Internet Research, 22*, 57–74. https://doi.org/10.1108/10662241211199960

Banks, D. (2011). Reproducible research: A range of response. *Statistics, Politics, and Policy, 2*(online). https://doi.org/10.2202/2151-7509.1023

Battle, J., Pastrana, A., & Harris, A. (2017a). *An examination of Black LGBT populations across the United States*. New York, NY: Palgrave.

Battle, J., Pastrana, A., & Harris, A. (2017b). *An examination of Asian and Pacific Islander LGBT populations across the United States*. New York, NY: Palgrave.

Battle, J., Pastrana, A., & Harris, A. (2017c). *An examination of Latinx LGBT populations across the United States*. New York, NY: Palgrave.

Bermúdez, J. M., Muruthi, B. A., & Jordan, L. S. (2016). Decolonizing research methods for family science: Creating space at the center. *Journal of Family Theory & Review, 8*, 192–206. https://doi.org/10.1111/jftr.12139

Biblarz, T. J., & Savci, E. (2010). Lesbian, gay, bisexual, and transgender families. *Journal of Marriage and Family, 72*, 480–497. https://doi.org/10.1111/j.1741-3737.2010.00714.x

Blackwell, L., Hardy, J., Ammari, T., Veinot, T., Lampe, C., & Schoenebeck, S. (2016). LGBT parents and social media: Advocacy, privacy, and disclosure during shifting social movements. *Proceedings of* the 2016 CHI Conference on Human Factors in Computing Systems - CHI '16, 610–622. https://doi.org/10.1145/2858036.2858342

Bowleg, L. (2008). When black + lesbian + woman ≠ black lesbian woman: The methodological challenges of qualitative and quantitative intersectionality research. Sex Roles, 59, 312–325. https://doi.org/10.1007/s11199-008-9400-z

Carroll, M. (2018). Gay fathers on the margins: Race, class, marital status, and pathway to parenthood. Family Relations, 67, 104–117. https://doi.org/10.1111/fare.12300

Charmaz, K. (2006). Constructing grounded theory. Thousand Oaks, CA: Sage.

Charmaz, K. (2014). Constructing grounded theory (2nd ed.). Thousand Oaks, CA: Sage.

Chung, G., Oswald, R., & Wiley, A. (2006). Good daughters. Journal of GLBT Family Studies, 2, 101–124. https://doi.org/10.1300/J461v02n02_05

Cohler, B. J. (2005). Life course social science perspectives on the GLBT family. Journal of GLBT Family Studies, 1, 69–95. https://doi.org/10.1300/J461v01n01_06

Cokley, K. (2007). Critical issues in the measurement of ethnic and racial identity: A referendum on the state of the field. Journal of Counseling Psychology, 54, 224–234. https://doi.org/10.1037/0022-0167.54.3.224

Compton, D. (2018). How many (Queer) cases do I need? Thinking through research design. In D. Compton, T. Meadow, & K. Schilt (Eds.), Other, please specify: : Queer methods in sociology (pp. 185–200). Oakland, CA: University of California Press.

DeBlaere, C., Brewster, M. E., Sarkees, A., & Moradi, B. (2010). Conducting research with LGB people of color: Methodological challenges and strategies. The Counseling Psychologist, 38, 331–362. https://doi.org/10.1177/0011000009335257

Demers, J. (2018, June 12). The Facebook boost post button: How to use it and get results. Retrieved from https://blog.hootsuite.com/how-does-facebook-boost-posts-work/

Diemer, M. A., Mistry, R. S., Wadsworth, M. E., López, I., & Reimers, F. (2013). Best practices in conceptualizing and measuring social class in psychological research: Social class measurement. Analyses of Social Issues and Public Policy, 13, 77–113. https://doi.org/10.1111/asap.12001

Duggan, M., Lenhart, A., Lampe, C., & Ellison, N. B. (2015, July 16). Parents and social media. Retrieved from http://www.pewinternet.org/2015/07/16/parents-and-social-media/

Duncan, D. T., & Hatzenbuehler, M. L. (2014). Lesbian, gay, bisexual, and transgender hate crimes and suicidality among a population-based sample of sexual-minority adolescents in Boston. American Journal of Public Health, 104, 272–278. https://doi.org/10.2105/AJPH.2013.301424

Elder, G. H., Jr. (1978). Family history and the life course. In T. Hareven (Ed.), Family history and the life course

perspective (pp. 17–64). New York, NY: Academic Press.

Farr, R. H., Tasker, F., & Goldberg, A. E. (2016). Theory in highly cited studies of sexual minority parent families: Variations and implications. Journal of Homosexuality, 64, 1143–1179. https://doi.org/10.1080/00918369.2016.1242336

Few-Demo, A. L., Humble, Á. M., Curran, M. A., & Lloyd, S. A. (2016). Queer theory, intersectionality, and LGBT-parent families: Transformative critical pedagogy in family theory. Journal of Family Theory & Review, 8, 74–94. https://doi.org/10.1111/jftr.12127

Fish, J., & Karban, K. (Eds.). (2015). Lesbian, gay, bisexual, and trans health inequalities: International perspectives in social work. Chicago, IL: The University of Chicago Press.

Fish, J. N., & Russell, S. T. (2018). Queering methodologies to understand queer families. Family Relations, 67, 12–25. https://doi.org/10.1111/fare.12297

Fulcher, M., Sutfin, E. L., & Patterson, C. J. (2008). Individual differences in gender development: Associations with parental sexual orientation, attitudes, and division of labor. Sex Roles: A Journal of Research, 58(5–6), 330–341. https://doi.org/10.1007/s11199-007-9348-4

Garcia, C. (2017). In defense of Latinx. Composition Studies, 45(2), 210–211.

Gartrell, N., Banks, A., Hamilton, J., Reed, N., Bishop, H., & Rodas, C. (1999). The National Lesbian Family Study: 2. Interviews with mothers of toddlers. American Journal of Orthopsychiatry, 69, 362–369. https://doi.org/10.1037/h0080410

Gartrell, N., Hamilton, J., Banks, A., Mosbacher, D., Reed, N., Sparks, C. H., & Bishop, H. (1996). The National Lesbian Family Study: 1. Interviews with prospective mothers. American Journal of Orthopsychiatry, 66, 272–281. https://doi.org/10.1037/h0080178

Gartrell, N., Rodas, C., Deck, A., Peyser, H., & Banks, A. (2006). The USA National Lesbian Family Study: Interviews with Mothers of 10-Year-Olds. Feminism & Psychology, 16(2), 175–192. https://doi.org/10.1177/0959-353506062972

Gates, G. J. (2013). LGBT Parenting in the United States (p. 6). Retrieved from Williams Institute website: http://williamsinstitute.law.ucla.edu/wp-content/uploads/LGBT-Parenting.pdf

Gates, G. J. (2017). In U.S., more adults identifying as LGBT. Retrieved from https://news.gallup.com/poll/201731/lgbt-identification-rises.aspx

Gatlin, T. K., & Johnson, M. J. (2017). Two case examples of reaching the hard-to-reach: Low income minority and LGBT individuals. Journal of Health Disparities Research and Practice, 10(3), 153–163.

Gelinas, L., Pierce, R., Winkler, S., Cohen, I. G., Lynch, H. F., & Bierer, B. E. (2017). Using social media as a research recruitment tool: Ethical issues and recommendations. The American Journal of Bioethics, 17(3), 3–14. https://doi.org/10.1080/15265161.2016.1276644

Goldberg, A. (2012). *Gay dads: Transitions to adoptive fatherhood*. New York, NY: NYU Press.

Goldberg, A. E. (2010). *Lesbian and gay parents and their children: Research on the family life cycle*. Washington, DC: American Psychological Association.

Goldberg, A E., & Allen, K. R. (2013). Donor, dad, or ...? Young adults with lesbian parents' experiences with known donors. Family Process, 52, 338–350. https://doi.org/10.1111/famp.12029

Goldberg, A. E., & Allen, K. R. (2015). Communicating qualitative research: Some practical guideposts for scholars. *Journal of Marriage and Family, 77*, 3–22. https://doi.org/10.1111/jomf.12153

Goldberg, A. E., Gartrell, N. K., & Gates, G. J. (2014). *Research report on LGB-parent families*. Retrieved from https://escholarship.org/uc/item/7gr4970w

Goldberg, A. E., Weber, E. R., Moyer, A. M., & Shapiro, J. (2014). Seeking to adopt in Florida: Lesbian and gay parents navigate the legal process. *Journal of Gay & Lesbian Social Services, 26*, 37–69. https://doi.org/10.1080/10538720.2013.865576

Guillory, J., Wiant, K. F., Farrelly, M., Fiacco, L., Alam, I., Hoffman, L., ... Alexander, T. N. (2018). Recruiting hard-to-reach populations for survey research: Using Facebook and Instagram advertisements and in-person intercept in LGBT bars and nightclubs to recruit LGBT young adults. *Journal of Medical Internet Research, 20*, e197. https://doi.org/10.2196/jmir.9461

Halberstam, J. (2005). *In a queer time and place: Transgender bodies, subcultural lives*. New York, NY: NYU Press.

Harris, A., & Battle, J. (2013). Unpacking civic engagement: The sociopolitical involvement of same-gender loving Black women. *Journal of Lesbian Studies, 17*, 195–207. https://doi.org/10.1080/10894160.2012.711679

Hartwell, E. E., Serovich, J. M., Grafsky, E. L., & Kerr, Z. Y. (2012). Coming out of the dark: Content analysis of articles pertaining to gay, lesbian, and bisexual issues in couple and family therapy journals. *Journal of Marital and Family Therapy, 38*(s1), 227–243. https://doi.org/10.1111/j.1752-0606.2011.00274.x

Heldman, A. B., Schindelar, J., & Weaver, J. B. (2013). Social media engagement and public health communication: Implications for public health organizations being truly "social.". *Public Health Reviews, 35*, 13. https://doi.org/10.1007/BF03391698

Hiscott, R. (2013). *The beginner's guide to the hashtag*. Retrieved from https://mashable.com/2013/10/08/what-is-hashtag/

Hughes, J. P., Emel, L., Hanscom, B., & Zangeneh, S. (2016). Design issues in transgender studies. *Journal of Acquired Immune Deficiency Syndromes, 72*(Suppl 3), S248–S251. https://doi.org/10.1097/QAI.0000000000001077

King, D. B., O'Rourke, N., & DeLongis, A. (2014). Social media recruitment and online data collection: A beginner's guide and best practices for accessing low-prevalence and hard-to-reach populations. *Canadian Psychology, 55*, 240–249. https://doi.org/10.1037/a0038087

Kinsey, A. C., Pomeroy, W. B., & Martin, C. E. (1948). *Sexual behavior in the human male*. Bloomington, IN: Indiana University Press.

Koerber, A., & McMichael, L. (2008). Qualitative sampling methods: A primer for technical communicators. *Journal of Business and Technical Communication, 22*, 454–473. https://doi.org/10.1177/1050651908320362

Korczynski, M. (2003). Access. In M. Lewis-Beck, A. E. Bryman, & T. F. Liao (Eds.), *The SAGE encyclopedia of social science research methods* (Vol. 1, pp. 2–3). Thousand Oaks, CA: Sage.

Kosinski, M., Matz, S. C., Gosling, S. D., Popov, V., & Stillwell, D. (2015). Facebook as a research tool for the social sciences: Opportunities, challenges, ethical considerations, and practical guidelines. *The American Psychologist, 70*, 543–556. https://doi.org/10.1037/a0039210

Laumann, E. O., Gagnon, J. H., Michael, R. T., & Michaels, S. (2000). *The social organization of sexual practices in the United States*. Chicago, IL: University of Chicago Press.

Lavender-Stott, E. S., Grafsky, E. L., Nguyen, H. N., Wacker, E., & Steelman, S. M. (2018). Challenges and strategies of sexual minority youth research in southwest Virginia. *Journal of Homosexuality, 65*, 691–704. https://doi.org/10.1080/00918369.2017.1364104

Lewis, J. A., & Neville, H. A. (2015). Construction and initial validation of the Gendered Racial Microaggressions Scale for Black women. *Journal of Counseling Psychology, 62*, 289–302. https://doi.org/10.1037/cou0000062

Lin, Y.-C., Yeh, C.-H., & Wei, C.-C. (2013). How will the use of graphics affect visual aesthetics? A user-centered approach for web page design. *International Journal of Human-Computer Studies, 71*, 217–227. https://doi.org/10.1016/j.ijhcs.2012.10.013

Martinez, O., Wu, E., Shultz, A. Z., Capote, J., López Rios, J., Sandfort, T., ... Rhodes, S. D. (2014). Still a hard-to-reach population? Using social media to recruit Latino gay couples for an HIV intervention adaptation study. *Journal of Medical Internet Research, 16*, e113. https://doi.org/10.2196/jmir.3311

Mays, V. M., Chatters, L. M., Cochran, S. D., & Mackness, J. (1998). African American families in diversity: Gay men and lesbians as participants in family networks. *Journal of Comparative Family Studies, 29*, 73–87.

Meyer, I., & Wilson, P. (2009). Sampling lesbian, gay, and bisexual populations. *Journal of Counseling Psychology, 56*, 23–31. https://doi.org/10.1037/a0014587

Meyer, I. H., Schwartz, S., & Frost, D. M. (2008) Social patterning of stress and coping: Does disadvantaged social statuses confer more stress and fewer coping resources?. *Social Science & Medicine 67*(3):368–379

Miner, M. H., Bockting, W. O., Romine, R. S., & Raman, S. (2012). Conducting internet research with the transgender population: Reaching broad samples and collecting valid data. *Social Science Computer Review, 30,* 202–211. https://doi.org/10.1177/0894439311404795

Minkler, M. (Ed.). (2012). *Community organizing and community building for health and welfare* (3rd ed.). New Brunswick, NJ: Rutgers University Press.

Moore, M. (2011). *Invisible families: Gay identities, relationships, and motherhood among black women.* Berkeley, CA: University of California Press.

Moore, M. (2018a). Challenges, triumphs, and praxis: Collecting qualitative data on less visible and marginalized populations. In D. Compton, T. Meadow, & K. Schilt (Eds.), *Other, please specify:_____: Queer methods in sociology* (pp. 169–184). Oakland, CA: University of California Press.

Moore, M. (2018b). *Keynote address from lesbian, gay, bisexual, transgender, and queer research symposium: An interdisciplinary symposium on LGBTQ research in the social sciences.* Urbana-Champaign, IL.

Moore, M. R., & Stambolis-Ruhstorfer, M. (2013). LGBT sexuality and families at the start of the twenty-first century. *Annual Review of Sociology, 39,* 491–507. https://doi.org/10.1146/annurev-soc-071312-145643

Newberry, C. (2017). *The Twitter algorithm: What you need to know to boost organic reach.* Retrieved from https://blog.hootsuite.com/twitter-algorithm/

Neyman, J. (1934). On the two different aspects of the representative method: The method of stratified sampling and the method of purposive selection. *Journal of the Royal Statistical Society, 97,* 558–625. https://doi.org/10.2307/2342192

Norris, P. (2001). *Digital divide: Civic engagement, information poverty, and the internet world-wide.* Cambridge, MA: Cambridge University Press.

Noy, C. (2008). Sampling knowledge: The hermeneutics of snowball sampling in qualitative research. *International Journal of Social Research Methodology, 11,* 327–344. https://doi.org/10.1080/13645570701401305

Orel, N. A. (2014). Investigating the needs and concerns of lesbian, gay, bisexual, and transgender older adults: The use of qualitative and quantitative methodology. *Journal of Homosexuality, 61,* 53–78. https://doi.org/10.1080/0091369.2013.835236

Oswald, R. F., Blume, L. B., & Marks, S. R. (2005). Decentering heteronormativity: A model for family studies. In V. L. Bengtson, A. C. Acock, K. R. Allen, P. Dilworth-Anderson, & D. M. Klein (Eds.), *Sourcebook of family theory and research* (pp. 143–165). Thousand Oaks, CA: Sage.

Oswald, R. F., & Culton, L. S. (2003). Under the rainbow: Rural gay life and its relevance for family providers. *Family Relations, 52,* 72–81. https://doi.org/10.1111/j.1741-3729.2003.00072.x

Oswald, R. F., & Lazarevic, V. (2011). "You live where?!" Lesbian mothers' attachment to nonmetropolitan communities. *Family Relations, 60,* 373–386. https://doi.org/10.1111/j.1741-3729.2011.00663.x

Panozzo, D. (2015). Child care responsibility in gay male-parented families: Predictive and correlative factors.

*Journal of GLBT Family Studies, 11,* 248–277. https://doi.org/10.1080/1550428X.2014.947461

Patterson, C. J. (2000). Family relationships of lesbians and gay men. *Journal of Marriage and the Family, 62,* 1052–1069. https://doi.org/10.1111/j.1741-3737.2000.01052.x

Patterson, J. G., Jabson, J. M., & Bowen, D. J. (2017). Measuring sexual and gender minority populations in health surveillance. *LGBT Health, 4,* 82–105. https://doi.org/10.1089/lgbt.2016.0026

Peterson, A., Wahlström, M., & Wennerhag, M. (Eds.). (2018). *Pride parades and LGBT movements: Political participation in an international comparative perspective.* New York, NY: Routledge.

Pew Research Institute. (2018). *Demographics of social media users and adoption in the United States.* Retrieved from http://www.pewinternet.org/fact-sheet/social-media/

Potter, D., & Potter, E. C. (2017). Psychosocial well-being in children of same-sex parents: A longitudinal analysis of familial transitions. *Journal of Family Issues, 38,* 2303–2328. https://doi.org/10.1177/0192513X16646338

Potter, E. C., & Allen, K. R. (2016). Agency and access: How gay fathers secure health insurance for their families. *Journal of GLBT Family Studies, 12,* 300–317. https://doi.org/10.1080/1550428X.2015.1071678

QuickSprout. (2019, January 28). *How to increase Twitter engagement by 324%* [Blog]. Retrieved Quick Sprout website: https://www.quicksprout.com/twitter-engagement/

Rainie, L. (2016). *Digital divides 2016.* Retrieved from Pew Research Center website: http://www.pewinternet.org/2016/07/14/digital-divides-2016/

Rainie, L. (2017). *Digital divides – Feeding America.* Retrieved from Pew Research Center website: http://www.pewinternet.org/2017/02/09/digital-divides-feeding-america/

Ridolfo, H., Miller, K., & Maitland, A. (2012). Measuring sexual identity using survey questionnaires: How valid are our measures? *Sexuality Research and Social Policy, 9,* 113–124. https://doi.org/10.1007/s13178-011-0074-x

Rosenfeld, M. J. (2010). Nontraditional families and childhood progress through school. *Demography, 47,* 755–775. https://doi.org/10.1353/dem.0.0112

Rosenfeld, M. J. (2013). Reply to Allen et al. *Demography, 50,* 963–969. https://doi.org/10.1007/s13524-012-0170-4

Ross, L., Epstein, R., Goldfinger, C., Steele, L., Anderson, S., & Strike, C. (2008). Lesbian and queer mothers navigating the adoption system: The impacts on mental health. *Health Sociology Review, 17,* 254–266. https://doi.org/10.5172/hesr.451.17.3.254

Rostosky, S. S., & Riggle, E. D. B. (2017). Same-sex couple relationship strengths: A review and synthesis of the empirical literature (2000–2016). *Psychology of Sexual Orientation and Gender Diversity, 4,* 1–13. https://doi.org/10.1037/sgd0000216

Saines, S. (2017). *Using social media: Recruiting research participants via Twitter*. Office for Scholarly Communication. Retrieved from https://blogs.kent.ac.uk/osc/2017/11/03/twitter-recruiting-research-participants/

Sarno, E. L., Mohr, J. J., Jackson, S. D., & Fassinger, R. E. (2015). When identities collide: Conflicts in allegiances among LGB people of color. *Cultural Diversity & Ethnic Minority Psychology, 21*, 550–559. https://doi.org/10.1037/cdp0000026

Sayegh, P., & Knight, B. G. (2011). The effects of familism and cultural justification on the mental and physical health of family caregivers. *The Journals of Gerontology Series B: Psychological Sciences and Social Sciences, 66B*, 3–14. https://doi.org/10.1093/geronb/gbq061

Schneebaum, A., & Badgett, M. V. L. (2019). Poverty in US lesbian and gay couple households. *Feminist Economics, 25*, 1–30. https://doi.org/10.1080/13545701.2018.1441533

Schumm, W. R., & Crawford, D. W. (2018). How have other journals compared to "the top seven" journals in family social science with respect to LGBT-related research and reviews? A comment on "A content analysis of LGBT research in top family journals 2000–2015"? An editorial analysis. *Marriage & Family Review, 54*, 521–530. https://doi.org/10.1080/01494929.2018.1460145

Semlyen, J., & Hagger-Johnson, G. (2017). Sampling frame for sexual minorities in public health research. *Journal of Public Health, 39*, 644–644. https://doi.org/10.1093/pubmed/fdw078

Shadish, W. R., Cook, T. D., & Campbell, D. T. (2002). *Experimental and quasi-experimental designs for generalized causal inference*. Boston, MA: Houghton, Mifflin and Company.

Smith, A., & Anderson, M. (2018, March 1). *Social media use 2018: Demographics and statistics*. Retrieved from http://www.pewinternet.org/2018/03/01/social-media-use-in-2018/

Solomon, S. E., Rothblum, E. D., & Balsam, K. F. (2004). Pioneers in partnership: Lesbian and gay male couples in civil unions compared with those not in civil unions and married heterosexual siblings. *Journal of Family Psychology, 18*, 275–286. https://doi.org/10.1037/0893-3200.18.2.275

Stack, C., & Burton, L. (1994). Kinscripts: Reflections on family, generation, and culture. In E. N. Glenn, G. Chang, & L. R. Forcey (Eds.), *Mothering: Ideology, experience, and agency* (pp. 33–44). New York, NY: Routledge.

Stone, A. L. (2018). The geography of research on LGBTQ Life: Why sociologists should study the South, rural queers, and ordinary cities. *Sociology Compass, 12*, e12638. https://doi.org/10.1111/soc4.12638

Sullivan, G., & Losberg, W. M. (2003). A study of sampling in research in the field of lesbian and gay studies. *Journal of Gay & Lesbian Social Services, 15*, 147–162. https://doi.org/10.1300/J041v15n01_10

Tasker, F., & Delvoye, M. (2015). Moving out of the shadows: Accomplishing bisexual motherhood. *Sex Roles, 73*, 125–140. https://doi.org/10.1007/s11199-015-0503-z

Tasker, F., & Patterson, C. J. (2007). Research on gay and lesbian parenting. *Journal of GLBT Family Studies, 3*(2–3), 9–34. https://doi.org/10.1300/J461v03n02_02

Teddlie, C., & Tashakkori, A. (2010). Overview of contemporary issues in mixed method research. In A. Tashakkori & C. Teddlie (Eds.), *Handbook of mixed methods in social and behavioral research* (2nd ed., pp. 1–41). Thousand Oaks, CA: Sage.

Thorlacius, L. (2007). The role of aesthetics in web design. *Nordicom Review, 28*, 63–76. https://doi.org/10.1515/nor-2017-0201

Tourangeau, K., Le, T., Nord, C., & Sorongon, A. (2009). *ECLS-K eighth grade methodology report (No. 2009-003)* (p. 445). Washington, DC: National Center for Education Statistics, Institute of Education Sciences, U.S. Department of Education.

Tourangeau, R., Edwards, B., Johnson, T., Wolter, K., & Bates, N. (Eds.). (2014). *Hard-to-survey populations*. Cambridge, UK: Cambridge University Press.

U.S. Census Bureau. (2018). *LGBT pride month: June 2018*. Retrieved from https://www.census.gov/newsroom/stories/2018/lgbt.html

Vaccaro, A. (2010). Toward inclusivity in family narratives: Counter-stories from queer multi-parent families. *Journal of GLBT Family Studies, 6*, 425–446. https://doi.org/10.1080/1550428X.2010.511086

van Eeden-Moorefield, B., & Chauveron, L. (2016). Big data bias and LGBT research. In A. E. Goldberg (Ed.), *The SAGE encyclopedia of LGBTQ studies* (pp. 112–115). Thousand Oaks, CA: Sage.

van Eeden-Moorefield, B., Few-Demo, A. L., Benson, K., Bible, J., & Lummer, S. (2018). A content analysis of LGBT research in top family journals 2000-2015. *Journal of Family Issues, 39*, 1374–1395. https://doi.org/10.1177/0192513X17710284

Veldorale-Griffin, A. (2014). Transgender parents and their adult children's experiences of disclosure and transition. *Journal of GLBT Family Studies, 10*, 475–501. https://doi.org/10.1080/1550428X.2013.866063

Ward, J. (2008). White normativity: The cultural dimensions of whiteness in a racially diverse LGBT organization. *Sociological Perspectives, 51*, 563–586. https://doi.org/10.1525/sop.2008.51.3.563

Weathington, B. L., Cunningham, C. J. L., & Pittenger, D. J. (2017). *Research methods for the behavioral and social sciences*. Hoboken, NJ: Wiley.

Williams Institute. (2009). *Best practices for asking questions about sexual orientation on surveys*. Retrieved from https://williamsinstitute.law.ucla.edu/research/census-lgbt-demographics-studies/best-practices-for-asking-questions-about-sexual-orientation-on-surveys/

Williams Institute. (2014). *Best practices for asking questions to identify transgender and other gender minority respondents on population-based surveys*. Retrieved from https://williamsinstitute.law.ucla.

edu/research/census-lgbt-demographics-studies/geniuss-report-sept-2014/

Wilson, R. E., Gosling, S. D., & Graham, L. T. (2012). A review of Facebook research in the social sciences. *Perspectives on Psychological Science, 7*, 203–220. https://doi.org/10.1177/1745691612442904

Window, M. (2018, July 24). *5 data-driven tips for scroll stopping video*. Retrieved from Twitter Business website: https://business.twitter.com/en/blog/5-data-driven-tips-for-scroll-stopping-video.html

Wright, L. A., King, D. K., Retrum, J. H., Helander, K., Wilkins, S., Boggs, J. M., … Gozansky, W. S. (2017). Lessons learned from community-based participatory research: Establishing a partnership to support lesbian, gay, bisexual and transgender ageing in place. *Family Practice, 34*, 330–335. https://doi.org/10.1093/fampra/cmx005

Yang, K., & Banamah, A. (2014). Quota sampling as an alternative to probability sampling? An experimental study. *Sociological Research Online, 19*, 1–11. https://doi.org/10.5153/sro.3199

Yang, K. S., & Yeh, K. H. (2005). The psychology and behavior of filial piety among Chinese. In K. S. Yang, K. K. Hwang, & C. F. Yang (Eds.), *Chinese indigenized psychology* (pp. 293–330). Taipei, China: Yuan-Liou.

Zickuhr, K., & Smith, A. (2012, April). *Digital differences*. Retrieved from Pew Research Institute website: http://pewinternet.org/Reports/2012/Digital-differences.aspx

# Index

CPSIA information can be obtained
at www.ICGtesting.com
Printed in the USA
LVHW021411240520
656463LV00005B/185